Recent Results in Cancer Research

Volume 201

For further volumes:
http://www.springer.com/series/392

Uwe M. Martens
Editor

Small Molecules in Oncology

Second Edition

Springer

Editor
Uwe M. Martens
Cancer Center Heilbronn-Franken
SLK-Kliniken Heilbronn GmbH
Academic Teaching Hospital
Ruprecht-Karls-University Heidelberg
Heilbronn
Germany

ISSN 0080-0015 ISSN 2197-6767 (electronic)
ISBN 978-3-662-51925-7 ISBN 978-3-642-54490-3 (eBook)
DOI 10.1007/978-3-642-54490-3
Springer Heidelberg New York Dordrecht London

Softcover reprint of the hardcover 2nd edition 2014

Springer is part of Springer Science+Business Media (www.springer.com)

Preface

The past decade has resulted in major breakthroughs in the treatment of cancer. Even though conventional chemotherapy currently remains the backbone of most treatment regimens, the paradigm of cancer therapy is shifting unambiguously towards more selective, mechanism-based strategies.

With the tremendous advances in our recent understanding of aberrant signalling pathways in various types of cancer—including such as leukemia, breast and lung cancer and melanoma—plenty of crucial regulators of malignant behavior in cancer cells have emerged as promising candidates for molecular target-based cancer therapies. Specific alterations in key signalling molecules driving the progression of individual cancers can now precisely be targeted by small low-molecular-weight compounds. This new class of rationally designed anticancer agents is able to induce striking regressions in molecularly defined subsets of patients.

One of the early pioneers has been Imatinib mesylate (Glivec®) that showed remarkable efficacy for the treatment of patients with Philadelphia chromosome-positive CML, changing the course of this formerly deadly disease profoundly. Since then, numerous new small molecules have already been approved for the treatment of many types of cancer—and even more are currently investigated in clinical trials. With the second edition of "Small Molecules in Oncology" we aim to give you a comprehensive survey of both, already established drugs as well as promising new substances. Therefore, all 25 chapters of this book have been contributed by renowned scientists and clinicians, offering first-hand insight into this exciting and rapidly evolving field of targeted cancer therapies.

Heilbronn — Uwe M. Martens

Contents

Imatinib Mesylate

Cornelius F. Waller

Abstract

Imatinib mesylate (Gleevec, Glivec [Novartis, Basel, Switzerland], formerly referred to as STI571 or CGP57148B) represents the paradigm of a new class of anticancer agents, so-called small molecules. They have a high selectivity against a specific molecular target known to be the cause for the establishment and maintenance of the malignant phenotype. Imatinib is a rationally designed oral signal transduction inhibitor that specifically targets several protein tyrosine kinases, Abl, Arg (*Abl*-related gene), the stem cell factor receptor (c-KIT), platelet-derived growth factor receptor (PDGF-R), and their oncogenic forms, most notably BCR-ABL. Imatinib has been shown to have remarkable clinical activity in patients with chronic myeloid leukemia (CML) and malignant gastrointestinal stroma tumors (GIST) leading to its approval for treatment of these diseases. Treatment with imatinib is generally well tolerated with a low incidence of severe side effects. The most common adverse events include mild to moderate edema, muscle cramps, diarrhea, nausea, skin rashes, and myelosuppression. Several mechanisms of resistance have been identified. Clonal evolution, amplification, or overexpression of BCR-ABL as well as mutations in the catalytic domain, P-loop, and other mutations have been demonstrated to play a role in primary and secondary resistance to imatinib, respectively. Understanding of the underlying mechanisms of resistance has led to the development of new second- and third-generation tyrosine kinase inhibitors (see chapters on dasatinib, nilotinib, bosutinib, and ponatinib).

C. F. Waller (✉)
Department of Hematology and Oncology, University of Freiburg Medical Center,
Hugstetter Street 55, 79106 Freiburg, Germany
e-mail: cornelius.waller@uniklinik-freiburg.de

U. M. Martens (ed.), *Small Molecules in Oncology*, Recent Results in Cancer Research 201, DOI: 10.1007/978-3-642-54490-3_1,

Contents

1 Introduction

Chronic myeloid leukemia (CML) is a clonal disorder of the hematopoietic stem cell. The clinical presentation often includes granulocytosis, a hypercellular bone marrow and splenomegaly. The natural course of the disease involves three sequential phases—chronic phase (CP), progressing often through an accelerated phase (AP) into the terminal blast crisis (BC). The duration of CP is several years, while AP and BC usually last only for months. In the past, prior to the introduction of TKIs into the treatment of CML, median survival was in the range of 4–5 years (Hehlmann et al. 2007b; Sawyers 1999).

CML is characterized by the presence of the Philadelphia chromosome (Ph), a unique reciprocal translocation between the long arms of chromosomes 9 and 22, t(9:22), which is present in >90 % of patients with CML and approximately 15–30 % of ALL (Nowell and Hungerford 1960; Rowley 1973). On the molecular level, t(9:22) results in the generation of an oncogene, the BCR-ABL fusion gene, encoding the BCR-ABL protein which has constitutive tyrosine kinase activity (Konopka et al. 1984; Fig. 1).

Its causal role in the development of CML has been demonstrated in vitro as well as in several animal models (Daley et al. 1990; Heisterkamp et al. 1990; Lugo et al. 1990; Voncken et al. 1995).

The pathological effects of BCR-ABL include increased proliferation, protection from programmed cell death, altered stem cell adhesion and possibly genetic instability that leads to disease progression (Deininger and Goldman 1998; Deininger et al. 2000).

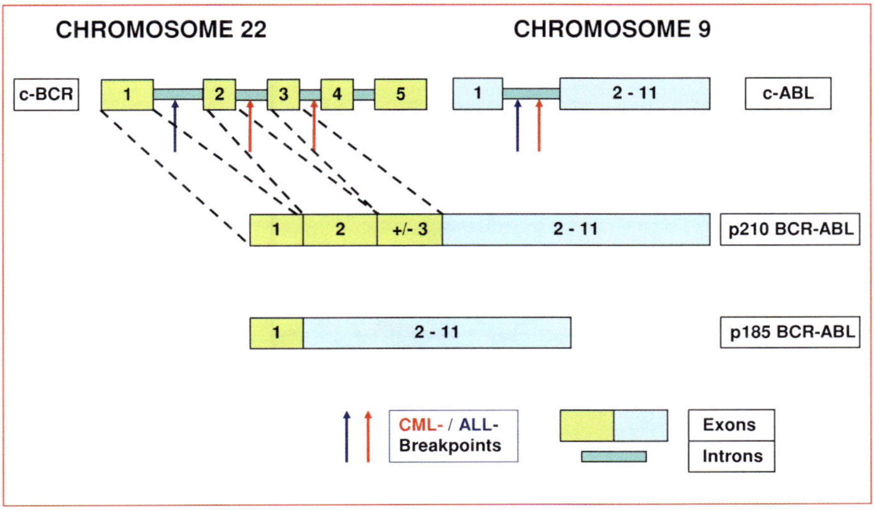

Fig. 1 Common breakpoints in CML and Ph$^+$ ALL: In CML, *BCR* breakpoints occur after the second or third exon, whereas in Ph$^+$ ALL, breaks can occur after the first exon. In *c-ABL*, a break occurs between the first and second exon (CML and Ph$^+$ ALL)

Before the introduction of imatinib, standard therapy of CML was interferon-α alone or in combination with cytarabine (ara-C) leading to hematologic remissions in the majority of patients, but major cytogenetic responses—i.e., <35 % Ph$^+$ metaphases—were only seen in 6–25 % of patients (Hehlmann et al. 2007b). The only curative treatment of CML is allogeneic stem cell transplantation from an HLA-compatible donor. However, it is only an option for a part of the patients and still associated with considerable morbidity and mortality (Gratwohl et al. 1998; Hehlmann et al. 2007a).

The presence of BCR-ABL in >90 % of CML patients and the identification of its essential role in the pathogenesis of the disease provided the rationale of targeting this fusion protein for treatment of CML.

In the nineties of the twentieth century, first data of compounds with an effect on tyrosine kinases were published (Levitzky and Gazit 1995). Tyrphostins and other similar compounds were shown to inhibit the ABL- as well as the BCR-ABL tyrosine kinase at micromolar concentrations but had only limited specificity (Anafi et al. 1993a, b; Carlo-Stella et al. 1999). This led to the rational design of further TKI with selective activity against the ABL tyrosine kinase, one of which was a 2-phenylaminopyrimidine called CGP57148B, later called STI571 or imatinib mesylate (Buchdunger et al. 1995, 1996; Druker and Lydon 2000; Druker et al. 1996).

After demonstration of specificity in vitro, in cell-based systems as well as in different animal models, this compound was tested in several phase I and phase II studies (Druker et al. 2001a; Kantarjian et al. 2002a, b). Imatinib was shown to have very high rates of hematologic remissions in CP-CML patients previously treated with interferon-α as well as in advanced stages of the disease. Cytogenetic remissions were achieved in a considerable portion of patients. Based on these good results, imatinib was approved for treatment of CML patients in CP after treatment failure with interferon-α and the advanced stages, i.e., AP and BC (Cohen et al. 2002b).

The phase III (IRIS) trial led to establishment of imatinib as standard for first-line therapy of CP-CML (Cohen et al. 2009; Dagher et al. 2002). Currently, several trials investigate the effect of stopping imatinib in patients reaching a very good long-lasting remission based upon the results of the so-called STIM trial where it could be shown that a part of patients stayed in a very good molecular remission after the end of the therapy (Mahon et al. 2010).

Other molecular targets of imatinib are the stem cell factor receptor (c-KIT) and platelet-derived growth factor receptor (PDGF-R) (Buchdunger et al. 1995, 1996, 2000; Heinrich et al. 2002a, b).

c-KIT is expressed in a variety of human cancers, including germ cell tumors, neuroblastoma, melanoma, small cell lung cancer, breast and ovarian cancers, acute myeloid leukemia, mast cell disorders as well as malignant gastrointestinal stroma tumors (GIST). While in most of these diseases, the exact role of c-KIT expression is not defined in mastocytosis and GISTs activating mutations of c-KIT have been identified.

Based upon data of a single open-label phase II trial and two large phase III trials by the EORTC and SWOG, imatinib received approval for treatment of metastatic/ unresectable GIST (Cohen et al. 2009; Dagher et al. 2002). In addition, the role of adjuvant treatment with imatinib after successful resection of primary GIST has been clearly demonstrated and led to the adjuvant label (Joensuu et al. 2012).

Furthermore, imatinib has been successfully used in diseases with aberrant PDGF receptors. They have been shown to deregulate the growth of a variety of cancers, such as GIST; myeloproliferative disorders (Pardanani and Tefferi 2004), e.g., in hypereosinophilic syndrome (FIP1L1/PDGFRα-rearrangement), chronic myelomonocytic leukemia (CMML), harboring the activating translocations involving the PDGF receptor beta locus on chromosome 5q33 (FIP1/PDGFR-translocation); carcinomas; melanoma; gliomas; and sarcomas, including dermatofibrosarcoma protuberans (Barnhill et al. 1996; Greco et al. 2001).

In addition, in several non-malignant diseases, e.g., pulmonary hypertension, and autoimmune disease, the effect of imatinib has been investigated (Hoeper et al. 2013; Moinzadeh et al. 2013).

2 Structure and Mechanisms of Action

Imatinib mesylate is designated chemically as 4-[(4-methyl-1-piperazinyl)methyl]-*N*-[4-methyl-3-[[4-(3-pyridinyl)-2-pyrimidinyl] aminophenyl] benzamide methanesulfonate. Its molecular formula is $C_{29}H_{31}N_7O \cdot CH_4SO_3$, and its relative molecular mass is 589.7 (Fig. 2).

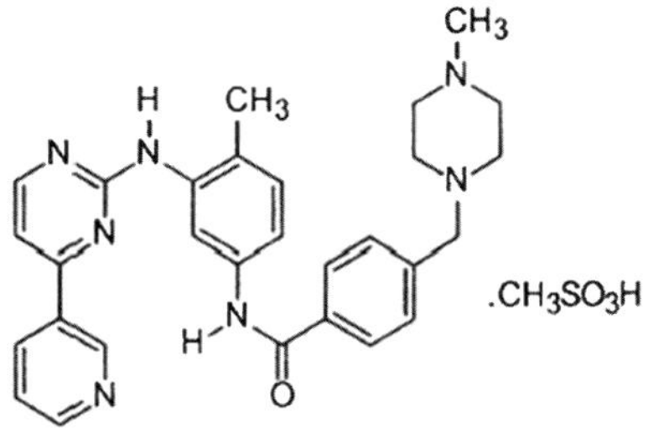

Fig. 2 Structure of imatinib mesylate (formerly STI 571 bzw. CGP57148)

Imatinib functions as a specific competitive inhibitor of ATP. It binds with high affinity at the ATP binding site in the inactive form of the kinase domain, blocks ATP binding, and thereby inhibits kinase activity by interrupting the transfer of phosphate from ATP to tyrosine residues on substrate proteins (Cohen et al. 2002a, b, 2005; Lyseng-Williamson and Jarvis 2001; Mauro et al. 2002).

Imatinib selectively inhibits all the ABL tyrosine kinases, including BCR-ABL, cellular homologue of the Abelson murine leukemia viral oncogene product (c-ABL), v-ABL, TEL-ABL, and Abelson-related gene (ARG). In addition, it was found to potently inhibit the tyrosine kinase activity of the α- and β-platelet-derived growth factor receptors (PDGFR) and the receptor for stem cell factor (c-KIT; CD117). The concentrations required for a 50 % kinase inhibition were in the range of 0.025 μM in in vitro kinase assays and approximately 0.25 μM in intact cells. Extensive screening did not show activity against other tyrosine kinases or serine/threonine kinases (Buchdunger et al. 1995, 1996, 2000, 2001; Deininger et al. 2005; Druker and Lydon 2000; Druker et al. 1996; Heinrich et al. 2002a; Okuda et al. 2001; Table 1).

3 Preclinical Data

In vitro studies demonstrated specific inhibition of myeloid cell lines expressing BCR-ABL without killing the parental cell lines from which they were derived (Deininger et al. 1997; Druker et al. 1996; Gambacorti-Passerini et al. 1997). Continuous treatment with imatinib inhibited tumor formation in syngeneic mice as well as in a nude mouse model after inoculation of BCR-ABL-expressing cells in a dose-dependent manner, treated intraperitoneally or with oral administration of STI571, respectively (Druker et al. 1996; le Coutre et al. 1999). Activity on primary CML cells could be demonstrated, and a >90 % reduction of BCR-ABL-expressing colonies in colony-forming assays from peripheral blood or bone marrow from CML patients was achieved at a concentration of imatinib of 1 μM while normal colonies did not show growth inhibition (Deininger et al. 1997; Druker et al. 1996; Gambacorti-Passerini et al. 1997).

Table 1 Inhibition of protein kinases by imatinib mesylate (formerly STI 571 bzw. CGP57148) (adapted from Deininger et al. 2005)

Protein kinase	Substrate phosphorylation IC50[a] (μM)	Cellular tyrosine phosphorylation IC50[a] (μM)
c-abl	0.2; 0.025	ND
v-abl	0.038	0.1–0.3
$p210^{BCR\text{-}ABL}$	0.025	0.25
$p185^{BCR\text{-}ABL}$	0.025	0.25
TEL-ABL	ND	0.35
PDGF-Rα and β	0.38 (PDGF-Rβ)	0.1
Tel-PDGF-R	ND	0.15
c-KIT	0.41	0.1
FLT-3	>10	>10
Btk	>10	ND
c-FMS	ND	>10
v-FMS	ND	>10
c-SRC	>100	ND
v-SRC	ND	>10
c-LYN	>100	ND
c-FGR	>100	ND
LCK	9.0	ND
SYK (TPK-IIB)	>100	ND
JAK-2	>100	>100
EGF-R	>100	>100
Insulin receptor	>10	>100
IGF-IR	>10	>100
FGF-R1	31.2	ND
VEGF-R1 (FLT-1)	19.5	ND
VEGF-R2 (KDR)	10.7	ND
VEGF-R3 (FLT-4)	5.7	ND
TIE-2 (TEK)	>50	ND
c-MET	>100	ND
PKA	>500	ND
PPK	>500	ND
PKC α, $\beta 1$, γ, δ, ε, ξ, η	>100	ND

(continued)

Table 1 (continued)

Protein kinase	Substrate phosphorylation IC50[a] (μM)	Cellular tyrosine phosphorylation IC50[a] (μM)
Protein kinase CK-1, CK-2	>100	ND
PKB	>10	ND
P39	>10	ND
PDK1	>10	ND
c-RAF-1	0.97	ND
CDC2/cyclin B	>100	ND

Imatinib concentrations causing a 50 % reduction in kinase activity (IC50) are given
ND not done, *PDGF-R* platelet-derived growth factor receptor, *Btk* Bruton tyrosine kinase, *TPK* tyrosine-protein kinase, *EGF-R* epidermal growth factor receptor, *IGF-IR* insulin-like growth factor receptor I, *FGF-R1* fibroblast growth factor receptor 1, *VEGF-R* vascular endothelial growth factor receptor, *PKA* cAMP-dependent protein kinase, *PPK* phosphorylase kinase; *PKC* protein kinase C, *CK* casein kinase, *PKB* protein kinase B (also known as Akt), *PKD1* 3-phosphoinoside-dependent protein kinase 1
[a]IC50 was determined in immunocomplex assays

4 Clinical Data in CML

4.1 Phase I Trials

In 1998, a phase I clinical trial with imatinib was initiated. This study was a dose escalation trial designed to determine the maximally tolerated dose, with clinical benefit as a secondary endpoint. 83 patients with CP CML who had failed standard therapy with interferon-α (IFN-α) or were intolerant to it were enrolled. One-third of patients had signs of early progression to AP. They received escalating oral doses of imatinib, ranging from 25 to 1,000 mg/day. Clinical features of patients were typical of the disease. Dose-limiting toxicity was not reached, although a higher frequency of severe toxicities was encountered at imatinib doses >750 mg/day. The most common adverse events were nausea (43 %), myalgia (41 %), edema (39 %), and diarrhea (25 %). After 29 patients were enrolled, therapeutic doses of 300 mg or more per day were reached. 53 of 54 patients achieved a complete hematologic response, reaching normal blood counts typically within four weeks of treatment. 51 of these 53 patients maintained normal blood counts after one year of therapy. Furthermore, these patients had a 31 % rate of major cytogenetic responses (MCyR; <35 % Ph^+ metaphases) and a 13 % rate of complete cytogenetic responses (CCyR; eradication of Ph^+ bone marrow cells) (Druker 2008; Druker et al. 2001b).

In another phase I trial, patients with myeloid and lymphoid blast crisis and patients with relapsed or refractory Ph^+ lymphoblastic leukemia (ALL) were treated with daily doses of 300–1,000 mg of imatinib. 55 % of patients with myeloid blast crisis responded to therapy (45 % of patients with <5 % blasts in the bone marrow, and 11 % reached a complete remission with full recovery of peripheral blood counts, respectively) but only in 18 % response was maintained longer than one year.

Of 20 patients with Ph^+ ALL or lymphoid blast crisis, 70 % responded, 20 % reached a complete hematologic remission. Nevertheless, all but one relapsed between days 45 and 117 (Druker et al. 2001a).

Based on the results of the phase I trials, the use of imatinib was expanded to large phase II and phase III clinical trials.

4.2 Phase II Studies

Three open-label, single-arm phase II studies using imatinib as a single agent were conducted in patients with Ph^+ CML in three clinical settings: CML-CP after IFN-α failure or with intolerance to the drug, CML-AP, and CML-BC. Imatinib was administered orally once daily. Initially, all patients received 400 mg/day. Early in the study, however, the imatinib dose was increased to 600 mg daily for CML-AP and CML-BC trials. Patients with resistant or progressive disease receiving a dose of 400 or 600 mg/day could receive doses of 600 or 800 mg daily (administered as 400 mg twice daily).

In 532 patients with CP CML who had failed IFN-α therapy, 95 % of patients reached a complete hematologic response, with CCR rates of 41 % and major cytogenetic remission (MCR) of 60 %. The estimated rates of freedom from progression to accelerated or blastic phase and overall survival at 6 years were 61 and 76 %, respectively (Druker 2008; Hochhaus et al. 2008; Kantarjian et al. 2002a).

For patients in BC and with Ph^+ ALL, the studies confirmed the results of the phase I trial. Response rates were also high; however, relapses were seen frequently. The majority of patients in BC relapsed during the first year of treatment. Hematologic responses were observed in 52 % of patients ($n = 260$) with myeloid BC, with a median response duration of 10 months. Interestingly, 48 % of patients in this trial developed new cytogenetic abnormalities during treatment, demonstrating clonal evolution (Druker et al. 2001a; Ottmann et al. 2002; Sawyers et al. 2002).

The efficacy in patients with AP CML was intermediate between CP and BC. Of 181 patients with AP, 82 % showed a hematologic response, 53 % reached a CHR which was sustained in 69 %. Major cytogenetic remissions were seen in 24 % of patients with a CCR rate of 17 % (Talpaz et al. 2002).

The treatment results in advanced phase CML and Ph^+ ALL underline the necessity of combination therapies with conventional chemotherapy as well as the use of second-generation tyrosine kinase inhibitors.

The results of the phase I and phase II trials led to the approval by the Food and Drug Administration (FDA) of imatinib for the treatment of CML in advanced phase and after failure of IFN therapy (Cohen et al. 2002b; Deininger et al. 2005; Druker 2008).

4.3 Phase III Study (IRIS Trial)

In a landmark phase III study, the International Randomized Study of Interferon and STI571 (IRIS) trial, imatinib and the combination of IFN plus cytarabine were compared in newly diagnosed CP CML patients. More than 1,000 patients were accrued in less than 7 months. 553 patients were randomized to each of the two treatments, imatinib at 400 mg per day or interferon-α plus Ara-C. There were no significant differences in prognostic or clinical features between the two treatment arms. After a median follow-up of 19 months, patients randomized to imatinib had significantly better results for CHR, MCR, and CCR, as well as progression-free survival than patients treated with interferon-α plus Ara-C (O'Brien et al. 2003a, b).

The remarkable superiority of imatinib led to early disclosure of study results. Thereafter, most patients were crossed over from interferon-α plus Ara-C to the imatinib arm.

The IRIS trial is now a long-term follow-up study of patients who received imatinib as initial therapy. After a follow-up of 5 years, the overall survival for newly diagnosed CP patients treated with imatinib was 89 %. An estimated 93 % of imatinib-treated patients remain free from disease progression to the AP or BC. The estimated annual rate of treatment failure was 3.3 % in the first year, 7.5 % in year two, 4.8 % in year three, 1.5 % in year four, and 0.9 % in year five. The progression rate did not increase over time (Druker et al. 2006; Fig. 3).

Most of the side effects of imatinib were mild to moderate, with the most common being edema, muscle cramps, diarrhea, nausea, skin rashes, and myelosuppression (Druker et al. 2006). Quality of life was far better in patients treated with imatinib (Hahn et al. 2003). Rates of hematologic and cytogenetic responses are shown in Table 2. A recent update at 7 years showed an estimated overall survival of 86 and of 94 % considering only CML-related deaths, respectively. The estimated EFS at 7 years was 81 % and the estimated rate without progression to AP or BC is 93 %. A CCR was achieved by 456 of 553 (82 %) of patients on first-line imatinib (O'Brien et al. 2008).

Monitoring of residual disease by quantitative RT-PCR in complete cytogenetic responders showed that the risk of disease progression was inversely correlated with the reduction of BCR-ABL mRNA compared with pre-therapeutic levels (Hughes et al. 2003). The rates of major molecular remissions as well as the depth of molecular responses increase over time with a downward trend of relapse (O'Brien et al. 2008).

Investigation of pharmacokinetics in the imatinib-treated patients showed a correlation between imatinib trough plasma concentrations with clinical responses, EFS and adverse events. Patient with high imatinib exposure had better rates of CCR, major molecular responses, and event-free survival (Larsen et al. 2008).

The results of the IRIS trial have led to FDA approval of imatinib for first-line treatment of patients with CP CML in 2002 (Cohen et al. 2002b, 2005; Druker et al. 2001b).

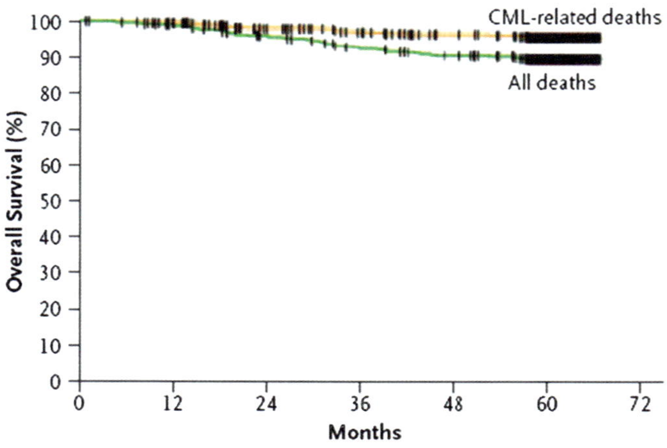

	12	24	36	48	60
No. of Deaths					
Related to CML	3	11	16	19	23
All deaths	6	22	41	52	57
No. at Risk					
Related to CML	536	498	474	450	322
All deaths	542	518	492	475	333

Fig. 3 IRIS trial: overall survival for newly diagnosed patients with CML treated with imatinib at 5-year follow-up (Druker et al. 2006). The estimated overall survival rate at 60 months was 89 %. After the censoring of data for patients who died from causes unrelated to CML or transplantation, the estimated overall survival was 95 % at 60 months (adapted from Druker et al. 2006)

5 Treatment Recommendations for the Use of Imatinib in Chronic Phase CML

Based upon the results achieved in the phase I, II, and III trials with imatinib, expert panels of the European Leukemia Net and the NCCN have developed guidelines for monitoring and treatment of CP-CML with imatinib (http://www.nccn.org/professionals/physician_gls/PDF/cml.pdf; Baccarani et al. 2013; http://www.nccn.org/professionals/physician_gls/PDF/cml.pdf; Table 3).

In case of suboptimal response, imatinib dosage should be increased and the option of allogeneic stem cell transplantation should be considered. In addition, in patients with failure of imatinib therapy, second- and third-generation tyrosine kinase inhibitors such as dasatinib, nilotinib, bosutinib or ponatinib have been approved (see according chapters). Further, TKI are currently under investigation.

Table 2 Results from the IRIS trial (Druker et al. 2006; O'Brien et al. 2003a, b)

Timepoint of follow-up	First-line treatment	Estimated cumulative rate of CHR (%)	Estimated cumulative rate of MCR (%)	Estimated cumulative rate of CCR (%)	Progression-free survival (PFS) (%)	Freedom from progression to AP or BC (%)	OAS (%)	References
18 months	IFN + Ara-C $n = 553$	55.5	22.1	8.5	73.5	91.5		O'Brien et al. (2003a, b)
	Imatinib $n = 553$	95.3*	85.2*	73.8*	92.1	96.7		O'Brien et al. (2003a, b)
60 months	Imatinib	98	92	87	83	93	89	Druker et al. (2006)

*Statistically significant difference to treatment with IFN + Ara-C ($p = 0.001$)
**OAS 94 % considering only CML-related deaths

Table 3 Response definitions to first-line treatment with TKIs (any TKI) (adapted from Baccarani et al. 2013)

Timepoint	Optimal response	Warning	Treatment failure
Baseline	NA	High risk or CCA /Ph+ Major Route	NA
3 months	BCR-ABL1 ≤10 % and/or Ph+ ≤35 %	BCR-ABL1 >10 % and/or Ph+ 36–95 %	Non-CHR and/or Ph+ >95 %
6 months	BCR-ABL1 <1 % and/or Ph+ 0	BCR-ABL1 1–10 % and/or Ph+ 1–35 %	BCR-ABL1 >10 % and/or Ph+ >35 %
12 months	BCR-ABL1 ≤0.1 %	BCR-ABL1 >0.1–1 %	BCR-ABL1 >1 % and/or Ph+ >0
Any time point	BCR-ABL1 ≤0.1 %	CCA/Ph− (−7, or 7q−)	Loss of CHR/CCgR
			Confirmed loss of MMR§
			Mutation
			CCA/Ph+

CHR complete hematologic response
CCgR complete cytogenetic response (absence of Ph^{+})
MMR major molecular response (ratio BCR-ABL/ABL >0,10)
CCA/Ph+ clonal chromosome abnormalities in Ph+ cells
CCA/Ph− clonal chromosome abnormalities in Ph− cells
§ In 2 consecutive tests, of which one with a BCR-ABL1 transcripts level ≥1 %

6 Imatinib in Combination with Other Drugs

In order to further optimize the efficacy of imatinib in CML, a number of approaches have been investigated in phase II trials. Increase in the dose of imatinib monotherapy to 800 mg/d in CP-CML has shown earlier complete cytogenetic responses but is associated with more side effects. However, the importance of faster responses has not been clear yet (Cortes et al. 2003). In addition, imatinib in combination with other agents, such as interferon-α, cytarabine, and homoharringtonine, has been examined. Patients treated with combination therapy reached faster cytogenetic remission, but also experienced higher rates of toxicity, in particular myelotoxicity (Baccarani et al. 2003, 2004; Gardembas et al. 2003). Several major phase III trials have been initiated which compare standard dose imatinib with increased doses and combinations with cytarabine or interferon. In these trials, the induction of faster cytogenetic as well as molecular remissions could be shown in patients receiving higher dosages of imatinib. However, the increased dosage if imatinib as well as when used in combination with cytarabine was more toxic than standard dose (Hehlmann et al. 2011; Preudhomme et al. 2010).

7 Imatinib: Other Targets

Other molecular targets of imatinib are the platelet-derived growth factor receptor (PDGF-R) and the stem cell factor receptor (c-KIT) (Buchdunger et al. 1995, 2000; Heinrich et al. 2002a).

Aberrant PDGF receptors have been shown to deregulate the growth of a variety of cancers, such as myeloproliferative disorders (Pardanani and Tefferi 2004), e.g., in hypereosinophilic syndrome (FIP1L1/PDGFR-rearrangment) (Jovanovic et al. 2007), CMML involving the 5q33 translocations (Jovanovic et al. 2007), carcinomas, melanoma, gliomas, and sarcomas, including dermatofibrosarcoma protuberans (Barnhill et al. 1996; Greco et al. 2001).

c-KIT is expressed in a variety of human malignancies, including germ cell tumors, neuroblastoma, melanoma, small cell lung cancer, breast and ovarian cancer, acute myeloid leukemia, mast cell disorders and malignant GIST.

In most of these diseases, the exact role of c-KIT expression is not defined in mastocytosis and GISTs activating mutations of c-KIT have been identified (Heinrich et al. 2003a, b).

In approximately 60 % of cases of GIST, there are mutations in *c-kit*[105] in the juxtamembrane domain. In most of the remaining cases, mutations in exon 13 and exon 9 have been found. The mutations lead to constitutive activation of the receptor without its ligand (Lux et al. 2000). Imatinib was investigated in 147 patients with histologically and immunohistochemically confirmed metastatic and/or unresectable GIST in a single, open-label trial involving one European center and three centers in the United States. Seventy-three patients were randomized to receive 400 mg of imatinib daily, and 74 patients received 600 mg daily. An objective response was confirmed in 56 patients with an overall response rate for the combined study arms of 38 % (95 % confidence interval, 30–46 %). All responses were partial responses. Adverse events were similar to CML patients and included edema, fluid retention, nausea, vomiting, diarrhea, myalgia, skin rash, bone marrow suppression, bleeding, and elevations in aspartate aminotransferase, alanine aminotransferase, or bilirubin. Gastrointestinal bleeding or intratumoral hemorrhage occurred in seven patients (5 %) and was not correlated with thrombocytopenia or tumor bulk. The pharmacokinetics of imatinib in GIST patients were similar to those of CML patients (Demetri 2002; Demetri et al. 2002). Imatinib mesylate at a recommended dose of 400 or 600 mg daily was approved by the United States FDA for the treatment of malignant metastatic and/or unresectable GISTs in 2001 (Dagher et al. 2002).

Following approval, two open-label, controlled, multicenter, randomized phase III studies were performed by the EORTC ($N = 946$) and the other by SWOG ($N = 746$). Both studies compared imatinib at a dosage of 400 mg/day and 800 mg/day, respectively. Combined analysis of the two studies was prospectively defined by both groups. Objective responses were achieved in >50 % of patients receiving either imatinib dose. Median PFS was approximately 20 months and median OS was approximately 49 months, respectively. In the combined analysis,

347 patients crossed over to imatinib 800 mg/day at the time of progression according to the protocol. Median OS after crossover was 14.3 months (Blanke et al. 2008; Heinrich et al. 2008).

After approval of imatinib in metastatic GIST, the role of adjuvant treatment after successful resection was investigated. The ACOSOG Z9001 trial could demonstrate a significantly improved recurrence-free survival following surgical resection of primary GIST, resulting in the adjuvant label for imatinib. An improved 5-year RFS and overall survival by extending the duration of adjuvant imatinib treatment to 3 years could be shown in a further large phase III trial (Joensuu et al. 2012).

8 Side Effects/Toxicity

Hematologic side effects of imatinib are shown in Tables 4 and 5. Grade 3 or 4 neutropenia, thrombocytopenia, or anemia was seen in all phase II trials and the phase III study. While grade 3/4 neutropenia occured in first-line treatment of CP CML in about 17 %, in accelerated and blastic phase, it could be detected in approximately 60 % of patients. In addition, in advanced phase, CML thrombocytopenia and anemia are more frequently than in CP-CML (first or second line).

Typical non-hematologic side effects in phase II trials of imatinib in CML are shown in Table 4 (Cohen et al. 2002b, 2005; Guilhot 2004). In the IRIS trial, most of the side effects of imatinib were mild to moderate, with the most common being edema, muscle cramps, diarrhea, nausea, skin rashes, and myelosuppression *as shown in* Table 5 (Druker et al. 2006; O'Brien et al. 2003b).

Recently, it has been suggested that imatinib may cause cardiotoxicity (Kerkela et al. 2006). However, a preexisting condition predisposing to congestive heart failure (CHF) could not be excluded in these patients. Furthermore, a follow-up examination of the Novartis database of imatinib clinical trials including >5,600 years of exposure to imatinib found an incidence of CHF in imatinib recipients of 0.2 % cases per year with a possible or probable relationship to the drug. In the IRIS trial, the incidence of cardiac failure and left ventricular dysfunction was estimated at 0.04 % per year in the imatinib arm compared to 0.75 % in interferon-a- and ara-C-treated patients (Hatfield et al. 2007).

In an early trial in GIST, adverse events were similar to CML patients and included edema, fluid retention, nausea, vomiting, diarrhea, myalgia, skin rash, bone marrow suppression, bleeding, and elevations in aspartate aminotransferase, alanine aminotransferase, or bilirubin. Gastrointestinal bleeding or intratumoral hemorrhage occurred in 7 patients (5 %) and was not correlated with thrombocytopenia or tumor bulk. Other non-hematologic side effects included fatigue and gastrointestinal complaints which were usually mild to moderate. The most common laboratory abnormality was anemia. Fluid retention and skin rash were reported more often in patients treated with 800 mg/day. Based upon these data, escalation of imatinib dosing up to 800 mg/day for patients with progressive disease was approved (Blanke et al. 2008; Heinrich et al. 2008).

Table 4 Adverse events ≥10 % in the phase II CML trials (Guilhot 2004; Cohen et al. 2002a, b)

Reported or specified term	CML-CP[1] after IFN-failure/ intolerance		CML-AP[2]		CML-myeloid BC[2]	
	$N = 532$		$N = 235$		$N = 260$	
	Dosage: 400 mg		Dosage 600 mg: $n = 158$		Dosage 600 mg: $n = 223$	
			Dosage 400 mg: $n = 77$		Dosage 400 mg: $n = 37$	
	All grades (%)	Grades 3/4 %	All grades (%)	Grades 3/4 %	All grades (%)	Grades 3/4 %
Hematologic adverse events						
Anemia		4		36		50
Neutropenia		33		58		62
Thrombocythemia		16		42		58
Non-hematologic AEs						
Nausea	60	2	71	5	70	4
Fluid retention	66	3	73	6	71	12
Superficial edema	64	2	71	4	67	5
Other fluid retention	7	2	7	2	22	8
Muscle cramps	55	1	42	0.4	27	0.8
Diarrhea	43	2	55	4	42	2
Vomiting	32	1	56	3	54	4
Hemorrhage	22	2	44	9	52	19
GI hemorrhage	2	0.4	5	3	8	3
CNS hemorrhage	1	1	2	0.9	7	5
Musculoskeletal pain	35	2	46	9	43	9
Skin rash	42	3	44	4	35	5
Headache	34	0.2	30	2	27	5
Fatigue	40	1	41	4	29	3
Arthralgia/joint pain	36	1	31	6	25	4
Dyspepsia	24	0	21	0	11	0
Myalgia	25	0.2	22	2	8	0
Weight gain	30	5	14	3	5	0.8
Pyrexia	17	1	39	8	41	7
Abdominal pain	29	0.6	33	3	31	6

(continued)

Table 4 (continued)

Reported or specified term	CML-CP[1] after IFN-failure/ intolerance		CML-AP[2]		CML-myeloid BC[2]	
	$N = 532$		$N = 235$		$N = 260$	
	Dosage: 400 mg		Dosage 600 mg: $n = 158$		Dosage 600 mg: $n = 223$	
			Dosage 400 mg: $n = 77$		Dosage 400 mg: $n = 37$	
	All grades (%)	Grades 3/4 %	All grades (%)	Grades 3/4 %	All grades (%)	Grades 3/4 %
Cough	17	0	26	0.9	14	0.8
Dyspnea	9	0.6	20	7	14	4
Anorexia	6	0	17	2	14	2
Constipation	6	0.2	15	0.9	15	2
Nasopharyngitis	18	0.2	16	0	8	0
Night sweats	10	0.2	14	1	12	0.8
Pruritus	12	0.8	13	0.9	8	1
Epistaxis	5	0.2	13	0	13	3
Hypokalemia	5	0.2	8	2	13	4
Petechiae	1	0	5	0.9	10	2
Pneumonia	3	0.8	8	6	12	6
Weakness	7	0.2	9	3	12	3
Upper respiratory tract infection	15	0	9	0.4	3	0
Dizziness	13.0	0.2	12	0	11	0.4
Insomnia	13	0.2	13	0	10	0
Sore throat	11	0	11	0	8	0
Ecchymosis	2	0	6	0.9	11	0.4
Rigors	8	0	11	0.4	10	0
Asthenia	6	0	11	2	5	2
Influenza	10	0.2	6	0	0.8	0.4

Abbreviations CP chronic phase, *AP* accelerated phase; *BC* blast crisis, *AE* adverse event
[1]Adverse events considered possibly related to treatment
[2]All adverse events regardless of relationship to treatment

Table 5 Most frequently reported AEs: first-line imatinib at 7-year follow-up: (Druker et al. 2006; O'Brien et al. 2008)

Most common adverse events (by 5 years)	All grade AEs patients (%)	Grade 3/4 AEs patients (%)
Superficial edema	60	2
Nausea	50	1
Muscle cramps	49	2
Musculoskeletal pain	47	5
Diarrhea	45	3
Rash/Skin problems	40	3
Fatigue	39	2
Headache	37	<1
Abdominal pain	37	4
Joint pain	31	3
Elevated liver enzymes	5	5
Hematologic toxicity		
Neutropenia	60.8	17
Thrombocytopenia	56.6	9
Anemia	44.6	4

Only serious adverse events (SAEs) were collected after 2005. Grade 3/4 adverse events decreased in incidence after years 1–2

9 Clinical Pharmacology and Drug Interactions

Imatinib AUC is dose proportional at the recommended daily dose range of 400 and 600 mg. Within 7 days, approximately 81 % of the dose is eliminated, 68 % in feces, and 13 % in urine.

Cytochrome P450 (CYP3A4) is the major enzyme responsible for imatinib metabolism, and both imatinib and CGP74588 appear to be potent in vitro CYP2D6 inhibitors. Imatinib plasma concentrations may be altered when the drug is administered with inhibitors or inducers of CYP3A4. When CYP3A4 inhibitors, e.g., itroconazole, ketoconazole, erythromycin, or clarithromycin, are co-administered with imatinib, its metabolization may be decreased. CYP3A4 inducers, such as dexamethasone, phenytoin, rifampicin, carbamazepine, phenobarbital, may increase imatinib metabolism. Furthermore, increased plasma concentrations of drugs which are substrates of CYP3A4, e.g., simvastatin, cyclosporine and others, may be the result of imatinib use (Cohen et al. 2002b, 2005; Lyseng-Williamson and Jarvis 2001; Mauro et al. 2002).

In a small number of children with Ph^+ ALL imatinib, plasma levels as well as of its metabolite CGP74588 were measured. Imatinib plasma levels were similar to those in adult patients. However, AUC of CGP74588 was only 5–24 % of the parent drug's AUC, and it was eliminated much faster than in adults indicating a lesser role of the metabolite in antileukemic activity (Marangon et al. 2009).

In the phase-III-(IRIS) trial, the correlation of imatinib pharmacokinetics and the response to treatment as well as to side effects could be shown (Larsen et al. 2008).

10 Biomarkers

10.1 CML

Disease progression and imatinib resistance

Resistance to imatinib includes de novo resistance and relapse after an initial response. The frequent and durable responses in CP-CML are caused by the selective inhibition of BCR-ABL by imatinib. In accelerated and blastic phase CML as well as in Ph^+ ALL, the combination of high numbers of proliferating tumor cells and genomic instability may lead to secondary genetic alterations, independent of BCR-ABL (von Bubnoff et al. 2003). In the majority of patients who respond to imatinib and then relapse, reactivation of the BCR-ABL tyrosine kinase could be shown. This indicates that BCR-ABL-dependent mechanisms either prevent imatinib from reaching its target or render the target insensitive to BCR-ABL. In the former category are mechanisms such as increased drug efflux through the multidrug resistance gene or protein binding of imatinib while the latter include mutations in the catalytic domain, the P-loop, and other mutations (Druker 2008; Gorre et al. 2001). Over 70 point mutations have been demonstrated to play a role in primary and secondary resistance to imatinib, respectively (Hochhaus et al. 2011; Fig. 4).

Gene amplification or overexpression of BCR-ABL as reason for resistance is seen occasionally (Shah et al. 2008; Shah and Sawyers 2003).

Understanding the underlying mechanisms of resistance has led to the development and investigation of new second- and third-generation tyrosine kinase inhibitors (Mueller 2009; Schiffer 2007) (see chapters bosutinib, dasatinib, nilotinib, and ponatinib).

10.2 GIST

Other molecular targets of imatinib are the platelet-derived growth factor receptor (PDGF-R) and the stem cell factor receptor (c-KIT) (Buchdunger et al. 1995, 2000; Heinrich et al. 2002a).

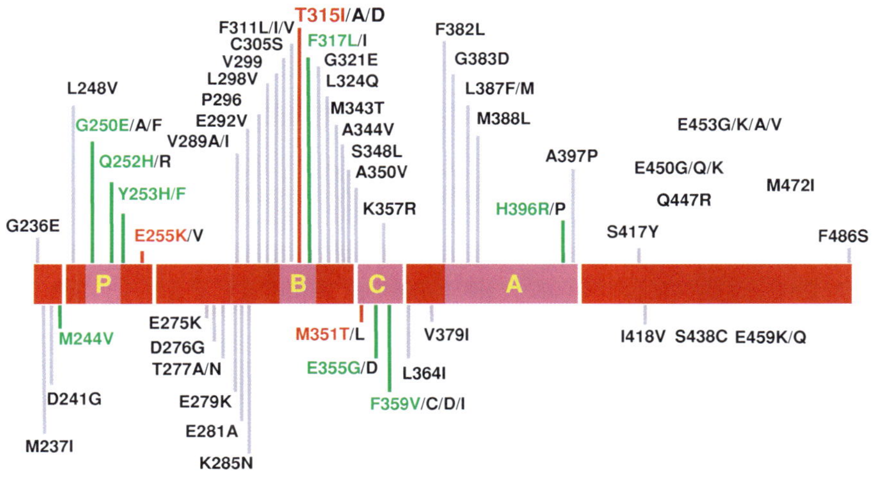

Fig. 4 Map of BCR-ABL kinase domain mutations associated with clinical resistance to imatinib (adapted from Branford 2006). *Abbreviations P* P-loop, *B* imatinib binding site, *C* catalytic domain, *A* activation loop. Amino acid substitutions in *green indicate* mutations detected in 2–10 % and in *red* in >10 % of patients with mutations (adapted with permission from Dr. Susan Branford, IMVS, Adelaide, Australia.)

In GISTs, activating mutations of c-KIT and PDGF-R have been identified (Heinrich et al. 2003a, b).

In approximately 60 % of cases of GIST, there are mutations in *c-kit*[105] in the juxtamembrane domain. In most of the remaining cases, mutations in exon 13 and exon 9 have been found. The mutations lead to constitutive activation of the receptor without its ligand (Lux et al. 2000). The mutational status is being used for the choice and duration of adjuvant therapy. In case of a PDGF-RA D842V mutation, no adjuvant therapy is indicated. In the presence of wild-type kit, the situation has to be discussed on an individual base. In exon-11 and all mutations except exon-9 mutations, adjuvant therapy should be performed with 400 mg imatinib while in the presence of exon-9-mutations, 800 mg/d should be used (Joensuu et al. 2012).

11 Summary and Perspectives

The development of imatinib mesylate resembles the progress made in molecular biology over the past 30 years and has changed the landscape of cancer treatment leading toward causative treatment not only of CML and GIST but also for other malignancies.

After identification of the critical role of BCR-ABL in the pathogenesis of CML, less than 15 years went by until the development of imatinib which is now the standard of care for patients in CP CML. It has specific activity against a limited number of targets and has been shown to be highly effective not only in CML but also in other hematologic malignancies and solid tumors such as GIST. Side effects of treatment are mild to moderate. The understanding of mechanisms of resistance and disease progression has further lead to the development of second- and third-generation tyrosine kinase inhibitors.

References

Anafi M, Gazit A, Gilon C, Neriah YB, Levitzki A (1993a) Tyrphostin-induced differentiation of mouse erythroleukemia cells. FEBS Lett 330:260–264

Anafi M, Gazit A, Zehavi A, Ben-Neriah Y, Levitzki A (1993b) Tyrphostin-induced inhibition of p210bcr-abl tyrosine kinase activity induces K562 to differentiate. Blood 82:3524–3529

Baccarani M, Russo D, Rosti G, Martinelli G (2003) Interferon-alfa for chronic myeloid leukemia. Semin Hematol 40:22–33

Baccarani M, Martinelli G, Rosti G, Trabacchi E, Testoni N, Bassi S, Amabile M, Soverini S, Castagnetti F, Cilloni D et al (2004) Imatinib and pegylated human recombinant interferon-alpha2b in early chronic-phase chronic myeloid leukemia. Blood 104:4245–4251

Baccarani M, Deininger MW, Rosti G, Hochhaus A, Soverini S, Apperley JF, Cervantes F, Clark RE, Cortes JE, Guilhot F et al (2013) European LeukemiaNet recommendations for the management of chronic myeloid leukemia: 2013. Blood 122:872–884

Barnhill RL, Xiao M, Graves D, Antoniades HN (1996) Expression of platelet-derived growth factor (PDGF)-A, PDGF-B and the PDGF-alpha receptor, but not the PDGF-beta receptor, in human malignant melanoma in vivo. Br J Dermatol 135:898–904

Blanke CD, Rankin C, Demetri GD, Ryan CW, von Mehren M, Benjamin RS, Raymond AK, Bramwell VH, Baker LH, Maki RG et al (2008) Phase III randomized, intergroup trial assessing imatinib mesylate at two dose levels in patients with unresectable or metastatic gastrointestinal stromal tumors expressing the kit receptor tyrosine kinase: S0033. J Clin Oncol 26:626–632

Buchdunger E, Zimmermann J, Mett H, Meyer T, Muller M, Regenass U, Lydon NB (1995) Selective inhibition of the platelet-derived growth factor signal transduction pathway by a protein-tyrosine kinase inhibitor of the 2-phenylaminopyrimidine class. Proc Natl Acad Sci U S A 92:2558–2562

Buchdunger E, Zimmermann J, Mett H, Meyer T, Muller M, Druker BJ, Lydon NB (1996) Inhibition of the Abl protein-tyrosine kinase in vitro and in vivo by a 2-phenylaminopyrimidine derivative. Cancer Res 56:100–104

Buchdunger E, Cioffi CL, Law N, Stover D, Ohno-Jones S, Druker BJ, Lydon NB (2000) Abl protein-tyrosine kinase inhibitor STI571 inhibits in vitro signal transduction mediated by c-kit and platelet-derived growth factor receptors. J Pharmacol Exp Ther 295:139–145

Buchdunger E, Matter A, Druker BJ (2001) Bcr-Abl inhibition as a modality of CML therapeutics. Biochim Biophys Acta 1551:M11–M18

Carlo-Stella C, Regazzi E, Sammarelli G, Colla S, Garau D, Gazit A, Savoldo B, Cilloni D, Tabilio A, Levitzki A, Rizzoli V (1999) Effects of the tyrosine kinase inhibitor AG957 and an Anti-Fas receptor antibody on CD34(+) chronic myelogenous leukemia progenitor cells. Blood 93:3973–3982

Cohen MH, Dagher R, Griebel DJ, Ibrahim A, Martin A, Scher NS, Sokol GH, Williams GA, Pazdur R (2002a) US Food and Drug Administration drug approval summaries: imatinib mesylate, mesna tablets, and zoledronic acid. Oncologist 7:393–400

Cohen MH, Williams G, Johnson JR, Duan J, Gobburu J, Rahman A, Benson K, Leighton J, Kim SK, Wood R et al (2002b) Approval summary for imatinib mesylate capsules in the treatment of chronic myelogenous leukemia. Clin Cancer Res 8:935–942

Cohen MH, Johnson JR, Pazdur R (2005) U.S. Food and Drug Administration drug approval summary: conversion of imatinib mesylate (STI571; Gleevec) tablets from accelerated approval to full approval. Clin Cancer Res 11:12–19

Cohen MH, Farrell A, Justice R, Pazdur R (2009) Approval summary: imatinib mesylate in the treatment of metastatic and/or unresectable malignant gastrointestinal stromal tumors. Oncologist

Cortes J, Giles F, O'Brien S, Thomas D, Garcia-Manero G, Rios MB, Faderl S, Verstovsek S, Ferrajoli A, Freireich EJ et al (2003) Result of high-dose imatinib mesylate in patients with Philadelphia chromosome-positive chronic myeloid leukemia after failure of interferon-alpha. Blood 102:83–86

Dagher R, Cohen M, Williams G, Rothmann M, Gobburu J, Robbie G, Rahman A, Chen G, Staten A, Griebel D, Pazdur R (2002) Approval summary: imatinib mesylate in the treatment of metastatic and/or unresectable malignant gastrointestinal stromal tumors. Clin Cancer Res 8:3034–3038

Daley GQ, Van Etten RA, Baltimore D (1990) Induction of chronic myelogenous leukemia in mice by the P210bcr/abl gene of the Philadelphia chromosome. Science 247:824–830

Deininger MW, Goldman JM (1998) Chronic myeloid leukemia. Curr Opin Hematol 5:302–308

Deininger MW, Goldman JM, Lydon N, Melo JV (1997) The tyrosine kinase inhibitor CGP57148B selectively inhibits the growth of BCR-ABL-positive cells. Blood 90:3691–3698

Deininger MW, Goldman JM, Melo JV (2000) The molecular biology of chronic myeloid leukemia. Blood 96:3343–3356

Deininger M, Buchdunger E, Druker BJ (2005) The development of imatinib as a therapeutic agent for chronic myeloid leukemia. Blood 105:2640–2653

Demetri GD (2002) Identification and treatment of chemoresistant inoperable or metastatic GIST: experience with the selective tyrosine kinase inhibitor imatinib mesylate (STI571). Eur J Cancer 38(Suppl 5):S52–S59

Demetri GD, von Mehren M, Blanke CD, Van den Abbeele AD, Eisenberg B, Roberts PJ, Heinrich MC, Tuveson DA, Singer S, Janicek M et al (2002) Efficacy and safety of imatinib mesylate in advanced gastrointestinal stromal tumors. N Engl J Med 347:472–480

Druker BJ (2008) Translation of the Philadelphia chromosome into therapy for CML. Blood 112:4808–4817

Druker BJ, Lydon NB (2000) Lessons learned from the development of an abl tyrosine kinase inhibitor for chronic myelogenous leukemia. J Clin Invest 105:3–7

Druker BJ, Tamura S, Buchdunger E, Ohno S, Segal GM, Fanning S, Zimmermann J, Lydon NB (1996) Effects of a selective inhibitor of the Abl tyrosine kinase on the growth of Bcr-Abl positive cells. Nat Med 2:561–566

Druker BJ, Sawyers CL, Kantarjian H, Resta DJ, Reese SF, Ford JM, Capdeville R, Talpaz M (2001a) Activity of a specific inhibitor of the BCR-ABL tyrosine kinase in the blast crisis of chronic myeloid leukemia and acute lymphoblastic leukemia with the Philadelphia chromosome. N Engl J Med 344:1038–1042

Druker BJ, Talpaz M, Resta DJ, Peng B, Buchdunger E, Ford JM, Lydon NB, Kantarjian H, Capdeville R, Ohno-Jones S, Sawyers CL (2001b) Efficacy and safety of a specific inhibitor of the BCR-ABL tyrosine kinase in chronic myeloid leukemia. N Engl J Med 344:1031–1037

Druker BJ, Guilhot F, O'Brien SG, Gathmann I, Kantarjian H, Gattermann N, Deininger MW, Silver RT, Goldman JM, Stone RM et al (2006) Five-year follow-up of patients receiving imatinib for chronic myeloid leukemia. N Engl J Med 355:2408–2417

Gambacorti-Passerini C, Le Coutre P, Mologni L, Fanelli M, Bertazolli C, Marchesi E, Di Nicola M, Biondi A, Corneo GM, Belotti D et al (1997) Inhibition of the ABL kinase activity blocks the proliferation of BCR/ABL+ leukemic cells and induces apoptosis. Blood Cells Mol Dis 23:380–394

Gardembas M, Rousselot P, Tulliez M, Vigier M, Buzyn A, Rigal-Huguet F, Legros L, Michallet M, Berthou C, Cheron N et al (2003) Results of a prospective phase 2 study combining imatinib mesylate and cytarabine for the treatment of Philadelphia-positive patients with chronic myelogenous leukemia in chronic phase. Blood 102:4298–4305

Gorre ME, Mohammed M, Ellwood K, Hsu N, Paquette R, Rao PN, Sawyers CL (2001) Clinical resistance to STI-571 cancer therapy caused by BCR-ABL gene mutation or amplification. Science 293:876–880

Gratwohl A, Hermans J, Goldman JM, Arcese W, Carreras E, Devergie A, Frassoni F, Gahrton G, Kolb HJ, Niederwieser D et al (1998) Risk assessment for patients with chronic myeloid leukaemia before allogeneic blood or marrow transplantation. Chronic leukemia working party of the European group for blood and marrow transplantation. Lancet 352:1087–1092

Greco A, Roccato E, Miranda C, Cleris L, Formelli F, Pierotti MA (2001) Growth-inhibitory effect of STI571 on cells transformed by the COL1A1/PDGFB rearrangement. Int J Cancer 92:354–360

Guilhot F (2004) Indications for imatinib mesylate therapy and clinical management. Oncologist 9:271–281

Hahn EA, Glendenning GA, Sorensen MV, Hudgens SA, Druker BJ, Guilhot F, Larson RA, O'Brien SG, Dobrez DG, Hensley ML, Cella D (2003) Quality of life in patients with newly diagnosed chronic phase chronic myeloid leukemia on imatinib versus interferon alfa plus low-dose cytarabine: results from the IRIS Study. J Clin Oncol 21:2138–2146

Hatfield A, Owen S, Pilot PR (2007) In reply to 'Cardiotoxicity of the cancer therapeutic agent imatinib mesylate'. Nat Med 13, 13: author reply 15–16

Hehlmann R, Berger U, Pfirrmann M, Heimpel H, Hochhaus A, Hasford J, Kolb HJ, Lahaye T, Maywald O, Reiter A et al (2007a) Drug treatment is superior to allografting as first-line therapy in chronic myeloid leukemia. Blood 109:4686–4692

Hehlmann R, Hochhaus A, Baccarani M (2007b) Chronic myeloid leukaemia. Lancet 370:342–350

Hehlmann R, Lauseker M, Jung-Munkwitz S, Leitner A, Muller MC, Pletsch N, Proetel U, Haferlach C, Schlegelberger B, Balleisen L et al (2011) Tolerability-adapted imatinib 800 mg/d versus 400 mg/d versus 400 mg/d plus interferon-alpha in newly diagnosed chronic myeloid leukemia. J Clin Oncol 29:1634–1642

Heinrich MC, Blanke CD, Druker BJ, Corless CL (2002a) Inhibition of KIT tyrosine kinase activity: a novel molecular approach to the treatment of KIT-positive malignancies. J Clin Oncol 20:1692–1703

Heinrich MC, Rubin BP, Longley BJ, Fletcher JA (2002b) Biology and genetic aspects of gastrointestinal stromal tumors: KIT activation and cytogenetic alterations. Hum Pathol 33:484–495

Heinrich MC, Corless CL, Demetri GD, Blanke CD, von Mehren M, Joensuu H, McGreevey LS, Chen CJ, Van den Abbeele AD, Druker BJ et al (2003a) Kinase mutations and imatinib response in patients with metastatic gastrointestinal stromal tumor. J Clin Oncol 21:4342–4349

Heinrich MC, Corless CL, Duensing A, McGreevey L, Chen CJ, Joseph N, Singer S, Griffith DJ, Haley A, Town A et al (2003b) PDGFRA activating mutations in gastrointestinal stromal tumors. Science 299:708–710

Heinrich MC, Owzar K, Corless CL, Hollis D, Borden EC, Fletcher CD, Ryan CW, von Mehren M, Blanke CD, Rankin C et al (2008) Correlation of kinase genotype and clinical outcome in the North American Intergroup Phase III Trial of imatinib mesylate for treatment of advanced gastrointestinal stromal tumor: CALGB 150105 Study by Cancer and Leukemia Group B and Southwest Oncology Group. J Clin Oncol 26:5360–5367

Heisterkamp N, Jenster G, ten Hoeve J, Zovich D, Pattengale PK, Groffen J (1990) Acute leukaemia in bcr/abl transgenic mice. Nature 344:251–253

Hochhaus A, Druker B, Sawyers C, Guilhot F, Schiffer CA, Cortes J, Niederwieser DW, Gambacorti-Passerini C, Stone RM, Goldman J et al (2008) Favorable long-term follow-up results over 6 years for response, survival, and safety with imatinib mesylate therapy in

chronic-phase chronic myeloid leukemia after failure of interferon-alpha treatment. Blood 111:1039–1043
Hochhaus A, La Rosee P, Muller MC, Ernst T, Cross NC (2011) Impact of BCR-ABL mutations on patients with chronic myeloid leukemia. Cell Cycle 10:250–260
Hoeper MM, Barst RJ, Bourge RC, Feldman J, Ghofrani HA, Galié N, Gómez-Sánchez MA, Grimminger F, Grünig E, Hassoun PM et al (2013) Imatinib mesylate as add-on therapy for pulmonary arterial hypertension results of the randomized IMPRES study. Circulation 127(10):1128–1138
Hughes TP, Kaeda J, Branford S, Rudzki Z, Hochhaus A, Hensley ML, Gathmann I, Bolton AE, van Hoomissen IC, Goldman JM, Radich JP (2003) Frequency of major molecular responses to imatinib or interferon alfa plus cytarabine in newly diagnosed chronic myeloid leukemia. N Engl J Med 349:1423–1432
Joensuu H, Eriksson M, Sundby Hall K, Hartmann JT, Pink D, Schutte J, Ramadori G, Hohenberger P, Duyster J, Al-Batran SE et al (2012) One vs three years of adjuvant imatinib for operable gastrointestinal stromal tumor: a randomized trial. JAMA 307:1265–1272
Jovanovic JV, Score J, Waghorn K, Cilloni D, Gottardi E, Metzgeroth G, Erben P, Popp H, Walz C, Hochhaus A et al (2007) Low-dose imatinib mesylate leads to rapid induction of major molecular responses and achievement of complete molecular remission in FIP1L1-PDGFRA-positive chronic eosinophilic leukemia. Blood 109:4635–4640
Kantarjian H, Sawyers C, Hochhaus A, Guilhot F, Schiffer C, Gambacorti-Passerini C, Niederwieser D, Resta D, Capdeville R, Zoellner U et al (2002a) Hematologic and cytogenetic responses to imatinib mesylate in chronic myelogenous leukemia. N Engl J Med 346:645–652
Kantarjian HM, O'Brien S, Cortes JE, Smith TL, Rios MB, Shan J, Yang Y, Giles FJ, Thomas DA, Faderl S et al (2002b) Treatment of philadelphia chromosome-positive, accelerated-phase chronic myelogenous leukemia with imatinib mesylate. Clin Cancer Res 8:2167–2176
Kerkela R, Grazette L, Yacobi R, Iliescu C, Patten R, Beahm C, Walters B, Shevtsov S, Pesant S, Clubb FJ et al (2006) Cardiotoxicity of the cancer therapeutic agent imatinib mesylate. Nat Med 12:908–916
Konopka JB, Watanabe SM, Witte ON (1984) An alteration of the human c-abl protein in K562 leukemia cells unmasks associated tyrosine kinase activity. Cell 37:1035–1042
Larsen RA, Druker BJ, Guilhot F, O'Brien SG, Riviere GJ, Krahnke T, Gathmann I, Wang Y et al (2008) Imatinib pharmacokinetics and its correlation with response and safety in chronic phase chronic myeloid leukemia: a subanalysis of the IRIS study. Blood 111:4022–4028
Le Coutre P, Mologni L, Cleris L, Marchesi E, Buchdunger E, Giardini R, Formelli F, Gambacorti-Passerini C (1999) In vivo eradication of human BCR/ABL-positive leukemia cells with an ABL kinase inhibitor. J Natl Cancer Inst 92:163–168
Levitzky A, Gazit A (1995) Tyrosine kinase inhibition: an approach to drug development. Science 267:1782–1788
Lugo TG, Pendergast AM, Muller AJ, Witte ON (1990) Tyrosine kinase activity and transformation potency of bcr-abl oncogene products. Science 247:1079–1082
Lux ML, Rubin BP, Biase TL, Chen CJ, Maclure T, Demetri GD, Xiao S, Singer S, Fletcher CD, Fletcher JA (2000) Kit extracellular and kinase domain mutations in gastrointestinal stromal tumors. Am J Pathol 156:791–795
Lyseng-Williamson K, Jarvis B (2001) Imatinib. Drugs 61:1765–1774
Mahon FX, Rea D, Guilhot J, Guilhot F, Huguet F, Nicolini F, Legros L, Charbonnier A, Guerci A, Varet B et al (2010) Discontinuation of imatinib in patients with chronic myeloid leukaemia who have maintained complete molecular remission for at least 2 years: the prospective, multicentre Stop Imatinib (STIM) trial. Lancet Oncol 11:1029–1035
Marangon E, Citterio M, Sala F, Barisone E, Lippi AA, Rizzari C, Biondi A, D'Incalci M, Zucchetti M (2009) Pharmacokinetic profile of imatinib mesylate and N-demethyl-imatinib (CGP74588) in children with newly diagnosed Ph+ acute leukemias. Cancer Chemother Pharmacol 63:563–566

Mauro MJ, O'Dwyer M, Heinrich MC, Druker BJ (2002) STI571: a paradigm of new agents for cancer therapeutics. J Clin Oncol 20:325–334
Moinzadeh P, Hunzelmann N, Krieg T (2013) Pharmacology and rationale for imatinib in the treatment of scleroderma. J Exp Pharmacol 5:15–22
Mueller BA (2009) Imatinib and its successors: how modern chemistry has changed drug development. Curr Pharm Design 15:120–133
NCCN Practice Guidelines in Oncology, v.1.2014. (http://www.nccn.org/professionals/physician_gls/PDF/cml.pdf)
NCCN_Practice_Guidelines_in_Oncology, v.3.2008. http://www.nccn.org/professionals/physician_gls/PDF/cml.pdf
Nowell PC, Hungerford DA (1960) A minute chromosome in human chronic granulocytic leukemia. Science 132:1497
O'Brien SG, Guilhot F, Goldman J, Hochhaus A, Hughes T, Radich J, Rudoltz M, Filian J, Gathmann I, Druker B et al (2008) International randomized study of interferon versus STI571 (IRIS) 7-year follow-up: sustained survival, low rate of transformation and increased rate of major molecular response (MMR) in patients (pts) with newly diagnosed chronic myeloid leukemia in chronic phase (CML-CP) treated with imatinib (IM). Blood 112:76
O'Brien S, Giles F, Talpaz M, Cortes J, Rios MB, Shan J, Thomas D, Andreeff M, Kornblau S, Faderl S et al (2003a) Results of triple therapy with interferon-alpha, cytarabine, and homoharringtonine, and the impact of adding imatinib to the treatment sequence in patients with Philadelphia chromosome-positive chronic myelogenous leukemia in early chronic phase. Cancer 98:888–893
O'Brien SG, Guilhot F, Larson RA, Gathmann I, Baccarani M, Cervantes F, Cornelissen JJ, Fischer T, Hochhaus A, Hughes T et al (2003b) Imatinib compared with interferon and low-dose cytarabine for newly diagnosed chronic-phase chronic myeloid leukemia. N Engl J Med 348:994–1004
Okuda K, Weisberg E, Gilliland DG, Griffin JD (2001) ARG tyrosine kinase activity is inhibited by STI571. Blood 97:2440–2448
Ottmann OG, Druker BJ, Sawyers CL, Goldman JM, Reiffers J, Silver RT, Tura S, Fischer T, Deininger MW, Schiffer CA et al (2002) A phase 2 study of imatinib in patients with relapsed or refractory Philadelphia chromosome-positive acute lymphoid leukemias. Blood 100:1965–1971
Pardanani A, Tefferi A (2004) Imatinib targets other than bcr/abl and their clinical relevance in myeloid disorders. Blood 104:1931–1939
Preudhomme C, Guilhot J, Nicolini FE, Guerci-Bresler A, Rigal-Huguet F, Maloisel F, Coiteux V, Gardembas M, Berthou C, Vekhoff A et al (2010) Imatinib plus peginterferon alfa-2a in chronic myeloid leukemia. N Engl J Med 363:2511–2521
Rowley JD (1973) A new consistent abnormality in chronic myelogenous leukaemia identified by quinacrine fluorescence and Giemsa staining. Nature 243:290–293
Sawyers CL (1999) Chronic myeloid leukemia. N Engl J Med 340:1330–1340
Sawyers CL, Hochhaus A, Feldman E, Goldman JM, Miller CB, Ottmann OG, Schiffer CA, Talpaz M, Guilhot F, Deininger MW et al (2002) Imatinib induces hematologic and cytogenetic responses in patients with chronic myelogenous leukemia in myeloid blast crisis: results of a phase II study. Blood 99:3530–3539
Schiffer CA (2007) BCR-ABL tyrosine kinase inhibitors in chronic myelogenous leukemia. N Engl J Med 357:258–265
Shah NP, Sawyers CL (2003) Mechanisms of resistance to STI571 in Philadelphia chromosome-associated leukemias. Oncogene 22:7389–7395
Shah NP, Kantarjian HM, Kim DW, Rea D, Dorlhiac-Llacer PE, Milone JH, Vela-Ojeda J, Silver RT, Khoury HJ, Charbonnier A et al (2008) Intermittent target inhibition with dasatinib 100 mg once daily preserves efficacy and improves tolerability in imatinib-resistant and intolerant chronic-phase chronic myeloid leukemia. J Clin Oncol 26:3204–3212

Talpaz M, Silver RT, Druker BJ, Goldman JM, Gambacorti-Passerini C, Guilhot F, Schiffer CA, Fischer T, Deininger MW, Lennard AL et al (2002) Imatinib induces durable hematologic and cytogenetic responses in patients with accelerated phase chronic myeloid leukemia: results of a phase 2 study. Blood 99:1928–1937
von Bubnoff N, Peschel C, Duyster J (2003) Resistance of Philadelphia-chromosome positive leukemia towards the kinase inhibitor imatinib (STI571, Glivec): a targeted oncoprotein strikes back. Leukemia 17:829–838
Voncken JW, Kaartinen V, Pattengale PK, Germeraad WT, Groffen J, Heisterkamp N (1995) BCR/ABL P210 and P190 cause distinct leukemia in transgenic mice. Blood 86:4603–4611

Dasatinib

Markus Lindauer and Andreas Hochhaus

Abstract

Dasatinib is an orally available short-acting dual ABL/SRC tyrosine kinase inhibitor (TKI). It potently inhibits BCR-ABL and SRC family kinases (SRC, LCK, YES, FYN), but also c-KIT, PDGFR-α and PDGFR-β, and ephrin receptor kinase. Dasatinib is an effective treatment for chronic myeloid leukemia (CML) and Philadelphia chromosome positive acute lymphoblastic leukemia (Ph+ ALL). Both diseases are characterized by a constitutively active tyrosine kinase; BCR-ABL. Dasatinib inhibits BCR-ABL with greater potency compared with other BCR-ABL inhibitors and is active in CML resistant or intolerant to imatinib. Dasatinib is approved for the treatment of CML (all phases) and for the treatment of Ph+ ALL, resistant or intolerant to prior imatinib treatment. Randomized trial data in CML show that first-line dasatinib provides superior responses compared with imatinib and enables patients to achieve early, deep responses, correlated with improved longer-term outcomes. A once-daily dose of 100 mg in chronic phase CML results in high hematologic and molecular remission rates and prolongation of survival. In accelerated and blastic phase of CML, as well as in Ph+ ALL, complete hematologic and cytogenetic remissions frequently occur. Remissions however are very short. In these patients, once-daily 140 mg is the recommended dose. The effect of dasatinib in other malignancies including solid

M. Lindauer (✉)
III. Medizinische Klinik, Klinikum am Gesundbrunnen, Am Gesundbrunnen 20–24, 74078 Heilbronn, Germany
e-mail: markus.lindauer@slk-kliniken.de

A. Hochhaus
Abteilung Hämatologie/Onkologie, Klinik für Innere Medizin II, Universitätsklinikum Jena, Erlanger Allee 101, 07740 Jena, Germany
e-mail: andreas.hochhaus@med.uni-jena.de

U. M. Martens (ed.), *Small Molecules in Oncology*, Recent Results in Cancer Research 201, DOI: 10.1007/978-3-642-54490-3_2,

tumors is subject of clinical studies. Regardless of many clinical trials in different tumor types and in different combinations of dasatinib with other agents, the role of dasatinib in the treatment of solid tumors has not yet been defined. Side effects of dasatinib are frequent but mostly moderate and manageable and include cytopenias and pleural effusions. The review presents the preclinical and clinical activity of dasatinib with a focus on clinical studies in CML.

Contents

1 Introduction

Chronic myeloid leukemia (CML) is a malignant clonal disorder of hematopoietic stem cells caused by a chromosomal aberration, the Philadelphia (Ph) chromosome. The Ph chromosome is formed by the chromosomal translocation t(9;22)(q34;q11). This translocation juxtaposes the ABL gene (chromosome 9) and the BCR gene (chromosome 22) creating a BCR-ABL fusion gene. The resulting chimeric protein is a constitutively active ABL tyrosine kinase (Hehlmann et al. 2007). Knowledge of the molecular pathogenesis of CML has allowed development of molecular targeted therapy, which has considerably changed the management and outcome of patients (Wong and Witte 2004; Hehlmann et al. 2007). Treatment options for CML include BCR-ABL tyrosine kinase inhibitors (TKIs), interferon alpha, chemotherapy, stem cell transplantation, or clinical trials of novel therapies (Baccarani et al. 2013; NCCN v4 2013).

Dasatinib is a potent multikinase inhibitor targeting BCR-ABL, the SRC family of kinases (SRC, LCK, HCK, YES, FYN, FGR, BLK, LYN, FRK), receptor tyrosine kinases (c-KIT, PDGFR, DDR1 and 2, c-FMS, ephrin receptors), and TEC family kinases (TEC and BTK). Most important is dasatinib's potent, short-acting inhibition of BCR-ABL. Dasatinib demonstrates activity against most imatinib-resistant BCR-ABL mutations (Karaman et al. 2008; Shah et al. 2004; Branford et al. 2009). The compound is indicated for the treatment of adults with newly diagnosed Philadelphia-chromosome-positive (Ph+) CML in all phases of the disease, e.g., chronic (CP), accelerated (AP), blast phase (BP; myeloid or lymphoid) Ph+ CML, and Ph+ ALL with resistance or intolerance to prior therapy, including imatinib (Sprycel® BMS 2012; EMA 2012; Hochhaus and Kantarjian 2013).

In malignancies, in which BCR-ABL is not the critical kinase, the role of dasatinib has still to be defined. Dasatinib inhibits the c-KIT receptor tyrosine kinase, which is involved in proliferation, differentiation, and survival of cells. Activating mutations of c-KIT are associated with different human neoplasms, including the majority of patients with systemic mast cell disorders, acute myelogenous leukemia (AML), and gastrointestinal stromal tumors (GISTs). Gain-of-function mutations of c-KIT are inhibited by dasatinib (Schittenhelm et al. 2006). Clinical studies to explore the clinical relevance of c-KIT inhibition by dasatinib are underway in acute myeloid leukemia.

SRC family kinases, involved in signal transduction, are potently inhibited by dasatinib. The drug blocks cell duplication, migration, and invasion, and it triggers apoptosis of tumor cells. It also diminishes metastatic spread of tumor cells and acts on the tumoral microenvironment. In addition, it sensitizes and resensitizes tumor cells to chemotherapy, antiangiogenetic, antihormonal, or epidermal growth factor receptor (EGFR) inhibitor therapy (Montero et al. 2011). The effect of dasatinib monotherapy in clinical trials is modest. Many clinical studies with dasatinib in solid tumors in different treatment lines and combinations are ongoing. Results are summarized in this review.

2 Structure and Mechanism of Action

Dasatinib (former BMS 354825), or *N*-(2-chloro-6-methyl-phenyl)-2-(6-(4-(2-hydroxyethyl)-piperazin-1-yl)-2-methylpyrimidin-4-ylamino)thiazole-5-carboxamide monohydrate (C22H26ClN7O2S), is an orally available small-molecule multitargeted kinase inhibitor (Fig. 1). Dasatinib was discovered by and named after Jagabandhu Das (Lombardo et al. 2004; Das et al. 2006) as part of an effort to develop potent inhibitors of SRC family kinases (SFKs).

The compound targets the SRC family of kinases (SRC, LCK, HCK, YES, FYN, FGR, BLK, LYN, FRK). In addition, and clinically more significant, dasatinib inhibits BCR-ABL with greater potency compared to other BCR-ABL inhibitors.

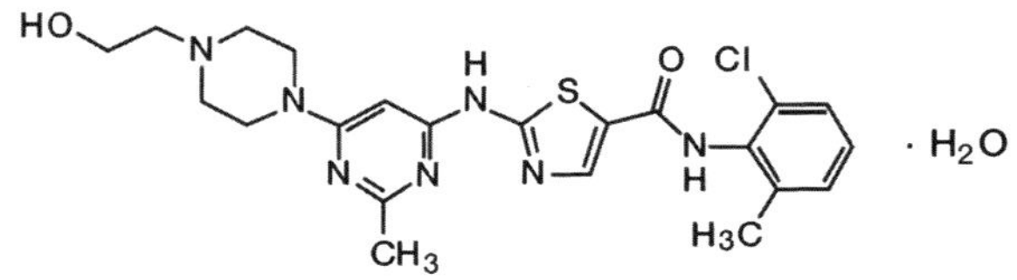

Fig. 1 Chemical structure of dasatinib

Table 1 Inhibitory activity of dasatinib on selected tyrosine kinases and potential clinical applications

Kinase	IC_{50} (nmol)	Neoplasias
Nonreceptor tyrosine kinases		
ABL	0.6	CML, Ph+ ALL
SRC	0.5	Several tumors, hematopoietic neoplasias
BTK	5	CLL, B-cell lymphomas
TEC	14	
Receptor tyrosine kinases		
c-kit	5–10	GIST, CML, breast cancer, AML, systemic mastocytosis
Ephrin A2 receptor kinase	17	Breast cancer, lung cancer
PDGFR-β	4	GIST, breast cancer, head and neck cancer
		chronic eosinophilic leukemia, hypereosinophilic syndrome

It also inhibits receptor tyrosine kinases (c-KIT, PDGFR, DDR1 and 2, c-FMS, ephrin receptors) and TEC family kinases (TEC and BTK) (Table 1).

Preclinical studies suggest that dasatinib induces apoptosis in only a small subset of cell lines. Inhibition of migration, invasion, and cell adhesion by dasatinib is reported more frequently (Johnson et al. 2005; Nam et al. 2005; Serrels et al. 2006). It has been demonstrated that dasatinib induces defects in spindle generation, cell cycle arrest, and centrosome alterations in leukemic cells, tumor cell lines, and also in normal cells. These effects are not attributable to the inhibition of a single kinase; rather it is expression of nonspecific effects on multiple kinases (Fabarius et al. 2008).

In a nude mouse model of prostate cancer, tumor growth and the development of lymph node metastasis were inhibited by dasatinib (Park et al. 2008). In addition, Dasatinib acts also on the tumoral microenvironment, especially in bone, where dasatinib inhibits osteoclastic activity and favors osteogenesis, exerting a bone-protecting effect (Metcalf et al. 2002).

Although immunosuppressive effects were initially observed in preclinical studies of dasatinib, recent evidence suggests that dasatinib may activate and mobilize antileukemic immune responses which may improve efficacy. These immunomodulatory effects may also be implicated in the clinically relevant side effects observed with dasatinib treatment (Mustjoki et al. 2010; 2011; 2013; Kreutzman et al. 2010; 2011).

3 Preclinical Data

3.1 Inhibition of ABL

Abelson kinase (ABL) is the constitutively active tyrosine kinase of the BCR-ABL fusion protein. It is a cytoplasmic nonreceptor tyrosine kinase. Human ABL has a number of structural domains critical for its activity. The major isoform of c-ABL has three SRC homology (SH) domains. SH1 domain contains the tyrosine kinase activity, while SH2 and SH3 domains allow interaction with other proteins. Under normal conditions, the activity of the ABL tyrosine kinase is tightly regulated.

Like many tyrosine kinases, ABL regulates its catalytic activity via conformational changes, switching between active and inactive forms by opening and closing an activation loop. The sequence available for binding in the inactive conformation varies dramatically between different kinases and provides a potential for binding specificity.

As demonstrated by X-ray crystallography, dasatinib, unlike imatinib, nilotinib, and ponatinib, binds the ATP-binding pocket of the SH domain 1 of BCR-ABL in both the active and inactive conformations (Tokarski et al. 2006; Vajpai et al. 2008; O'Hare et al. 2005; 2009; Weisberg et al. 2005; Levinson and Boxer 2012; Zhou et al. 2011; Radaelli et al. 2009; Cortes et al. 2010a).

Dasatinib has been shown to be 325-fold more potent than Imatinib for inhibiting unmutated BCR-ABL. The concentration required for 50 % inhibition [IC50] is 0.6 nmol/L for dasatinib and 280 nmol/L for imatinib (O'Hare et al. 2005). It is suggested that this stronger binding activity of dasatinib over imatinib is at least partially due to its ability to bind to active and inactive conformations of the ABL protein.

Crystal structures of the inhibitors bound to ABL show that dasatinib has fewer interactions with the P-loop, the activation loop, and α-helix compared with imatinib (Tokarski et al. 2006). Mutations resistant to imatinib but sensitive to dasatinib can be found in these regions (Tokarski et al. 2006). This is the basis for the activity of the drug in imatinib-resistant disease, caused by mutated BCR-ABL. Dasatinib demonstrates activity against most imatinib-resistant BCR-ABL mutations (Karaman et al. 2008; Shah et al. 2004; Branford et al. 2009).

Based on in vitro assays, outcomes in patients treated with second-line dasatinib after developing a BCR-ABL mutation on imatinib, and emergence of mutations during dasatinib treatment, dasatinib has little or no activity against T315I/A

F317L/I/C/V, or V299L, and lower activity against Q252H, E255V/K, and possibly G250E (O'Hare et al. 2005; Redaelli et al. 2009; Branford et al. 2009; Hochhaus et al. 2012a; Müller et al. 2009; Soverini et al. 2009; Shah et al. 2007; Cortes et al. 2007b).

ABL inhibition has a role also in chronic lymphocytic leukemia (CLL). Resistance to alkylating agents in CLL cells is accompanied by relatively high ABL levels. Dasatinib, through inhibition of ABL, sensitizes CLL cells to chlorambucil and fludarabine (Amrein et al. 2008). In addition, CD40-induced anti-apoptotic pathways in CLL are mediated by LYN (Ren et al. 1994) and ABL (Hallaert et al. 2008). Since ABL and LYN are targets for dasatinib, the drug is expected to be active in CLL. Clinical trials with dasatinib in CLL so far have shown only moderate activity (Amrein et al. 2011).

3.2 Inhibition of SRC

SRC is a member of a nine-gene family that includes YES, FYN, LYN, LCK, HCK, FGR, BLK, and YRK.

SRC family kinases are membrane-associated and involved in signal transduction. They integrate and regulate signaling from multiple transmembrane receptor-associated tyrosine kinases, such as the EGFR receptor family or PDGFR.

SRC family kinases (SFK) consist of a unique NH2-terminal region, two SRC homology domains (SH2 and SH3), a highly conserved kinase domain, and a COOH-terminal tail containing a negative regulatory tyrosine residue. SRC and SFK cooperate in several cellular processes including migration, adhesion, invasion, angiogenesis, proliferation, differentiation, and immune function. They play a major role in the development, growth, progression, and metastasis of a wide variety of human cancers (Kopetz et al. 2007; Montero et al. 2011).

Elevated levels of SRC kinase activity and/or protein expression levels have been found in a variety of human epithelial cancers, including colon, breast, pancreatic and lung carcinomas, in brain tumors, but also in osteosarcomas and Ewing sarcomas. The levels of expression or activation generally correlate with disease progression.

Dasatinib inhibits SRC with an IC_{50} of 0.5 nmol/L (Lombardo et al. 2004). Inhibition of SRC activation by dasatinib can suppress tumor growth in human breast cancer cell lines, in human prostate cancer cells, in head and neck, in lung cancer, and in osteosarcoma cell lines (Johnson et al. 2005; Finn et al. 2007; Shor et al. 2007). Pathologic SRC family kinase activity may contribute to BCR-ABL-independent imatinib resistance in CML (Donato et al. 2003; Pene-Dumitrescu and Smithall 2010).

Nuclear translocation of EGFR is mediated by SRC family kinases and may contribute to acquired resistance to cetuximab in solid tumors. Dasatinib treatment of cetuximab-resistant lung cancer cell line samples was found to be associated with loss of nuclear EGFR and resensitization to cetuximab (Li et al. 2009). In a similar manner, SRC is involved in coordinating signaling from the steroid receptors, including estrogen and androgen receptors. SRC inhibition may overcome endocrine resistance in hormonally driven cancers (Mayer and Krop 2010). Akin, dasatinib improves p53-mediated targeting of human acute myeloid stem cells by chemotherapy (Dos Santos et al. 2013).

Regarding the tumor microenvironment, SRC is involved in bone metabolism. Increased SRC activity has a net bone resorption result, as a consequence of inhibition of osteoclast generation, together with osteoclast stimulation (Metcalf et al. 2002; Garcia-Gomez et al. 2012).

3.3 Inhibition of KIT

KIT (CD117) is a 145-kD transmembrane glycoprotein, which is a member of the type III receptor tyrosine kinase family. Following ligand binding, the receptor dimerizes, is phosphorylated, and activates downstream signaling pathways involved in proliferation, differentiation, and survival. Normally, c-KIT is activated when bound to its ligand, the stem cell factor (SCF). Ligand-independent activation of c-KIT can be caused by gain-of-function mutations that have been reported in several malignancies, including GIST (Hirota et al. 1998), systemic mastocytosis (SM), acute myeloid leukemia (AML) especially core binding factor-AML (CBF-AML), lymphomas, and germ cell tumors (Schittenhelm et al. 2006). Imatinib, which is a potent inhibitor of KIT, has become the treatment of choice for advanced GIST. Comparable with its binding properties to ABL, imatinib only binds the inactive conformation of KIT.

Imatinib-resistant KIT mutants are frequent and often occur in the activation loop of KIT, resulting in a constitutive active conformation of c-KIT, to which imatinib cannot bind. These mutations have relevance in mast cell disorders, seminoma, and AML and are always resistant to imatinib. Dasatinib inhibits c-KIT 10–20-fold stronger than imatinib with an IC_{50} for inhibition of autophosphorylation and cellular proliferation of 5–10 nmol/L (Schittenhelm et al. 2006). In addition, dasatinib is a potent inhibitor of many clinically relevant mutated forms of c-KIT, including imatinib-resistant KIT activation loop mutations in vitro (Shah et al. 2006). In core binding factor (CBF)-AML, KIT mutations cluster most frequently within exon 17, which encodes the KIT activation loop in the kinase domain. In addition, CBF-AML is characterized by a higher KIT expression compared with other AML subgroups (Bullinger et al. 2004). Clinical trials with dasatinib in CBF-AML are ongoing.

3.4 Inhibition of Platelet-Derived Growth Factor Receptor (PDGFR) α and β Tyrosine Kinases

PDGFR-α and PDGFR-β are receptor tyrosine kinases. They are activated by binding of platelet-derived growth factor (PDGF). PDGF-signaling has a significant role in the formation of connective tissue and is also important during wound healing in the adult. PDGFR-α and PDGFR-β are expressed mainly on fibroblasts and smooth muscle cells (Heldin and Westmark 1999). Dasatinib inhibits PDGFR-β with an IC_{50} of 4 nmol/L (Chen et al. 2006).

PDGFR-α tyrosine kinase activating mutations have been described in the pathogenesis of some GISTs (Heinrich et al. 2003). Fusion proteins consisting of the fibroblast growth factor receptor 1 (FGFR1) and PDGFR-α and PDGFR-β receptor tyrosine kinases have constitutive transforming activity. They are found in a subgroup of myeloproliferative disorders associated with eosinophilia (Cross and Reiter 2008). In intima sarcoma, amplification of PDGFR-α is a common finding. Dasatinib was shown to inhibit PDGFR-α in intima sarcoma in vitro (Dewaele et al. 2010).

3.5 Inhibition of Ephrin Receptor Tyrosine Kinases

The ephrin family of receptor tyrosine kinases constitutes the largest subfamily of receptor tyrosine kinases. They are divided into two subclasses (ephrin A and ephrin B) based on sequence similarity and their preferential binding to ligands, which are tethered to the cell surface either by a glycosylphosphatidylinositol-anchor (ephrin A) or by a single transmembrane domain (ephrin B) (Kullander and Klein 2002). Eph receptor tyrosine kinases have important functions in development and diseases. In tumorigenesis, they have been implicated in cellular transformation, metastasis, and angiogenesis. EphA2 is frequently overexpressed and functionally altered in many invasive cancers including metastatic melanoma, as well as cancers of the mammary gland, cervix, ovary, prostate, colon, lung, kidney, esophagus, and pancreas.

Dasatinib was shown to be a potent inhibitor of ephrin A2 receptor kinase with an IC_{50} of 17 nmol/L in various cell lines (Huang et al. 2007; Chang et al. 2008).

3.6 Inhibition of TEC Family Kinases and BTK

TEC kinases are a large group of nonreceptor TKs and are closely related to SRC and ABL. TEC kinases play a pivotal role in the development and signaling of hematopoietic cells (Smith et al. 2001). Bruton tyrosine kinase (BTK) is a member of the TEC family kinases with a well-characterized role in B-cell receptor signaling and B-cell activation. Dasatinib has been shown to inhibit BTK with an IC_{50} of 5 nM and TEC with an IC_{50} of 14 nM (Hantschel et al. 2007). The irreversible strong BTK inhibitor ibrutinib, former PCI-32765, with an IC_{50} of 0.5 nM (Pan et al. 2007) has been shown to be very effective in CLL in a phase I–II clinical trial (Byrd et al. 2013). Clinical trials with dasatinib in CLL are ongoing.

4 Clinical Data

4.1 Pharmacokinetic Profile

Dasatinib is administered orally. The drug is rapidly absorbed, peak plasma concentrations occur 0.5–3 h after administration. The intake of food is not relevant for pharmacokinetics of dasatinib. In a dose range of 25–120 mg twice daily, the area under the plasma concentration–time curve (AUC) increased proportionally. The drug is extensively metabolized in the liver, predominantly by cytochrome P 450 (CYP) 3A4, only 30 % remain unchanged. The metabolites of the compound are unlikely to play a pharmacologic role. There were linear elimination characteristics over the above-mentioned dose range with a terminal elimination half-life of 5–6 h.

Elimination occurs mostly in the feces (85 %) only little in urine (4 %). Dasatinib is excreted as metabolites, only 19% of a dose was recovered as unchanged drug in the feces (Sprycel® BMS 2012).

4.2 Clinical Trials with Dasatinib

More than 200 clinical trials in almost all tumor entities have been performed so far with dasatinib, about 70 are still ongoing. Dasatinib treatment is most effective in the BCR-ABL-driven diseases CML and Ph+ ALL. Dasatinib is approved for the treatment of all phases of CML and Ph+ ALL, and therefore, treatment of these diseases will be discussed in more detail, followed by an overview of trials in other malignancies.

4.3 Clinical Trials with Dasatinib in CML Patients: Overview

The clinical efficacy of dasatinib in CML patients resistant or intolerant to imatinib was assessed in a phase I trial (Talpaz et al. 2006). Five phase II trials, termed START (**S**RC-ABL **T**yrosine kinase inhibition **A**ctivity **R**esearch **T**rials), were consecutively performed in all phases of CML in patients resistant or intolerant to imatinib (Kantarjian et al. 2007; Hochhaus et al. 2007; Ottmann et al. 2007; Guilhot et al. 2007a; Cortes et al. 2007a).

Dose-optimization phase III trials have been performed in chronic phase CML (Shah et al. 2008a) and in advanced phases of the disease (Kantarjian et al. 2009b, Saglio et al. 2010).

First-line treatment of CML patients with dasatinib was assessed in two phase II trials (Pemmaraju et al. 2011; Radich et al. 2012) and one phase III trial (Kantarjian et al. 2010; 2012).

4.3.1 Phase I Clinical Trial of Dasatinib in CML, All Phases and Ph+ ALL

The efficacy of oral dasatinib was first assessed in a phase I, open-label, dose-escalation study. Patients ($n = 84$) with various phases of CML or Ph+ ALL intolerant or resistant to imatinib, received oral dasatinib (15−240 mg/d) once or twice daily in 4-week treatment cycles (Talpaz et al. 2006). Dasatinib had clinical activity in all CML phases and Ph+ ALL. Complete hematologic response (CHR) was achieved in 92 % of patients (37/40) with CML-CP, and major hematologic response (MHR) was seen in 70 % of patients (31/44) with CML-AP, CML-BP, or Ph+ ALL. The rates of major cytogenetic response (MCyR) were 45 % in patients with CML-CP (18/40) and 43 % in patients with CML-AP (19/44), CML-BP, or Ph+ ALL. Of note, imatinib-associated side effects including muscle cramps and nausea were infrequently observed with dasatinib and patients intolerant to i-matinib did not have recurrence of the same nonhematologic adverse events (AEs) (e.g., rash and live-function abnormalities) with dasatinib treatment. The major AE associated with dasatinib was reversible myelosuppression.

4.3.2 Phase II Clinical Trials in Chronic Phase CML

A series of phase II trials, the pivotal START trial program, followed the phase I dose-escalation study. The primary objective for these trials was to treat patients with resistance or intolerance to imatinib treatment and who therefore had a life-threatening medical need. As the pharmacokinetics of the dasatinib 70 mg twice-daily regimen were better understood, it was selected for these trials. These open-label, multicenter trials established the efficacy and safety of second-line dasatinib (70 mg twice-daily) in the treatment of imatinib-resistant or imatinib-intolerant patients with CML (all phases) or Ph+ ALL (Table 2). Data from this program led to the initial approval of dasatinib in these indications.

Two START studies assessed second-line dasatinib 70 mg twice daily in patients with CML-CP. START-C trial was a single-arm study and START-R was a randomized, parallel-arm study of dasatinib versus high-dose imatinib (800 mg/day) in patients resistant to standard dose imatinib (Hochhaus et al. 2008; Kantarjian et al. 2009c). In START-C ($n = 387$), dasatinib-induced MCyR (primary endpoint) in 62 % of patients after a minimum follow-up of 24 months (Mauro et al. 2008). The corresponding CCyR rate was 53 %. In START-R, rates of MCyR were 53 % in the dasatinib 70 mg twice daily arm ($n = 101$) and 33 % in the high-dose imatinib arm ($n = 49$) ($P = 0.017$) after a minimum follow-up of 24 months (Kantarjian et al. 2009a). CCyR rates were 44 and 18 %, respectively ($P = 0.0025$). Although no formal statistical comparison between the study arms was planned, the data are suggestive of better efficacy for dasatinib compared with imatinib (Kantarjian et al. 2009a). These responses were also durable, as a pooled analysis ($n = 387$) of the START-C and START-R studies showed that 90 % of patients achieving a CCyR maintained this level of response after 24 months (Baccarani et al. 2008).

Table 2 Efficacy of dasatinib in chronic phase CML second line

Trial	No. patients/ Type of treatment	CHR (%)	MCyR (%)	CCyR (%)	MMR (%)	OS	PFS (%)	Reference
START-C[a]	387 (dasatinib 70 mg BID)	90	62	53	–	94 %	80	Hochhaus et al. (2008)
START-R[a]	101 (dasatinib 70 mg BID)	93	53	44	29	nr	86	Kantarjian et al. (2009c)
	49 (high-dose imatinib 400 mg BID)	82	33	18	12	nr	65	
CA180-034[a]	167 (dasatinib 100 mg QD)	92	63	50	37	71 %[b]	49[b]	Shah et al. (2008a), (2010), Rea et al. (2012)
	168 (dasatinib 70 mg BID)	88	61	53	43	70 %[b]	47[b]	
	167 (dasatinib 140 mg QD)	87	63	50	42	77 %[b]	40[b]	
	168 (dasatinib 50 MG BID)	92	61	49	41	74 %[b]	51[b]	

QD once daily; *BID* twice daily, *CHR* complete hematologic remission, *MCyR* major cytogenetic response: <= 35 % Ph+ cells in metaphase in bone marrow, *CCyR* complete cytogenetic response: 0% Ph+ cells in metaphase in bone marrow, *MMR* major molecular response: defined as a BCR-ABL transcript level of 0.1 % or lower, corresponding to a reduction in the BCR-ABL transcript level by at least 3 log from the standardized baseline level, *OS* overall survival, *PFS* progression-free survival, [a]at 2-year follow-up, [b]at 6-year follow-up

4.3.3 Dose-Optimization Study

The recommended starting dose for dasatinib in patients with CML in chronic phase is 100 mg once daily (Sprycel® BMS 2012; EMA 2012). This dose is the result of a phase III dose-optimization study (NCT00123474; CA180-034) showing that 100 mg once daily was associated with similar efficacy as the twice daily regimen, but with a reduction in toxicity (Shah et al. 2008a). The rationale for this study was based on observations from the phase I study that once-daily and twice-daily dose schedules were associated with similar response rates (Talpaz et al. 2006). Although dasatinib has a half-life of 3–5 h (Sprycel® BMS 2012), transient exposure of CML cell lines to dasatinib has been demonstrated to induce apoptosis (Shah et al. 2008b), supporting once-daily dosing. Furthermore, due to dose reductions in the START-C and START-R studies, the median total daily dose delivered to patients approximated 100 mg/day (Hochhaus et al. 2007; Kantarjian et al. 2007). It was therefore proposed to compare the 100 mg once schedule with other schedules. In this dose-optimization study, patients ($n = 670$) were randomized to receive dasatinib at 100 mg once daily ($n = 167$), 140 mg once daily ($n = 167$), 50 mg twice daily ($n = 168$), or 70 mg twice daily ($n = 168$) (Shah et al. 2008a) (Table 2). After a minimum follow-up of 2 years, rates of CCyR and MMR were similar across the different dosing schedules (CCyR 50–54 %; MMR 37–38 %) (Shah et al. 2010). In the 100 mg once daily arm, the 24-month rates of CCyR and MMR were 50 and 37 %, respectively. Rates of progression-free survival (PFS), overall survival (OS), and transformation to AP/BP by 24 months were 80, 91, and 3 %, respectively. The 100 mg once daily arm was associated with improved safety. Rates of all-grade pleural effusion ($P = 0.049$), grade ≥ 3 thrombocytopenia ($P = 0.003$), all-grade neutropenia ($P = 0.034$), and all-grade leukocytopenia ($P = 0.017$) were significantly lower for patients treated with dasatinib 100 mg once daily compared with other schedules (Shah et al. 2010). After a minimum follow-up of 6 years, PFS, OS, and rates of transformation to AP/BP were 49, 71, and 5 %, respectively, in the 100 mg once daily arm (Shah et al. 2012).

4.3.4 First-Line Treatment of CML with Dasatinib

First-line treatment of CML with dasatinib was investigated in the MDACC phase II trial (Pemmaraju et al. 2011), one phase III study (Kantarjian et al. 2010; 2012), and a second randomized phase II trial, the SWOG S0325 study (Radich et al. 2012) (Table 3).

The first trial investigating dasatinib as first-line treatment was a phase II, open-label study (Cortes 2010b). Patients with newly diagnosed CML-CP were randomized to receive dasatinib 100 mg once daily ($n = 66$) or 50 mg twice daily ($n = 33$) (Pemmaraju et al. 2011). Because of results from a phase III multinational randomized study of first-line dasatinib (discussed in the previous section) and trends in favor of the 100 mg once-daily schedule of dasatinib seen in this study, the 50 mg twice daily arm of this trial was closed after 66 patients were enrolled and all subsequent patients were randomized to the 100 mg once daily arm. The study continued with the once daily schedule (Cortes et al. 2010b; Pemmaraju et al. 2011). After a median follow-up of 29 months, in patients with ≥ 3 months follow-up ($n = 87$), rates of CCyR and MMR were 95 and 86 %, respectively. BCR-ABL levels of ≤ 0.0032 % (≥ 4.5 log reduction; $MR^{4.5}$) were achieved in 67 % of patients. Responses were achieved rapidly with 94 and 95 % of patients achieving a CCyR after 6 and 12 months, respectively. Similarly, MMR rates at 6 and 12 months were 68 and 73 %, respectively. These data compare favorably with historic response data for imatinib (Pemmaraju et al. 2011).

Dasatinib in the first-line setting was further investigated in the pivotal, open-label, multinational, randomized phase III trial of Dasatinib versus Imatinib Study in Treatment-Naïve CML Patients (DASISION) (Kantarjian et al. 2010). In this study, 519 patients newly diagnosed with CML-CP were randomized to receive dasatinib 100 mg once daily ($n = 259$) or imatinib 400 mg once daily ($n = 260$) (Kantarjian et al. 2010). Efficacy data are shown in Table 4. The primary endpoint of this study was confirmed CCyR (cCCyR; CCyR on two consecutive assessments) by 12 months. For the dasatinib versus imatinib arms, the rate of cCCyR by 12 months was 77 versus 66 % ($P = 0.007$), respectively (Kantarjian et al. 2010). Cumulative CCyR, MMR, and $MR^{4.5}$ rates were higher for dasatinib across a

Table 3 Efficacy of dasatinib in chronic myeloid leukemia as first-line treatment

Trial	n	Treatment	CHR	CCyR (%)	MMR (%)	OS (%)	PFS (%)	Reference
MDACC	31	Dasatinib 50 mg BID	98 %	95	73	100	100	Pemmaraju et al. (2011)
(3-year follow-up)	62	Dasatinib 100 mg QD						
DASISION	295	Dasatinib 100 mg QD	nr	80	64	95	94	Kantarjian et al. (2012)
(2-year follow-up)	265	Imatinib 400 mg QD	nr	74	46	95	92	
SWOG-S0325	123	Dasatinib 100 mg QD	81 %	84	59	97	93	Radich et al. (2012)
(3-year follow-up)	123	Imatinib 400 mg QD	82 %	69	44	97	90	

QD once daily, *BID* twice daily, *CHR* complete hematologic remission, *CCyR* complete cytogenetic remission, *MMR* major molecular response: defined as a BCR-ABL transcript level of 0.1 % or lower, corresponding to a reduction in the BCR-ABL transcript level by at least 3 log from the standardized baseline level, *OS* overall survival, *PFS* progression-free survival

24-month period ($P = 0.0002$, $P < 0.0001$, and $P = 0.002$, respectively) (Kantarjian et al. 2012). Responses to dasatinib were rapid and prolonged; median times to CCyR were 3.2 and 6.0 months and median times to MMR were 15 and 36 months in the dasatinib and imatinib arms, respectively (Kantarjian al. 2012). At 24 months, for dasatinib versus imatinib, cumulative rates of MMR were 64 versus 46 % ($P < 0.0001$), rates for BCR-ABL $\leq$0.01 % (MR^4) were 29 versus 19 % ($P = 0.0053$), and rates of $MR^{4.5}$ were 17 versus 8 % ($P = 0.0032$) (Hochhaus et al. 2012a; Kantarjian et al. 2012). After 2-year follow-up, transformation to AP/BP throughout study follow-up (including on study and after discontinuation) occurred in nine patients (3.5 %) receiving dasatinib and 15 (5.8 %) receiving imatinib (Hochhaus et al. 2012a; Kantarjian et al. 2012). At 2-year follow-up, survival data for this study remain immature. No difference was observed between dasatinib and imatinib for PFS (93.7 and 92.1 %) and OS (95.3 and 95.2 %). A small difference in failure-free survival for dasatinib versus imatinib was observed (including protocol defined progression; 91.2 vs. 87.8 %) (Hochhaus et al. 2012a; Kantarjian et al. 2012).

Rapid molecular responses were associated with lower transformation rates and better long-term outcomes. An early molecular response (BCR-ABL levels of $\leq$10 %) at 3 months was associated with lower transformation rates (dasatinib 1.5 vs. 8.1 %; imatinib 2.6 vs. 9.4 %), better long-term outcomes (24-month PFS: dasatinib 97 vs. 83 %, imatinib 96 vs. 85 %) and improved response (24-month MMR rates: dasatinib 76 vs. 16 %, imatinib 66 vs. 19 %) in both treatment arms (Hochhaus et al. 2012b). Deeper levels of response were achieved earlier with dasatinib compared with imatinib as equivalent BCR-ABL levels were achieved

Table 4 Efficacy of dasatinib second line after imatinib in phase II single-arm clinical studies in advanced stages of CML including blast crisis and Ph+ ALL (START trials)

Trial	Disease/ Phase	n	Follow-up (months)	Mutated BCR-ABL (% pts.)	Response (% of patients)				Survival				References
					MHR	CHR	MCyR	CCyR	1 year PFS (%)	1 year OS (%)	Median PFS (mo)	Median OS (mo)	
Start-A	Accelerated phase	174	14.1		64	45	39	32	66	82			Guilhot et al. (2007a)
													Apperley et al. (2009)
Start-B	Myeloid blast phase	109	>12	42	34	27	33	26			6.7	11.8	Cortes et al. (2008)
Start-L	Lymphoid blast phase	49	>12	65	35	29	52	46			3.0	5.3	Cortes et al. (2008)
Start-L	Ph+ ALL	46	>12	78	41	35	57	54				3	Porkka et al. (2007)
													Ottmann et al. (2007)

CHR complete hematologic response: normal white blood cell count, platelets <450.000/μl, no blasts or promyelocytes in peripheral blood, <5 % myelocytes and metamyelocytes in peripheral blood, normal basophil count, no extramedullary involvement, *MHR* major hematologic response: CHR or neutrophil count between 500 and 1,000/μl, and/or platelets between 20.000 and 100.000/μl, *MCyR* major cytogenetic response: <= 35 % Ph+ cells in metaphase in bone marrow, *CCyR* complete cytogenetic response: 0 % Ph+ cells in metaphase in bone marrow, *PFS* progression-free survival, *OS* overall survival

6 months earlier with dasatinib and a higher proportion of patients receiving dasatinib achieved BCR-ABL levels of $\leq$10 % at 3 months compared with patients receiving imatinib (84 vs. 64 %) (Hochhaus et al. 2012b; Saglio et al. 2012).

In total, 23 % of dasatinib-treated patients and 25 % of imatinib-treated patients discontinued treatment in DASISION; 5 and 7 % due to study-defined disease progression (defined as any of the following: doubling of white cell count to >20 × 10^9/L in absence of CHR; loss of CHR; increase in Ph-positive metaphases to >35 %; transformation to AP/BP; death from any cause), 3 and 4 % due to treatment failure, and 7 and 5 % due to drug-related AEs, respectively (Kantarjian et al. 2012). In patients who discontinued treatment, BCR-ABL mutations were found in 10 patients in each arm with a narrower spectrum of mutations seen with dasatinib versus imatinib (three versus nine different amino acids affected). Mutations associated with discontinuation in the dasatinib arm were T315I ($n = 7$), F317L ($n = 2$), and F317I/V299L ($n = 1$) (Kantarjian et al. 2012).

Similar levels of response have been observed in additional studies of first-line dasatinib. In the SWOG S0325 phase II study, newly diagnosed patients were randomized to receive dasatinib 100 mg once daily ($n = 123$) or imatinib 400 mg once daily ($n = 123$) (Radich et al. 2012). At 12 months, median reductions in BCR-ABL transcript levels were greater with dasatinib compared with imatinib (3.3 vs. 2.8 log, $P = 0.063$), as were the rates of >3-log BCR-ABL reductions (59 vs. 44 %, $P = 0.059$). Rate of CCyR was significantly different between the dasatinib and imatinib arms (84 and 69 %, respectively, $P = 0.040$), although cytogenetic responses were only assessed in 53 % of patients (Radich et al. 2012).

In the phase II OPTIM study, association of dasatinib (100 mg once daily) pharmacokinetics with safety and response is being investigated. Dose adjustments were made as needed to achieve optimal minimal dasatinib concentrations (C_{min}) in order to reduce the rates of AEs. Interim data for the first 125 patients are available (Rousselot et al. 2012). For all patients enrolled with at least 12 months follow-up, the rates of CCyR at 3, 6, and 12 months were 60, 82, and 95 %, and rates of MMR were 21, 46, and 62 %, respectively. At 12 months, the rate of $MR^{4.5}$ was 25 %, of which 80 % had undetectable BCR-ABL transcript levels (Rousselot et al. 2010; 2012).

4.3.5 Treatment of Advanced Stages of CML

Three studies out of the START program, assessing dasatinib in imatinib-resistant disease, were dedicated to advanced stages of CML. START-A, START-B, and START-L were single-arm studies of second-line dasatinib 70 mg twice daily in patients with CML-AP, CML-BP, and CML-BP/Ph+ ALL, respectively (Apperley et al. 2009; Guilhot et al. 2007b; Cortes et al. 2008; Porkka et al. 2007; Ottmann et al. 2007; Saglio et al. 2008). In the START-A trial, including 174 patients with CML in accelerated phase (CML-AP), after a median follow-up of 14.1 months, 64 % of patients achieved the primary endpoint of MHR (Apperley et al. 2009). START-B included patients with myeloid blast phase (CML-BP) ($n = 109$) and START-L included patients with lymphoid CML-BP ($n = 48$) and a subset of patients with Ph+ ALL (Cortes et al. 2008; Porkka et al. 2007; Ottmann et al. 2007). After a minimum follow-up of 24 months, a CHR was achieved in 26 % of patients with myeloid CML-BP, in 29 % of patients with lymphoid CML-BP, and in 35 % of patients with Ph+ ALL. The median overall survival in myeloid blast phase, lymphoid blast phase, and Ph+ ALL was 11.8 months, 5.3 months, and 3 months, respectively (Table 4).

A phase III dose-optimization study in patients with CML-AP (Kantarjian 2009b) and CML-BP (Saglio et al. 2010) led to a recommended dasatinib dose of 140 mg once daily in these indications (Sprycel® BMS 2012; EMA 2012). Patients were randomized to receive dasatinib 70 mg twice daily (n = 159, AP; n = 74, myeloid BP; n = 28, lymphoid BP) or 140 mg once daily (n = 158, AP; n = 75 MBP; n = 33, LBP). In patients with CML-AP, similar rates of MHR (68 vs. 66 %) and MCyR (43 vs. 39 %) were observed in both treatment arms after a median follow-up of 15 months. Significantly fewer patients in the once-daily arm had pleural effusion compared with the twice-daily arm ($P < 0.001$) (Kantarjian et al. 2009b). After 2 years of follow-up, for patients with myeloid BP, the MHR rates in both arms were 28 %; for those with lymphoid BP, the corresponding rates were 42 % in the once-daily arm and 32 % in the twice-daily arm. AE rates were suggestive of improved safety for dasatinib 140 mg once daily (Saglio et al. 2010).

4.4 Dasatinib in Ph+ Acute Lymphoblastic Leukemia (Ph+ ALL)

The effect of dasatinib in the treatment of Ph+ ALL was examined further in two phase II studies. Two more phase III studies with dasatinib in children with PH+ ALL are still active.

One phase II study in adults evaluated the combination of dasatinib with alternating hyper-CVAD (hyper-fractioned cyclophosphamide, doxorubicin, vincristine, and dexamethasone) and high-dose cytarabine and methotrexate. Dasatinib was administered for the first 14 days of 8 cycles.

Thirty-five patients were treated with a median age of 53 years and 94 % of them achieved complete remission, whereas two patients died due to infections before the evaluation of response. Twenty-seven patients achieved a cytogenetic response after the first cycle, whereas four patients had persistent Ph+ metaphases. Twenty patients achieved complete molecular remission at a median of 14 weeks, and additional sevev patients achieved a MMR at a median time of 11 weeks. Monitoring of residual disease was negative by flow cytometry in 29 of 33 patients at a median of 3 weeks. After a median follow-up of 14 months, median disease-free survival and median OS were not reached with an estimated 2-years OS of 64 % (Ravandi et al. 2010). Side effects included 16 episodes of bleeding and 8 episodes of pleural effusions, in addition infections, deep vein thrombosis and pulmonary emboli, diarrhea and metabolic abnormalities.

In a second study, dasatinib as single agent was combined with steroids for 84 days and free post-remission therapy (Foa et al. 2011). Of 53 evaluable patients, all achieved complete hematologic remission, of which 92.5 % at day 22 and at this time point, 10 patients achieved 3-log reduction in the BCR-ABL transcript. Twenty-months OS and DFS were 69 and 51 %, with better results in terms of DFS for patients who showed a molecular response at day 22. No deaths or relapses occurred during induction therapy: 23 out of 53 patients relapsed after completing induction and of these 12 with the T315I mutation, resistant to most TKIs. Overall, treatment was well tolerated: four patients discontinued due to toxicity (only one case of pleural effusion grades 1–2). Another case of pleural effusion was recorded in one patient who continued therapy with the drug (Foa et al. 2011).

Central nervous system disease of Ph+ blast phase CML or Ph+ ALL

Substantial activity of dasatinib in patients with Ph+ ALL or blast phase CML and central nervous system (CNS) involvement has been shown. Eleven adult and pediatric patients were treated with dasatinib as first-line treatment for CNS leukemia, whereas three patients experienced a CNS relapse while on dasatinib therapy for other reasons. All of the eleven patients responded with seven complete responders, four after dasatinib monotherapy. Three patients achieved a partial response. Responses were generally durable, and response durations of more than 26 months have been reported (Porkka et al. 2008).

4.5 Dasatinib in Philadelphia-Chromosome-Negative Acute and Chronic Myeloid Diseases, Including Systemic Mastocytosis

Few studies have been reported with dasatinib in Philadelphia-chromosome-negative myeloid diseases. The largest study included a total number of 67 patients, with various hematologic disorders including 33 patients with SM, nine patients with AML, six patients with myelodysplastic syndromes, five patients with hypereosinophilic syndrome (HES), three patients with chronic eosinophilic leukemia (CEL), and 11 patients with primary myelofibrosis (PMF) (Verstovsek et al. 2008).

Most patients with SM presented with the D816V KIT mutation, which confers imatinib resistance. Since dasatinib has been shown to be active against the KIT D816V mutation in vitro, activity of the drug in SM was expected. The D816V was present in 28 of the 33 patients with SM. Patients were treated with dasatinib with different doses and schedules. In SM patients, an overall response rate of 33 % was reported, mostly symptomatic improvements including two complete responses, none of them with the D816V.

The authors concluded that it is questionable, whether the use of dasatinib provides any advantage over other treatment options in SM and that dasatinib therapy does not seem to have significant activity in patients with MDS, PMF, and HES/CEL (Verstovsek et al. 2008).

Table 5 Summary of phase II trials with dasatinib in hematologic malignancies other than CML and Ph+ ALL

Indication	No. of pts	Treatment	Outcome	Reference
Ph- acute and chronic myeloid disease, including systemic mastocytosis	67	Dasatinib 140 mg	Overall response rate in systemic mastocytosis 33 %	Verstofsek et al. (2008)
	33 with systemic mastocytosis		CR in AML and hyper-eosinophilic syndrome, no responses in MDS and myelofibrosis	
CLL	13	Dasatinib 50 mg twice daily	1 SD for 12 weeks	Garg et al. (2008)
CLL	15	Dasatinib 140 mg	PR in 3 of 15 Pts	Amrein et al. (2011)
			Additional 5 Pts with clinical response	
High-risk MDS	18	Dasatinib 100 mg	3 PR	Duong et al. (2008)
			4 SD	
			10 progressive disease	

However, complete remissions were reported in the same study for a patient with HES, and one patient with AML. The patient with HES had a complex karyotype with an aberrant signaling via PDGFR-β. The patient with AML was KIT mutation positive.

An additional case with HES, characterized by the FIP1L1-PDGFR-α gene fusion, intolerant to imatinib was successfully treated with dasatinib 20 mg/day (Imagawa et al. 2011).

Patients with high-risk MDS have been treated with dasatinib monotherapy in another phase II clinical study. Few responses to dasatinib monotherapy were reported (Table 5). The authors conclude that the treatment was save but with only limited clinical efficacy (Duong et al. 2008).

4.5.1 Dasatinib in the Treatment of Chronic Lymphocytic Leukemia (CLL)

Dasatinib monotherapy has modest clinical activity in CLL, as shown in two phase II studies and one case report, documenting dasatinib-induced CR in a CLL-patient (Garg et al. 2008; Pittini et al. 2009; Amrein et al. 2011). Clinical trials, combining dasatinib with alkylating agents in CLL, are still ongoing. One study requires dasatinib sensitivity in vitro as an inclusion criterion (NCT01441882).

4.5.2 Dasatinib in the Treatment of Acute Myeloid Leukemia (AML)

Since mutated c-KIT is overexpressed in 26 % of core binding factor (CBF)-AML and dasatinib inhibits both mutated and unmutated forms of KIT, clinical studies are ongoing evaluating dasatinib in CBF-AML. Individual cases have been reported so far with promising results (Ustun et al. 2009; Verstofsek et al. 2008). A phase II trial (NCT00850382) found beneficial effects by the addition of dasatinib to standard chemotherapy in CBF-AML. Based on these results, a phase III clinical trial in patients with CBF-AML is ongoing, randomizing patients to standard AML therapy with or without addition of dasatinib. Patients in the dasatinib arm will receive one year of dasatinib maintenance treatment.

4.6 Dasatinib in the Treatment of Solid Tumors

Up to now dasatinib is only approved for diseases where BCR-ABL is the critical kinase. Due to its ability to inhibit SRC family kinases and other kinases, dasatinib has been investigated in a huge number of phase I and phase II clinical trials in different cancers, few selected studies are summarized in Table 6. In Clinicaltrials.gov, more than 200 clinical trials with dasatinib are registered, with more than 70 studies still recruiting patients in various indications, the magnitude in solid tumors.

In summary, dasatinib as monotherapy has only modest activity in solid tumors. Combinations of dasatinib and other agents have been investigated intensively. Only few remissions have been reported in singular patients, even in combination with dasatinib and other treatments.

Since SRC is involved in bone metabolism and has the potency to resensitize tumor cells to antihormonal treatment, the SRC inhibitor dasatinib was expected to be effective in metastatic castration-resistant prostate cancer (CRPC). Results of a phase II clinical trial with dasatinib in combination with docetaxel have suggested clinical benefit with PSA decreases of more than 50 % from baseline for at least 6 weeks in almost half of the patients (Araujo et al. 2009, 2012).

Based on these data, the recently published multinational, double-blinded, placebo-controlled READY trial randomized 1,522 patients with metastatic CRPC 1:1 to receive either docetaxel 75 mg/m^2 every three weeks plus prednisone with dasatinib 100 mg every day ($n = 762$) or docetaxel plus prednisone with placebo ($n = 760$). The primary endpoint was overall survival (Table 7) (Araujo et al. 2013).

Despite the large number of patients, the study failed to show any significant improvement in dasatinib-treated patients with respect to overall survival, progression-free survival, or reduction of pain. Treatment-related AEs were more frequent in the dasatinib arm: 18 versus 9 % for placebo. Serious AEs were reported in 30 % of patients in both arms of the study. The rate of death occurring within 30 days of the last study drug was 10 % in the dasatinib arm versus 6 % in the placebo arm (Araujo et al. 2013). Results of this study were disappointing. Unselected patients with mCRPC did not have any advantage from the addition of dasatinib to standard treatment. The probability, that this would be the case in other cancers is fading, despite the large number of ongoing clinical trials. Eventually, there will be subgroups of patients with solid tumors, selected by appropriate biomarkers, benefitting from dasatinib.

Table 6 Clinical trials of dasatinib in solid tumors

Indication	Clinical phase	*n*	Treatment	Outcome	Reference
Breast cancer					
Advanced breast cancer	I	52	Capecitabine 1,000 mg/m2, d1-14, Dasatinib 100 mg daily	Clinical benefit in 56 % of patients	Somlo et al. (2013)
Metastatic breast cancer	I	15	Paclitaxel weekly 80 mg/m2 for 3 weeks Dasatinib 120 mg daily	Of 13 assessable patients responses in 4 (31 %)	Fornier et al. (2011)
Advanced HER2-positive and/or hormone receptor-positive breast cancer	II	70	Dasatinib 70 mg twice daily	Of 69 Pts, 3 PR, 6 SD, all 9 hormone receptor-positive Limited single agent activity	Mayer et al. (2011)
Triple-negative breast cancer	II	43	Dasatinib 70 mg twice daily, initially 100 mg twice daily	Overall response rate 4.7 % Limited activity	Finn et al. (2011)
Ovarian cancer					
Ovarian or primary peritoneal carcinoma	II	35	Dasatinib 100 mg	No objective responses	Schilder et al. (2012)
Advanced or recurrent ovarian cancer	I	20	Paclitaxel 175 mg/m2, Carboplatin AUC 6, Dasatinib 150 mg	Remission rate 40 %, SD 50 %, PFS 7.8 months, OS 16.2 months	Secord et al. (2012)
Colorectal cancer					
Advanced colorectal cancer, first line	I	13	Capecitabine 850 mg/m2, d1-14, every 3 weeks, oxaliplatin 130 mg/m2, bevacizumab 7.5 mg/kg, Dasatinib 70 mg	3 PR, 6 SD,	Starodub et al. (2011) Strickler et al. (2011)
Previously treated metastatic colorectal cancer	II	19	Dasatinib monotherapy	No activity in metastatic colorectal cancer	Sharma et al. (2012)

(continued)

Table 6 (continued)

Indication	Clinical phase	*n*	Treatment	Outcome	Reference
Lung cancer					
Advanced nonsmall cell lung cancer, first line	II	34	Dasatinib 100 mg twice daily, later due to toxicity 100 mg-0-50 mg	Activity of dasatinib lower than that observed with chemotherapy, however marked activity in one patient and prolonged SD in 4 pts	Johnson et al. (2010)
Lung adenocarcinoma resistant to gefitinib or erlotinib	II	21	Dasatinib 70 mg twice daily	No activity in patients with EGFR-mutant adenocarcinoma resistant to erlotinib and gefitinib	Johnson et al. (2011)
Chemosensitive relapsed lung cancer	II	45	Dasatinib 70 mg twice daily	No activity	Miller et al. (2010)
Advanced nonsmall cell lung cancer	I/II	34	Erlotinib Dasatinib	Disease control rate 63 %	Haura et al. (2010)
Glioma					
Recurrent glioblastoma	I/II	26	CCNU 90-110 mg/m2 Dasatinib 100-200 mg	Significant hematologic toxicities, suboptimal exposure to both agents	Franceschi et al. (2012)
Recurrent malignant Glioma	I	47	Erlotinib 150-450 mg Dasatinib 180 mg	No radiographic responses, only one Pt SD after 6 months	Reardon et al. (2012)
Melanoma					
Advanced melanoma	II	39	Initial 100 mg twice daily, decreased to 70 mg twice daily	No activity	Kluger et al. (2011)
Melanoma	I	29	Dacarbazine 800 mg/m2 Dasatinib 70 mg twice daily	Objective responses in 13.8 % 12-month overall survival 34.5 %	Algazi et al. (2012)

(continued)

Table 6 (continued)

Indication	Clinical phase	*n*	Treatment	Outcome	Reference
Prostate cancer					
Castration-resistant prostate cancer	I/II	I: 16	Docetaxel 75 mg/m2 Q3 weeks	Durable 50 % PSA-decline in 26 of 46 Pts (57 %)	Araujo et al. (2012)
		II: 30	Dasatinib 100 mg	18 of 30 Pts with measurable disease PR	
Other					
Previously treated mesothelioma	II	46	Dasatinib 70 mg BID	No activity in mesothelioma	Dudek et al. (2012)
Head and neck squamous cell carcinoma	II	15	Dasatinib monotherapy	No remissions despite proven SRC inhibition	Brooks et al. (2011)

5 Toxicity

Dasatinib has a unique safety profile and since early clinical trials some AEs have been consistently reported in patients receiving dasatinib including myelosuppression, fluid retention, pleural effusion, gastrointestinal disorders, fatigue, headache, musculoskeletal disorders, rash, and infection (Table 8). Some bleeding events have also been reported. More recently, cases of pulmonary arterial hypertension (PAH), a subcategory of pulmonary hypertension (PH), have been reported in a small number of patients receiving dasatinib (Galie et al. 2009; McLaughlin et al. 2009; Fang et al. 2012). In clinical trials of first-line and second-line dasatinib, most AEs occurred within 12–24 months of treatment and were managed with dose modifications (Kantarjian et al. 2012; Shah et al. 2012; Sprycel® BMS 2012).

In the early phase I, open-label, dose-escalation study, the major AE was reversible myelosuppression, leading to dose interruption in 60 % of patients (Talpaz et al. 2006). Grade 3–4 neutropenia and thrombocytopenia were seen in 45 and 35 % of patients with CML-CP, respectively. Nonhematologic AEs included diarrhea, nausea, and peripheral edema. Treatment-related pleural effusion occurred in 13 % of patients with CML-CP (Talpaz et al. 2006). Rates of AEs in this study may be expected to be elevated as some patients received doses of dasatinib considerably higher than the current recommended dose of 100 mg once daily (range of dasatinib dose received: 15–240 mg/day). A maximum tolerated dose was not determined in this study and no patient withdrew from treatment as a result of toxic effects (Talpaz et al. 2006).

Table 7 Phase III study of dasatinib in combination with docetaxel and prednisolon in the treatment of metastatic castration-resistant prostatic cancer (mCRPC) (READY trial)

	Docetaxel–prednisolon–dasatinib	Docetaxel–prednisolon–placebo	HR
No. of patients	762	766	
Median overall survival	21.5 months	21.2 months	0.99
Overall response rate	31.9 %	30.5 %	
PFS	11.8 months	11.1 months	0.92
Median time to PSA progression	8.0 months	7.6 months	0.91
Pain reduction	66.6 %	71.5 %	

Median follow-up 19 months (Araujo et al. 2013)

In the following START-C phase II trial, in which patients with CML-CP received second-line dasatinib 70 mg twice daily, 9 % of patients discontinued treatment because of study-drug toxicity after 8 months of follow-up (Hochhaus et al. 2007). Cytopenias were common (grade 3/4: thrombocytopenia 47 %, neutropenia 49 %), but generally reversible and manageable with dose adjustments. Pleural effusion was observed in 19 % of patients (grade 3/4 in 3 %) (Hochhaus et al. 2007). Similar results were seen in the START-R phase II trial of dasatinib 70 mg twice daily (Kantarjian et al. 2007). After a median follow-up of 15 months, 28 % of patients had discontinued treatment, 16 % due to study drug intolerance. Cytopenias were common (grade 3/4: thrombocytopenia 56 %, neutropenia: 61 %) but reversible and manageable with dose modification. Pleural effusion occurred in 17 % of patients and was successfully managed with dose interruption, diuretics, or pulse steroid therapy (Kantarjian et al. 2007). Most cases of pleural effusion observed across the START studies were uncomplicated and resolved with temporary dose interruption, diuretics, or pulse steroid therapy. In the START-C and START-R trials, patients received dasatinib at 70 mg twice daily which is higher than the current recommended dose for CML-CP (100 mg once-daily). It may therefore be expected that the frequency of AEs and the rate of discontinuation due to study-drug intolerance might be higher than expected in these trials compared with patients receiving the current recommended dose for CML-CP.

A single institution analysis of 138 patients treated with dasatinib in the phase I dose-escalation study and phase II START trials showed that 29 % of patients with CML-CP developed pleural effusion (Quintás-Cardama et al. 2007). Patients receiving dasatinib 100 mg once daily had a lower incidence of pleural effusion compared with patients receiving 50 or 70 mg twice daily, or 140 mg once daily, while efficacy remained consistent across all four dosing schedules. Furthermore, a separate analysis indicated that intermittent dosing of dasatinib at 100 mg per day for five days per week, including a weekend drug holiday where dasatinib was not taken, led to reductions in the rate and severity of AEs including fluid retention and

Table 8 Adverse drug reactions reported ≥5 % in clinical trials ($n = 2.182$)

	All grades	Grades 3/4
Gastrointestinal disorders		
Diarrhea	32	4
Nausea	22	1
Vomiting	13	1
Abdominal pain	10	1
Gastrointestinal bleeding	8	4
Mucosal inflammation (including mucositis/stomatitis)	7	<1
Dyspepsia	5	0
Abdominal distension	5	0
Respiratory, thoracic and mediastinal disorders		
Pleural effusion	25	6
Dyspnoea	21	4
Cough	10	< 1
Nervous system disorders		
Headache	25	1
Neuropathy (including peripheral neuropathy)	6	<1
Skin and subcutaneous tissue disorders		
Skin rash	22	1
Pruritus	7	<1
General disorders and administration site conditions		
Superficial edema	21	<1
Fatigue	21	2
Pyrexia	13	1
Pain	7	<1
Asthenia	9	1
Chest pain	5	1
Vascular disorders		
Hemorrhage	15	2
Musculoskeletal and connective tissue disorders		
Musculoskeletal pain	14	1
Arthralgia	8	1
Myalgia	8	<1

(continued)

Table 8 (continued)

	All grades	Grades 3/4
Infections and infestations		
Infection (including bacterial, viral, fungal, nonspecific)	10	3
Metabolism and nutrition disorders		
Anorexia	9	<1
Blood and lymphatic system disorders		
Febrile neutropenia	5	5

Percent of patients

pleural effusion while efficacy and disease control were maintained (La Rosée et al. 2013). An analysis of risk factors for pleural effusion in patients treated with second-line dasatinib identified prior history of cardiac disease ($P = 0.02$), hypertension ($P = 0.01$), and twice daily dosing schedule ($P = 0.05$), was associated with an increased risk of pleural effusion (Quintás-Cardama et al. 2007). In a separate analysis, older age was the only baseline characteristic associated with an increased risk of pleural effusion (Porkka et al. 2010). The development of lymphocytosis during dasatinib treatment was associated with a 1.7-fold increased risk of pleural effusion (95 % CI, 1.1–2.5) (Porkka et al. 2010).

The second-line, phase III dose-optimization study indicated that dasatinib 100 mg once daily was associated with reduced frequency of AEs in patients with CML-CP, while efficacy was maintained (Shah et al. 2008a; Porkka et al. 2010; Shah et al. 2012). With a minimum follow-up of 6 months, patients receiving dasatinib 100 mg once daily had lower rates of pleural effusion and grade 3–4 thrombocytopenia compared with patients receiving 70 mg twice daily (7 vs. 16 % and 22 vs. 37 %, respectively) (Shah et al. 2008a). Furthermore, fewer patients receiving dasatinib 100 mg once daily required dose interruptions (51 vs. 68 %), dose reductions (30 vs. 55 %), or discontinuation (16 vs. 23 %) (Shah et al. 2008a). With a minimum follow-up of 24 months, 14 % of patients receiving dasatinib 100 mg once daily developed pleural effusion, compared with 25 % of patients receiving 70 mg twice daily (Porkka et al. 2010). Improved tolerability of once-daily dosing may be due to intermittent dasatinib exposure, in comparison with continuous exposure achieved by twice-daily dosing (Porkka et al. 2010). After a minimum follow-up of 5 years, grade 3–4 hematologic AEs in the 100 mg once daily arm included neutropenia (36 %) and thrombocytopenia (24 %). Any-grade nonhematologic AEs included headache (33 %), diarrhea (28 %), fatigue (26 %), and pleural effusion (24 %) (Shah et al. 2012). Grade 3–4 cytopenias and any-grade nonhematologic AEs generally first occurred within 12–24 months of treatment (Shah et al. 2012).

In the first-line setting, similar AEs were observed. Treatment-related AEs led to the discontinuation of dasatinib in 7 % of patients (Kantarjian et al. 2012). Grade 3–4 hematologic AEs were common in patients with CML-CP receiving dasatinib (100 mg once daily) or imatinib (400 mg once daily) (neutropenia 24 vs. 21 %, thrombocytopenia 19 vs. 11 %, anemia 11 vs. 8 %) (Kantarjian et al. 2012). Severe biochemical abnormalities were uncommon with the exception of grade 3–4 hypophosphatemia (dasatinib arm 7 %, imatinib arm 25 %) (Kantarjian et al. 2012). The most common nonhematologic AEs in DASISION (all grades, dasatinib versus imatinib) were myalgia (22 vs. 39 %), diarrhea (19 vs. 21 %), pleural effusion (14 vs. 0 %), headache (13 vs. 11 %), superficial edema (11 vs. 36 %), rash (11 vs. 17 %), and nausea (10 vs. 23 %) (Kantarjian et al. 2012). Grade 3–4 nonhematologic AEs associated with dasatinib were uncommon at 0–2 % (fluid retention 2 %, pleural effusion 1 %, diarrhea <1 %, fatigue <1 %) (Kantarjian et al. 2012). In DASISION, at 1-year follow-up, 26 patients (10 %) had pleural effusion; all events were grade 1 (2 %) or grade 2 (8 %) (Kantarjian et al. 2010). By 2-year follow-up, pleural effusion events had occurred in 37 patients (14.3 %) and were generally mild-to-moderate in severity (grade 1: $n = 9$, 3.5 %; grade 2: $n = 26$, 10.1 %; grade 3: $n = 2$, 0.8 %) with no grade 4 events observed. Events were largely manageable with treatment interruption ($n = 30$), dose reduction ($n = 19$), or the use of diuretics ($n = 17$) or corticosteroids ($n = 15$). Four patients required a therapeutic thoracocentesis. At 2-year follow-up, five patients (1.9 %) had discontinued dasatinib due to pleural effusion. Notably, the occurrence and management of pleural effusion appeared not to affect the efficacy of dasatinib (Laneuville et al. 2011; Kantarjian et al. 2012).

In some patients receiving dasatinib, large granular lymphocyte (LGL) expansions carrying clonal T-cell receptor gene arrangements occur resulting in lymphocytosis (Kreutzman et al. 2010). Data from a retrospective analysis of patients enrolled in DASISION suggested that dasatinib-treated patients with lymphocytosis had higher rates of any-grade pleural effusion and lower rates of myalgias and arthralgias compared with patients without lymphocytosis (Schiffer et al. 2010a). In a separate analysis of pooled study data, 31 % of patients with CML-CP had lymphocytosis, which was associated with a higher rate of CCyR and longer PFS in patients with advanced disease (Schiffer et al. 2010b). However, no formal statistical testing has been reported for either of these analyses. A subanalysis of DASISION demonstrated no substantial effects of baseline cardiovascular conditions, other comorbidities, or use of baseline medications on the general safety profile of dasatinib (Khoury et al. 2010; Saglio et al. 2010c; Guilhot et al. 2010).

More recently, rare cases of PAH in patients receiving dasatinib for CML and Ph+ ALL have been reported in the literature ($n = 16$) (Mattei et al. 2009; Rasheed et al. 2009; Hennigs et al. 2011; Orlandi et al. 2011; Dumitrescu et al. 2011; Philibert et al. 2011; Montani et al. 2012; Sano et al. 2012). By 2-year follow-up of the phase III DASISION trial of dasatinib versus imatinib in newly diagnosed CML-CP, three patients receiving dasatinib developed PH; however, no cases of PAH diagnosed by RHC were recorded (Kantarjian et al. 2012). No patient in DASISION discontinued dasatinib therapy because of PH or PAH (Kantarjian et al. 2012). PAH observed in patients receiving dasatinib is not typical as this disease is normally progressive, including cases with a drug-induced etiology which do not reverse on treatment withdrawal (Galie et al. 2009; McLaughlin et al. 2009) To date, however, the typical clinical course for dasatinib-associated cases of PAH is improvement or complete resolution in the majority of cases upon withdrawal of treatment.

Most AEs occurring in patients receiving dasatinib treatment are manageable through dose interruption or dose reduction (Sprycel® BMS 2012). If hematologic AEs occur in patients receiving dasatinib, treatment should be interrupted until the absolute neutrophil count is $\geq 1.0 \times 10^9$/L and platelets $\geq 50 \times 10^9$/L. Dasatinib can then be resumed at the original dose if recovery occurs within 7 days or at a reduced dose of 80/50 mg/d if recovery takes longer than seven days or if the event was a second/third recurrence. Growth factor support may also be considered (Sprycel® BMS 2012). If a severe nonhematologic AE (grade 3/4) develops dasatinib should be withheld until resolution or improvement. Treatment can then be resumed at a reduced dose dependent on initial severity of the event (Sprycel® BMS 2012). Pleural effusion events are largely manageable through dose reduction or interruption, and/or corticosteroids and diuretics. Once resolved a reduced dasatinib dose can be resumed. Rare cases of severe pleural effusion may require thoracentesis and oxygen therapy (Laneuville et al. 2011; Kantarjian et al. 2012). Other fluid retention events can be managed with diuretics and supportive care. To reduce the risk of PAH, patients should be evaluated for signs and symptoms of underlying cardiopulmonary disease before initiating dasatinib treatment. Upon confirmation of a PAH diagnosis based on RHC, dasatinib should be permanently discontinued (Sprycel® BMS 2012). PAH may be at least partially reversible upon treatment discontinuation. For bleeding events, management steps include dose interruption and transfusion (Quintás-Cardama et al. 2009; Sprycel® BMS 2012). Rash may be managed with topical or systemic steroids in addition to dose reduction, interruption, or discontinuation. In cases of gastrointestinal upset, the NCCN guidelines suggest that dasatinib be taken with a meal and a large glass of water. Specific supportive medication is also indicated in case of headache and diarrhea (Sprycel® BMS 2012; NCCN v4 2013). A subanalysis of DASISION showed that dose modifications taken to manage AEs had no apparent effect on response (Jabbour et al. 2011).

6 Drug Interactions

Dasatinib is a substrate and an inhibitor of CYP3A4. Therefore, there is a potential for interaction with other concomitantly administered drugs that are metabolized primarily by or modulate the activity of CYP3A4.

Systemic exposure to dasatinib is increased if it is coadministered with drugs that are inhibitors of CYP 3A4 (e.g., clarithromycin, erythromycin, itraconazole, ketoconazole).

If coadministered with drugs that induce CYP 3A4 (e.g., dexamethasone, phenytoin, carbamazepine, rifampicin, phenobarbital or *Hypericum perforatum*, also known as St. John's Wort), dasatinib AUC is reduced. It was reduced by 82 % when coadministered with rifampicin.

Dasatinib AUC was reduced when coadministered with H2-blockers/proton-pump inhibitors, or antacids. Concomitant administration of famotidin reduced dasatinib AUC by 61 %, coadministration of aluminum hydroxide by 55 %.

Dasatinib is an inhibitor of CYP3A4. Substrates of CYP3A4 with a narrow therapeutic index should be administered with caution in patients receiving dasatinib. Drugs that rank among that list are alfentanil, astemizole, terfenadine, cyclosporine, fentanyl, pimozide, quinidine, sirolimus, tacrolimus, or ergot alkaloid (ergotamine, dihydroergotamine) (Sprycel® BMS 2012).

7 Biomarkers

Valid biomarkers that may predict the sensitivity of a disease to dasatinib are important.

In the case of the BCR-ABL-positive diseases CML and Ph+ ALL, the presence of the fusion gene not only determines the diagnosis. BCR-ABL transcript levels under TKI treatment are a good biomarker for prognosis. In chronic phase CML scheduled response, checkpoints have been published, describing minimal requirements, expressed as BCR-ABL transcript levels or the extent of cytogenetic response at a given time. Treatment results are categorized as "optimal response" or "failure," in between an intermediate warning zone. Warnings imply that the patient should be monitored very carefully and may become eligible for other treatments. Failure implies that the patient should be moved to other treatments whenever available (Baccarani et al. 2013).

In diseases, where KIT plays a major role, KIT expression can be detected immunohistologically by the presence of the CD117 antigen. Moreover, the identification of activating KIT mutations might predict the efficacy of dasatinib.

Definition of an SRC oncogenic pathway signature can predict sensitivity to dasatinib (Bild et al. 2006; Huang et al. 2007). Attempts to find markers of dasatinib sensitivity and/or resistance have been carried out by analyzing gene expression profiles in 23 breast cancer cell lines. A six-gene profile was identified that predicted dasatinib sensitivity in breast and lung cancer cell lines. In addition, a gene expression signature related to dasatinib resistance was described (Huang et al. 2007). A SRC pathway activity index has been defined to establish patients that may respond to dasatinib (Moulder et al. 2010). In CLL, the activity of SYK and phospholipase Cγ2 (PLCγ2) correlates with sensitivity to dasatinib (Song et al. 2010).

8 Summary and Perspectives

Dasatinib has superior efficacy over imatinib and an acceptable safety profile in first- and second-line treatment of patients with CML. The potent, multitargeted activity of dasatinib may contribute to the depth and speed of response achieved with this agent. Dasatinib's potential immune activity may play a role in the observed potency and requires further investigation. These factors may also play a role in the unique safety profile and the AEs observed in patients receiving dasatinib.

In exploratory analyses, a greater proportion of patients achieved early, deep molecular responses ($\leq$10 % BCR-ABL at 3 months) associated with improved response and survival, and decreased transformation to AP/BP, with dasatinib compared with imatinib. With significantly deeper levels of molecular response achieved at all time points with up to 2-years follow-up in DASISION; more patients receiving dasatinib versus imatinib may achieve undetectable levels of BCR-ABL transcripts and a complete molecular response. Second-generation BCR-ABL inhibitors have also demonstrated some activity against CML stem cells, providing support for future investigation of dasatinib in achieving a functional cure (Mustjoki et al. 2011; Bocchia et al. 2010; Hiwase et al. 2010).

With changing treatment goals supporting earlier, deeper responses, it is reasonable to suggest that dasatinib and other second-generation BCR-ABL inhibitors are likely to be used more frequently as a first-line treatment option in patients with newly diagnosed disease, dependent on existing patient comorbidities and BCR-ABL mutation status (if known). The speed of response achieved with second-generation BCR-ABL inhibitors may also allow the early identification of a subset of patients resistant to BCR-ABL inhibitor treatment who may benefit from alternate TKI, stem cell transplant or clinical trials.

The loss of patent exclusivity for imatinib in 2015 (US) and 2016 (EU) is likely to influence first-line treatment selection. With the potential for increased use of imatinib, it will be important to closely monitor patient response to ensure early milestones are achieved. Data are emerging to support a change in treatment for patients failing to reach certain levels of response ($\leq$10 % BCR-ABL by 3 months) (Marin et al. 2012; Hanfstein et al. 2012; Neelakantan et al. 2013). A phase II study comparing dasatinib 100 mg once daily to imatinib standard of care in patients failing to achieve an optimal response of $\leq$10 % BCR-ABL after 3 months of imatinib 400 mg/day is currently in progress. This study will prospectively test the hypothesis that changing to dasatinib treatment in this patient population will induce an improved response rate (primary endpoint, MMR at 12 months) compared with continuing imatinib at any dose.

With the growing number of BCR-ABL inhibitors available for patients with CML-CP and the lack of head-to-head clinical trials with second-generation BCR-ABL inhibitors, choosing a treatment requires consideration on a patient-to-patient basis and therefore information regarding the efficacy and use of these agents in the real-world setting is of increasing interest. An observational 5-year prospective cohort study (SIMPLICITY: NCT01244750) has been initiated to further understand the use of dasatinib, imatinib, and nilotinib in patients with newly diagnosed CML-CP including real-world response, outcomes, treatment adherence, and patient quality of life. Data are anticipated to provide additional information to help guide initial treatment selection for CML patients.

The role of dasatinib in the treatment of other malignancies is not yet defined. The drug has only moderate effects on cell proliferation, but due to its activity on several TKIs, it is supposed to sensitize or resensitize tumors to chemotherapy, antiangiogenetic treatment, EGFR-inhibitor treatment or antihormonal treatment. The moderate effect in monotherapy studies was to be expected. By adding dasatinib to standard treatment in different tumors and lines of treatment, only few additional patients responding have been reported. The negative results of the first large phase III study with dasatinib in solid tumors, the READY-study, treating 1,522 patients with metastatic CRPC with standard chemotherapy in combination with dasatinib, dampen the expectations to treat other malignancies, not dependent on BCR-ABL, with dasatinib in the near future.

Studies are ongoing in AML and CLL, but also in several solid tumors including breast cancer and colorectal cancer. Testing for dasatinib sensitivity prior to study entry might be a way to select a patient population benefitting from dasatinib.

Signal transduction in solid tumors is getting more important for the choice of treatment, for example the use of EGF inhibitors in colorectal cancer dependent on K-RAS status (Van Cutsem et al. 2009) or the treatment of melanoma dependent on the B-RAF mutation status (Flaherty et al. 2012). In a concept of personalized medicine, the focus might switch from the histology of a given tumor to the oncogenic pathways involved in malignant transformation. Since dasatinib is a potent inhibitor of several TKs involved in oncogenic pathways, it is possible, that some patients might benefit from dasatinib, if their pattern of activated or overexpressed TKs is sensitive to dasatinib.

References

Algazi AP, Weber JS, Andrews SC (2012) Phase I clinical trial of the Src inhibitor dasatinib with dacarbazine in metastatic melanoma. Br J Cancer 106:85–91

Amrein L, Hernandez TA, Ferrario C et al (2008) Dasatinib sensitizes primary chronic lymphocytic leukaemia lymphocytes to chlorambucil and fludarabine in vitro. Br J Haematol 143:698–706

Amrein PC, Attar EC, Takvorian T et al (2011) Phase II study of dasatinib in relapsed or refractory chronic lymphocytic leukemia. Clin Cancer Res 17:2977–2986

Apperley JF, Cortes JE, Kim DW et al (2009) Dasatinib in the treatment of chronic myeloid leukemia in accelerated phase after imatinib failure: the START a trial. J Clin Oncol 27:3472–3479

Araujo J, Armstrong AJ, Braud EL et al (2009) Dasatinib and docetaxel combination treatment for patients with castration-resistant progressive prostate cancer: a phase I/II study (CA180086). J Clin Oncol 27(Suppl):5061

Araujo J, Mathew P, Armstrong AJ et al (2012) Dasatinib combined with docetaxel for castration-resistant prostate cancer. Results from a phase 1-2 study. Cancer 118:63–71

Araujo J, Trudel GC, Saad F et al (2013) Overall survival (OS) and safety of dasatinib/docetaxel versus docetaxel in patients with metastatic castration-resistant prostate cancer (mCRPC): results from the randomized phase III READY trial. J Clin Oncol 31(Suppl 6):abstract LBA8

Baccarani M, Deininger MW, Rosti G et al (2013) European LeukemiaNet recommendations for the management of chronic myeloid leukemia: 2013. Blood 122:872–884

Bild AH, Yao G, Chang JT et al (2006) Oncogenic pathway signatures in human cancers as a guide to targeted therapies. Nature 439:353–357

Baccarani M, Rosti G, Saglio G et al (2008) Dasatinib time to and durability of major and complete cytogenetic response (MCyR and CCyR) in patients with chronic myeloid leukemia in chronic phase (CML-CP). Blood 112(Suppl):450

Bocchia M, Defina M, Ippoliti M et al (2010) Evaluation of residual CD34+/Ph+ stem cells in chronic myeloid leukemia patients in complete cytogenetic response during first line nilotinib therapy. Blood 116:1398

Branford S, Melo JV, Hughes TP (2009) Selecting optimal second-line tyrosine kinase inhibitor therapy for chronic myeloid leukemia patients after imatinib failure: does the BCR-ABL mutation status really matter? Blood 114:5426–5435

Brooks HD, Glisson BS, Bekele BN et al (2011) Phase 2 study of dasatinib in the treatment of head and neck squamous cell carcinoma. Cancer 117:2112–2119

Bullinger L, Döhner K, Bair E et al (2004) Use of gene expression profiling to identify prognostic subclasses in adult acute myeloid leukemia. New Engl J Med 350:1605–1616

Byrd JC, Furman RR, Coutre SE et al (2013) Targeting BTK with ibrutinib in relapsed chronic lymphocytic leukemia. N Engl J Med 369:32–42

Chang Q, Jorgensen C, Pawson T, Hedley DW (2008) Effects of dasatinib on EphA2 receptor tyrosine kinase activity and downstream signaling in pancreatic cancer. Br J Cancer 99:1074–1082

Chen Z, Lee FY, Bhalla KN et al (2006) Potent inhibition of platelet-derived growth factor-induced responses in vascular smooth muscle cells by BMS-354825 (Dasatinib). Mol Pharmacol 69:1527–1533

Cortes J, Jabbour E, Kantarjian H et al (2007a) Dynamics of BCR-ABL kinase domain mutations in chronic myeloid leukemia after sequential treatment with multiple tyrosine kinase inhibitors. Blood 110:4005–4011

Cortes J, Kim DW, Raffoux E et al (2008) Efficacy and safety of dasatinib in imatinib-resistant or intolerant patients with chronic myeloid leukemia in blast phase. Leukemia 22:2176–2183

Cortes J, Rousselot P, Kim DW et al (2007b) Dasatinib induces complete hematologic and cytogenetic responses in patients with imatinib-resistant or—intolerant chronic myeloid leukemia in blast crisis. Blood 109:3207–3213

Cortes J, Talpaz M, Bixby D et al (2010a) A phase 1 trial of oral ponatinib (AP24534) in patients with refractory chronic myelogenous leukemia (CML) and other hematologic malignancies: Emerging safety and clinical response findings. Blood 116(suppl) (abs 210)

Cortes JE, Jones D, O'Brien S et al (2010b) Results of dasatinib therapy in patients with early chronic-phase chronic myeloid leukemia. J Clin Oncol 28:398–404

Cross NCP, Reiter A (2008) Fibroblast growth factor receptor and platelet-derived growth factor receptor abnormalities in eosinophilic myeloproliferative disorders. Acta Haematol 119:199–206

Das J, Chen P, Norris D et al (2006) 2-aminothiazole as a novel kinase inhibitor template. Structure-activity relationship studies toward the discovery of N-(2-chloro-6-methylphenyl)-2-[[6-[4-(2-hydroxyethyl)-1-piperazinyl)]-2-methyl-4-pyrimidinyl]amino)]-1,3-thiazole-5-carboxamide (dasatinib, BMS-354825) as a potent pan-Src kinase inhibitor. J Med Chem 49:6819–6832

Dewaele B, Floris G, Finalet-Ferreiro J et al (2010) Coactivated platelet-derived growth factor receptor alpha and epidermal growth factor receptor are potential therapeutic targets in intimal sarcoma. Cancer Res 70:7304–7314
Donato NJ, Wu JY, Stapley G et al (2003) BCR-ABL independence and LYN kinase overexpression in chronic myelogenous leukemia cells selected for resistance to ST571. Blood 101:690–698
Dos Santos C, McDonald T, Ho YW et al (2013) The Src and c-Kit kinase inhibitor dasatinib enhances p53-mediated targeting of human acute myeloid leukemia stem cell by chemotherapeutic agents. Blood. July 29 (Epub ahead of print)
Dudek AZ, Pang H, Kratzke RA et al (2012) Phase II study of dasatinib in patients with previously treated malignant mesothelioma (cancer and leukemia group B 30601): a brief report. J Thorac Oncol 7:755–759
Dumitrescu D, Seck C, Ten FH et al (2011) Fully reversible pulmonary arterial hypertension associated with dasatinib treatment for chronic myeloid leukaemia. Eur Respir J 38:218–220
Duong VH, Jaglal MV, Zhang L et al (2008) Phase II pilot study of oral dasatinib in patients with higher-risk myelodysplastic syndrome (MDS) who failed conventional therapy. Blood 112(Suppl) (abstract 4197)
European Medicines Agency (2012) Sprycel (dasatinib) summary of product characteristics. Uxbridge, UK, Bristol-Myers Squibb Pharma EEIG. Nov 2012. http://www.ema.europa.eu/docs/en_GB/document_library/EPAR_-_Product_Information/human/000709/WC500056998.pdf
Fabarius A, Giehl M, Rebacz B et al (2008) Centrosome aberrations and G1 phase arrest after in vitro and in vivo treatment with the SRC/ABL inhibitor dasatinib. Haematologica 93:1145–1154
Fang JC, DeMarco T, Givertz MM et al (2012) World Health Organization pulmonary hypertension group 2: pulmonary hypertension due to left heart disease in the adult–a summary statement from the pulmonary hypertension council of the international society for heart and lung transplantation. J Heart Lung Transplant 31:913–933
Finn RS, Dering J, Ginther C et al (2007) Dasatinib, an orally active small molecule inhibitor of both the src and abl kinases, selectively inhibits growth of basal-type/"triple-negative" breast cancer cell lines growing in vitro. Breast Cancer Res Treat 105:319–326
Finn RS, Bengala C, Ibrahim N et al (2011) Dasatinib as a single agent in triple-negative breast cancer: results of an open-label phase 2 study. Clin Cancer Res 17(21):6905–6913
Flaherty KD, Robert C, Hersey P et al (2012) Improved survival with MEK inhibition in BRAF-mutated melanoma. N Engl J Med 367:107–114
Foa R, Vitale A, Vignetti M et al (2011) Dasatinib as first-line treatment for adult patients with Philadelphia chromosome-positive acute lymphoblastic leukemia. Blood 118:6521–6528
Fornier MN, Morris PG, Abbruzzi A et al (2011) A phase I study of dasatinib and weekly paclitaxel for metastatic breast cancer. Ann Oncol 22:2575–2581
Franceschi E, Stupp R, van den Bent MJ et al (2012) EORTC 26083 phase I/II trial of dasatinib in combination with CCNU in patients with recurrent glioblastoma. Neuro Oncol 14:1503–1510
Galie N, Hoeper MM, Humbert M et al (2009) Guidelines for the diagnosis and treatment of pulmonary hypertension: the task force for the diagnosis and treatment of pulmonary hypertension of the European Society of Cardiology (ESC) and the European Respiratory Society (ERS), endorsed by the International Society of Heart and Lung Transplantation (ISHLT). Eur Heart J 30:2493–2537; Eur Respir J 34:1219–1263
Garcia-Gomez A, Ocio EM, Crusoe E et al (2012) Dasatinib as a bone-modifying agent: anabolic and anti-resorptive effects. PLoS ONE 7(4):e34914
Garg RJ, Wierda W, Fayad L et al (2008) Phase II study of dasatinib in patients with relapsed CLL abstract. Blood 112(Suppl) (abstract 4197)
Guilhot F, Apperley J, Kim D-W et al (2007a) Dasatinib induces significant hematologic and cytogenetic responses in patients with imatinib-resistant or—intolerant chronic myeloid leukemia in accelerated phase. Blood 109:4143–4150

Guilhot F, Apperley JF, Kim DW et al (2007b) Efficacy of dasatinib in patients with. Accelerated-phase chronic myelogenous leukemia with resistance or intolerance to imatinib: 2-year follow-up data from START-A (CA180-005). Blood 110(Suppl) (abstract 470)

Guilhot F, Kantarjian H, Shah NP et al (2010) Dasatinib (versus imatinib) in patients (pts) with newly diagnosed chronic myeloid leukemia in chronic phase (CML-CP): analysis of safety and efficacy by use of baseline medications in the DASISION trial. Blood 116(Suppl) (abstract 2295)

Hallaert DYH, Jaspers A, van Noesel CJ et al (2008) c-Abl kinase inhibitors overcome CD40-mediated drug resistance in CLL: implications for therapeutic targeting of chemoresistant niches. Blood 112:5141–5149

Hanfstein B, Muller MC, Hehlman R et al (2012) Early molecular and cytogenetic response is predictive for long-term progression-free and overall survival in chronic myeloid leukemia (CML). Leukemia 26:2096–2102

Hantschel O, Rix U, Schmidt U et al (2007) The Btk tyrosine kinase is a major target of the Bcr-Abl inhibitor dasatinib. Proc Natl Acad Sci USA 104:13283–13288

Haura EB, Tanvetyanon T, Chiappori A et al (2010) Phase I/II study of the Src inhibitor dasatinib in combination with erlotinib in advanced non-small-cell lung cancer. J Clin Oncol 28:1387–1394

Hehlmann R, Hochhaus A, Baccarani M (2007) Chronic myeloid leukaemia. Lancet 370:342–350

Heinrich MC, Corless CL, Duensing A et al (2003) PDGFRA activating mutations in gastrointestinal stromal tumors. Science 299:708–710

Heldin CH, Westermark B (1999) Mechanism of action and in vivo role of platelet-derived growth factor. Physiol Rev 79:1283–1316

Hennigs JK, Keller G, Baumann HJ et al (2011) Multi tyrosine kinase inhibitor dasatinib as novel cause of severe pre-capillary pulmonary hypertension? BMC Pulm Med 11:30

Hirota S, Isozaki K, Moriyama Y et al (1998) Gain-of-function mutations of c-kit in human gastrointestinal stromal tumors. Science 279:577–580

Hiwase DK, White DL, Powell JA et al (2010) Blocking cytokine signaling along with intense Bcr-Abl kinase inhibition induces apoptosis in primary CML progenitors. Leukemia 24:771–778

Hochhaus A, Baccarani M, Deininger M et al (2008) Dasatinib induces durable cytogenetic responses in patients with chronic myelogenous leukemia in chronic phase with resistance or intolerance to imatinib. Leukemia 22:1200–1206

Hochhaus A, Boqué C, Bradley Garelik MB et al (2012b) Molecular response kinetics and BCR-ABL reductions in patients with newly diagnosed chronic myeloid leukemia in chronic phase (CML-CP) receiving dasatinib versus imatinib: DASISION 3-year follow-up. Haematologica 97(Suppl 1) (abstract 1537)

Hochhaus A, Kantarjian HM (2013) The development of dasatinib as a treatment for chronic myeloid leukemia (CML): from initial studies to application in newly diagnosed patients. J Cancer Res Clin Oncol. Aug 13 (Epub ahead of print)

Hochhaus A, Kantarjian HM, Baccarani M et al (2007) Dasatinib induces notable hematologic and cytogenetic responses in chronic-phase chronic myeloid leukemia after failure of imatinib therapy. Blood 109:2303–2309

Hochhaus A, Shah NP, Cortes JE et al (2012a) Dasatinib versus imatinib in newly diagnosed chronic myeloid leukemia in chronic phase (CML-CP): DASISION 3-year follow-up. J Clin Oncol 30(Suppl) (abstract 6504)

Huang F, Reeves K, Han X et al (2007) Identification of candidate molecular markers predicting sensitivity in solid tumors to dasatinib: rationale for patient selection. Cancer Res 67:2226–2238

Imagawa J, Harada Y, Yoshida T et al (2011) Successful treatment with low-dose dasatinib in a patient with chronic eosinophilic leukemia intolerant to imatinib. Rinsho Ketsueki 52:546–550

Jabbour E, Kantarjian HM, Quintás-Cardama A et al (2011) Impact of dose reductions and interruptions due to adverse events (AEs) on efficacy in newly diagnosed chronic myeloid leukemia in chronic phase (CML-CP) patients (pts) receiving either dasatinib (D) or imatinib (IM): analysis of the DASISION trial. Blood 118(Suppl) (abstract 2768)

Johnson FM, Agrawal S, Burris H et al (2010) Phase 1 pharmacokinetic and drug-interaction study of dasatinib in patients with advanced solid tumors. Cancer 116:1582–1591

Johnson FM, Saigal B, Talpaz M et al (2005) Dasatinib (BMS-354825) tyrosine kinase inhibitor suppresses invasion and induces cell cycle arrest and apoptosis of head and neck squamous cell carcinoma and non-small cell lung cancer cells. Clin Cancer Res 11:6924–6932

Johnson ML, Riely GJ, Rizvi NA et al (2011) Phase II trial of dasatinib for patients with acquired resistance to treatment with the epidermal growth factor receptor tyrosine kinase inhibitors erlotinib or gefitinib. J Thorac Oncol 6:1128–1131

Kantarjian H, Cortes J, Kim D-W et al (2009a) Phase 3 study of dasatinib 140 mg once daily versus 70 mg twice daily in patients with chronic myeloid leukemia in accelerated phase resistant or intolerant to imatinib: 15-month median follow-up. Blood 113:6322–6329

Kantarjian H, Pasquini R, Levy V et al (2009b) Dasatinib or high-dose imatinib for chronic-phase chronic myeloid leukemia resistant to imatinib at a dose of 400 to 600 milligrams daily: two-year follow-up of a randomized phase 2 study (START-R). Cancer 115:3935–3942

Kantarjian H, Pasquini R, Lévy V et al (2009c) Dasatinib or high-dose imatinib for chronic-phase chronic myeloid leukemia resistant to imatinib at a dose of 400 to 600 milligrams daily. Cancer 115:4136–4147

Kantarjian H, Shah NP, Hochhaus A et al (2010) Dasatinib versus imatinib in newly diagnosed chronic-phase chronic myeloid leukemia. N Engl J Med 362:2260–2270

Kantarjian HM, Pasquini R, Hamerschlak N et al (2007) Dasatinib or high-dose imatinib for chronic-phase chronic myeloid leukemia after failure of first-line imatinib: a randomized phase 2 trial. Blood 109:5143–5150

Kantarjian HM, Shah NP, Cortes JE et al (2012) Dasatinib or imatinib in newly diagnosed chronic phase chronic myeloid leukemia: 2-year follow-up from a randomized phase 3 trial (DASISION). Blood 119:1123–1129

Karaman MW, Herrgard S, Treiber DK et al (2008) A quantitative analysis of kinase inhibitor selectivity. Nat Biotechnol 26:127–132

Khoury HJ, Cortes JE, Kantarjian H et al (2010) Safety and efficacy of dasatinib (DAS) versus imatinib (IM) by baseline comorbidity in patients with chronic myeloid leukemia in chronic phase (CML-CP): analysis of the DASISION trial. Blood 116(Suppl) (abstract 3421)

Kluger HM, Dudek AZ, McCann C et al (2011) A phase 2 trial of dasatinib in advanced melanoma. Cancer 117:2202–2208

Kopetz S, Shah AN, Gallick GE (2007) Src continues aging: Current and future clinical directions. Clin Cancer Res 13:7232–7236

Kreutzman A, Juvonen V, Kairisto V et al (2010) Mono/oligoclonal T and NK cells are common in chronic myeloid leukemia patients at diagnosis and expand during dasatinib therapy. Blood 116:772–782

Kreutzman A, Ladell K, Koechel C et al (2011) Expansion of highly differentiated CD8þ T-cells or NK-cells in patients treated with dasatinib is associated with cytomegalovirus reactivation. Leukemia 25:1587–1597

Kullander K, Klein R (2002) Mechanisms and functions of Eph and ephrin signalling. Nat Rev Mol Cell Biol 3:475–486

La Rosée P, Martiat P, Leitner, A et al (2013) Improved tolerability by a modified intermittent treatment schedule of dasatinib for patients with chronic myeloid leukemia resistant or intolerant to imatinib. Ann Hematol. April 28 (Epub ahead of print)

Laneuville P, Baccarani M, Cortes J et al (2011) Analysis of patients (pts) with chronic-phase chronic myeloid leukemia (CML-CP) who develop pleural effusion on first-line dasatinib: management and outcomes. J Clin Oncol 29(Suppl) (abstract 6605)

Levinson NM, Boxer SG (2012) Structural and spectroscopic analysis of the kinase inhibitor bosutinib and an isomer of bosutinib binding to the Abl Tyrosine Kinase Domain. PLoS One 7:e29828

Li C, Lida M, Dunn EF et al (2009) Nuclear EGFR contributes to acquired resistance to cetuximab. Oncogene 28:3801–3813

Lombardo LJ, Francis YL, Chen P et al (2004) Discover of N-(2-Chloro-6-methyl-phenyl)-2-(6-(4-(2-hydroxyethyl)-piperazin-1-yl)-2-methylpyrimidin-4-ylamino)thiazole-5-carboxamide (BMS-354825), a dual Src/Abl kinase inhibitor with potent antitumor activity in preclinical assays. J Med Chem 47:6658–6661

Marin D, Hedgley C, Clark RE et al (2012) The predictive value of early molecular response in chronic phase CML patients treated with dasatinib first line therapy. Blood 120:291–294

Mattei D, Feola M, Orzan F et al (2009) Reversible dasatinib-induced pulmonary arterial hypertension and right ventricle failure in a previously allografted CML patient. Bone Marrow Transplant 43:967–968

Mauro MJ, Baccarani M, Cervantes F et al (2008) Dasatinib 2-year efficacy in patients with chronic-phase chronic myelogenous leukemia (CML-CP) with resistance or intolerance to imatinib (START-C). J Clin Oncol 26(Suppl) (abstract 7009)

Mayer EL, Krop IE (2010) Advances in targeting Src in the treatment of breast cancer and other solid malignancies. Clin Cancer Res 16:3526–3532

Mayer EL, Baurain JF, Sparano J et al (2011) A phase 2 trial of dasatinib in patients with advanced HER2-positive and/or hormone receptor-positive breast cancer. Clin Cancer Res 17(21):6897–6904

McLaughlin VV, Archer SL, Badesch DB et al (2009) ACCF/AHA 2009 expert consensus document on pulmonary hypertension a report of the American College of Cardiology Foundation task force on expert consensus documents and the American Heart Association developed in collaboration with the American College of Chest Physicians; American Thoracic Society, Inc.; and the Pulmonary Hypertension Association. J Am Coll Cardiol 53:1573–1619; Circulation 119:2250–2294

Metcalf CA 3rd, van Schravendijk MR, Dalgarno DC, Sawyer TK (2002) Targeting protein kinases for bone disease: discovery and development of Src inhibitors. Curr Pharm Des 8:2049–2075

Miller AA, Pang H, Hodgson L et al (2010) A phase II study of dasatinib in patients with chemosensitive relapsed small cell lung cancer (Cancer and Leukemia Group B 30602). J Thorac Oncol 5:380–384

Montani D, Bergot E, Gunther S (2012) Pulmonary arterial hypertension in patients treated by dasatinib. Circulation 125:2128–2137

Montero JS, Seoane S, Ocaña A et al (2011) Inhibition of Src family kinases and receptor tyrosine kinases by dasatinib: possible combinations in solid tumors. Clin Cancer Res 17:5546–5552

Moulder S, Yan K, Huang F et al (2010) Development of candidate genomic markers to select breast cancer patients for dasatinib therapy. Mol Cancer Ther 9:1120–1127

Müller MC, Cortes JE, Kim DW et al (2009) Dasatinib treatment of chronic-phase chronic myeloid leukemia: analysis of responses according to preexisting BCR-ABL mutations. Blood 114:4944–4953

Mustjoki S, Auvinen K, Kreutzman A et al (2013) Rapid mobilization of cytotoxic lymphocytes induced by dasatinib therapy. Leukemia 27:914–924

Mustjoki S, Richter J, Barbany G et al (2011) Favorable therapeutic responses in newly diagnosed CML-CP patients induced by dasatinib are reflected at the CD34+CD38+ progenitor cell but not at the CD34+CD38—stem cell level: results from randomized NordCML006 study. Blood 118(Suppl) (abstract 784)

Mustjoki S, Rousselot P, Jalkanen S et al (2010) Dasatinib induces a rapid, dose-controllable mobilization of cytotoxic lymphocytes: a novel immunomodulatory effect associated with prolonged therapy responses in advanced leukemia. Blood 116(Suppl) (abstract 1204)

Nam S, Kim D, Cheng JQ et al (2005) Action of the Src family kinase inhibitor, dasatinib (BMS-354825), on human prostate cancer cells. Cancer Res 65:9185–9189

National Comprehensive Cancer Network. NCCN Clinical Practice Guidelines in Oncology™. Chronic myelogenous leukemia v.4.2013. http://www.nccn.org/professionals/physician_gls/f_guidelines.asp#site

Neelakantan P, Gerrard G, Lucas C et al (2013) Combining BCR-ABL1 transcript levels at 3 and 6 months in chronic myeloid leukemia: implications for early intervention strategies. Blood 121:2739–2742

O'Hare T, Shakespeare WC, Zhu X et al (2009) AP24534, a pan-BCR-ABL inhibitor for chronic myeloid leukemia, potently inhibits the T315I mutant and overcomes mutation-based resistance. Cancer Cell 16:401–412

O'Hare T, Walters DK, Stoffregen EP et al (2005) In vitro activity of Bcr-Abl inhibitors AMN107 and BMS-354825 against clinically relevant imatinib-resistant Abl kinase domain mutants. Cancer Res 65:4500–4505

Orlandi EM, Rocca B, Pazzano AS et al (2011) Reversible pulmonary arterial hypertension likely related to long-term, low-dose dasatinib treatment for chronic myeloid leukaemia. Leuk Res 36(1):e4–e6

Ottmann O, Dombret H, Martinelli G et al (2007) Dasatinib induces rapid hematologic and cytogenetic responses in adult patients with Philadelphia chromosome positive acute lymphoblastic leukemia with resistance or intolerance to imatinib: interim results of a phase 2 study. Blood 110:2309–2315

Pan Z, Scheerens H, Li SJ et al (2007) Discovery of selective irreversible inhibitors for Bruton's tyrosine kinase. ChemMedChem 2:58–61

Park SI, Zhang JZ, Phillips KA et al (2008) Targeting Src family kinases inhibits growth and lymph node metastases of prostate cancer in an orthotopic nude mouse model. Cancer Res 68:3323–3333

Pemmaraju N, Kantarjian H, Luthra R et al (2011) Results of a phase II trial of dasatinib as frontline therapy for chronic myeloid leukemia (CML) in chronic phase (CP). Blood 118(Suppl) (abstract 1700)

Pene-Dumitrescu T, Smithall TE (2010) Expression of a Src family kinase in chronic myelogenous leukemia cells induces resistance to imatinib in a kinase-dependent manner. J Biol Chem 285:21446–21457

Philibert L, Carzola C, Peyriere H et al (2011) Pulmonary arterial hypertension induced by dasatinib: positive reintroduction with nilotinib. Fundam Clin Pharmacol 25(Suppl):95 (abstract 476)

Pittini V, Arrigo C, Altavilla G. et al (2009) Dasatinib induces a response in chronic lymphocytic leukemia. Blood 113(Suppl) (abstract 498)

Porkka K, Khoury HJ, Paquette RL et al (2010) Dasatinib 100 mg once daily minimizes the occurrence of pleural effusion in patients with chronic myeloid leukemia in chronic phase and efficacy in unaffected in patients who develop pleural effusion. Cancer 116:377–386

Porkka K, Koskenvesa P, Lundan T et al (2008) Dasatinib crosses the blood-brain barrier and is an efficient therapy for central nervous system Philadelphia chromosome–positive leukaemia. Blood 112:1005–1012

Porkka K, Simonsson B, Dombret H et al (2007) Efficacy of dasatinib in patients with Philadelphia-chromosome-positive acute lymphoblastic leukemia who are resistant or intolerant to imatinib: 2-year follow-up data from START-L (CA180-015). Blood 110(Suppl) (abstract 2810)

Quintás-Cardama A, Kantarjian H, O'Brien S et al (2007) Pleural effusion in patients with chronic myelogenous leukemia treated with dasatinib after imatinib failure. J Clin Oncol 25:3908–3914

Quintás-Cardama A, Kantarjian H, Ravandi F et al (2009) Bleeding diathesis in patients with chronic myelogenous leukemia receiving dasatinib therapy. Cancer 115:2482–2490

Radich JP, Kopecky KJ, Applebaum FR et al (2012) A randomized trial of dasatinib 100 mg versus imatinib 400 mg in newly diagnosed chronic phase chronic myeloid leukemia in chronic phase (CML-CP). Blood 120:3898–3905
Rasheed W, Flaim B, Seymour JF (2009) Reversible severe pulmonary hypertension secondary to dasatinib in a patient with chronic myeloid leukemia. Leuk Res 33:861–864
Ravandi F, O'Brien S, Thomas D et al (2010) First report of phase 2 study of dasatinib with hyper-CVAD for the frontline treatment of patients with Philadelphia chromosome-positive (Ph+) acute lymphoblastic leukemia. Blood 116:2070–2077
Rea D, Vellenga E, Junghan C et al (2012) Six-year follow-up of patients with imatinib-resistant or imatinib-intolerant chronic phase chronic myeloid leukemia (CML-CP) receiving dasatinib. Haematologica 97(Suppl 1) (abstract 199)
Reardon DA, Vredenburgh JJ, Desjardins A et al (2012) Phase 1 trial of dasatinib plus erlotinib in adults with recurrent malignant glioma. J Neurooncol 108:499–506
Redaelli S, Piazza R, Rostagno R et al (2009) Activity of bosutinib, dasatinib and nilotinib against 18 imatinib-resistant BCR/ABL mutants. J Clin Oncol 27:469–471
Ren CL, Morio T, Fu SM, Geha RS (1994) Signal transduction via CD40 involves activation of lyn kinase and phosphatidylinositol-3-kinase, and phosphorylation of phospholipase C gamma 2. J Exp Med 179:673–680
Rousselot P, Boucher S, Etienne G et al (2010) Pharmacokinetics of dasatinib as a first line therapy in newly diagnosed CML patients (OPTIM dasatinib trial): correlation with safety and response. Blood 116(Suppl) (abstract 3432)
Rousselot P, Mollica L, Etienne G et al (2012) Pharmacologic monitoring of dasatinib as first line therapy in newly diagnosed chronic phase chronic myelogenous leukemia (CP-CML) identifies patients at higher risk of pleural effusion: a sub-analysis of the OPTIM-dasatinib trial. Blood 120(Suppl) (abstract 3770)
Saglio G, Dombret H, Rea D et al (2008) Dasatinib efficacy in patients with imatinib-resistant/-intolerant chronic myeloid leukemia in blast phase: 24-month data from the START program. Haematologica 93 (abstract 0880)
Saglio G, Hochhaus A, Cortes JE et al (2010c) Safety and efficacy of dasatinib versus imatinib by baseline cardiovascular comorbidity in patients with chronic myeloid leukemia in chronic phase (CML-CP): analysis of the DASISION trial. Blood 116(Suppl) (abstract 2286)
Saglio G, Hochhaus A, Goh YT et al (2010) Dasatinib in imatinib-resistant or imatinib-intolerant chronic myeloid leukemia in blast phase after 2 years of follow-up in a phase 3 study. Cancer 116:3852–3861
Saglio G, Kantarjian HM, Shah N et al (2012) Early response (molecular and cytogenetic) and long-term outcomes in newly diagnosed chronic myeloid leukemia in chronic phase (CML-CP): exploratory analysis of DASISION 3-year data. Blood 120(Suppl) (abstract 1675)
Sano M, Saotome M, Urushida T et al (2012) Pulmonary arterial hypertension caused by treatment with dasatinib for chronic myeloid leukemia: critical alert. Intern Med 51:2337–2340
Schiffer CA, Cortes JE, Saglio G et al (2010a) Lymphocytosis following first-line treatment for CML in chronic phase with dasatinib is associated with improved responses: a comparison with imatinib. Blood 116(Suppl) (abstract 358)
Schiffer CA, Cortes JE, Saglio G et al (2010b) Lymphocytosis following treatment with dasatinib is associated with improved response and outcome. J Clin Oncol 28:15s (abstract 6553)
Schittenhelm MM, Shiraga S, Schroeder A et al (2006) Dasatinib (BMS-354825), a dual SRC/ABL kinase inhibitor, inhibits the kinase activity of wild-type, juxtamembrane, and activation loop mutant KIT isoforms associated with human malignancies. Cancer Res 66:473–481
Schilder RJ, Brady WE, Lankes HA et al (2012) Phase II evaluation of dasatinib in the treatment of recurrent or persistent epithelial ovarian or primary peritoneal carcinoma: a gynecologic oncology group (GOG) trial. Gynecol Oncol 127:70–74

Secord AA, Teoh DK, Barry WT et al (2012) A phase I trial of dasatinib, an SRC-family kinase inhibitor, in combination with paclitaxel and carboplatin in patients with advanced or recurrent ovarian cancer. Clin Cancer Res 18:5489–5498

Serrels A, Macpherson IRJ, Evans TRJ et al (2006) Identification of potential biomarkers for measuring inhibition of Src kinase activity in colon cancer cells following treatment with dasatinib. Mol Cancer Ther 5:3014–3022

Shah NP, Kantarjian H, Kim DW et al (2012) Six-year follow-up of patients with imatinib-resistant or—intolerant chronic-phase chronic myeloid leukemia receiving dasatinib. J Clin Oncol 30(Suppl) (abstract 6506)

Shah NP, Kantarjian HM, Kim DW et al (2008a) Intermittent target inhibition with dasatinib 100 mg once daily preserves efficacy and improves tolerability in imatinib-resistant and—intolerant chronic-phase chronic myeloid leukemia. J Clin Oncol 26:3204–3212

Shah NP, Kasap C, Weier C et al (2008b) Transient potent BCR-ABL inhibition is sufficient to commit chronic myeloid leukemia cells irreversibly to apoptosis. Cancer Cell 14:485–493

Shah NP, Kim DW, Kantarjian H et al (2010) Potent, transient inhibition of BCR-ABL with dasatinib 100 mg daily achieves rapid and durable cytogenetic responses and high transformation-free survival rates in chronic phase chronic myeloid leukemia patients with resistance, suboptimal response or intolerance to imatinib. Haematologica 95:232–240

Shah NP, Lee FY, Luo R et al (2006) Dasatinib (BMS-354825) inhibits KITD816V, an imatinib-resistant activating mutation that triggers neoplastic growth in most patients with systemic mastocytosis. Blood 108:286–291

Shah NP, Skaggs BJ, Branford S et al (2007) Sequential ABL kinase inhibitor therapy selects for compound drug-resistant BCR-ABL mutations with altered oncogenic potency. J Clin Invest 117:2562–2569

Shah NP, Tran C, Lee FY et al (2004) Overriding imatinib resistance with a novel ABL kinase inhibitor. Science 305:399–401

Sharma MR, Wroblewski K, Polite BN et al (2012) Dasatinib in previously treated metastatic colorectal cancer: a phase II trial of the University of Chicago Phase II Consortium. Invest New Drugs 30:1211–1215

Shor AC, Keschman EA, Lee FY et al (2007) Dasatinib inhibits migration and invasion in diverse human sarcoma cell lines and induces apoptosis in bone sarcoma cells dependent on Src kinase for survival. Cancer Res 67:2800–2808

Smith CI, Islam TC, Mattsson PT et al (2001) The Tec family of cytoplasmic tyrosine kinases: mammalian Btk, Bmx, Itk, Tec, Txk and homologs in other species. BioEssays 23:436–446

Somlo G, Atzori F, Strauss LC et al (2013) Dasatinib plus capecitabine for advanced breast cancer: safety and efficacy in phase I study CA180004. Clin Cancer Res 19:1884–1893

Song Z, Lu P, Furman RR et al (2010) Activities of SYK and PLCg2 predict apoptotic response of CLL cells to SRC tyrosine kinase inhibitor dasatinib. Clin Cancer Res 16:587–599

Soverini S, Gnani A, Colarossi S et al (2009) Philadelphia-positive patients who already harbor imatinib-resistant Bcr-Abl kinase domain mutations have a higher likelihood of developing additional mutations associated with resistance to second- or third-line tyrosine kinase inhibitors. Blood 114:2168–2171

Sprycel® (dasatinib) capsules prescribing information. Princeton, NJ, Bristol-Myers Squibb Company, Nov 2012. http://packageinserts.bms.com/pi/pi_sprycel.pdf

Starodub A, Cohn AL, Arrowood C et al (2011) Phase I study of dasatinib in combination with capecitabine, oxaliplatin, and bevacizumab followed by an expanded cohort in previously untreated metastatic colorectal cancer. J Clin Oncol 29(Suppl) (abstract 513)

Strickler JH, Cohn AL, Arrowood C et al (2011) Phase I study of dasatinib in combination with capecitabine, oxaliplatin and bevacizumab followed by an expanded cohort in previously untreated metastatic colorectal cancer. J Clin Oncol 29(Suppl) (abstract 3586)

Talpaz M, Shah NP, Kantarjian H et al (2006) Dasatinib in imatinib-resistant Philadelphia chromosome-positive leukemias. N Engl J Med 354:2531–2541

Tokarski JS, Newitt JA, Chang CY et al (2006) The structure of dasatinib (BMS-354825) bound to activated ABL kinase domain elucidates its inhibitory activity against imatinib-resistant ABL mutants. Cancer Res 66:5790–5797

Ustun C, Corless CL, Savage N et al (2009) Chemotherapy and dasatinib induce long-term hematologic and molecular remission in systemic mastocytosis with acute myeloid leukemia with KIT D816V. Leuk Res 33:735–741

Vajpai N, Strauss A, Fendrich G et al (2008) Solution conformations and dynamics of ABL kinase-inhibitor complexes determined by NMR substantiate the different binding modes of imatinib/nilotinib and dasatinib. J Biol Chem 283:18292–18302

Van Cutsem E, Kohne C-H, Hitre E et al (2009) Cetuximab and chemotherapy as initial treatment for metastatic colorectal cancer. N Engl J Med 360:1408–1417

Verstovsek S, Tefferi A, Cortes J et al (2008) Phase II study of dasatinib in Philadelphia chromosome-negative acute and chronic myeloid diseases, including systemic mastocytosis. Clin Cancer Res 14:3907–3915

Weisberg E, Manley PW, Breitenstein W et al (2005) Characterization of AMN107, a selective inhibitor of native and mutant Bcr-Abl. Cancer Cell 7:129–141

Wong S, Witte ON (2004) The BCR-ABL story: bench to bedside and back. Annu Rev Immunol 22:247–306

Zhou T, Commodore L, Huang W-S et al (2011) Structural mechanism of the pan-BCR-ABL inhibitor ponatinib (AP24534): lessons for overcoming kinase inhibitor resistance. Chem Biol Drug Des 77:1–11

Nilotinib

Benjamin N. Ostendorf, Philipp le Coutre, Theo D. Kim and Alfonso Quintás-Cardama

Abstract

Targeted therapy of Philadelphia chromosome-positive chronic myeloid leukemia (CML) using the tyrosine kinase inhibitor imatinib mesylate has been one of the most striking achievements in modern cancer medicine. However, while imatinib can establish long-term remission in many cases, resistance to or intolerance of imatinib is eventually experienced by a substantial number of patients. Subsequent advances have led to the development of novel tyrosine kinase inhibitors (TKIs). One such inhibitor, nilotinib, was rationally designed to increase its affinity and specificity for the oncogenic tyrosine kinase Bcr-Abl compared with imatinib and has been shown to be effective after imatinib failure. Recently, nilotinib has been shown to be more effective when used as first-line therapy of chronic phase CML.

Contents

B. N. Ostendorf (✉) · P. le Coutre · T. D. Kim
Campus Virchow-Klinikum, Medical Department, Division of Hematology, Oncology and Tumor Immunology, Charité – Universitätsmedizin Berlin, Augustenburger Platz 1, 13353 Berlin, Germany
e-mail: benjamin.ostendorf@charite.de

A. Quintás-Cardama
Department of Leukemia, MD Anderson Cancer Center, 1515 Holcombe Blvd, Houston, TX 77030, USA
e-mail: aquintas@mdanderson.org

U. M. Martens (ed.), *Small Molecules in Oncology*, Recent Results in Cancer Research 201, DOI: 10.1007/978-3-642-54490-3_3,

1 Introduction

Philadelphia chromosome-positive chronic myeloid leukemia (CML) cells are addicted to the oncogenic activity of tyrosine kinase Bcr-Abl, the molecular correlate of the Philadelphia chromosome (Druker et al. 1996). Imatinib mesylate (formerly STI571 or CGP5148B) is a specific inhibitor of Bcr-Abl and quickly replaced former therapy regimes as first-line therapy for CML in chronic phase (CP) because of its considerable antiproliferative activity against Bcr-Abl expressing cells (Druker et al. 2006). However, follow-up data in the landmark IRIS trial revealed a significant portion of patients to develop disease resistance to imatinib with an overall failure rate of 17 % after 5 years (Druker et al. 2006).

Secondary resistance most commonly arises as a consequence of point mutations within the kinase domain of Bcr-Abl (Gorre et al. 2001; O'Hare et al. 2007), with other mechanisms being less well-characterized (Apperley 2007). Over 100 mutations conferring varying degrees of resistance to imatinib have been detected in patients with CML, although seven mutations account for the majority of imatinib refractory cases (Ernst et al. 2011; Shah et al. 2002). In addition to secondary resistance, some patients never meet optimum response criteria to imatinib therapy. Moreover, patients in accelerated phase (AP) and blast phase (BP) are frequently resistant to imatinib and when they respond, responses are usually short-lived (Sawyers et al. 2002; Talpaz et al. 2002).

The high frequency with which CML recurs after discontinuation of therapy suggests that only a minute CML patient population might achieve a cure or at least long-term remission with tyrosine kinase inhibitors (TKIs) (Cortes et al. 2004; Mahon et al. 2010). Thus, prolonged therapy is required in most cases. However, despite its targeted mechanism imatinib therapy is not devoid of relevant side effects, sometimes compromising long-term therapy. The IRIS study showed imatinib discontinuation for various reasons in 30 % after 5 years (Druker et al. 2006), and Deininger and colleagues showed discontinuation of imatinib therapy due to adverse effects in 10 % of patients (Deininger et al. 2003).

Primary and secondary resistance to imatinib treatment as well as intolerance of therapy prompted the development of new generation TKIs. Recently, the second-generation TKIs nilotinib (Tasigna®) and dasatinib (Sprycel®) have been approved for first-line therapy of CML in chronic phase.

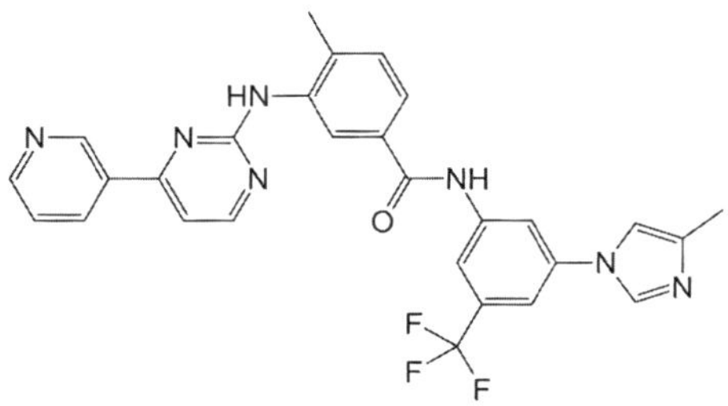

Chemical name:	4-Methyl-3-((4-(3-pyridinyl)-2-pyrimidinyl)amino)-N-(5-(4-methyl-1H-imidazol-1-yl)-3-(trifluoromethyl)phenyl)benzamide
Synonym:	AMN107
Molecular weight:	529.52
Molecular formula:	$C_{28}H_{22}F_3N_7O$

Fig. 1 Molecular structure and chemical characteristics of nilotinib

2 Structure and Mechanism of Action

Crystallographic analysis of the interaction between imatinib and the Abl kinase domain led to the rational development of nilotinib (formerly AMN107) by replacing an N-methylpiperazine group in imatinib (Manley et al. 2004; Weisberg et al. 2005) (for molecule structure see Fig. 1). Similar to imatinib, nilotinib is an orally bioavailable ATP-competitive inhibitor of the Abl kinase domain. It was shown to have a 10- to 50-fold increased potency against unmutated Bcr-Abl compared with imatinib. Importantly, nilotinib also has considerable activity against most imatinib-resistant Bcr-Abl mutations (Weisberg et al. 2005).

Nilotinib exerts its inhibitory activity on Bcr-Abl by binding to an inactive conformation of the kinase and preventing its change to an active conformation. In addition to Bcr-Abl, nilotinib also inhibits tyrosine kinases KIT, platelet-derived growth factor receptor (PDGFR), and discoidin domain receptor 1 (DDR1). Nilotinib was also found to inhibit the non-tyrosine kinase NAD(P)H:quinone oxidoreductase (NQO2) (Rix et al. 2007). Whether these interactions impact clinical activity or the toxicity profile of nilotinib remains unknown.

3 Preclinical Data

Nilotinib was shown to be more potent than imatinib at inhibiting proliferation of Bcr-Abl expressing murine and human cells in culture. Autophosphorylation of Bcr-Abl in cells exposed to nilotinib was lower than in cells exposed to imatinib (Golemovic et al. 2005; Weisberg et al. 2005). Consistently, nilotinib was shown

Table 1 Categorized sensitivity to nilotinib of clinically relevant Bcr-Abl mutations recovered in unbiased mutational screens

Sensitivity	IC_{50} (nM)	Bcr-Abl mutations
High	100	M237I, M244V, K247N, G250A, G250E[a], G250V, Q252H, E255D, E255R, L273F, E275K, D276G[a], E281K, E285N, K285N, V289L, E292K[a], N297T, F311L, F317C, F317L[a], FF317V[a], D325N, S348L, M351T, E355A, E355G, H375P, V379I, L387F, M388L, L387F, L387M, H396P, H396R, T406I, W430L, E431G
Medium	200	L284V[a], G250E[a], Y253F, E255K[a], D276G[a], E282K, E292K[a], F311, F317L[a], F317R, F359, A380S, F486S
Low	1,000	L248V[a], Y253C, Y253H[a], E255K[a], E255V[a], K285, F317V[a], F359C, F359I[a]
None	>2,000	T315I, T315V, L248R

Of note, the extent of sensitivity depends not only on the position of the mutation but also on the specific substitution

[a]Denotes mutations that fall into two different categories, based on different values reported. Values are from references (Bradeen et al. 2006; von Bubnoff et al. 2006; O'Hare et al. 2005; Ray et al. 2007; Redaelli et al. 2012; Weisberg et al. 2006)

to significantly prolong survival and reduce tumor burden in a CML mouse model (Golemovic et al. 2005; Weisberg et al. 2005).

Importantly, nilotinib retained its inhibitory activity against most Bcr-Abl mutants resistant to imatinib with the exception of the T315I-, T315V-, and L248R-mutations (Table 1).

4 Clinical Data

4.1 Nilotinib Phase I Trial

A phase I dose escalation study showed higher steady-state levels when nilotinib was administered twice daily (Kantarjian et al. 2006). The median time to peak concentration was three hours after administration, reaching a mean peak concentration of 3.6 μM at steady-state level at 400 mg twice daily. Increase in steady-state levels was dose-dependent and achieved by day 8 with a mean serum trough level at steady state of 1.7 μM at 400 mg twice daily and of 2.3 μM at 600 mg twice daily. These trough levels exceeded the 50 % inhibitory concentration for phosphorylation of unmutated Bcr-Abl as well as of 32 out of 33 Bcr-Abl mutants. The half-life of nilotinib was 16 h. Nilotinib absorption but not elimination was shown to be increased when taken after a light or high-fat meal (Tanaka et al. 2009). Results were consistent with pharmacokinetic analyses in healthy volunteers (Kagan et al. 2005; Tanaka et al. 2009).

Table 2 Efficacy of nilotinib in chronic phase (*CP*), accelerated phase (*AP*), myeloid blastic phase (*MBP*), and lymphoid blastic phase (*LBP*) of Ph-positive chronic myeloid leukemia (*CML*) with imatinib resistance or intolerance

	CP (n = 321)	AP (n = 137)	MBP (n = 105)	LBP (n = 31)
Overall HR (%) (CHR + MR/NEL + RTC)	–	55	54	59
CHR (%)	–	31	24	21
MR/NEL (%)	–	12	–	–
RTC (%)	–	12	–	–
MCyR (CCyR + PCyR) (%)	59	32	38	52
CCyR (%)	45	21	30	32
PCyR (%)	14	11	8	20
Continuous HR (%)	–	49	51	21
Continuous MCyR (%)	–	66	44	0
Progression-free survival (%)	57	33	–	–
Overall survival (%)	78	70	32	10

Numbers are based on references (Giles et al. 2012, 2013; le Coutre et al. 2012). Time of analysis was 48 months after initiation of nilotinib therapy for CML in CP and 24 months for CML in AP or BP. *HR* hematologic response; *CHR* complete hematologic response; *MR/NEL* marrow response/no evidence of leukemia; *RTC* return to chronic phase; *MCyR* major cytogenetic response; *CCyR* complete cytogenetic response; *PCyR* partial cytogenetic response;—not reported/applicable

4.2 Nilotinib Second- and Third-Line Therapy

Nilotinib was first used as second-line therapy in the context of imatinib resistance or intolerance (Kantarjian et al. 2006). Phase II trials have been conducted to study nilotinib administration in patients with CML in CP, AP, or BC resistant to or intolerant of imatinib (Table 2).

The first phase II trial published in 2007 included patients with CML in CP (Kantarjian et al. 2007). The last update reported on 321 patients, 70 % of which were resistant to and 30 % intolerant of imatinib (Giles et al. 2013). Median CML duration before study entry was 58 months (range, 5–275). Mean duration of prior imatinib treatment was 32 months (range, <1–94), and median follow-up was 1,555 days. Seventy percent of patients had discontinued nilotinib at 48 months, mostly due to disease progression (n = 96, 30 %) or adverse events (n = 66, 21 %). At 24 months, 190 patients (59 %) had achieved a major cytogenetic response (MCyR) (Kantarjian et al. 2011a), and no additional patients achieved a MCyR between months 24 and 48 (Giles et al. 2013). Remission rates in patients resistant to and intolerant of imatinib were comparable. Most patients achieving a MCyR also achieved a complete cytogenetic response (CCyR) (45 %). Progression-free survival at 48 months was 57 % (95 % CI, 51–64 %) with only very few patients progressing to AP or BP (3 %). The estimated overall survival rate at

48 months was 78 %, and a median survival time was not reached. The median administered nilotinib dose of 789 mg/day (range, 151–1,110) was close to the planned initial dose of 800 mg/day, indicating excellent tolerability.

Another phase II trial analyzed the efficacy of nilotinib after failure of both imatinib and dasatinib in 39 patients with CML in CP (Giles et al. 2010). The median CML duration before initiation of nilotinib therapy was 89 months. Complete hematological response (CHR) and MCyR were achieved in 79 and 43 %, respectively. Although most patients in the study were included due to intolerance to dasatinib treatment (67 %), most had also failed to attain a MCyR (79 %), despite a median duration of dasatinib exposure of 7 months. The estimated overall survival at 18 months was 86 %.

The efficacy of nilotinib in patients with CML in AP and imatinib resistance or intolerance was also studied in a phase II study (le Coutre et al. 2008). Overall, 137 patients with a follow-up of at least 24 months or after early discontinuation were evaluated (le Coutre et al. 2012). The majority of patients were imatinib resistant (80 %), while 20 % had imatinib intolerance. The median duration of CML was 71 months, and the median duration of prior imatinib therapy was 28 months. Nilotinib was administered for a median of 264 days (range, 2–1,160), and the median dose intensity was 780 mg/day (range, 150–1,149). A hematologic response was confirmed in 55 % of patients with 31 % attaining a CHR and 32 % a MCyR (most of which were complete). At 24 months, 49 and 66 % of responders had maintained a hematological and MCyR, respectively. Response rates were similar in patients with resistance and intolerance. The estimated OS and PFS at 24 months were 70 and 33 %, respectively. At the time of analysis, 85 % of patients had discontinued nilotinib treatment, mostly due to disease progression (44 %) with only 10 % discontinuing due to drug-related AEs.

The efficacy of nilotinib in patients with CML in BP was analyzed in 136 patients enrolled in a phase II study (Giles et al. 2008), 105 of which were in myeloid blastic phase (MBP) and 31 in lymphoid blastic phase (LBP). The median duration of prior imatinib therapy was 490 days (range, 1–3,267), and the majority of patients were enrolled due to imatinib resistance (82 %). At 24 months, major hematologic responses were observed in 60 and 59 % of patients in MBP and LBP, respectively, with corresponding figures for MCyR of 38 and 52 % (Giles et al. 2012). The median respective duration of MCyR was 10.8 and 3.2 months. Overall survival was 27 % (MPP 32 %, LBP 10 %). In conclusion, nilotinib was shown to have significant efficacy in patients with CML after failure of imatinib therapy, including patients with advanced phase CML, although in such cases response rates and duration were significantly lower compared with CML in CP.

4.3 Nilotinib First-Line Therapy

The randomized, open-label, multicenter phase III trial Evaluating Nilotinib Efficacy and Safety in Clinical Trials Newly Diagnosed Patients (ENESTnd) evaluated nilotinib as first-line therapy in patients with CML in CP (Saglio et al. 2010) by comparing imatinib 400 mg once daily to nilotinib 300 mg twice daily or nilotinib 400 mg twice daily in 283, 282, and 281 patients, respectively. In the most recent update with a follow-up time of 4 years significantly more patients treated with nilotinib 400 mg twice daily (73 %) and nilotinib 300 mg twice daily (76 %) had reached a major molecular response (MMR) than patients treated with imatinib (56 %). The molecular response at 4 years was also deeper in patients on nilotinib 300 mg and nilotinib 400 mg than in patients on imatinib, with 56 and 50 % versus 32 % of patients achieving a molecular response of Bcr-Abl $\leq$ 0.01 % expressed on the international scale (Bcr-Abl^{IS}; MR^{4}), respectively. Similarly, rates of Bcr-Abl $\leq$ 0.0032 % (MR$^{4.5}$) were significantly higher in patients on nilotinib 300 mg and nilotinib 400 mg than in the imatinib arm (40 and 37 % vs. 23 %, respectively). The difference in depth of molecular response across arms became more apparent on longer follow-up (Kantarjian et al. 2011b; Larson et al. 2012, 2013). Rates of progression to AP or BP were significantly lower in patients on nilotinib 300 mg and nilotinib 400 mg than in patients on imatinib (3.3, 2.2, and 6.9 %, respectively). While not statistically significant, overall survival was higher in both nilotinib arms compared with the imatinib arm (94.3, 96.7, and 93.3 % of patients on nilotinib 300 mg twice daily, nilotinib 400 mg twice daily, and imatinib 400 mg once daily, respectively).

In conclusion, nilotinib has shown superior efficacy to imatinib in first-line therapy of CML in CP.

4.4 Resistance to Nilotinib

In vitro screening assays showed nilotinib to render a reduced spectrum of mutant clones compared with imatinib (Bradeen et al. 2006; von Bubnoff et al. 2006; Ray et al. 2007). In the majority of cases, resistance was conferred by mutations within the P-loop of the Bcr-Abl kinase domain, only partly overlapping with the spectrum of mutations conferring resistance to other TKIs. This is reflected in the significant efficacy of nilotinib after previous failure of other TKIs (Giles et al. 2013).

Recently, the Bcr-Abl mutational profile during nilotinib versus imatinib treatment was assessed in 846 patients treated in the ENESTnd trial (Hochhaus et al. 2013). No mutations were detected at baseline in either group. Significantly more patients treated with imatinib developed Bcr-Abl mutations at 3 years than patients treated with nilotinib. Most mutations in the imatinib group retained sensitivity to nilotinib. The most frequent mutations in the nilotinib group were Y253H-, E255K/V-, and F359C/V. Notably, T315I, which is resistant to either agent, was acquired at comparable rates in both groups. Of note, fewer patients treated with nilotinib progressed to advanced disease or lost response to treatment compared with those treated with imatinib.

In conclusion, nilotinib is a potent inhibitor of the majority of imatinib-resistant Bcr-Abl mutant isoforms, with the exception of T315I and some mutations mapping to the P-loop.

5 Toxicity

In phase II and phase III studies investigating nilotinib efficacy, a high dose intensity was reached and discontinuation of nilotinib due to grade 3 and 4 adverse events was rare (Table 3), indicating that nilotinib has an overall favorable toxicity profile (Giles et al. 2012, 2013; Larson et al. 2012; le Coutre et al. 2012).

Among the most frequently reported, non-hematological events of any grade were rash and headache. Grade 3 and 4 adverse events were uncommon, with rash being the only non-hematological grade 3/4 adverse event observed in more than 2 % of patients. Notably, rates of drug-related fluid retention syndromes and gastrointestinal events were higher with imatinib than with nilotinib. Also, grade 3 and 4 neutropenia were more frequent in the imatinib group. With regard to already known toxicities, the safety profile of nilotinib showed only minimal change over a 4 year follow-up period (Larson et al. 2013).

In patients receiving nilotinib as second-line therapy, adverse events were expectedly higher, with grade 3 and 4 abnormalities mainly consisting of hematological toxicities. In patients treated with second-line nilotinib 400 mg twice daily for CML in CP, AP, and BP rates of grade 3/4 anemia were 11, 27, and 47 %, respectively. Rates of grade 3/4 neutropenia were 32, 42, and 68 %, respectively. Grade 3/4 thrombocytopenia was documented in 30, 42, and 63 % of patients, respectively (Giles et al. 2012, 2013; le Coutre et al. 2012).

Non-hematological biochemical laboratory abnormalities included lipase, alanine transaminase, and bilirubin elevations as well as hyperglycemia. These were often self-limited, rarely leading to treatment interruption or discontinuation.

In preclinical analyses, nilotinib was shown to prolong QTc-duration, making frequent ECG-monitoring mandatory. In particular, caution is warranted when drugs either inhibiting CYP3A4 or causing QTc prolongation themselves such as amiodarone or digoxin are administered. However, after 4 years of follow-up in the ENESTnd study, nilotinib induced no QTc prolongation $\geq$500 ms and no episodes of Torsade de Pointes were reported (Larson et al. 2013), thus markedly minimizing the risk previously adjudicated to nilotinib regarding QTc interval prolongation.

An alarming and new finding made after long follow-up of nilotinib-treated patients was an increase in the incidence of peripheral artery occlusive disease (PAOD). In patients treated with nilotinib 300 and 400 mg twice daily as first-line therapy for CML in CP 1.4 and 1.8 % of patients developed PAOD compared with 0 % in the imatinib group (Larson et al. 2013). PAOD did not lead to study discontinuation, and most patients had preexisting risk factors for PAOD at study entry. These data are confirmatory of the initial reports by Aichberger et al. and our groups showing severe cases of PAOD in nilotinib-treated patients (Aichberger et al. 2011; le Coutre et al. 2011; Quintás-Cardama et al. 2012). In addition, a higher proportion of nilotinib-treated patients as compared with imatinib-treated patients developed cardiac and cerebrovascular events, indicating a general risk of atherosclerosis in the context of nilotinib treatment. Recently, a prospective

Table 3 Adverse events (%) with nilotinib 300 mg twice daily, nilotinib 400 mg twice daily, and imatinib 400 mg once daily as reported from patients with CML in CP treated in a phase III trial with a minimum follow-up of 3 years (Larson et al. 2012)

	Nilotinib 300 mg twice daily	Nilotinib 400 mg twice daily	Imatinib 400 mg once daily
Study drug-related AEs	91.0	96.4	93.6
AEs leading to discontinuation	10.0	14.1	11.4
Study drug-related AEs leading to discontinuation	9.3	12.6	10.4
AEs leading to dose reduction/ interruption	57.3	66.4	50.0
Hematologic toxicity grade 3/4			
Anemia	3.9	4.7	5.7
Neutropenia	11.8	10.8	21.4
Thrombocytopenia	10.4	12.3	8.9
Non-hematologic toxicity (any grade)			
Symptomatic QT prolongation	1.8	1.4	2.5
Pancreatitis	1.8	2.2	0.7
Hepatotoxicity	1.4	4.0	2.5
Fluid retention	18.6	23.5	56.4
Effusions	1.8	0.7	1.8
Rash	41.2	46.9	22.1
Significant bleeding	2.9	4.3	1.4
CNS hemorrhage	0.4	0.7	0.4
Gastrointestinal hemorrhage	2.5	4.0	1.1
Ischemic heart disease	3.2	4.0	1.1
Peripheral arterial occlusive disease	1.4	1.1	0
Grade 3/4 laboratory abnormalities			
AST elevation	1.4	2.9	1.4
ALT elevation	4.3	9.4	2.5
Bilirubin (total) elevation	3.9	7.9	0.4
Lipase (plasma) elevation	7.5	7.9	3.9
Glucose elevation	6.1	5.4	0
QTc prolongation			

(continued)

Table 3 (continued)

	Nilotinib 300 mg twice daily	Nilotinib 400 mg twice daily	Imatinib 400 mg once daily
Absolute QTcF $\geq$ 480 ms	0	0.4	0.7
Absolute QTcF $\geq$ 500 ms	0	0	0.4
QTcF $\geq$ 60 ms change from baseline	0.4	1.1	0.4

Abbreviations AE adverse event; *CNS* central nervous system; *ALT* alanine aminotransferase; *AST* aspartate aminotransferase

analysis compared the rates of PAOD in nilotinib- versus imatinib-treated patients (Kim et al. 2013). Significantly more patients on nilotinib first- and second-line therapy than on first-line imatinib therapy showed a pathological ankle-brachial index (26, 35.7, and 6.3 %, respectively). Clinically obvious PAOD was documented only in patients exposed to nilotinib. In addition, elevation of both cholesterol and LDL levels was observed in patients receiving nilotinib. Thus, noninvasive monitoring for PAOD as well as careful assessment of risk factors is warranted in patients treated with nilotinib. In detail, we presently recommend pretherapy ankle-brachial-index testing as well as control of biochemical risk factors and to repeat these tests annually.

In summary, nilotinib has a favorable safety profile with few severe adverse events, most of which can be controlled by dose reduction or interruptions. Caution is warranted especially in patients at increased cardiovascular risk due to a small but sizeable risk of PAOD.

6 Drug Interactions

Therapy with TKIs usually requires prolonged, if not lifelong administration to maintain CML remission, which increases the risk of drug–drug interactions over the course of the lives of patients with CML. This becomes particularly relevant for those patients that require additional therapy for other comorbidities.

Nilotinib is metabolized by the cytochrome P450 enzyme CYP3A4. Thus, inhibitors of CYP3A4 can result in higher nilotinib exposure, as shown when co-administered with ketoconazole or grapefruit juice (Tanaka et al. 2011; Yin et al. 2010). Conversely, drugs inducing expression of CYP3A4 such as rifampicin lead to significantly lower nilotinib exposure (Tanaka et al. 2011).

Nilotinib itself inhibits CYP2C8, CYP2C9, CYP2D6, CYP3A4, UGT1A1, and Pgp. Therefore, caution should be exercised when drugs metabolized by these enzymes, including vitamin K-antagonists, are administered with nilotinib (Haouala et al. 2011).

7 Biomarkers

Several endpoints have been used in trials studying the efficacy of TKIs for treatment of CML, including hematological, cytogenetic, and molecular response. Monitoring guidelines suggested by The European Leukemia Net define an optimal response to imatinib therapy as reaching CHR at 3 months and a partial cytogenetic response (PCyR) at 6 months. At 12 months, a CCyR should be reached and at 18 months an optimum response is defined as reaching an MMR (Baccarani et al. 2009). Importantly, similar criteria are not available to monitor response to second-generation TKIs such as nilotinib. Several studies suggest that more stringent criteria for both cytogenetic and molecular response at early time points (e.g., 3 months) are best suited to define optimal response and failure to nilotinib or dasatinib therapy in the frontline setting (Jain et al. 2013).

A topical issue regarding TKI therapy in CML is the possibility of treatment discontinuation in patients achieving very deep levels of response (e.g., Bcr-Abl undetectability). This has been demonstrated in patients receiving imatinib therapy. A prospective trial assessed discontinuation of imatinib in patients achieving long-term complete molecular remission (Mahon et al. 2010). At 12 months follow-up, 41 % of patients remained in complete molecular remission. All patients that required re-initiation of therapy due to molecular relapse remained sensitive to imatinib. Another trial included 40 patients with CML in CP who had sustained undetectable minimal residual disease for at least 2 years (Ross et al. 2013). At 24 months, 47.1 % remained in stable treatment-free remission. These data indicate that it is safe to discontinue TKI therapy in patients who have maintained deep molecular remission over an extended period of time (Mahon 2012). Given the opportunity of achieving deeper and faster molecular responses with second-generation TKIs, this issue may be even more relevant in patients starting CML therapy with nilotinib. Preliminary data indicate that similar conclusions might be drawn regarding discontinuation of second-generation TKIs, but larger studies are warranted (Rea et al. 2011).

8 Summary and Perspectives

In summary, nilotinib is a rationally designed second-generation TKI with significant efficacy in treating patients with CML. It is currently approved for patients with CML both newly diagnosed as well as after imatinib failure.

An unsolved issue is how individual risk factors, disease status, comorbidities, and Bcr-Abl mutation status should guide the choice of TKI therapy given the fact that several of them in addition to nilotinib are currently approved for the same indication. Data from the ENESTnd study indicate that nilotinib appears to be superior both from an efficacy and tolerability point of view compared with imatinib, most strikingly, in preventing progression to AP or BP. As therapy for advanced phase CML is still very deficient, most efforts when treating patients with CML in CP should be focused on preventing progression to AP or BP. A potential added benefit of using nilotinib over imatinib as frontline therapy in CML in CP is the induction of deep and fast molecular responses in a larger number of patients, which might facilitate future TKI interruption strategies.

References

Aichberger KJ, Herndlhofer S, Schernthaner G-H et al (2011) Progressive peripheral arterial occlusive disease and other vascular events during nilotinib therapy in CML. Am J Hematol 86:533–539

Apperley JF (2007) Part I: mechanisms of resistance to imatinib in chronic myeloid leukaemia. Lancet Oncol 8:1018–1029

Baccarani M, Cortes J, Pane F (2009) Chronic myeloid leukemia: an update of concepts and management recommendations of European LeukemiaNet. J Clin Oncol 27:6041–6051

Bradeen HA, Eide CA, O'Hare T et al (2006) Comparison of imatinib mesylate, dasatinib (BMS-354825), and nilotinib (AMN107) in an N-ethyl-N-nitrosourea (ENU)-based mutagenesis screen: high efficacy of drug combinations. Blood 108:2332–2338

Cortes J, O'Brien S, Kantarjian H (2004) Discontinuation of imatinib therapy after achieving a molecular response. Blood 104:2204–2205

Deininger MWN, O'Brien SG, Ford JM et al (2003) Practical management of patients with chronic myeloid leukemia receiving imatinib. J Clin Oncol 21:1637–1647

Druker BJ, Guilhot F, O'Brien S et al (2006) Long-term benefits of imatinib (IM) for patients newly diagnosed with chronic myelogenous leukemia in chronic phase (CML-CP): the 5-year update from the IRIS study. J Clin Oncol 24:338S–338S

Druker BJ, Tamura S, Buchdunger E, Ohno S (1996) Effects of a selective inhibitor of the Abl tyrosine kinase on the growth of Bcr-Abl positive cells. Nat Med 2:561–566

Ernst T, La Rosee P, Mueller MC, Hochhaus A (2011) Bcr-Abl mutations in chronic myeloid leukemia. Hematol Oncol Clin North Am 25:997–1008

Giles FJ, Abruzzese E, Rosti G et al (2010) Nilotinib is active in chronic and accelerated phase chronic myeloid leukemia following failure of imatinib and dasatinib therapy. Leukemia 24:1299–1301

Giles FJ, Kantarjian HM, le Coutre PD et al (2012) Nilotinib is effective in imatinib-resistant or -intolerant patients with chronic myeloid leukemia in blastic phase. Leukemia 26:959–962

Giles FJ, Larson RA, Kantarjian HM (2008) Nilotinib in patients with Philadelphia chromosome-positive chronic myelogenous leukemia in blast crisis (CML-BC) who are resistant or intolerant to imatinib—Giles et al. 26 (15 Supplement): 7017—ASCO Meeting Abstracts. J Clin Oncol 26:7017

Giles FJ, le Coutre PD, Pinilla-Ibarz J et al (2013) Nilotinib in imatinib-resistant or imatinib-intolerant patients with chronic myeloid leukemia in chronic phase: 48-month follow-up results of a phase II study. Leukemia 27:107–112

Golemovic M, Verstovsek S, Giles F et al (2005) AMN107, a novel aminopyrimidine inhibitor of Bcr-Abl, has in vitro activity against imatinib-resistant chronic myeloid leukemia. Clin Cancer Res 11:4941–4947

Gorre ME, Mohammed M, Ellwood K et al (2001) Clinical resistance to STI-571 cancer therapy caused by Bcr-Abl gene mutation or amplification. Science 293:876–880

Haouala A, Widmer N, Duchosal MA et al (2011) Drug interactions with the tyrosine kinase inhibitors imatinib, dasatinib, and nilotinib. Blood 117:E75–E87

Hochhaus A, Saglio G, Larson RA et al (2013) Nilotinib is associated with a reduced incidence of Bcr-Abl mutations vs imatinib in patients with newly diagnosed chronic myeloid leukemia in chronic phase. Blood 121:3703–3708

Jain P, Kantarjian H, Nazha A et al (2013) Early responses predicts for better outcomes in patients with newly diagnosed CML: results with four TKI modalities. Blood 121:4867–4874

Kagan M, Tran P, Fischer V et al (2005) Safety, pharmacokinetics (PK), metabolism, and mass balance of [C-14]-AMN107, a novel aminopyrimidine inhibitor of Bcr-Abl tyrosine kinase, in healthy subjects. Blood 106:302B–302B

Kantarjian H, Giles F, Wunderle L et al (2006) Nilotinib in imatinib-resistant CML and Philadelphia chromosome-positive ALL. N Engl J Med 354:2542–2551

Kantarjian HM, Giles F, Gattermann N et al (2007) Nilotinib (formerly AMN107), a highly selective Bcr-Abl tyrosine kinase inhibitor, is effective in patients with Philadelphia chromosome-positive chronic myelogenous leukemia in chronic phase following imatinib resistance and intolerance. Blood 110:3540–3546

Kantarjian HM, Giles FJ, Bhalla KN et al (2011a) Nilotinib is effective in patients with chronic myeloid leukemia in chronic phase after imatinib resistance or intolerance: 24-month follow-up results. Blood 117:1141–1145

Kantarjian HM, Hochhaus A, Saglio G et al (2011b) Nilotinib versus imatinib for the treatment of patients with newly diagnosed chronic phase, Philadelphia chromosome-positive, chronic myeloid leukaemia: 24-month minimum follow-up of the phase 3 randomised ENESTnd trial. Lancet Oncol 12:841–851

Kim TD, Rea D, Schwarz M et al (2013) Peripheral artery occlusive disease in chronic phase chronic myeloid leukemia patients treated with nilotinib or imatinib. Leukemia 27:1316–1321

Larson RA, Hochhaus A, Hughes TP et al (2012) Nilotinib vs imatinib in patients with newly diagnosed Philadelphia chromosome-positive chronic myeloid leukemia in chronic phase: ENESTnd 3-year follow-up. Leukemia 26:2197–2203

Larson RA, Hochhaus A, Saglio G et al. (2013) Nilotinib vs imatinib in patients with newly diagnosed chronic myeloid leukemia in chronic phase (CML-CP): ENESTnd 4-year update. J Clin Oncol (suppl) 31:abstr. 7052

le Coutre P, Ottmann OG, Giles F et al (2008) Nilotinib (formerly AMN107), a highly selective Bcr-Abl tyrosine kinase inhibitor, is active in patients with imatinib-resistant or -intolerant accelerated-phase chronic myelogenous leukemia. Blood 111:1834–1839

le Coutre P, Rea D, Abruzzese E et al (2011) Severe peripheral arterial disease during nilotinib therapy. J Natl Cancer Inst 103:1347–1348

le Coutre PD, Giles FJ, Hochhaus A et al (2012) Nilotinib in patients with Ph+ chronic myeloid leukemia in accelerated phase following imatinib resistance or intolerance: 24-month follow-up results. Leukemia 26:1189–1194

Mahon F-X (2012) Is going for cure in chronic myeloid leukemia possible and justifiable? Hematology Am Soc Hematol Educ Program 2012:122–128

Mahon F-X, Rea D, Guilhot J et al (2010) Discontinuation of imatinib in patients with chronic myeloid leukaemia who have maintained complete molecular remission for at least 2 years: the prospective, multicentre stop imatinib (STIM) trial. Lancet Oncol 11:1029–1035

Manley PW, Breitenstein W, Brüggen J et al (2004) Urea derivatives of STI571 as inhibitors of Bcr-Abl and PDCFR kinases. Bioorg Med Chem Lett 14:5793–5797

O'Hare T, Eide CA, Deininger MWN (2007) Bcr-Abl kinase domain mutations, drug resistance, and the road to a cure for chronic myeloid leukemia. Blood 110:2242–2249

O'Hare T, Walters DK, Stoffregen EP et al (2005) In vitro activity of Bcr-Abl inhibitors AMN107 and BMS-354825 against clinically relevant imatinib-resistant Abl kinase domain mutants. Cancer Res 65:4500–4505

Quintás-Cardama A, Kantarjian H, Cortes J (2012) Nilotinib-associated vascular events. Clin Lymphoma Myeloma Leuk 12:337–340

Ray A, Cowan-Jacob SW, Manley PW et al (2007) Identification of Bcr-Abl point mutations conferring resistance to the Abl kinase inhibitor AMN107 (nilotinib) by a random mutagenesis study. Blood 109:5011–5015

Rea D, Rousselot P, Nicolini FE et al (2011) Discontinuation of dasatinib or nilotinib in chronic myeloid leukemia (CML) patients (pts) with stable undetectable Bcr-Abl transcripts: results from the French CML group (FILMC). ASH Annual Meeting Abstracts 118:604
Redaelli S, Mologni L, Rostagno R et al (2012) Three novel patient-derived BCR/ABL mutants show different sensitivity to second and third generation tyrosine kinase inhibitors. Am J Hematol 87:E125–E128
Rix U, Hantschel O, Duernberger G et al (2007) Chemical proteomic profiles of the Bcr-Abl inhibitors imatinib, nilotinib, and dasatinib, reveal novel kinase and nonkinase targets. Blood 110:4055–4063
Ross DM, Branford S, Seymour JF et al (2013) Safety and efficacy of imatinib cessation for CML patients with stable undetectable minimal residual disease: results from the TWISTER study. Blood 122:515–522
Saglio G, Kim D-W, Issaragrisil S et al (2010) Nilotinib versus imatinib for newly diagnosed chronic myeloid leukemia. N Engl J Med 362:2251–2259
Sawyers CL, Hochhaus A, Feldman E et al (2002) Imatinib induces hematologic and cytogenetic responses in patients with chronic myelogenous leukemia in myeloid blast crisis: results of a phase II study. Blood 99:3530–3539
Shah NP, Nicoll JM, Nagar B et al (2002) Multiple Bcr-Abl kinase domain mutations confer polyclonal resistance to the tyrosine kinase inhibitor imatinib (STI571) in chronic phase and blast crisis chronic myeloid leukemia. Cancer Cell 2:117–125
Talpaz M, Silver RT, Druker BJ (2002) Imatinib induces durable hematologic and cytogenetic responses in patients with accelerated phase chronic myeloid leukemia: results of a phase 2 study. Blood 99:1928–1937
Tanaka C, Yin OQP, Sethuraman V et al (2009) Clinical pharmacokinetics of the Bcr–Abl tyrosine kinase inhibitor nilotinib. Clin Pharmacol Ther 87:197–203
Tanaka C, Yin OQP, Smith T et al (2011) Effects of rifampin and ketoconazole on the pharmacokinetics of nilotinib in healthy participants. J Clin Pharmacol 51:75–83
von Bubnoff N, Manley PW, Mestan J et al (2006) Bcr-Abl resistance screening predicts a limited spectrum of point mutations to be associated with clinical resistance to the Abl kinase inhibitor nilotinib (AMN107). Blood 108:1328–1333
Weisberg E, Manley P, Mestan J et al (2006) AMN107 (nilotinib): a novel and selective inhibitor of Bcr-Abl. Br J Cancer 94:1765–1769
Weisberg E, Manley PW, Breitenstein W et al (2005) Characterization of AMN107, a selective inhibitor of native and mutant Bcr-Abl. Cancer Cell 7:129–141
Yin OQP, Gallagher N, Li A et al (2010) Effect of grapefruit juice on the pharmacokinetics of nilotinib in healthy participants. J Clin Pharmacol 50:188–194

Bosutinib: A Novel Second-Generation Tyrosine Kinase Inhibitor

Susanne Isfort, Gunhild Keller-v. Amsberg, Philippe Schafhausen, Steffen Koschmieder and Tim H. Brümmendorf

Abstract

Bosutinib (SKI-606) is a 4-anilino-3-quinoline carbonitrile, which acts as a dual inhibitor of Src and ABL kinases. In addition, the BCR-ABL fusion gene product, a constitutively activated tyrosine kinase which is crucial for the development of chronic myeloid leukemia (CML), is highly sensitive to bosutinib. Interestingly, distinctly lower concentrations of bosutinib are required to ablate BCR-ABL phosphorylation when compared to the first-generation tyrosine kinase inhibitor imatinib (IM). Bosutinib is a potent inhibitor of CML cell proliferation in vitro and has demonstrated promising activity in CML patients resistant or intolerant to IM as well as in newly diagnosed patients with chronic phase CML (CML-CP). Remarkably, bosutinib has been found to be capable of overcoming the majority of IM-resistant BCR-ABL mutations. Bosutinib has the potency to induce deep and fast responses in second- and third-/fourth-line treatment, and as a consequence, the drug has recently been licensed for patients previously treated with one or more tyrosine kinase inhibitor(s) and for whom imatinib, nilotinib, and dasatinib are not considered appropriate treatment options. Due to its potency and differing toxicity profile, it promises to be a good therapeutic option for a defined cohort of patients. The most common side effects are gastrointestinal with most of the patients suffering from nausea, vomiting, or diarrhea. For the most part, these gastrointestinal symptoms occur early after treatment initiation, are

S. Isfort · S. Koschmieder · T. H. Brümmendorf (✉)
Department of Hematology, Oncology and Stem Cell Transplantation, University Hospital RWTH Aachen, Pauwelsstraße 30, 52074, Aachen, Germany
e-mail: tbruemmendorf@ukaachen.de

G. K. Amsberg · P. Schafhausen
Department of Oncology and Hematology, Hubertus Wald Tumorzentrum-Universitäres Cancer Center Hamburg (UCCH), Martinistraße 52, 20246, Hamburg, Germany

U. M. Martens (ed.), *Small Molecules in Oncology*, Recent Results in Cancer Research 201, DOI: 10.1007/978-3-642-54490-3_4,

manageable, and often self-limiting. Continuous monitoring of liver enzymes upon treatment initiation is necessary during bosutinib treatment. In addition to CML treatment, bosutinib has shown some efficacy in selected patients suffering from advanced-stage solid tumors. In conclusion, bosutinib is a promising novel small molecule inhibitor approved now for targeted therapy of CML and in clinical development for other malignancies.

Contents

1 Structure and Mechanism of Action

1.1 Chemical Structure

Bosutinib (SKI-606), 4-[(2,4-dichloro-5-methoxyphenyl)amino]-6-methoxy-7-[3-(4-methyl-1-piperazinyl) propoxy]-3-quinolinecarbonitrile monohydrate, is a competitive inhibitor of both Src and ABL tyrosine kinases. It was originally synthesized as an inhibitor of the Src kinase family. The small molecule inhibitor is of low weight (548.46 kDa) and orally bioavailable (Boschelli et al. 2001).

1.2 Mechanism of Action (Target Profile)

Bosutinib is a potent dual inhibitor of the Src and ABL tyrosine kinases (Puttini et al. 2006). In addition, more than 45 other tyrosine and serine/threonine kinases have been identified as potential targets of bosutinib.

1.3 SRC Kinase Inhibition

The tyrosine kinase Src is a member of a family of related kinases known as the Src family kinases (SFKs) that share a common structural organization and function as key regulators of signal transduction pathways triggered by a wide variety of surface receptors, including receptor tyrosine kinases, integrins, G-protein-coupled receptors, and antigen receptors (Thomas and Brugge 1997). Various studies and clinical observations point to a key role of Src kinases in malignant cell transformation, tumor progression, and metastatic spread as a consequence of changes in protein expression and/or kinase activity (Summy and Gallick 2003; Johnson and Gallick 2007; Li 2008). Indeed, overexpression of Src kinases has been detected in several human malignancies, including carcinomas of the breast, lung, colon, esophagus, skin, pancreas, cervix as well as gastric tissues (Mazurenko et al. 1992; Ottenhoff-Kalff et al. 1992; Verbeek et al. 1996; Lutz et al. 1998; Jallal et al. 2007; Zhang et al. 2007). Bosutinib is capable of inhibiting Src kinase at nanomolar concentrations; an IC50 of 1.2 nM has been reported in an enzymatic assay. Inhibition of Src-dependent protein tyrosine phosphorylation can be detected at comparable or lower concentrations (Boschelli et al. 2001). In addition, bosutinib successfully inhibited the growth of Src-transformed fibroblasts and Src overexpressing HT29 colon tumors subcutaneously transplanted into athymic nu/nu mice (Compound 31a) (Boschelli et al. 2001).

1.4 ABL and BCR-ABL Inhibition

c-ABL belongs to an evolutionary conserved protein family and encodes a ubiquitously expressed non-receptor protein tyrosine kinase localized in the cytoplasm and the nucleus (Laneuville 1995; Pendergast 1996). Oncogenic transformation mediated by different genomic alterations of the c-ABL proto-oncogene results in abnormal cellular development and suppression of apoptosis (Chung et al. 1996). This was first observed with chromosomal translocations in human leukemia. Recently, activation of c-ABL was not only found to be linked to chromosomal translocations but rather driven by enhanced ABL expression which has been described in solid-tumor-derived cancer cells (Greuber et al. 2013).

In chronic myeloid leukemia (CML) and Philadelphia chromosome-positive (Ph+) acute lymphocytic leukemia (ALL), a reciprocal translocation of the proto-oncogene *c-ABL* from chromosome 9 to the breakpoint cluster region (*BCR*) of chromosome 22 results in the expression of a constitutively activated tyrosine kinase which phosphorylates a broad range of substrates, many of which are crucial in cellular signal transduction (Sattler and Griffin 2003). However, while the efficacy between IM and bosutinib as inhibitors of v-ABL phosphorylation is within the same range, substantially lower concentrations of the dual Src/ABL inhibitor are required to ablate BCR-ABL phosphorylation. Thus, bosutinib virtually abolishes tyrosine phosphorylation of BCR-ABL at concentrations between 25 and 50 nM, whereas v-ABL phosphorylation in the immunoprecipitates does not decrease to this extent until a concentration of 200 nM is achieved. This indicates that tyrosine phosphorylation of v-ABL is less sensitive to bosutinib than BCR-ABL (Golas et al. 2003).

Bosutinib inhibits bacterially expressed ABL kinase and growth of ABL-MLV-transformed fibroblasts with similar IC50 values obtained for the tyrosine kinase inhibitor imatinib (IM) (IC50 of 1 nM and IC50 of 90 nM, respectively). The extent of tyrosine phosphorylation inhibition by bosutinib in ABL-MLV-transformed fibroblasts correlates with the degree of anti-proliferative activity. In addition, incubation of ABL-MLV-transformed Rat 2 fibroblasts with comparable concentrations of bosutinib and IM results in quantitatively similar reductions in tyrosine phosphorylation of cellular proteins (Golas et al. 2003).

The treatment of CML with TKIs such as IM (and later nilotinib, dasatinib, or bosutinib) led to the new prominent clinical problem of TKI resistance, mediated by specific mutations in BCR-ABL that confer varying degrees of resistance to 1st (IM), 2nd (nilotinib, dasatinib, and bosutinib), and third-generation (ponatinib) TKIs.

The in vitro resistance profile of bosutinib and other TKIs, as studied in Ba/F3 cell lines, are shown in Fig. 1 (Redaelli et al. 2012).

Levinson et al. (2012) identified the specific structure of bosutinib by structural and spectroscopic analysis. These data can now be used to explain the efficacy in most imatinib-resistant mutants and the lack of efficacy in T315I-mutational status.

Furthermore, ATP-binding cassette transporters (ABC transporters) are known mediators of drug resistance in cancer. While the mechanisms are not fully understood, Hegedus et al. (2009) were able to identify a significant difference between second-generation TKIs dasatinib and nilotinib in comparison with bosutinib, as neither ABCB1 nor ABCG2 induced resistance to bosutinib. The possible clinical impact of this finding has to be further evaluated.

2 Preclinical Data

2.1 BCR-ABL-Dependent Diseases

The anti-proliferative activity of bosutinib has been demonstrated in different BCR-ABL expressing leukemia cell lines. In fact, the efficacy of bosutinib is superior to IM with IC50 values ranging from 1 to 20 nM when compared to IM with 51–221 nM, respectively (Golas et al. 2003; Puttini et al. 2006). In addition, bosutinib successfully inhibits growth of IM-resistant human cell lines, such as Lama84R, KCL22R, and K562R (Golas et al. 2003). In line with these findings, inhibition of proliferation of murine pro-B Ba/F3 cells, stably transformed by p210 BCR-ABL WT or four imatinib-resistant point mutants (D276G, Y253F, E255K, and T315I), is more pronounced under bosutinib than under IM. Thus, WT, D276G, and Y253F transfectants are inhibited in the low nanomolar range by the dual Src/ABL kinase inhibitor. However, the T315I BCR-ABL mutant requires concentrations of bosutinib that are one to two orders of magnitude higher when

		IC50 fold increase (WT = 1)				
		Imatinib	Bosutinib	Dasatinib	Nilotinib	Ponatinib
	Parental	10.8	38.3	568.3	38.4	570.0
	WT	1	1	1	1	1
P-Loop	M244V	0.9	0.9	2.0	1.2	3.2
	L248R	14.6	22.9	12.5	30.2	6.2
	L248V	3.5	3.5	5.1	2.8	3.4
	G250E	6.9	4.3	4.4	4.6	6.0
	Q252H	1.4	0.8	3.1	2.6	6.1
	Y253F	3.6	1.0	1.6	3.2	3.7
	Y253H	8.7	0.6	2.6	36.8	2.6
	E255K	6.0	9.5	5.6	6.7	8.4
	E255V	17.0	5.5	3.4	10.3	12.9
C-Helix	D276G	2.2	0.6	1.4	2.0	2.1
	E279K	3.6	1.0	1.6	2.0	3.0
	E292L	0.7	1.1	1.3	1.8	2.0
ATP-binding region (drug contact sites)	V299L	1.5	26.1	8.7	1.3	0.6
	T315A	1.7	6.0	58.9	2.7	0.4
	T315I	17.5	45.4	75.0	39.4	3.0
	T315V	12.2	29.3	738.8	57.0	2.1
	F317L	2.6	2.4	4.5	2.2	0.7
	F317R	2.3	33.5	114.8	2.3	4.9
	F317V	0.4	11.5	21.3	0.5	2.3
SH2-contact	M343T	1.2	1.1	0.9	0.8	0.9
	M351T	1.8	0.7	0.9	0.4	1.2
Substrate binding region (drug contact sites)	F359I	6.0	2.9	3.0	16.3	2.9
	F359V	2.9	0.9	1.5	5.2	4.4
A-Loop	L384M	1.3	0.5	2.2	2.3	2.2
	H396P	2.4	0.4	1.1	2.4	1.4
	H396R	3.9	0.8	1.6	3.1	5.9
C-terminal lobe	F486S	8.1	2.3	3.0	1.9	2.1
	L248R + F359I	11.7	39.3	13.7	96.2	17.7

Sensitive	≤2
Moderately resistant	2.01 - 4
Resistant	4.01 – 10
Highly resistant	> 10

Fig. 1 Resistance profile of bosutinib, imatinib, nilotinib, dasatinib, and ponatinib. *Source* Redaelli et al. (2012)

compared with wt BCR-ABL cells (Puttini et al. 2006), suggesting inactivity against this mutation since these levels are unlikely to be achieved in patients. In in-vivo experiments, bosutinib administered at 75 mg/kg twice daily or 150 mg/kg once daily results in a complete regression of human K562 xenografts for up to 40 days (Golas et al. 2003). Remarkably, while IM is unable to eradicate KU812 human tumor xenografts with a relapse rate of 30 % at experimental day 8, bosutinib treatment initiated at day 8 and 15 after leukemic cell injection leads to a complete eradication of disease with all animals remaining tumor-free for up to experimental day 210 (Puttini et al. 2006). In mice injected s.c. with Ba/F3 BCR-ABL + xenografts containing WT or mutant BCR-ABL (E255K, Y253F, and D276G) and treated with bosutinib 1 day after tumor cell injection, the dual Src/ABL kinase inhibitor induces a statistically significant decrease in tumor growth and a prolonged event-free survival. However, in animals with a delayed initiation of bosutinib therapy, relapse of disease is found in the majority of mice. Furthermore, bosutinib does not influence proliferation of highly IM-resistant T315I xenografts (Puttini et al. 2006). The combination of imatinib with bosutinib was further evaluated by Redaelli et al. (2010) who could demonstrate synergistic effects of this combination in different CML cell lines and in primary CML patient cells.

Konig et al. (2008) evaluated bosutinib efficacy on hematopoietic progenitor cells in CML. Bosutinib was able to inhibit CML progenitor growth with relatively low side effects on normal progenitors; however, induction of apoptosis in CML progenitor cells was not more efficient than by the use of other TKIs like imatinib. This strategy has to be further evaluated.

2.2 Potential New Hematologic Diseases/Targets

As mentioned before, more than 45 other tyrosine and serine/threonine kinases have been identified as potential targets of bosutinib. Among these, STE20 and CAMK2G have been described to be associated with myeloid leukemia cell proliferation and apoptosis (Remsing et al. 2009).

As also Lyn and BTK are possible targets of bosutinib (Gleixner et al. 2011) and these pathways are involved in KIT-independent aggressive systemic mastocytosis, this could open more treatment options for this rare but clinically severe disease.

2.3 Breast Cancer

Bosutinib causes a decrease in cell proliferation, migration, and invasion of breast cancer cell lines accompanied by an increase in cell-to-cell adhesions and a membrane localization of beta-catenin, a phosphoprotein that functions as both a structural component of the cell adhesion/actin cytoskeleton network and a signaling molecule when localized in the nucleus. Analysis of downstream effectors of Src reveals an inhibition of mitogen-activated protein kinase (MAPK) and Akt phosphorylation as well as a reduced phosphorylation of focal adhesion kinase (FAK), proline-rich tyrosine kinase 2 (Pyk2), and Crk-associated substrate (p130Cas). Thus, bosutinib inhibits signaling pathways involved in cell proliferation and malignant transformation as well as tumor cell motility and invasion (Jallal et al. 2007; Vultur et al. 2008). Proliferation of MDA-MB-231 cells inoculated into the mammary fat pads of female BALB/c nu/nu mice is significantly suppressed secondary to bosutinib therapy when compared with control animals receiving only the vehicle solution. In addition, analysis of lung, liver, and spleen specimen have shown a significant reduction in metastatic spread in animals treated with the small molecule inhibitor at a well-tolerated dose.

2.4 Colorectal Cancer

Bosutinib decreases tumor growths of subcutaneous colorectal cancer xenograft models generated with different tumor cell lines (HT29, Colo205, HCT116, and DLD1) and causes substantial reduction in Src autophosphorylation at Tyr418 (Golas et al. 2005). In addition, it prevents Src-dependent activation of beta-catenin. However, protein levels of beta-catenin remain substantially unchanged by bosutinib, a cytosolic/membranous retention of beta-catenin is promoted instead. The bosutinib-mediated relocalization of beta-catenin increases its binding affinity to E-cadherin and adhesion of colorectal cancer cells resulting in reduced cell motility (Coluccia et al. 2006). A decreased cell motion as well as the ability of bosutinib to reduce VEGF-mediated vascular permeability and tumor cell extravasation combined with the effect of Src inhibition in stromal cells may be responsible for the superior activity of bosutinib in vivo when compared with the attained effects in cell culture experiments.

2.5 Non-small Cell Lung Cell Cancer

Immunohistochemical analyses of non-small cell lung cell cancer (NSCLC) biopsy samples reveal an upregulation of Src kinase in 33 % of the tumors. In NSCLC cell lines with increased Src kinase activity, treatment with bosutinib induces apoptosis and causes a cleavage of caspase-3 and PARP (Zhang et al. 2007).

2.6 Polycystic Kidney Disease

In polycystic kidney disease (PKD), the precise functions of the cystoprotein products remain unknown. Recent data suggest that multimeric cystoprotein complexes lead to aberrant signaling cascades involving c-Src kinases. In two different animal models, greater Src activity was found to correlate with disease progression in PKD. Inhibition of Src activity via bosutinib resulted in amelioration of renal cyst formation and biliary ductal abnormalities in both animal models, suggesting this strategy may provide therapeutic benefit in PKD (Sweeney and von Vigier 2008).

3 Clinical Data

In spring of 2013, bosutinib has been conditionally approved for treatment in CML in chronic phase (CP), accelerated phase (AP), and blast crisis (BC) in Europe for patients after first-line therapy with first- or second-generation TKI for whom imatinib, nilotinib, or dasatinib are not considered appropriate treatment options. This approval was based on data published by Cortes et al. in 2011 and Khoury et al. in 2012 on their phase I/II trial, evaluating bosutinib in second-line and third-/fourth-line treatment upon intolerance or resistance to imatinib and/or intolerance or resistance to a second-generation TKI. In addition, a randomized, open-label, phase III clinical trial comparing the efficacy of bosutinib and IM in first-line therapy of CML-CP (the BELA trial) was published by Cortes et al. in October 2012.

The phase I/II clinical trial in Philadelphia chromosome-positive leukemia had recruited 288 patients with imatinib resistance or intolerance between January 2006 and July 2008 where bosutinib was given as second-line treatment. In addition, another 118 patients pre-treated with IM and at least one additional second-generation TKI were included.

In the phase I part of this trial (17 patients), dose-limiting toxicity (grade 3 rash, nausea, and vomiting) was found to occur at 600 mg daily. Therefore, a treatment dose of 500 mg daily was chosen for the phase II part of the study, investigating the efficacy and safety of bosutinib in CML patients (pts) in different patient cohorts. Two hundred and sixty-one patients with CP CML after first-line treatment with imatinib were included in this part of the study that was published by Cortes et al. in (2011, Blood). Another 118 patients received imatinib and at least one additional second-generation TKI before study inclusion. Moreover, 134 patients in AP or BC or Ph+ ALL were recruited as a third cohort of this study.

3.1 Bosutinib in Treatment-Resistant/-Intolerant CML

3.1.1 Bosutinib as Second-Line Treatment (Cortes et al. 2011)

The study population included IM-resistant or -intolerant patients: IM resistance has been defined by no hematologic improvement within 4 weeks, no complete hematologic response (CHR) after 12 weeks, no cytogenetic response after 24 weeks, and/or no major cytogenetic response (MCR) after 12 months of therapy with an IM dose of at least 600 mg daily. Acquired resistance was defined as a loss of a MyCR or any hematologic response. Individuals have been considered to be intolerant to IM if toxicities grade 4 lasted longer than 7 days, if imatinib-related non-hematologic toxicities grade 3 or higher occurred or persistent toxicities grade

Table 1 Patient characteristics of chronic phase (*CP*) CML patients in the second-line setting

Characteristics	IM resistant (n = 200)	IM intolerant (n = 88)	Total (n = 288)
Median age: years (range)	51.0	54.5	53 (18–91)
Median duration of disease in years (range)	4.0 (0.1–15.1)	2.8 (0.1–13.6)	3.6 (0.1–15.1)
Number of previous treatments			
1 (%)	131 (66)	65 (74)	196 (68)
2 (%)	69 (35)	23 (26)	92 (32)
Previous IFN (%)	69 (35)	23 (26)	92 (32)
Previous SCT (%)	6 (3)	2 (2)	8 (3)
1 or more BCR-ABL mutations detected	57/83	8/32	65/115

Source Cortes et al. (2011)

2 not responding to adequate management and/or dose adjustments appeared. In addition, patients in whom dose reductions were necessary due to toxicities and who subsequently lost their response to treatment were considered IM intolerant as well. Patients' characteristics are listed in Table 1. In total, 288 patients have been included in this part of the study with 69.4 % exhibiting resistance and 20.6 % intolerance to IM. In addition to prior treatment with IM, a subset of patients received interferon (92 pts). Eight patients had undergone stem cell transplantation. Median duration of bosutinib treatment was 14.9 months (range 0.2–49.2); the median dose intensity for IM-resistant and IM-intolerant patients was 484.9 and 394.1 mg/d, respectively. Hematologic and cytogenetic responses were evaluated for all 288 patients; molecular responses could only be assessed in a fraction of the patients as molecular monitoring was not universally available. 86 % (247 pts) had a CHR; 53 % (140 pts) achieved an MCR with a complete cytogenetic response (CCyR) in 41 % (110 pts). In addition, the MMR rate was 41 % and the CMR rate was 34 % among all the patients whose data were available for molecular response. In 115 pts., the mutation status was assessed before initiation of bosutinib therapy. Response analysis by individual mutations revealed hematologic and cytogenetic responses similar to patients without any mutation at baseline except for patients with T315I-mutational status.

3.1.2 Bosutinib After Failure of Second-Line Therapy (Khoury et al. 2012)

In the same study, 118 patients pre-treated with IM and at least one other second-generation TKI had been recruited. Bosutinib was administered in the 500 mg dose established in the phase I of the same trial. Among those, 118 patients who had previously been treated with IM 37 were dasatinib resistant and 50 dasatinib intolerant. In addition, 27 were nilotinib resistant, and one patient was intolerant to nilotinib. Three patients had been treated with all 3 TKIs and failed. Median

Table 2 Response by mutation status in CP CML after at least two lines of treatment

		Cumulative response, n/n evaluable (%)	
Mutation status	*n*	CHR	MCyR
No mutation	44	34/44 (77)	15/43 (35)
Any mutation	39	26/39 (67)	11/35 (31)
>1 mutation	9	3/9 (33)	2/9 (22)
Mutation type			
P-loop	14	9/14 (64)	4/13 (31)
G250E	6	3/6	0/5
Y253H	6	5/6	4/6
E255K	1	0/1	0/1
E255V	1	1/1	0/1
Non-P-loop	29	18/29 (62)	9/26 (35)
M244V	3	3/3	2/3
V299L	2	1/2	0/2
Q300R	1	1/1	1/1
T315I	7	2/7	0/6
F317L	8	4/8	1/7
N336S	1	1/1	0/1
M351T	1	1/1	0/1
F359C	2	2/2	1/2
F359I	2	2/2	2/2
F359V	2	0/2	1/2
L387F	1	1/1	0/1
H396R	1	0/1	0/1
E453A	1	1/1	0/0
C475V	1	1/1	1/1
F486S	1	0/1	0/1

Source Khoury et al. (2012)

follow-up was 28.5 months (range 0.3–56.2); median dose intensity was 478 mg/d (185–563 mg/d). MCyR rate was 32 % among all patients with 24 % ($n = 26$) achieving a CCyR; among them was one of the 3 patients being treated with all 3 TKIs before. Median time to MCyR among responders was 12.4 weeks (ranges 3.9–88.4 weeks). Molecular responses was assessed in 105 patients; among these, 16 (15 %) achieved a MMR, including 12 (11 %) with a CMR. Thirty-three patients had known mutations at the beginning of treatment with bosutinib; the results of these patients are summarized in Table 2.

Table 3 Response to bosutinib treatment in AP/BC CML and Ph+ ALL

Response	ADV cohort	
	Aged ≥65 years ($N = 30$)	Aged <65 years ($n = 135$)
Hematologic response		
Evaluable patients, n	29	123
MHR, n (%)	8 (28)	38 (31)
CHR	4 (14)	31 (25)
2-y probability of maintaining a MHR (%)	71	54
2-y probability of maintaining a CHR (%)	75	54
Cytogenetic response		
Evaluable patients, n	26	117
MCyR, n (%)	8 (31)	45 (39)
CCyR	7 (27)	24 (29)
2-y probability of maintaining a MCyR (%)	43	34

Source Bruemmendorf et al. (2013)

3.1.3 Accelerated Phase (AP CML), Blast Phase (BP CML), and Ph+ ALL

An update of data on patients with AP ($n = 77$) and BP CML ($n = 64$) and Ph+ ALL ($n = 24$) with an open-label continuous daily dosing schedule (bosutinib 500 mg/day) as part of the above-mentioned phase I/II trial was presented at the 2013 ASCO Annual Meeting (Bruemmendorf et al. 2013). In this analysis, patients were split into two different cohorts regarding their age (<65 years vs. ≥65 years). All patients included were previously treated with IM plus/minus other TKIs and exhibited IM resistance or intolerance. Hematologic and cytogenetic response data are shown in Table 3.

3.2 Bosutinib in CML First-Line Treatment

In the BELA trial published in 2012 by Cortes et al. (2012, JCO), bosutinib was evaluated in the first-line setting against imatinib in patients with CML in CP. The primary end point of this trial was the CCyR rate at 12 months which was the standard primary end point in first-line trials at that time, since standardized molecular analysis was not available in all countries.

502 pts were randomized in a 1:1 manner to each arm, median duration of treatment in both study arms was 13.8 months, and median dose intensity was 489 mg/d for bosutinib and 400 mg/d for imatinib. In the IIT population, the CCyR rate at 12 months was similar in both treatment groups (70 % for bosutinib vs. 68 % for imatinib; $p = 0.601$). However, time to CCyR was significantly

shorter with bosutinib (12.9 weeks vs. 24.6 weeks; $p < 0.001$) with higher rates for CCyR for bosutinib at months 3, 6, and 9. Molecular responses were also significantly higher in the bosutinib group; in detail, MMR rate at 12 months was 41 % versus 27 % ($p < 0.001$). Transformation to AP/BC CML on treatment occurred less frequently among the bosutinib-treated patients (4.2 % vs. 10.4 %).

3.3 Bosutinib in Solid Tumors

Daud et al. (2012) published their phase I trial in patients with advanced solid tumor malignancies. This trial was conducted in two parts, a dose escalation part where 400 mg/d could be identified as recommended dose for phase II. In the second part, approximately 30 patients each with refractory colorectal, pancreas, or NSCLC were treated. A partial response (breast) and unconfirmed complete response (pancreas) were observed; 8 of 112 evaluable patients had stable disease for 22–101 weeks. However, the primary efficacy end points for part 2 were not met.

Campone et al. (2012) performed a phase II study which evaluated single-agent bosutinib in pretreated patients with locally advanced or metastatic breast cancer in 73 patients. The primary end point was the progression-free survival (PFS) rate at 16 weeks. For the intent-to-treat population, the PFS rate at 16 weeks was 39.6 %. Unexpectedly, all responding patients ($n = 4$) were hormone receptor positive. The 2-year overall survival rate was 26.4 %.

4 Toxicity

While the general toxicity profile was very similar in hematologic trials and studies in solid tumors, there were some expected differences in hematologic adverse events.

In the phase II trial of bosutinib after imatinib failure, the most common non-hematologic adverse events included diarrhea, nausea, rash, abdominal pain, and vomiting. Diarrhea and other gastrointestinal AEs were of low grade in the majority of the cases, typically restricted to the period after treatment initiation and typically self-limiting. Fluid retention was observed in only 15 % of the patients and only 4 % of the patients showing pleural effusions. In 9 patients receiving bosutinib as third- or fourth-line treatment (Khoury et al. 2012), pleural effusions occurred, mostly grade 1 and 2. With regard to these latter, only one patient suffered from pleural effusion of grade 3 and none of grade 4. The events of hematologic toxicity were moderate with grade 3/4 neutropenia, thrombocytopenia, and anemia in 18, 24, and 13 %, respectively, in second-line patients. Hematologic toxicity was equally prominent in patients with bosutinib as third- or fourth-line treatment, with grade 3/4 anemia reported in 8 %, thrombocytopenia in 25 %, and neutropenia in 19 % of the treated individuals.

In contrast to the hematologic malignancies, myelosuppression in solid tumor studies was minimal. This might be explained by the fact that hematologic toxicity of TKI treatment in CML is not only a reflection of inhibition of normal hematopoiesis but at least in part mediated by suppression of the leukemic population itself by the TKI.

In part one of the solid tumor study, dose-limiting toxicities of grade 3 diarrhea (two patients) and grade 3 rash occurred with bosutinib 600 mg/day and the maximum tolerated dose identified was 500 mg/day. However, the majority of patients treated with 500 mg/day had grade 2 or greater gastrointestinal toxicity. The most common bosutinib-related adverse events were nausea (60 % patients), diarrhea (47 %), vomiting (40 %), fatigue (38 %), and anorexia (36 %).

Among breast cancer patients, the main toxic effects were diarrhea (66 %), nausea (55 %), and vomiting (47 %). Grade 3–4 laboratory aminotransferase increases occurred in 14 (19 %) patients.

5 Drug Interactions

Simultaneous medication with strong or intermediate inhibitors of CYP3A4 liver enzymes should be avoided because of the danger of increasing bosutinib plasma concentrations. Strong or intermediate inducers of CYP3A4 activity such as Rifampicin or St. John's worth decrease the plasma concentration of bosutinib and must be avoided as well.

As the solubility of bosutinib in water is pH dependent, the intake of antacids should be performed several hours apart to avoid decreased absorption of bosutinib.

Bosutinib might increase plasma levels of substrates of p-Glykoproteins such as Digoxin or Tacrolimus.

Special attention should be paid to patients who have to take other medication which could cause QT prolongation.

6 Biomarkers

In CML, BCR-ABL transcript monitoring is essential as with any TKI treatment. According to international guidelines (i.e., ELN guidelines Baccarani et al. 2013), BCR-ABL measuring should be performed every 3 months. The primary goal is to achieve at least a reduction in BCR-ABL to less than 1 % after 12 months at the latest. After 6 months, CCyR should be achieved. Early achievement of molecular remission becomes increasingly important, as more and more scientific groups showed that rapid decrease in BCR-ABL transcripts such as a BCR-ABL to ABL ratio of below 10 % after three months of treatment is associated with improved 5-year survival as compared to patients who do not achieve this goal (Hanfstein et al. 2012).

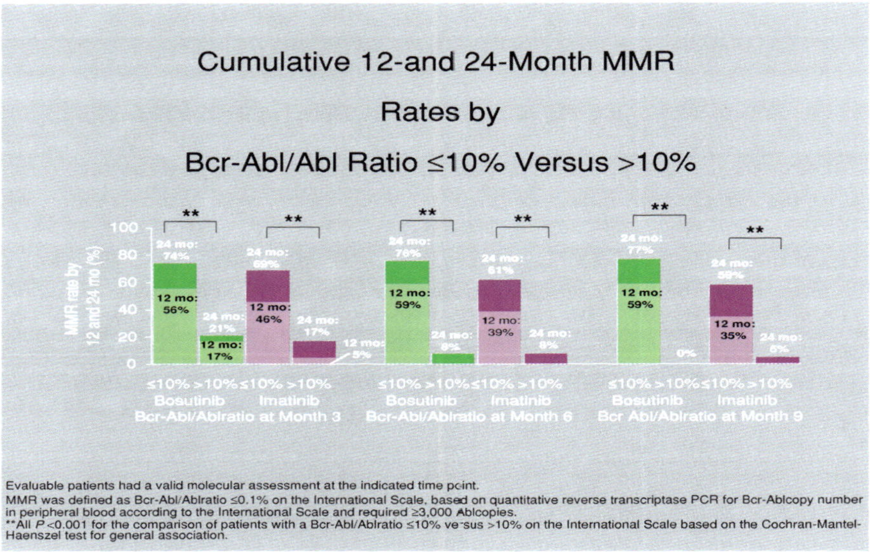

Fig. 2 Cumulative 12- and 24-month MMR rates by Bcr-Abl ratio ≤ 10 % versus >10 %. *Source* Bruemmendorf et al. (2012)

In the BELA trial testing bosutinib versus imatinib in the first-line setting in patients with newly diagnosed CP CML (Bruemmendorf et al. 2012), the rate of molecular response was generally higher at all time points for bosutinib versus imatinib. Bosutinib was associated with deeper cytogenetic and molecular responses compared with imatinib. For both bosutinib and imatinib, reduction in BCR-ABL/ABL ratio to ≤ 1 or ≤ 10 % at months 3, 6, and 9 was associated with higher rates of CCyR and MMR by 12 and 24 months (see Fig. 2). Overall, these results suggest that patients with early reduction in BCR-ABL/ABL ratio during bosutinib or imatinib therapy have a higher likelihood of experiencing better long-term outcomes.

Generally, it is very important to perform these measurements according to international standards in a well-experienced laboratory following their recommendations for national standardization for quality assurance (Mueller et al. 2009). Due to the established converting factor to the international scale, follow-up monitoring has not to be performed in the same laboratory as before in order to guarantee comparable results.

7 Summary and Perspectives

In conclusion, bosutinib is a novel dual Src/ABL kinase inhibitor with high activity against IM-resistant CML as well as solid tumors overexpressing the Src kinase. Its profile of activity is specific with a limited number of molecular targets outside the ABL and Src kinase family. When compared with other second-generation tyrosine kinase inhibitors and with IM, bosutinib shows differing toxicity profile and therefore might be of advantage for a certain cohort of patients based on their pretreatment, toxicities, and/or preexisting comorbidities. Indeed, presumably PDGFR and/or KIT-mediated side effects such as inhibition of normal hematopoiesis typically observed with other TKIs used in BCR-ABL-positive leukemias (Bartolovic et al. 2004) may possibly occur less frequent in patients treated with bosutinib. However, designation of adverse non-hematologic side effects such as edema, muscle cramps, and skin rash to an individual off-target is rarely possible.

The reciprocal translocation of chromosome 9 and 22 resulting in the *BCR-ABL* fusion gene is a key event in the malignant transformation of CML. However, different studies point to an important role of SFKs in disease progression. Thus, overexpression and/or activation of Hck and Lyn has been observed during CML progression (Donato et al. 2003). In addition, the transition of CP CML to lymphoid BC in mice requires the presence of Lyn, Hck, and Fgr (Hu et al. 2006). Remarkably, downregulation of Lyn expression by siRNA induces apoptosis in BCR-ABL-positive blasts, in particular, of lymphoid blasts (Ptasznik et al. 2004). With respect to these findings, the dual inhibition of BCR-ABL and SFK (also and first being followed as part of the development of bosutinib) may provide a promising strategy in CML treatment.

In solid tumors, different treatment combinations including bosutinib are currently being tested mainly in breast cancer. The value of bosutinib in this field has to be further evaluated as until now the clear definition of the patient collective which is benefitting from bosutinib is still missing.

References

Baccarani M, Cortes J et al (2013) European Leukemia Net recommendations for the management of chronic myeloid leukemia: 2013 Blood 2013 prepublished online 26 June 2013. doi:10.1182/blood-2013-05-501569

Bartolovic K, Balabanov S et al (2004) Inhibitory effect of imatinib on normal progenitor cells in vitro. Blood 103(2):523–529

Boschelli DH, Ye F et al (2001) Optimization of 4-phenylamino-3-quinolinecarbonitriles as potent inhibitors of Srckinaseactivity. J Med Chem 44(23):3965–3977

Boschelli F (2008) Activity of bosutinib, dasatinib, and nilotinibagainst 18 imatinib-resistantBcr/Ablmutants. doi:10.1200/JCO.2008.19.8853

Bruemmendorf TH, Kantarjian HM et al (2012) Assessment of early molecular response as a predictor of long-term clinical outcomes in the phase 3 BELA study. Blood (ASH Annual Meeting Abstracts), Nov 2012, 120:69

Bruemmendorf TH, Gambacorti-Passerini C et al (2013) Efficacy and Safety of bosutinib for Philadelphia chromosome-positive leukaemia in older versus younger patients. J Clin Oncol ASCO Annual Meeting abstract, 2013 (suppl; abstr 6511)

Campone M, Bondarenko I et al (2012) Phase II study of single-agent bosutinib, a Src/Abl tyrosine kinase inhibitor, in patients with locally advanced or metastatic breast cancer pretreated with chemotherapy. Ann Oncol 23(3):610–617

Chung SW, Daniel R et al (1996) The ABL genes in normal and abnormal cell development. CritRevOncog 7(1–2):33–48

Coluccia AM, Benati D et al (2006) SKI-606 decreases growth and motility of colorectal cancer cells by preventing pp 60(c-Src)-dependent tyrosine phosphorylation of beta-catenin and its nuclear signaling. Cancer Res 66(4):2279–2286

Cortes JE, Kantarjian HM et al (2011) Safety and efficacy of bosutinib (SKI-606) in chronic phase Philadelphia chromosome-positive chronic myeloid leukemia patients with resistance or intolerance to imatinib. Blood 118(17):4567–4576

Cortes JE, Kim D-W et al (2012) Bosutinib versus Imatinib in newly diagnosed chronic-phase chronic myeloid leukemia; results from the BELA trial. J Clin Oncol 30(28):3486–3492

Daud AI, Krishnamurthi SS et al (2012) Phase I study of bosutinib, a src/abl tyrosine kinase inhibitor, administered to patients with advanced solid tumors. Clin Cancer Res 18(4)

Donato NJ, Wu JY et al (2003) BCR-ABL independence and LYN kinase overexpression in chronic myelogenous leukemia cells selected for resistance to STI571. Blood 101(2):690–698

Gleixner KV, Mayerhofer M et al (2011) KIT-D816V–independant oncogenic signalling in neoplastic cells in systemic mastocytosis: role of Lyn and Btk activation and disruption by dasatinib and bosutinib. Blood 118(7):1885–1898

Golas JM, Arndt K et al (2003) SKI-606, a 4-anilino-3-quinolinecarbonitrile dual inhibitor of Src and Abl kinases, is a potent antiproliferative agent against chronic myelogenous leukemia cells in culture and causes regression of K562 xenografts in nude mice. Cancer Res 63(2):375–381

Golas JM, Lucas J et al (2005) SKI-606, a Src/Abl inhibitor with in vivo activity in colon tumor xenograft models. Cancer Res 65(12):5358–5364

Greuber EK, Smith-Pearson P, Wang J, Pendergast AMet al. (2013) Role of ABL family kinases in cancer: from leukaemia to solid tumours. Nat Rev Cancer 13(8):559–571. doi:10.1038/nrc3563

Hanfstein B, Mueller C et al (2012) Early molecular and cytogenetic response is predictive for long-term progression-free and overall survival in chronic myeloid leukemia (CML). Leukemia 26(9):2096–2102

Hegedus C, Özvegy-Laczka C et al (2009) Interaction of nilotinib, dasatinib and bosutinib with ABCB1 and ABCG2: implications for altered anti-cancer effects and pharmacological properties. Br J Pharmacol 158(4):1153–1164

Hu Y, Swerdlow S et al (2006) Targeting multiple kinase pathways in leukemic progenitors and stem cells is essential for improved treatment of Ph+ leukemia in mice. Proc Natl Acad Sci USA 103(45):16870–16875

Jallal H, Valentino ML et al (2007) A Src/Abl kinase inhibitor, SKI-606, blocks breast cancer invasion, growth, and metastasis in vitro and in vivo. Cancer Res 67(4):1580–1588

Johnson FM, Gallick GE (2007) SRC family nonreceptor tyrosine kinases as molecular targets for cancer therapy. Anticancer Agents Med Chem 7(6):651–659

Khoury JH, Cortes JE et al (2012) Bosutinib is active in chronic phase chronic myeloid leukemia after imatinib and dasatinib and/or nilotinib therapy failure. Blood 119(15):3403–3412

Konig H, Holyoake TL, Bhatia R (2008) Effective and selective inhibition of chronic myeloid leukemia primitive hematopoetic progenitors by the dual Src/Abl kinase inhibitor SKI-606. Blood 111(4):2329–2338

Laneuville P (1995) Abl tyrosine protein kinase. Semin Immunol 7(4):255–266

Levinson NM, Boxer SG et al (2012) Structural and spectroscopic analysis of the kinase inhibitor bosutinib and an isomer of bosutinib binding to the Abl tyrosine kinase domain. PLoS One 7(4):e29828

Li S (2008) Src-family kinases in the development and therapy of Philadelphia chromosome-positive chronic myeloid leukemia and acute lymphoblastic leukemia. Leuk Lymphoma 49(1):19–26

Lutz MP, Esser IB et al (1998) Overexpression and activation of the tyrosine kinase Src in human pancreatic carcinoma. Biochem Biophys Res Commun 243(2):503–508

Mazurenko NN, Kogan EA et al (1992) Expression of pp 60c-src in human small cell and non-small cell lung carcinomas. Eur J Cancer 28(2–3):372–377
Mueller MC, Cross NCP et al (2009) Harmonization of molecular monitoring of CML therapy in Europe. Leukemia 23:1957–1963
Ottenhoff-Kalff AE, Rijksen G et al (1992) Characterization of protein tyrosine kinases from human breast cancer: involvement of the c-src oncogene product. Cancer Res 52(17):4773–4778
Pendergast AM (1996) Nuclear tyrosine kinases: from Abl to WEE1. Curr Opin Cell Biol 8(2):174–181
Ptasznik A, Nakata Y et al (2004) Short interfering RNA (siRNA) targeting the Lyn kinase induces apoptosis in primary, and drug-resistant, BCR-ABL1(+) leukemia cells. Nat Med 10(11):1187–1189
Puttini M, Coluccia AM et al (2006) In vitro and in vivo activity of SKI-606, a novel Src-Abl inhibitor, against imatinib-resistant Bcr-Abl+ neoplastic cells. Cancer Res 66(23):11314–11322
Redaelli S, Boschelli F et al (2010) Synergistic activity of the Src/Abl inhibitor bosutinib in combination with imatinib. Leukemia 24(6):1223–1227
Redaelli S, Mologni L et al (2012) Three novel patient-derived BCR/ABL mutants show different sensitivity to second and third generation tyrosine kinase inhibitors. Am J Hematol 87(11):E125–E128. doi:10.1002/ajh.23338. Epub 2012 Oct 9
Remsing LLR, Rix U et al (2009) Global target profile of the kinase inhibitor bosutinib in primary chronic myeloid leukemia cells. Leukemia 23(3):477–485
Sattler M, Griffin JD (2003) Molecular mechanisms of transformation by the BCR-ABL oncogene. Semin Hematol 40(2 Suppl 2):4–10
Summy JM, Gallick GE (2003) Src family kinases in tumor progression and metastasis. Cancer Metastasis Rev 22(4):337–358
Sweeney WE, von Vigier RO (2008) Src inhibition ameliorates polycystic kidney disease. J Am Soc Nephrol 19:1331–1341
Thomas SM, Brugge JS (1997) Cellular functions regulated by Src family kinases. Annu Rev Cell Dev Biol 13:513–609
Verbeek BS, Vroom TM et al (1996) c-Src protein expression is increased in human breast cancer. An immunohistochemical and biochemicalanalysis. J Pathol 180(4):383–388
Vultur A, Buettner R et al (2008) SKI-606 (bosutinib), a novel Src kinase inhibitor, suppresses migration and invasion of human breast cancer cells. Mol Cancer Ther 7(5):1185–1194
Zhang J, Kalyankrishna S et al (2007) SRC-family kinases are activated in non-small cell lung cancer and promote the survival of epidermal growth factor receptor-dependent cell lines. Am J Pathol 170(1):366–376

Ponatinib: A Third-Generation Inhibitor for the Treatment of CML

Julius Wehrle, Heike L. Pahl and Nikolas von Bubnoff

Abstract

The establishment of imatinib as the standard therapy for CML marked the beginning of a new era of treatment. Due to occurring intolerance and resistance against the drug, developing newer inhibitors was promoted. This led to the second-generation inhibitors dasatinib, nilotinib and bosutinib. Despite all achieved improvement, all first- and second-generation inhibitors are ineffective against the BCR-ABL T315I "gatekeeper" mutation. In order to overcome this issue and to further improve the inhibitory effect, the third-generation inhibitor ponatinib was developed. Various clinical trials have been launched to study the effect of ponatinib in the clinical setting. Based on positive phase 1 and phase 2 trials, ponatinib was approved for the second-line treatment of CML and Ph^+ ALL in December 2012 in the United States and in July 2013 in the European Union. Further trials investigate the potential effect of ponatinib in kinase-dependent subgroups of other malignancies. In conclusion, ponatinib has proved to be a powerful BCR-ABL inhibitor, which exhibits clinical activity both in BCR-ABL wild-type and mutant CML, including activity against the T315I mutation. Despite previous TKI failure, chronic-phase CML patients can achieve sustained remissions using the novel drug, offering a new therapeutic option in the treatment for CML.

J. Wehrle · H. L. Pahl · N. von Bubnoff (✉)
University of Freiburg - Medical Center - Department of Medicine I, Freiburg, Germany
e-mail: nikolas.bubnoff@uniklinik-freiburg.de

U. M. Martens (ed.), *Small Molecules in Oncology*, Recent Results in Cancer Research 201, DOI: 10.1007/978-3-642-54490-3_5,

Contents

1 Resistance to Treatment in CML

The establishment of imatinib as the standard therapy for CML in 2001 (Druker et al. 2001) fundamentally changed the clinical course of this disease. For many patients, CML became a chronic disorder and patients experiencing a major molecular response (MMR) might not face a loss in life expectancy (Jain et al. 2013). However, this favorable prognosis is not true for all patients. Around 20–30 % of patients treated with imatinib do not respond adequately to treatment (primary resistance) or relapse after initial response to imatinib (secondary resistance) (Druker et al. 2006; de Lavallade et al. 2008).

Resistance against imatinib or newer Abl inhibitors is caused by various mechanisms that can occur in combination especially in advanced stages of disease (von Bubnoff et al. 2005; Lahaye et al. 2005; Nicolini et al. 2007). Patient-related causes for primary as well as secondary resistance are mainly noncompliance to the treatment regime (Darkow et al. 2007). However, inadequate serum levels can arise despite proper compliance from individual differences in the activity of imatinib-metabolizing enzymes such as CYP3A4. In addition, these enzymes can be induced by co-medication and nutritional habits (Floyd et al. 2003).

At the cellular level, the ability of the malignant clone to transport drug out of the cell or to hinder drug influx can result in drug resistance. For example, the proteins ABCB1 and MDR-1 are considered responsible for the increased efflux of imatinib from CML cells (Kuwazuru et al. 1990; Mahon et al. 2003; Thomas et al. 2004).

Just as the BCR-ABL fusion protein represents the causative event for CML, it is also the main reason for the development of resistance (Shah and Sawyers 2003). Mutations of this fusion gene result in changes in critical amino acids, such that inhibitors become ineffective (Branford et al. 2003; Soverini et al. 2006). More than 90 different mutations of BCR-ABL in CML have been described in recent years (Soverini et al. 2011). However, the majority of observed mutations are limited to a small number of specific changes (one study found 14 mutations in 95 % of cases (Zhou et al. 2011) another 20 mutations in 88 % of cases (Branford et al. 2009)). Hence, these common mutations are clinically most relevant and have directed the development of second- and third-line inhibitors.

2 Second-Generation Inhibitors

After the approval of imatinib in 2002, second-generation BCR-ABL kinase inhibitors were developed. The need for these novel inhibitors became evident both from patients presenting with primary imatinib intolerance, or developing intolerance during treatment, and from the growing number of mutations in BCR-ABL, which confer imatinib resistance.

Based on the positive results of phase 2 trials, the second-generation inhibitors dasatinib and nilotinib were approved as second-line therapy in imatinib-resistant or imatinib-intolerant CML and Ph^+ ALL (Kantarjian et al. 2007; Talpaz et al. 2006). In March 2013, bosutinib was also approved for second-line treatment. Recently, phase 3 trials (DAISION for dasatinib; ENESTnd for nilotinib) reported earlier and deeper remissions compared to imatinib in newly diagnosed, chronic-phase CML patients, as well as lower rates of progression to accelerated phase or blast crisis along with good tolerability of the drugs (Kantarjian et al. 2010, 2011; Saglio et al. 2010). These trials consequently led to the approval of both second-generation inhibitors, dasatinib and nilotinib, for the first-line treatment of CML. Although all second-generation inhibitors proved to be effective against a variety of known mutations, each of these inhibitors still faces a distinct spectrum of mutations, whose resistances they cannot overcome (Zhou et al. 2011; Branford et al. 2009) (Table 1).

Most notably, despite their differences, all first- and second-generation inhibitors are ineffective against the BCR-ABL T315I mutation. The exchange of threonine at position 315 for the more bulky isoleucine leads to a steric hindrance, inhibiting binding of all these inhibitors. Unable to bind the kinase, most Abl inhibitors lose their ability to block the BCR-ABL function. Twenty percent of patients who are imatinib resistant because of a BCR-ABL mutation bear the T315I "gatekeeper" mutation (O'Hare et al. 2007).

3 Ponatinib: A New Third-Generation Inhibitor

The small molecule ponatinib was developed specifically to overcome resistance based on the T315I mutation. The integration of a linear carbon–carbon triple bond into the structure of the molecule to link two functional groups avoids the blocking effect of the isoleucine in the context of the T315I mutation (Fig. 1). Furthermore, sites for interaction between the inhibitor and the kinase were optimized and are distributed over a wide range of protein residues. This increases the affinity and thereby reduces the required serum drug level. In addition, increased binding affinity ensures effectiveness of the inhibitor, even in those cases where one of the drug-binding site is lost, due to a mutation (Zhou et al. 2011).

Initial preclinical studies of ponatinib—formerly referred to as AP24534—revealed the activity of the drug as a pan-BCR-ABL inhibitor in biochemical assays, in cell lines as well as in mouse models. In contrast to the previously

Table 1 Resistance of BCR-ABL-mutations against first-, second- and third-generation inhibitors

	imatinib	dasatinib	nilotinib	bosutinib	ponatinib
WT	1,0	1,0	1,0	1,0	1,0
M244V	0,9	2,0	1,2	0,9	3,2
L248R	14,6	12,5	30,2	22,9	6,2
L248V	3,5	5,1	2,8	3,5	3,4
G250E	6,9	4,4	4,6	4,3	6,0
Q252H	1,4	3,1	2,6	0,8	6,1
Y253F	3,6	1,6	3,2	1,0	3,7
Y253H	8,7	2,6	36,8	0,6	2,6
E255K	6,0	5,6	6,7	9,5	8,4
E255V	17,0	3,4	10,3	5,5	12,9
D276G	2,2	1,4	2,0	0,6	2,1
E279K	3,6	1,6	2,0	1,0	3,0
E292L	0,7	1,3	1,8	1,1	2,0
V299L	1,5	8,7	1,3	26,1	0,6
T315A	1,7	58,9	2,7	6,0	0,4
T315I	17,5	75,0	39,4	45,4	3,0
T315V	12,2	738,8	57,0	29,3	2,1
F317L	2,6	4,5	2,2	2,4	0,7
F317R	2,3	114,0	2,3	33,5	4,9
F317V	0,4	21,3	0,5	11,5	2,3
M343T	1,2	0,9	0,8	1,1	0,9
M351T	1,8	0,9	0,4	0,7	1,2
F359I	6,0	3,0	16,3	2,9	2,9
F359V	2,9	1,5	5,2	0,9	4,4
L384M	1,3	2,2	2,3	0,5	2,2
H396P	2,4	1,1	2,4	0,4	1,4
H396R	3,9	1,6	3,1	0,8	5,9
F486S	8,1	3,0	1,9	2,3	2,1
L248R & F359I	1,2	13,7	96,2	39,3	17,7
Generation:	1st gen	2nd gen			3th gen.

Relative activity ($IC50^{MUT}/IC50^{WT}$) of imatinib, dasatinib, nilotinib, bosutinib and ponatinib in the context of the respective mutation relative to the effectiveness against BCR-ABL^{WT}. Color code: *green* <2/sensitive; *yellow* 2, 1–4/moderately resistant; *orange* 4, 1–10/resistant; *red* >10/ highly resistant. Note that ponatinib is the only inhibitor displaying activity against the common "gatekeeper" T315I mutation. Modified from Redaelli et al. (Redaelli et al. 2012)

approved first- and second-generation inhibitors, the activity profile of the new inhibitor included the T315I mutation. In addition, so-called "compound mutants", defined by the co-occurrence of several concurrent mutations within the

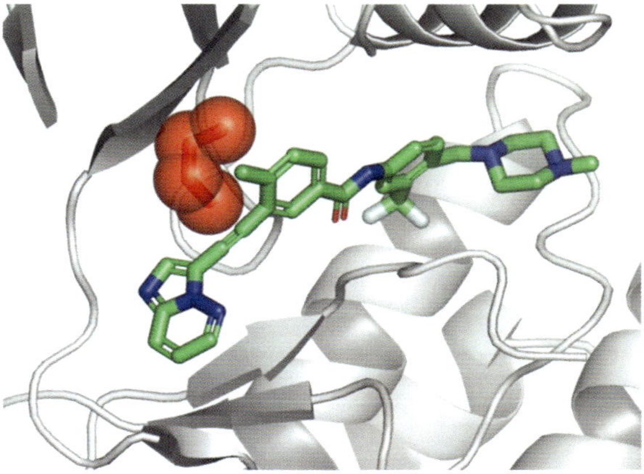

Fig. 1 Illustration of ponatinib in complex with the BCR-ABL protein. The *red spheres* represent the bulky side *chain* introduced by the T315I mutation. With kind permission of ARIAD Pharmaceuticals, Inc.

BCR-ABL fusion protein, were inhibited at a higher concentration by ponatinib (O'Hare et al. 2009).

In 2012, the first phase 1 trial for ponatinib in previously therapy-refractory patients was published (Cortes et al. 2012a). This study included 60 CML and 5 Ph^+ ALL patients. The CML cases included 43 patients in chronic phase (CP), 9 in accelerated phase (AP) and 8 in blast phase (BP) and represented a highly pretreated collective (59/60 $\geq$ 2 TKIs; 41/60 $\geq$ 3 TKIs). Ponatinib was given once daily at doses ranging from 2 to 60 mg. Among the CP-CML patients, 98 % achieved a complete hematologic remission (CHR), 72 % achieved a major cytogenetic response (MCyR) and 44 % achieved a major molecular response (MMR). Given the refractory nature of CML in these patients and the high degree of pretreatment, these numbers were quite remarkable.

It should be highlighted that 12 of the 43 CP patients (28 %) carried the T315I mutation and therefore were refractory to first- or second-generation inhibitors. Under ponatinib therapy, 100 % of these T315I patients achieved a major hematologic response (MHR), 92 % achieved a MCyR and 67 % achieved a MMR.

Of the 13 refractory CML cases, which lacked any BCR-ABL mutation, rates for CHR, MCyR and MMR of 100, 62 and 15 %, respectively, were observed.

Patients with advanced CML (AP, BP) were analyzed together with the Ph^+ ALL cohort in this study and responded to ponatinib as well. A MHR was achieved in 36 %, MCyR in 32 % and MMR in 9 % of patients. Thus, the novel third-generation inhibitor showed a clinically significant effect even in advanced-phase CML.

In order to further investigate the primary response rates to ponatinib (45 mg once daily) and its safety, a phase 2 trial (PACE trial) was launched (Cortes J, et al. 2012b). Patients in all phases of CML (CP, AP and BP) and Ph^+ ALL, resistant or intolerant to dasatinib or nilotinib or with a known T315I mutation, were enrolled. To date, the recruitment of 449 patients has been completed and the follow-up assessment is still ongoing. Interim results were presented in December 2012

(Cortes J, et al. 2012b). In CP-CML patients (n = 267), the primary endpoint (MCyR at 12 months) was achieved in 56 % of cases. In particular, patients carrying a T315I mutation responded better than those who were included because of resistance or intolerance (70 % vs. 51 %). In the CP-CML cohort, progression-free survival (PFS) and overall survival (OS) after twelve months were 80 and 94 %, respectively. Furthermore, the study revealed that the response rates for MCyR, CCyR and MMR of those patients decreased depending on the number of previously applied TKIs.

The primary endpoint (MHR after 12 months) was achieved in 57 % of the AP CML and in 34 % of the group containing BP CML and Ph^+. Altogether, the interim results of the PACE trial confirm the efficacy of ponatinib in second-generation TKI-resistant or TKI-intolerant CML and PH^+ ALL patients at a dose of 45 mg daily. Importantly, the results confirm the efficacy of this new inhibitor against the "gatekeeper" T315I mutation.

Based on the two above-mentioned trials, ponatinib was approved for the second-line treatment of CML and Ph^+ ALL in December 2012 in the United States and in July 2013 in the European Union. The approval in the EU covers patients in all phases of CML

- Who are resistant to dasatinib or nilotinib.
- Who are intolerant to dasatinib or nilotinib and for whom subsequent treatment with imatinib is not clinically appropriate.
- Who carry the T315I mutation.

The same terms apply to the approval for the use in Ph^+ ALL except that nilotinib is not considered here.

A phase 3 trial (EPIC trial) opened in July 2012 strives to compare ponatinib (45 mg daily) with imatinib (400 mg daily) in first-line therapy of newly diagnosed CML in CP. This trial aims to enroll 528 patients, and the MMR at 12 months is defined as primary endpoint. Depending on the results of this study, ponatinib will potentially be approved for first-line therapy in CML.

The growing number of patients treated with ponatinib during clinical trials has now increased the overall experience in terms of safety and adverse effects. The interim results of the PACE trial reported the following non-hematologic adverse reactions in descending order of frequency: rash, stomach aches, headaches, dry skin, constipation, fatigue, fever, nausea, arthralgia, hypertension, increased lipase, pancreatitis and amylase increase. Hematologic adverse effects have been observed more frequently compared to other Abl kinase inhibitors (thrombocytopenia > neutropenia > anemia). Focusing on the serious adverse events of grades 3 and 4, the increase in lipase (11 % of CP-CML patients) and hematologic adverse effects (thrombocytopenia 34 %, neutropenia 16 %, anemia 8 %) have to be highlighted and should receive special attention (Cortes et al. 2012b).

In addition to the use of ponatinib in CML and Ph^+ ALL, other diseases could potentially benefit from the treatment with this new drug as well. Preclinical studies reported that ponatinib inhibits not only BCR-ABL but also RET, FLT3, KIT, SCR, as well as members of receptor kinase families VEGFR, FGFR and

PDGFR (O'Hare et al. 2009). Following these findings, in vitro as well as in vivo studies investigated the effect of ponatinib on AML as well as on breast cancer cells and carcinoma of the endometrium, bladder, stomach, colon, lung and medullary thyroid. In these neoplasms, ponatinib was shown to inhibit proliferation and additionally to induce apoptosis in FLT3-ITD-driven AML. The effect of ponatinib on diverse cancer cells gives rise to the hope that ponatinib could potentially be applied to kinase-dependent subgroups of other malignancies and that this novel TKI may prove therapeutic in additional cancer entities (Falco et al. 2013; Gozgit et al. 2011, 2012; Zirm et al. 2012).

In conclusion, ponatinib constitutes a powerful BCR-ABL inhibitor and has been approved for the treatment of CML patients resistant or intolerant to imatinib, dasatinib or nilotinib. It displays clinical activity both in wild-type and in BCR-ABL mutant CML, including activity against the T315I mutation. Ponatinib induces high rates of remission and simultaneously exhibits a good overall safety profile. Despite previous TKI failure, chronic-phase CML patients can achieve sustained remissions using the novel drug. For patients in advanced CML or Ph^+ ALL, ponatinib therapy can successfully bridge the time to allogeneic stem cell transplantation.

References

Branford S, Rudzki Z, Walsh S, Parkinson I, Grigg A, Szer J et al (2003) Detection of BCR-ABL mutations in patients with CML treated with imatinib is virtually always accompanied by clinical resistance, and mutations in the ATP phosphate-binding loop (P-loop) are associated with a poor prognosis. Blood 102(1):276–283

Branford S, Melo JV, Hughes TP (2009) Selecting optimal second-line tyrosine kinase inhibitor therapy for chronic myeloid leukemia patients after imatinib failure: does the BCR-ABL mutation status really matter? Blood 114(27):5426–5435

Cortes JE, Kantarjian H, Shah NP, Bixby D, Mauro MJ, Flinn I et al (2012a) Ponatinib in refractory Philadelphia chromosome-positive leukemias. N Engl J Med 367(22):2075–2088

Cortes J, Kim D-W, Pinilla-Ibarz J, le Coutre P, Chuah C, Nicolini F, et al (2012b) A pivotal phase 2 trial of ponatinib in patients with CML and Ph+ ALL resistant or intolerant to dasatinib or nilotinib, or with the T315I BCR-ABL mutation: 12 month follow up of the PACE trial. Blood 120 ([Abstract 163] presented at ASH meeting 2012 in Atlanta)

Darkow T, Henk HJ, Thomas SK, Feng W, Baladi J-F, Goldberg GA et al (2007) Treatment interruptions and non-adherence with imatinib and associated healthcare costs: a retrospective analysis among managed care patients with chronic myelogenous leukaemia. Pharmacoeconomics 25(6):481–496

de Lavallade H, Apperley JF, Khorashad JS, Milojkovic D, Reid AG, Bua M et al (2008) Imatinib for newly diagnosed patients with chronic myeloid leukemia: incidence of sustained responses in an intention-to-treat analysis. J Clin Oncol 26(20):3358–3363

Druker BJ, Talpaz M, Resta DJ, Peng B, Buchdunger E, Ford JM et al (2001) Efficacy and safety of a specific inhibitor of the BCR-ABL tyrosine kinase in chronic myeloid leukemia. N Engl J Med 344(14):1031–1037

Druker BJ, Guilhot F, O'Brien SG, Gathmann I, Kantarjian H, Gattermann N et al (2006) Five-year follow-up of patients receiving imatinib for chronic myeloid leukemia. N Engl J Med 355(23):2408–2417

Falco VD, Buonocore P, Muthu M, Torregrossa L, Basolo F, Billaud M, et al. (2013) Ponatinib (AP24534) is a novel potent inhibitor of oncogenic RET mutants associated with thyroid cancer. J Clin Endocrinol Metab (Internet). 2013 Mar 22 (cited 2013 Apr 29); Available from: http://jcem.endojournals.org/content/early/2013/03/21/jc.2012-2672

Floyd MD, Gervasini G, Masica AL, Mayo G, George AL Jr, Bhat K et al (2003) Genotype-phenotype associations for common CYP3A4 and CYP3A5 variants in the basal and induced metabolism of midazolam in European- and African–American men and women. Pharmacogenetics 13(10):595–606

Gozgit JM, Wong MJ, Wardwell S, Tyner JW, Loriaux MM, Mohemmad QK et al (2011) Potent activity of ponatinib (AP24534) in models of FLT3-driven acute myeloid leukemia and other hematologic malignancies. Mol Cancer Ther 10(6):1028–1035

Gozgit JM, Wong MJ, Moran L, Wardwell S, Mohemmad QK, Narasimhan NI et al (2012) Ponatinib (AP24534), a multitargeted Pan-FGFR inhibitor with activity in multiple FGFR-amplified or mutated cancer models. Mol Cancer Ther 11(3):690–699

Jain P, Kantarjian H, Cortes J (2013) Chronic myeloid leukemia: overview of new agents and comparative analysis. Curr Treat Options Oncol 14(2):127–143

Kantarjian HM, Giles F, Gattermann N, Bhalla K, Alimena G, Palandri F et al (2007) Nilotinib (formerly AMN107), a highly selective BCR-ABL tyrosine kinase inhibitor, is effective in patients with Philadelphia chromosome–positive chronic myelogenous leukemia in chronic phase following imatinib resistance and intolerance. Blood 110(10):3540–3546

Kantarjian H, Shah NP, Hochhaus A, Cortes J, Shah S, Ayala M et al (2010) Dasatinib versus imatinib in newly diagnosed chronic-phase chronic myeloid leukemia. N Engl J Med 362(24):2260–2270

Kantarjian HM, Hochhaus A, Saglio G, De Souza C, Flinn IW, Stenke L et al (2011) Nilotinib versus imatinib for the treatment of patients with newly diagnosed chronic phase, Philadelphia chromosome-positive, chronic myeloid leukaemia: 24-month minimum follow-up of the phase 3 randomised ENESTnd trial. Lancet Oncol. 12(9):841–851

Kuwazuru Y, Yoshimura A, Hanada S, Ichikawa M, Saito T, Uozumi K et al (1990) Expression of the multidrug transporter, P-glycoprotein, in chronic myelogenous leukaemia cells in blast crisis. Br J Haematol 74(1):24–29

Lahaye T, Riehm B, Berger U, Paschka P, Müller MC, Kreil S et al (2005) Response and resistance in 300 patients with BCR-ABL–positive leukemias treated with imatinib in a single center. Cancer 103(8):1659–1669

Mahon F-X, Belloc F, Lagarde V, Chollet C, Moreau-Gaudry F, Reiffers J et al (2003) MDR1 gene overexpression confers resistance to imatinib mesylate in leukemia cell line models. Blood 101(6):2368–2373

Nicolini FE, Chabane K, Tigaud I, Michallet M, Magaud J-P, Hayette S (2007) BCR-ABL mutant kinetics in CML patients treated with dasatinib. Leuk Res 31(6):865–868

O'Hare T, Eide CA, Deininger MWN (2007) Bcr-Abl kinase domain mutations, drug resistance, and the road to a cure for chronic myeloid leukemia. Blood 110(7):2242–2249

O'Hare T, Shakespeare WC, Zhu X, Eide CA, Rivera VM, Wang F et al (2009) AP24534, a pan-BCR-ABL inhibitor for chronic myeloid leukemia, potently inhibits the T315I mutant and overcomes mutation-based resistance. Cancer Cell 16(5):401–412

Redaelli S, Mologni L, Rostagno R, Piazza R, Magistroni V, Ceccon M et al (2012) Three novel patient-derived BCR-ABL mutants show different sensitivity to second and third generation tyrosine kinase inhibitors. Am J Hematol 87(11):E125–E128

Saglio G, Kim D-W, Issaragrisil S, le Coutre P, Etienne G, Lobo C et al (2010) Nilotinib versus Imatinib for newly diagnosed chronic myeloid leukemia. N Engl J Med 362(24):2251–2259

Shah NP, Sawyers CL (2003) Mechanisms of resistance to STI571 in Philadelphia chromosome-associated leukemias. Oncogene 22(47):7389–7395

Soverini S, Colarossi S, Gnani A, Rosti G, Castagnetti F, Poerio A et al (2006) Contribution of ABL kinase domain mutations to imatinib resistance in different subsets of Philadelphia-

positive patients: by the GIMEMA Working Party on Chronic Myeloid Leukemia. Clin Cancer Res Off J Am Assoc Cancer Res 12(24):7374–7379
Soverini S, Hochhaus A, Nicolini FE, Gruber F, Lange T, Saglio G et al (2011) BCR-ABL kinase domain mutation analysis in chronic myeloid leukemia patients treated with tyrosine kinase inhibitors: recommendations from an expert panel on behalf of European LeukemiaNet. Blood 118(5):1208–1215
Talpaz M, Shah NP, Kantarjian H, Donato N, Nicoll J, Paquette R et al (2006) Dasatinib in imatinib-resistant Philadelphia chromosome-positive leukemias. N Engl J Med 354(24): 2531–2541
Thomas J, Wang L, Clark RE, Pirmohamed M (2004) Active transport of imatinib into and out of cells: implications for drug resistance. Blood 104(12):3739–3745
von Bubnoff N, Veach DR, van der Kuip H, Aulitzky WE, Sänger J, Seipel P et al (2005) A cell-based screen for resistance of Bcr-Abl-positive leukemia identifies the mutation pattern for PD166326, an alternative Abl kinase inhibitor. Blood 105(4):1652–1659
Zhou T, Commodore L, Huang W-S, Wang Y, Thomas M, Keats J et al (2011) Structural mechanism of the Pan-BCR-ABL inhibitor ponatinib (AP24534): lessons for overcoming kinase inhibitor resistance. Chem Biol Drug Des 77(1):1–11
Zirm E, Spies-Weisshart B, Heidel F, Schnetzke U, Böhmer F-D, Hochhaus A et al (2012) Ponatinib may overcome resistance of FLT3-ITD harbouring additional point mutations, notably the previously refractory F691I mutation. Br J Haematol 157(4):483–492

Erlotinib

M. Steins, M. Thomas and M. Geißler

Abstract

The epidermal growth factor receptor (EGFR) has been implicated in a multiplicity of cancer-related signal transduction pathways such as cellular proliferation, adhesion, migration, neoangiogenesis and apoptosis inhibition, all of them are important features of cancerogenesis and tumour progression. Its tyrosine kinase activity plays a central role in mediating these processes and has been intensely studied to exploit it as a therapeutic target. Inhibitors of this pathway have been developed and assessed in trials with significant efficacy in clinical applications. The current review focuses in particular on the clinical data of EGFR tyrosine kinase inhibition in different tumour entities, preferably non-small cell lung cancer and pancreatic cancer with emphasis to the approved small molecule *erlotinib*. Its clinical applications, evidence-based efficacy and toxicity as well as predictive markers of response are discussed.

Review on Erlotinib

M. Steins (✉) · M. Thomas (✉)
Clinic for Thoracic Diseases, University of Heidelberg, Amalienstr. 5, 69126, Heidelberg, Germany
e-mail: martin.steins@med.uni-heidelberg.de

M. Thomas
e-mail: michael.thomas@med.uni-heidelberg.de

M. Geißler
Department of Oncology, Gastroenterology and Internal Medicine, Städtische Kliniken Esslingen, Hirschlandstr. 97, 73730, Esslingen, Germany
e-mail: m.geissler@klinikum-esslingen.de

U. M. Martens (ed.), *Small Molecules in Oncology*, Recent Results in Cancer Research 201, DOI: 10.1007/978-3-642-54490-3_6,

Contents

1 Introduction

The development of small molecule inhibitors such as erlotinib, gefitinib, sorafenib, sunitinib or lapatinib evoked a new era of antineoplastic agents in cancer therapy besides conventional cytotoxic drugs. The principle of this novel anti-cancer treatment is based on the inhibition of receptor tyrosine kinases, which are essential components of the intracellular signalling apparatus. Several cellular receptors on the cell surface regulate their signalling via extracellular binding of ligands with consecutive activation of intracellular tyrosine kinase domains and tyrosine phosphorylation. One of these receptors, the epidermal growth factor receptor (EGFR), has gained considerable interest as a possible useful therapeutic target of tumour cells. EGFR is frequently overexpressed in solid tumours and plays a pivotal role in signal transduction pathways involved in cell proliferation, migration, adhesion, angiogenesis induction and apoptosis inhibition. Its overexpression correlates in some tumour entities with disease progression and poorer prognosis (Brabender et al. 2001).

In clinical practice, the use of the EGFR tyrosine kinase inhibitors (EGFR-TKI) erlotinib (Fig. 1) and gefitinib have been approved so far for patients with non-small cell lung cancer (NSCLC) for selected indications. In addition, erlotinib combined with gemcitabine has also gained approval for systemic treatment in advanced, non-operable pancreatic carcinoma. The TKI benefit is mainly based on tumour control and overall survival (OS) rather than rapid tumour responses and complete remission rates. In contrast to cytotoxic agents, these responses have been achieved by a specific molecular mechanism disturbing enzyme-mediated signal pathways in cancerogenesis.

2 Mechanism of Action

EGFR, the primary therapeutic target for erlotinib, belongs to the human epidermal growth factor receptor (HER) family 1, also known as erbB. The structure of this 170 kDa membrane-spanning glycoprotein consists of an extracellular cysteine-rich ligand-binding region, a transmembrane part and the cytoplasmic tyrosine kinase domain, which is the binding site for kinase inhibitors like erlotinib. Extracellular

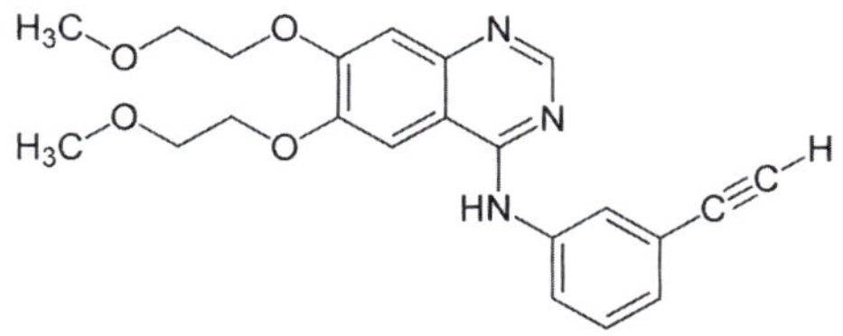

Fig. 1 Erlotinib. Chemical formula $C_{22}H_{23}N_3O_4$. Molecular mass 393.436 g/mol. Bioavailability 59 %, protein binding 95 %, half-life 36.2 h, excretion >90 % via faeces, 9 % via urine. Chemical structure

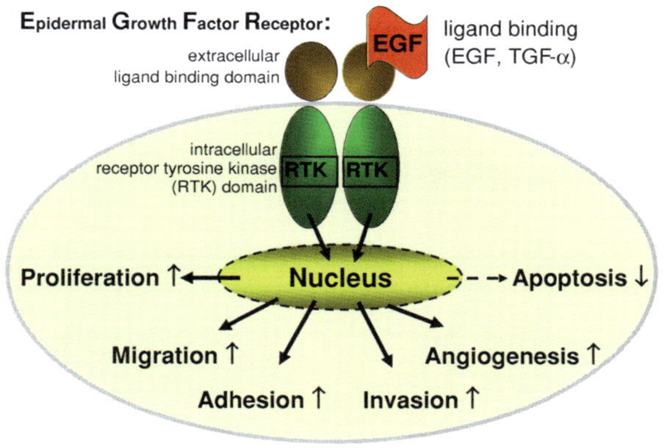

Fig. 2 Function of *epidermal growth factor receptor*: induction of signal transduction pathways by extracellular binding of ligands with consecutive activation of the receptor tyrosine kinase

binding of ligands such as the epidermal growth factor (EGF) and transforming growth factor-alpha (TGF-α) renders the receptor from inactive monomers to active homo- or heterodimers through confirmational changes with subsequent phosphorylation of tyrosine residues (Fig. 2). These phosphorylated tyrosine residues serve as binding sites for signal transducers with initiation of a cascade of signalling pathways, resulting in tumour growth and progression (Salomon et al. 1995; Alroy and Yarden 1997). In contrast, the small molecule TKIs inhibit the intracellular tyrosine kinase of EGFR by competitive and reversible docking at the ATP-binding site of the catalytic domain. Subsequently, the autophosphorylation of the receptor is prevented, which results in weakening of the downstream signalling pathways (Hynes and Lane 2005). Therefore, signals induced by extracellular ligand binding cannot be conveyed to the tumour cell nucleus where genes involved in cellular differentiation, proliferation and apoptosis are regulated. Consequences are on the one hand reduced potency for tumour cell migration and invasiveness, on the other hand induction of apoptosis (Fig. 3). This TKI mechanism differs from the active principle of anti-EGFR antibodies such as cetuximab or panitumumab, which function via a competitive binding to the extracellular domain. But it explains the striking efficacy of EGFR-TKIs in patients with somatic mutations of the EGFR kinase domain, as it targets a key protein in the tumorigenesis of these patients.

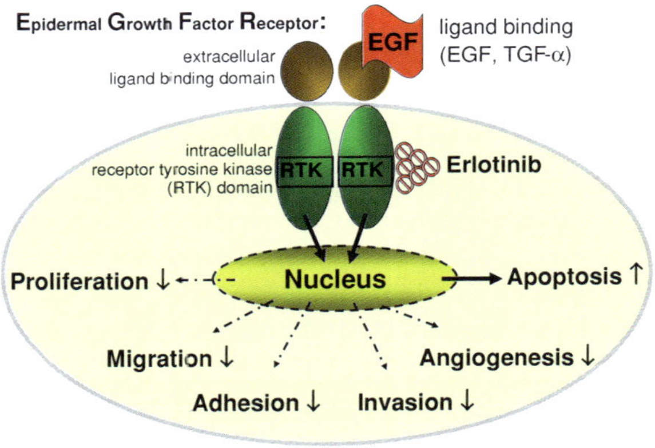

Fig. 3 Activity of *erlotinib*: binding to the intracellular tyrosine kinase domain of the epidermal growth factor receptor and blocking of its ATP-binding site. Subsequent disturbance of signal transduction to downstream cascades

3 Non-Small Cell Lung Cancer

Lung cancer does not only belong to the most frequent tumour entities in Western countries, it is also in cancer mortality statistics on the first range in men, and on the third (after breast and colorectal cancer) in women. This is the consequence of late detection due to delayed and unspecific symptoms in patients with locally advanced or metastasized disease at the time of first diagnosis. But also in earlier and locally limited tumour stages, the risks for relapse are quite high. Altogether, only 15 % of all lung cancer patients survive 5 years after diagnosis despite multimodal therapeutic concepts and new chemotherapeutic agents. Prognosis of the disease still remains serious. Therefore, the development of new agents with different efficacy mechanisms compared to conventional chemotherapy is necessary to expand the arsenal of systemic therapy. In the last years, these efforts have led to the emergence of the new group of TKIs with approvals of the EGFR inhibitors erlotinib and gefitinib in advanced NSCLC after failure of previously applicated chemotherapy. In unselected patients, these inhibitors have shown objective tumour responses in 8–19 % and prolongation of OS of 2 months (Fukuoka et al. 2003; Kris et al. 2003; Pérez-Soler et al. 2004; Shepherd et al. 2005). Especially, this last trial, the BR.21 study of Shepherd et al., has led to the approval of erlotinib in the USA and the European Community in the year 2004 and 2005, respectively, as a TKI for patients with advanced NSCLC who did not respond sufficiently to systemic chemotherapy or suffered a tumour relapse. Approval was based on the data of 731 patients in this randomised, placebo-controlled, multicenter phase III trial performed by the National Cancer Institute of Canada. Oral erlotinib was used as single agent in the 2nd or 3rd therapy line in patients with stage IIIb or IV according to UICC/AJCC. It demonstrated substantial advantage in terms of OS and significant release of disease-related symptoms such as dyspnoea, pain and cough (Bezjak et al. 2006). Whereas response rates in the erlotinib group comprise only 8.9 % with 0.4 month difference in progression-free survival (PFS), the OS—previously defined as the study's primary endpoint—was 2 months longer compared with the placebo group (6.7 vs. 4.7 months, hazard ratio (HR) 0.70, $p < 0.001$). According to the prolongation in median survival, 31 % of patients treated with erlotinib in this study were alive at 1 year versus 22 % in the placebo group. As independent clinical predictors for survival non-smoking status, female gender, adenocarcinoma histology and Asian ethnicity have been identified in the BR.21 trial (Tsao et al. 2005), which are often related to the presence of activating EGFR gene mutations. EGFR mutations of the tyrosine kinase domain have been found in 10 % up to 17 % of NSCLC patients, preferably with adenocarcinoma and non-smoking status (Marchetti et al. 2005; Pao and Miller 2005; Zhu et al. 2008).

These mutations, mainly within the exons 19 and 21 (exon 19 deletion, L858R mutation), are the most relevant biological factors associated with an improved response to erlotinib (Zhu et al. 2008). Various studies also with gefitinib have demonstrated that the presence of EGFR gene mutations within the kinase domain of the receptor correlates with TKI sensitivity (Lynch et al. 2004; Paez et al. 2004; Pao et al. 2004). In addition, analyses of EGFR copy numbers by fluorescence in situ hybridization (FISH) in the BR.21 study revealed high EGFR gene copy as a predictive marker of survival benefit from erlotinib.

On the other hand, erlotinib's efficacy for OS has also been described in patients not presenting the reported clinical characteristics, which are associated with the greatest degree of benefit such as non-smoking status, female gender or adenocarcinoma histology. Subset analyses of ever-smokers revealed significant survival advantages also for men and patients with squamous cell histology in the 2nd or 3rd therapy line despite very low response rates under erlotinib treatment (Clark et al. 2006). Additionally, prolonged PFS rates have been reported for erlotinib used as first-line maintenance therapy in patients who did not experience a tumour progression after conventional chemotherapy (Cappuzzo et al. 2010).

Gefitinib, another EGFR-TKI, was positively associated with clinical benefits, such as tumour response, health-related quality of life and increased survival, in two large randomised phase II studies (IRESSA Dose Evaluation in Advanced Lung Cancer IDEAL-1 and IDEAL-2) in pretreated NSCLC patients (Fukuoka et al. 2003; Natale 2004). However, it did not result in a statistically significant improvement in OS time in comparison with best supportive care in pretreated NSCLC patients of the ISEL (Iressa Survival Evaluation in Lung Cancer) trial, although in preplanned subgroup analyses a significant survival benefit was shown in never-smokers and Asian patients. Recently, the INTEREST trial (Iressa Non-small cell lung cancer Trial Evaluating REsponse and Survival against Taxotere) and the INVITE trial (open-label, parallel-group study compared gefitinib with vinorelbine in chemotherapy-naïve elderly patients) met the primary endpoint of demonstrating non-inferiority in terms of OS for gefitinib in comparison with docetaxel or vinorelbine (Kim et al. 2008; Crinó et al. 2008). Moreover, patients treated with gefitinib experienced a lower treatment-related toxicity and better improvement in quality of life. Nevertheless, a recently performed second-line trial comparing erlotinib and docetaxel showed significantly worse results in OS and PFS for the TKI applied in EGFR wild-type patients (Garassino et al. 2013).

On the other hand, small molecule EGFR-TKIs have class-specific adverse effects mainly including skin reactions such as xerosis, acneiform eruption and eczema or mucosa-associated toxicity like diarrhoea. Rash has been reported in up to 75 % of patients treated with these agents in phase II/III clinical trials. The rash that occurs with EGFR-targeted agents is generally mild to moderate; severe (grade 3/4) rash is rare (<10–15 % in NSCLC trials). In a number of clinical trials, a positive correlation between severity of rash (grade $\geq$ 2) and clinical outcome with EGFR-targeted therapy has been demonstrated (Dudek et al. 2006; Pérez-Soler 2006; Cedrés et al. 2009), suggesting rash as a surrogate marker for response. Other side effects have been reported rarely like liver dysfunction or interstitial lung disease (Sandler 2006).

For the first-line treatment of metastatic NSCLC, several phase II and III trials have been conducted utilising EGFR-TKIs in this setting. Patients with advanced NSCLC who are lifelong never-smokers, those with EGFR mutations and/or with bronchioloalveolar cell carcinoma histology seem to have promising efficacy with EGFR-TKI first-line therapy compared with unselected patients receiving the same agents. In fact, based on the data of the I-PASS (Iressa PanASia Study, Mok et al. 2009), the European Medicines Agency (EMA) has recommended the approval of gefitinib for mutation-positive NSCLC patients in all treatment lines including upfront therapy. This study performed in never or light former smokers yielded a statistically significant PFS for the gefitinib-treated patient group compared with carboplatin/paclitaxel in first-line therapy of EGFR-mutated NSCLC (HR 0.48, $p < 0.0001$). Similar therapeutic efficacy could be shown for erlotinib in EGFR mutation-positive Chinese (HR 0.16, $p < 0.0001$) and Caucasian (HR 0.37, $p < 0.0001$) patients (Zhou et al. 2011; Rosell et al. 2012). However, in contrast to PFS, no significant differences could be detected in OS when mutation-positive patients were treated with conventional chemotherapy at first and received TKI treatment as second-line therapy (Fukuoka et al. 2011). Nevertheless, quality of life and improvement of symptoms favoured TKI treatment compared with conventional chemotherapy procedures during first-line therapy (Thongprasert et al. 2011; Chen et al. 2013).

Generally, no improvement in survival could be demonstrated in phase III trials when EGFR-TKIs were directly combined with conventional platinum-based doublets, with the exception of subset analysis in non-smokers (Herbst et al. 2005; Gatzemeier et al. 2007).

The results have initiated further investigative activity to determine alterations in the EGFR-signalling pathway, but also to analyse clinical, immunohistologic, molecular and genetic issues to predict benefit from an EGFR tyrosine kinase inhibition. In general, the therapeutic aim should be to offer a personalised systemic therapy for NSCLC patients dependent on individual predictive parameters. Furthermore, in case of ineffectiveness against secondary mutations and acquired resistance, development of the 1st generation of TKIs with their reversible receptor binding should be continued including new agents with irreversible tyrosine kinase inhibition like afatinib. Combined EGFR targeting studies in this way revealed preliminary, but promising results encouraging ongoing trials (Janjigian et al. 2011).

4 Pancreatic Adenocarcinoma

Pancreatic cancer is the thirteenth most common cancer and the eighth leading cause of cancer death worldwide (Parkin et al. 2005). Only few patients with pancreatic cancer (15–20 %) present with resectable disease, where surgery offers a chance of cure. Following resection for operable pancreatic cancer, the median disease-free survival interval is 13.4 months for patients treated with adjuvant gemcitabine and 6.9 months for untreated patients. The longer median disease-free survival time associated with adjuvant gemcitabine has translated into a significant 5 year OS advantage (21 vs. 9 %) (Neuhaus et al. 2008). A much higher percentage of patients, however, present with metastatic disease (40–45 %) or unresectable locally advanced disease (40 %). These disease stages are characterised by median survival times of 3–6 months or 8–12 months, respectively. In locally advanced, unresectable disease, patients typically receive 5-fluorouracil (5-FU)-based chemoradiation or gemcitabine chemotherapy alone. The benefits of chemoradiation over chemotherapy alone in locally advanced disease have not been well established. Erlotinib has been evaluated in two phase I studies using a multimodal chemoradiation approach. One study examined erlotinib plus gemcitabine and paclitaxel plus radiation followed by maintenance with erlotinib and reported a partial response rate of 46 % and median survival time of 14 months (Iannitti et al. 2005). These results are supported by the other trial of erlotinib plus gemcitabine and radiation for patients with locally advanced, unresectable pancreatic cancer (Duffy et al. 2008). Single-agent gemcitabine is the standard first-line agent for the treatment of advanced inoperable pancreatic cancer with a marginally superior clinical benefit and survival compared with fluorouracil (FU) approximately 10 years ago (Burris et al. 1997). A number of randomised controlled trials performed over the last decade have aimed to demonstrate superiority of alternative cytotoxic agents and cytotoxic combinations over gemcitabine alone with mostly disappointing results. A recent meta-analysis, however, suggested a survival benefit with a reduction of 9 % in risk of death for gemcitabine-based combination chemotherapy (14 trials, 4,060 patients; HR = 0.91; 95 % CI, 0.85–0.97) (Sultana et al. 2007). In parallel, our understanding of the underlying genetic and molecular abnormalities that drive the development of pancreatic cancer has expanded significantly over the last decade (Schneider et al. 2008). Alterations to oncogenes and tumour suppressor genes, such as *KRas*, *TP53* and *p16INK4* are thought to play a critical role in the development of pancreatic cancer. In addition, expression of the human epidermal growth factor receptor (HER-1/EGFR) in pancreatic cancer cells is associated with the stimulation of tumour cell proliferation, poor disease outcomes and lower sensitivity to chemotherapy (Birk et al. 1999; Nicholson et al. 2001; Xiong and Abbruzzese 2002). These observations have allowed for the rational development of targeted therapies for this hard-to-treat disease. However, with the exception of erlotinib, the completed phase III trials have not confirmed an important clinical benefit (Van Cutsem et al. 2004; Moore et al. 2003; Bramhall et al. 2002; Moore et al. 2007; Kindler et al. 2010; Philip et al. 2007; Shapiro et al. 2005). Based on a phase III randomised, placebo-controlled trial (NCIC-CTG study), erlotinib in combination with gemcitabine received US Food and Drug Administration approval as treatment for chemotherapy-naïve locally advanced and metastatic pancreatic cancer in 2005 (Moore et al. 2007). The EMA subsequently licensed erlotinib in combination with gemcitabine restricted for the treatment of patients with metastatic pancreatic cancer only because there was no survival benefit in the locally advanced-stage (HR 0.94; 0.63–1.39). In total, 569 patients were randomly assigned in a 1:1 ratio to receive standard gemcitabine plus erlotinib (100 mg/day orally) or gemcitabine plus placebo in this double blind, international phase III trial. The primary endpoint of a longer OS time was achieved statistically with an HR of 0.82 (95 % CI, 0.69–0.99; $p = 0.038$) and a median survival duration of 6.24 versus 5.91 months. Secondary endpoint results from this trial showed a 1-year survival rate of 23 % in the erlotinib plus gemcitabine arm versus 17 % with gemcitabine monotherapy ($p = 0.023$). The PFS duration was also significantly longer with the combination regimen (3.75 vs. 3.55 months; HR, 0.77; $p = 0.004$). Objective response rates were not significantly different between the arms, although more patients on erlotinib had disease stabilization. The clinical significance of these efficacy results has been questioned by several investigators and treating physicians. A review of toxicities may further discourage the use of gemcitabine plus erlotinib. Patients receiving erlotinib and gemcitabine experienced higher frequencies of rash (72 %), diarrhoea (56 %), infection (43 %) and stomatitis (23 %), generally grade 1 or 2. Grade 3 or 4 toxicities were similar, except for diarrhoea and cutaneous rash, which were more frequent with the two-drug combination (6 % each). The six protocol-related deaths were all in the erlotinib–gemcitabine arm. Two were attributed to treatment complications (interstitial pneumonitis and sepsis), and four were attributed to a combination of cancer and protocol treatment complications (interstitial pneumonitis, sepsis, cerebrovascular accident and neutropenic sepsis). Interstitial lung disease was observed in seven patients receiving erlotinib plus gemcitabine and in one patient receiving placebo plus gemcitabine. In fact, there may be an interaction between gemcitabine and erlotinib contributing to increased pulmonary toxicity (Boeck et al. 2007).

An unplanned analysis of the NCIC-CTG study suggested the development of rash as a predictive marker for response to therapy with erlotinib. Patients with advanced pancreatic cancer who experienced grade 2 rash or higher ($n = 102$) had a reported median survival time of 10.5 months and a 1-year survival rate of 43 %. Rash development was linked to overall and PFS, and these correlations increased with grade (grade 1 vs. no rash: HR 0.47, $p < 0.001$; grade 2 or more vs. no rash: HR 0.29; $p < 0.001$). These data were supported by a combined analysis from two large phase III studies (National Cancer Institute of Canada Clinical Trials Group Studies BR.21 in non-small cell lung cancer and NCIC-CTG PA.3 in pancreatic cancer). Presence of rash strongly correlated with OS in both studies. Similar results were observed for PFS (Wacker et al. 2007). In addition, a retrospective exploratory analysis of the phase III AVITA study (gemcitabine + erlotinib + placebo vs. gemcitabine + erlotinib + bevacizumab) confirmed the results of the NCIC-CTG study (Van Cutsem et al. 2009). In the placebo arm, OS was only 4.3 months in patients without rash compared with 7.1 and 8.3 months in patients with grade 1 and grade > 1 rash, respectively ($p < 0.0001$). In the NCIC-CTG study, however, rash was also present in 18 % of placebo-taking patients with median survival 8.2 months (Moore et al. 2007). Placebo-taking patients who did not develop rash had a median survival of 4.7 months. In the combined treatment arm (gemcitabine plus erlotinib), 81 % of the patients developed a rash, compared with 30 % of patients in the control group. Since no reliable molecular predictive biomarker exists for the medical treatment of pancreatic cancer physicians and patients should view rash development as a positive event indicative of greater likelihood of clinical benefit. It is important to understand that the development of rash following erlotinib treatment is not an intrinsic effect of erlotinib itself but more likely correlated to individual differences in drug exposure, the integrity of the immune system or EGFR polymorphisms (Saif et al. 2008; Lynch et al. 2007). Further studies are required to identify patients most likely to develop rash and to determine if dose escalation to induce rash can improve efficacy.

How shall we use rash in daily practice? It has been suggested that the rash clinically improves with continuation of treatment. Nevertheless, severe rash development may be a determining cause of treatment discontinuation by patients on erlotinib outside clinical trials. If rash development is in fact a surrogate marker for treatment success, then patients discontinuing treatment are potentially stopping a life prolonging treatment. This is why it is crucial to exploit all means available in the treatment of the erlotinib-induced skin rash, in order to discourage patients from stopping it. Assessing the tumour response according to RECIST or WHO criteria remains the standard of care independent on the development of rash because there may exist responders without rash and, contrary, patients with a tumour progress despite the development of rash.

Since it is unclear if every patient with advanced pancreatic cancer has to be treated with a combination chemotherapy of gemcitabine and erlotinib, there may be a rationale for sequential therapeutic strategies. Several drugs have been examined as a second-line therapy (Kulke et al. 2007). The most promising chemotherapeutic regimen may be the OFF-protocol consisting of oxaliplatin, 5-FU and FA. In a randomised phase III study, this combination chemotherapy resulted in a significant survival advantage compared with 5-FU/FA alone (Pelzer et al. 2008). Another option in gemcitabine pre-treated patients would be the combination of erlotinib and capecitabine. In one single-arm phase II study with 32 patients, the median PFS time was 3.4 months, and the median OS time was 6.5 months (Kulke et al. 2007). One-year OS was 26 %. In contrast, disappointing results were reported in a retrospective analysis of 13 patients treated with single-agent erlotinib (Epelbaum et al. 2007). No responses and a median time to progression (TTP) of only 1 month were observed.

At the current time, gemcitabine, either alone or in combination with erlotinib, remains the only approved first-line treatment for advanced pancreatic carcinoma. Multiple trials are planned that will employ new and novel targeted and biological agents together with the search for predictive biomarkers.

5 Hepatocellular Carcinoma

Hepatocellular carcinoma (HCC) is the third largest cause of cancer-related death third to lung and colon cancers (Parkin et al. 2005). The incidence has increased in the Western world over the past 20 years primarily as a result of the prevalence of hepatitis C virus infection (El-Serag and Mason 1999). Management of HCC is complex and is guided by the Barcelona Liver Clinic (BCLC) staging system, which has important prognostic value (Llovet et al. 1999). The BCLC system is conceptually useful, because it helps to integrate liver function and tumour features into a classification that is meaningful from a standpoint of treatment options. For example, BCLC C patients are those best suited for systemic therapies or clinical trials. Systemic chemotherapy, however, has largely been disappointing in terms of palliation or cure. Cytotoxic chemotherapy has been shown to provide no survival benefit. With that background in mind, the multitargeted tyrosine kinase inhibitor sorafenib was studied in HCC. Patients with advanced-stage HCC who were not candidates for, or who had disease progression after locoregional therapy, were enrolled in the Sorafenib Hepatocellular Carcinoma Assessment Randomized Protocol (SHARP) trial (Llovet et al. 2008). The 1-year survival for the sorafenib group was 44 % and 33 % for the placebo group. The median survival for the sorafenib group was 10.7 months from enrollment compared with 7.9 months for those who received placebo. The survival benefit appeared to be correlated to a 2.7-month delay in radiologic progression (5.5 months for the sorafenib group vs. 2.8 months for the placebo group). A recent phase III study of sorafenib versus placebo in Asian patients reported a similar increase in survival (6.2 vs. 4.1 months) (Cheng et al. 2009). Sorafenib is now considered to be the standard medical treatment for patients with Child-Pugh stage A cirrhosis within the BCLC stage 3 group.

Epidermal growth factor receptor (EGFR) is frequently overexpressed in HCC (Buckley et al. 2008). In a phase II study, erlotinib was evaluated in 38 patients with unresectable or metastastic HCC (Philip et al. 2005). Most frequent grade 3–4 toxicities were skin rash (13 %), diarrhoea (8 %) and fatigue (8 %). There was a correlation between the severity (grade 3 or higher) of toxicity and Child-Pugh classification: only 22 % of the Child-Pugh A patients experienced severe toxicity compared with 70 % of Child-Pugh B patients ($p = 0.02$). Thirty-two per cent of the patients were progression-free after 24 weeks. The overall confirmed response rate was only 9 %. Seventeen patients (50 %) achieved stabilization of disease for a median of 3.8 months. There was no correlation between response and EGFR status. The median OS time was 13 months, with a probability of 33 % of patients alive at 18 months from entry into the study. In a second phase II study, 40 HCC patients were treated with erlotinib 150 mg daily for 16 weeks (Thomas et al. 2007). There were no complete or partial responses, however, 17 of 40 patients achieved stable disease at 16 weeks of continuous therapy. The PFS at 16 weeks was 43 %, and the median OS was 43 weeks (10.75 months). No patients required dose reductions in erlotinib. Again, no correlation between EGFR expression and outcome was found.

In contrast to lung cancer, the gain of function in EGFR signalling in HCC seems mediated through increase in ligand–receptor interaction, rather than by point mutations or amplifications (Llovet and Bruix 2008). Erlotinib treatment of HCC might inhibit the mitogen-activated protein (MAP)-kinase pathway and signal transducer of activation and transcription (STAT)-mediated signalling resulting in an altered expression of apoptosis and cell cycle-regulating genes (Huether et al. 2006). Overexpression of proapoptotic factors such as caspases and gadds associated with a downregulation of antiapoptotic factors such as Bcl-2, Bcl(XL) or jun-D might account for erlotinib's potency to induce apoptosis. In addition, downregulation of cell cycle regulators promoting the G_1/S-transition and overexpression of cyclin-dependent kinase inhibitors and gadds might contribute to the induction of a G_1/G_0-arrest of HCC cells in response to erlotinib. Together, erlotinib alone appears to have only modest activity against HCC, and further randomised studies are needed to evaluate the potential benefit of erlotinib in HCC patients.

There is scientific rationale for combining bevacizumab and erlotinib in HCC (Llovet and Bruix 2008). Overexpression of proangiogenic factors, such as vascular endothelial growth factor (VEGF), platelet-derived growth factor and angiopoietin-2, has been demonstrated in HCC (Llovet and Bruix 2008; Villanueva et al. 2007; Chiang et al. 2008). As mentioned above, there is also a rationale to abrogate EGFR signalling in HCC. Thomas et al. (2009) reported a single-arm phase II study with 40 HCC patients treated with the combination of bevacizumab (10 mg/kg every 14 days) and erlotinib (150 mg daily). Regarding efficacy, objective response rate was 25 %, and the median PFS and OS times were 9 and 15.6 months, respectively. The results are encouraging, but have to be interpreted with caution due to patient selection bias and the small sample size and short follow-up time.

Together, sorafenib is the standard of care in patients with advanced HCC as a result of robust data obtained in the setting of phase III investigations both in the West and Asia. The role of erlotinib and erlotinib combinations has to be explored in randomised phase II and III studies. In fact, a phase III study of erlotinib plus bevacizumab against sorafenib is under consideration within the North American GI Steering Committee Hepatobiliary Task Force.

6 Other Tumour Entities

Erlotinib has been examined in phase I and II studies in malignant glioma and colorectal, biliary, gastric, breast, ovarian, endometrial and renal cell cancer. Efficacy with respect to OS and response rates, however, was low. In contrast, single-agent erlotinib or erlotinib-based polychemotherapy may be promising in recurrent or metastatic squamous cell cancer of the head and neck. These studies are discussed in detail elsewhere (Tang et al. 2006).

References

Alroy I, Yarden Y (1997) The ErbB signaling network in embryogenesis and oncogenesis: signal diversification through combinatorial ligand-receptor interactions. FEBS Lett 410:83–86
Bezjak A, Tu D, Seymour L et al (2006) Symptom improvement in lung cancer patients treated with erlotinib: quality of life analysis of the National Cancer Institute of Canada Clinical Trials Group Study Br. 21. J Clin Oncol 24:3831–3837
Birk D, Gansauge F, Gansauge S (1999) Serum and correspondent tissue measurements of epidermal growth factor (EGF) and epidermal growth factor receptor (EGF-R). Clinical relevance in pancreatic cancer and chronic pancreatitis. Int J Pancreatol 25:89–96
Boeck S, Hausmann A, Reibke R et al (2007) Severe lung and skin toxicity during treatment with gemcitabine and erlotinib for metastatic pancreatic cancer. Anticancer Drugs 18:1109–1111
Brabender J, Danenberg KD, Metzger R et al (2001) Epidermal growth factor receptor and HER2-neu mRNA expression in non-small cell lung cancer is correlated with survival. Clin Cancer Res 7:1850–1855
Bramhall SR, Schulz J, Nemunaitis J (2002) A double-blind placebo-controlled, randomised study comparing gemcitabine and marimastat with gemcitabine and placebo as first line therapy in patients with advanced pancreatic cancer. Br J Cancer 87:161–167
Buckley AF, Burgart LJ, Sahai V et al (2008) Epidermal growth factor receptor expression and gene copy number in conventional hepatocellular carcinoma. Am J Clin Pathol 129:245–251
Burris HA 3rd, Moore MJ, Andersen J (1997) Improvements in survival and clinical benefit with gemcitabine as first-line therapy for patients with advanced pancreas cancer: a randomized trial. J Clin Oncol 15:2403–2413
Cappuzzo F, Cileanu T, Stelmakh L et al (2010) Erlotinib as maintenance treatment in advanced non-small cell lung cancer: a multicentre, randomised and placebo-controlled phase 3 study. Lancet Oncol 11:521–529
Cedrés S, Prat A, Martínez P et al (2009) Clinical surrogate markers of survival in advanced non-small cell lung cancer (NSCLC) patients treated with second-third line erlotinib. Lung Cancer 66:257–261
Chen G, Fen J, Zhou C et al (2013) Quality of life (QoL) analyses from OPTIMAL (CTONG-0802), a phase III, randomised, open-label study of first-line erlotinib versus chemotherapy in patients with advanced EGFR-mutation positive non-small cell lung cancer (NSCLC). Ann Oncol 24:1615–1622
Cheng AL, Kang YK, Chen Z et al (2009) Efficacy and safety of sorafenib in patients in the Asia-Pacific region with advanced hepatocellular carcinoma: a phase III randomised, double-blind, placebo-controlled trial. Lancet Oncol 10:25–34
Chiang D, Villanueva A, Peix J (2008) Focal VEGFA amplifications and molecular classification of hepatocellular carcinoma. Cancer Res 68:6779–6788
Clark GM, Zborowski DM, Santabarbara P et al (2006) Smoking history and epidermal growth factor receptor expression as predictors of survival benefit from erlotinib for patients with

non-small-cell lung cancer in the National Cancer Institute of Canada Clinical Trials Group study BR.21. Clin Lung Cancer 7:389–394

Crinó L, Cappuzzo F, Zatloukal P et al (2008) Gefitinib versus vinorelbine in chemotherapy-naive elderly patients with advanced non-small-cell lung cancer (INVITE): a randomized, phase II study. J Clin Oncol 26:4253–4260

Dudek AZ, Kmak KL, Koopmeiners J, Keshtgarpour M (2006) Skin rash and bronchoalveolar histology correlates with clinical benefit in patients treated with gefitinib as a therapy for previously treated advanced or metastatic non-small cell lung cancer. Lung Cancer 51:89–96

Duffy A, Kortmansky J, Schwartz GK et al (2008) A phase I study of erlotinib in combination with gemcitabine and radiation in locally advanced, non-operable pancreatic adenocarcinoma. Ann Oncol 19:86–91

El-Serag HB, Mason AC (1999) Rising incidence of hepatocellular carcinoma in the United States. N Engl J Med 340:745–750

Epelbaum R, Schnaider J, Gluzman A (2007) Erlotinib as a single-agent therapy in patients with advanced pancreatic cancer. ASCO Gastrointestinal Cancer Symposium, Orlando, FL, 19–21 Jan 2007

Fukuoka M, Wu YL, Thongprasert S et al (2011) Biomarker analyses and final overall survival results from a phase III randomized, open-label, first-line study of gefitinib versus carboplatin/paclitaxel in clinically selected patients with advanced non-small cell lung cancer in Asia (IPASS). J Clin Oncol 29:2866–2874

Fukuoka M, Yano S, Giaccone G et al (2003) Multi-institutional randomized phase II trial of gefitinib for previously treated patients with advanced non-small-cell lung cancer. J Clin Oncol 21:2237–2246

Garassino MC, Martelli O, Broggini M et al (2013) Erlotinib versus docetaxel as second-line treatment of patients with advanced non-small cell lung cancer and wild-type EGFR tumours (TAILOR): a randomised controlled trial. Lancet Oncol 14:981–988

Gatzemeier U, Pluzanska A, Szczesna A et al (2007) Phase III study of erlotinib in combination with cisplatin and gemcitabine in advanced non-small-cell lung cancer: the Tarceva lung cancer investigation trial. J Clin Oncol 25:1545–1552

Herbst RS, Prager D, Hermann R et al (2005) TRIBUTE: a phase III trial of erlotinib hydrochloride (OSI-774) combined with carboplatin and paclitaxel chemotherapy in advanced non-small-cell lung cancer. J Clin Oncol 23:5892–5899

Huether A, Hopfner M, Sutter AP et al (2006) Signaling pathways involved in the inhibition of epidermal growth factor receptor by erlotinib in hepatocellular cancer. World J Gastroenterol 12:5160–5167

Hynes NE, Lane HA (2005) ERBB receptors and cancer: the complexity of targeted inhibitors. Nat Rev Cancer 5:341–354

Iannitti D, Dipetrillo T, Akerman P (2005) Erlotinib and chemoradiation followed by maintenance erlotinib for locally advanced pancreatic cancer: a phase I study. Am J Clin Oncol 28:570–575

Janjigian YY, Groen HJ, Horn L et al (2011) Activity and tolerability of afatinib (BIBW 2992) and cetuximab in NSCLC patients with acquired resistance to erlotinib or gefitinib. J Clin Oncol 29(suppl) (abstr 7525)

Kim ES, Hirsh V, Mok T et al (2008) Gefitinib versus docetaxel in previously treated non-small cell lung cancer (INTEREST): a randomised phase III trial. Lancet 372:1809–1818

Kindler H, Niedzwiecki D, Hollis D et al (2010) Gemcitabine plus bevacizumab compared with gemcitabine plus placebo in patients with advanced pancreatic cancer: phase III trial of the cancer and Leukemia group B (CALGB 80303). J Clin Oncol 28:3617–3622

Kris MG, Natale RB, Herbst RS et al (2003) Efficacy of gefitinib, an inhibitor of the epidermal growth factor receptor tyrosine kinase, in symptomatic patients with non-small cell lung cancer: a randomized trial. JAMA 290:2149–2158

Kulke MH, Blaszkowsky LS, Ryan DP et al (2007) Capecitabine plus erlotinib in gemcitabine-refractory advanced pancreatic cancer. J Clin Oncol 25:4787–4792

Llovet JM, Brú C, Bruix J (1999) Prognosis of hepatocellular carcinoma: the BCLC staging classification. Semin Liver Dis 19:329–338
Llovet JM, Bruix J (2008) Molecular targeted therapies in hepatocellular carcinoma. Hepatology 48:1312–1327
Llovet JM, Ricci S, Mazzaferro V et al, SHARP Investigators Study Group (2008) Sorafenib in advanced hepatocellular carcinoma. N Engl J Med 359:378–390
Lynch TJ, Bell DW, Sordella R et al (2004) Activating mutations in the epidermal growth factor receptor underlying responsiveness of non-small-cell lung cancer to gefitinib. N Engl J Med 350:2129–2139
Lynch TJ Jr, Kim ES, Eaby B (2007) Epidermal growth factor receptor inhibitor-associated cutaneous toxicities: an evolving paradigm in clinical management. Oncologist 12:610–621
Marchetti A, Martella C, Felicioni L et al (2005) EGFR mutations in non–small-cell lung cancer: analysis of a large series of cases and development of a rapid and sensitive method for diagnostic screening with potential implications on pharmacologic treatment. J Clin Oncol 23:857–865
Mok T, Wu YL, Thongprasert S et al (2009) Gefitinib or carboplatin-paclitaxel in pulmonary adenocarcinoma. N Engl J Med 361:947–957
Moore MJ, Goldstein D, Hamm J (2007) Erlotinib plus gemcitabine compared with gemcitabine alone in patients with advanced pancreatic cancer: a phase III trial of the National Cancer Institute of Canada Clinical Trials Group. J Clin Oncol 25:1960–1966
Moore MJ, Hamm J, Dancey J (2003) Comparison of gemcitabine versus the matrix metalloproteinase inhibitor BAY12–9566 in patients with advanced or metastatic adenocarcinoma of the pancreas: a phase III trial of the National Cancer Institute of Canada Clinical Trials Group. J Clin Oncol 21:3296–3302
Natale RB (2004) Effects of ZD1839 (Iressa, gefitinib) treatment on symptoms and quality of life in patients with advanced non-small cell lung cancer. Sem Oncol 31(3 Suppl 9):23–30
Neuhaus P, Riess H, Post S et al (2008) CONKO-001: final results of the randomized, prospective, multicenter phase III trial of adjuvant chemotherapy with gemcitabine versus observation in patients with resected pancreatic cancer (PC). J Clin Oncol 26 (abstr LBA4504)
Nicholson RI, Gee JM, Harper ME (2001) EGFR and cancer prognosis. Eur J Cancer 37(suppl 4):S9–S15
Paez JG, Janne PA, Lee JC et al (2004) EGFR mutations in lung cancer: correlation with clinical response to gefitinib therapy. Science 304:1497–1500
Parkin DM, Bray F, Ferlay J (2005) Global cancer statistics, 2002. CA Cancer J Clin 55:74–108
Pao W, Miller V, Zakowski M et al (2004) EGF receptor gene mutations are common in lung cancers from "never smokers" and are associated with sensitivity of tumors to gefitinib and erlotinib. Proc Natl Acad Sci USA 101:13306–13311
Pao W, Miller VA (2005) Epidermal growth factor receptor mutations, small-molecule kinase inhibitors, and non-small cell lung cancer: current knowledge and future directions. J Clin Oncol 23:2556–2568
Pelzer U, Kubica K, Stieler J et al (2008) A randomized trial in patients with gemcitabine refractory pancreatic cancer. Final results of the CONKO 003 study. J Clin Oncol 26(suppl) (abstr 4508)
Pérez-Soler R, Chachoua A, Hammond LA et al (2004) Determants of tumour response and survival with erlotinib in patients with non-small-cell lung cancer: a randomized trial. J Clin Oncol 22:3238–3247
Pérez-Soler R (2006) Rash as a surrogate marker for efficacy of epidermal growth factor inhibitors in lung cancer. Clin Lung Cancer 8(Suppl 1):S7–14
Philip PA, Benedetti J, Fenoglio-Preiser C (2007) Phase III study of gemcitabine (G) plus cetuximab (C) versus gemcitabine in patients (Pts) with locally advanced or metastatic pancreatic adenocarcinoma (PC) SWOG S0205 study. J Clin Oncol 25(18 suppl) (LBA4509)
Philip PA, Mahoney MR, Allmer C (2005) Phase II study of erlotinib (OSI-774) in patients with advanced hepatocellular cancer. J Clin Oncol 23:6657–6663

Rosell R, Carcereny E, Gervais R et al (2012) Erlotinib versus standard chemotherapy as first-line treatment for European patients with advanced EGFR mutation-positive non-small cell lung cancer (EURTAC): a multicentre, open-label, randomised phase 3 trial. Lancet Oncol 13:239–246

Schneider G, Hamacher R, Eser S et al (2008) Molecular biology of pancreatic cancer—new aspects and targets. Anticancer Res 28(3A):1541–1550

Saif MW, Merikas I, Tsimboukis S et al (2008) Erlotinib-induced skin rash. Pathogenesis, clinical significance and management in pancreatic cancer patients. JOP 9:267–274

Salomon DS, Brandt R, Ciardiello F et al (1995) Epidermal growth factor-related peptides and their receptors in human malignancies. Crit Rev Oncol Hematol 19:183–232

Sandler AB (2006) Nondermatologic adverse events associated with anti-EGFR therapy. Oncology 20(5 Suppl 2):35–40

Shapiro J, Marshall J, Karasek P (2005) G17DT + gemcitabine (Gem) versus placebo + Gem in untreated subjects with locally advanced, recurrent, or metastatic adenocarcinoma of the pancreas: results of a randomized, double-blind, multinational, multicenter study. J Clin Oncol 23(16 suppl):4012

Shepherd FA, Pereira JR, Ciuleanu T et al, National Cancer Institute of Canada Clinical Trails Group (2005) Erlotinib in previously treated non-small-cell lung cancer. N Engl J Med 353:123–132

Sultana A, Smith CT, Cunningham D et al (2007) Meta-analyses of chemotherapy for locally advanced and metastatic pancreatic cancer. J Clin Oncol 20:2607–2615

Tang PA, Tsao MS, Moore MJ (2006) A review of erlotinib and its clinical use. Expert Opin Pharmacother 7:177–193

Thomas MB, Chadha R, Glover K (2007) Phase 2 study of erlotinib in patients with unresectable hepatocellular carcinoma. Cancer 110:1059–1067

Thomas MB, Morris JS, Chadha R et al (2009) Phase II trial of the combination of bevacizumab and erlotinib in patients who have advanced hepatocellular carcinoma. J Clin Oncol 27:843–850

Thongprasert S, Duffield E, Saijo N et al (2011) Health-related quality-of-life in a randomized first-line study of gefitinib versus carboplatin/paclitaxel in clinically selected patients from Asia with advanced NSCLC (IPASS). J Thorac Oncol 6:1872–1880

Tsao M-S, Sakurada A, Cutz J-C et al (2005) Erlotinib in lung cancer—molecular and clinical predictors of outcome. N Engl J Med 353:133–144

Van Cutsem E, Van de Velde H, Karasek P (2004) Phase III trial of gemcitabine plus tipifarnib compared with gemcitabine plus placebo in advanced pancreatic cancer. J Clin Oncol 22:1430–1438

Van Cutsem E, Vervenne WL, Bennouna J et al (2009) Rash as a marker for the efficacy of gemcitabine plus erlotinib-based therapy in pancreatic cancer: results from the AViTA study. ASCO gastrointestinal cancers symposium, p A117

Villanueva A, Newell P, Chiang D (2007) Genomics and signaling pathways in hepatocellular carcinoma. Semin Liver Dis 27:55–76

Wacker B, Nagrani T, Weinberg J et al (2007) Correlation between development of rash and efficacy in patients treated with the epidermal growth factor receptor tyrosine kinase inhibitor erlotinib in two large phase III studies. Clin Cancer Res 13:3913–3921

Xiong HQ, Abbruzzese JL (2002) Epidermal growth factor receptor-targeted therapy for pancreatic cancer. Semin Oncol 29(suppl 14):31–37

Zhou C, Wu YL, Chen G et al (2011) Erlotinib versus chemotherapy as first-line treatment for patients with advanced EGFR mutation-positive non-small cell lung cancer (OPTIMAL, CTONG-0802): a multicentre, open-label, randomizsed phase 3 trial. Lancet Oncol 12:735–742

Zhu C-Q, da Cunha Santos G, Ding K et al (2008) Role of KRAS and EGFR as biomarkers of response to erlotinib in National Cancer Institute of Canada Clinical Trials Group Study Br. 21. J Clin Oncol 26:4268–4275

Lapatinib

Minna Nolting, Tanja Schneider-Merck and Martin Trepel

Abstract

The human epidermal growth factor receptor (HER) family of receptor tyrosine kinases plays an important role in the biology of many cancers. In breast and gastric cancer, and maybe also additional tumor types, HER2 and its homo- or heterodimerization with HER1 or HER3 are essential for cancer cell growth and survival. Breast cancer patients overexpressing HER2 have a poor prognosis, which can be substantially improved upon HER2-targeted therapy using the monoclonal antibody trastuzumab. Lapatinib is a dual tyrosine kinase inhibitor (TKI), blocking HER1 and HER2 tyrosine kinase activity by binding to the ATP-binding site of the receptor's intracellular domain. This results in the inhibition of tumor cell growth. In patients, the drug is relatively well tolerated with mostly low-grade adverse effects. In particular and unlike to trastuzumab, it has very little, if any, adverse effects on cardiac function. In 2007, lapatinib has been approved in combination with capecitabine in patients with advanced HER2-positive breast cancer upon progressive disease following standard therapy with anthracyclines, taxanes, and trastuzumab. In 2010, the approval was extended to the treatment of postmenopausal women with advanced, hormone receptor- and HER2-positive breast cancer, for whom hormonal therapy is indicated. Ongoing and future studies will explore its role in the (neo)adjuvant therapy setting, in further drug combinations as well as in the treatment of HER2-positive tumors other than breast cancer.

M. Nolting · T. Schneider-Merck · M. Trepel (✉)
Department of Oncology and Hematology, Hubertus Wald Cancer Center, University Medical Center Hamburg-Eppendorf, Martinistr. 52, 20246 Hamburg, Germany
e-mail: m.trepel@uke.de

U. M. Martens (ed.), *Small Molecules in Oncology*, Recent Results in Cancer Research 201, DOI: 10.1007/978-3-642-54490-3_7,

Contents

1 Introduction

1.1 The Epidermal Growth Factor Receptor Family of Tyrosine Kinases

The human epidermal growth factor receptor family (HER, EGFR, ErbB) is comprised of four receptor tyrosine kinases (RTKs): HER1 (=EGFR1 or ErbB1), HER2 (=HER2/c-neu or ErbB2), HER3 (=ErbB3), and HER4 (=ErbB4) (Yarden and Sliwkowski 2001; Citri and Yarden 2006). RTKs consist of an extracellular ligand-binding domain with specific docking sites for various adapter proteins and ligands, a transmembrane domain and an intracellular cytoplasmic domain containing the tyrosine kinase catalytic site. Upon ligand binding, various downstream signaling pathways, which are linked to cell proliferation, survival, and apoptosis, are activated (Stern 2000; Danielsen and Maihle 2002). The receptors are not fixed in the lipid bilayer of the plasma membrane. Therefore, dimerization can and does occur upon ligand binding to the extracellular domain. Such dimers can be homodimers or heterodimers comprised of two different members of the same RTK family (Fig. 1) (Mendelsohn and Baselga 2003). The type of dimerization (homo- or heterodimerization) has an important impact on the downstream signaling pathways in terms of growth, proliferation, and transformation (Olayioye et al. 2000; Prenzel et al. 2001). While homodimers are either inactive (like HER3 homodimers) or provide only weak signaling, HER2-containing heterodimers have attributes that prolong and enhance downstream signaling (Sliwkowski 2003). When HER2 is overexpressed in cancer, it appears to be the preferred dimerization partner for all members of the HER family (Graus-Porta et al. 1997).

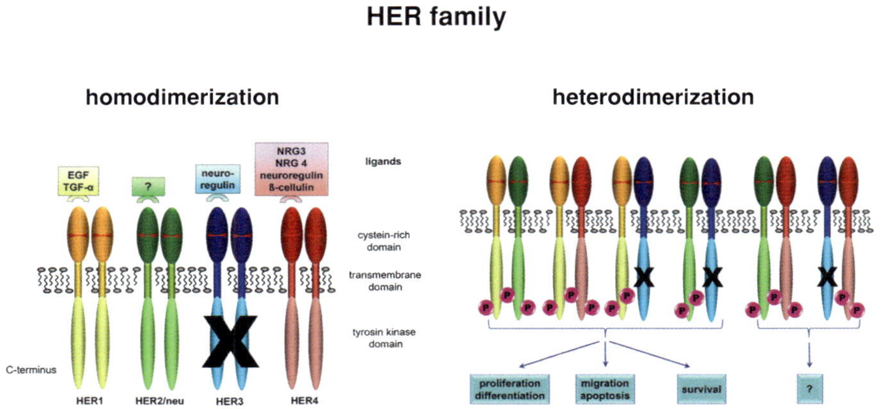

Fig. 1 Organizational principle of the epidermal growth factor receptor family and some dimerization possibilities with corresponding downstream biological events. The *left* half panel shows the names of the HER family members, depicted as homodimers. The *right* panel shows heterodimers and downstream effects upon dimerization. *P* symbolizes phosphorylation. Ligands are shown as *semicircles* (names in *rectangles*) and in the color corresponding to the suitable receptor. Note that HER2 does not have a known ligand, and it presumably acts mostly as a combination partner for heterodimers. Also note that HER3 homodimers lack tyrosine kinase activity (indicated by *X*), but upon ligand binding, the receptor can initiate signal transduction as heterodimer (mainly with the preferred dimerization partner HER2) through the other HER family member's intracellular domain, resulting in multiple downstream effects influencing cell growth and survival

1.2 Human Epidermal Growth Factor Receptors and Their Inhibition in Cancer

Numerous in vitro and in vivo studies indicated the functional importance of the HER family in a wide range of cancers as they are often overexpressed in tumor cells and thus promote their cell proliferation (e.g., Klapper et al. 2000; Nahleh 2008; Rapidis et al. 2008; Horn and Lovly 2012; Hong et al. 2013). This prompted the development of agents that target these receptors, including monoclonal antibodies like cetuximab, or small molecule inhibitors of the receptor tyrosine kinase (TKIs) such as erlotinib and gefitinib (Rivera et al. 2008; Kohler and Schuler 2013).

In breast cancer, overexpression of HER1 (27–30 % of cases) and HER2 (20–25 % of cases) is clearly associated with poor prognosis (Nahta et al. 2003; Witton et al. 2003). The outcome of early and advanced HER2-positive breast cancer patients has been substantially improved upon the addition of trastuzumab, a monoclonal antibody binding to the extracellular domain of HER2, thus inhibiting heterodimerization of HER2 and subsequent activation signals in cancer cells (Stebbing et al. 2000; Piccart-Gebhart et al. 2005; Romond et al. 2005). Unlike in breast cancer, the prognostic relevance of HER2 status in gastric cancer (16 % of cases) is still unclear (Chen et al. 2013). Yet, a survival benefit has been achieved by adding trastuzumab to standard first-line chemotherapy in HER2-positive advanced gastroesophageal cancer (Bang et al. 2010).

In view of the downstream signaling characteristics within the HER family, it is reasonable to assume that agents affecting more than one member of the HER family, like lapatinib inhibiting tyrosine kinase of HER1 and HER2, may suppress cancer cell growth and survival more effectively: First, simultaneous inhibition of HER1 and HER2 may overcome escape mechanisms mediated by redundancy in cell signaling pathways, a form of resistance observed in single tyrosine kinase inhibition, in which upregulation of other members of the HER family occurs (Lin and Winer 2004; Stern 2012). Second, synergistic inhibition of cancer cell growth has been demonstrated upon simultaneous targeting of HER1 and HER2, resulting in a more potent repression of cell growth or greater apoptotic effect compared with targeting either HER1 or HER2 alone (Burris 2004). Third, a dual HER1/HER2 TKI may be a useful substrate in a wider range of patients, in view of the impact of heterodimerization in the progression of a variety of cancer types (Olayioye et al. 2000; Xia et al. 2005).

Therefore, the dual HER TKI lapatinib was expected to have superior activity compared to monotarget TKIs, and even though lapatinib has been primarily developed for and evaluated in breast cancer, its potential goes far beyond this disease.

2 Structure and Mechanism of Action

Lapatinib ditosylate (Fig. 2) is an orally applicable, dual receptor TKI targeting two members of the HER family receptors: HER1 (EGFR1/ErbB1) and HER2/c-neu (ErbB2) (Nelson and Dolder 2006; Medina and Goodin 2008). Lapatinib acts intracellularly, interacting with the tyrosine kinase domain of the receptor (Fig. 3). Hereby, it binds reversibly to the cytoplasmic ATP-binding site of the kinase domain, blocking phosphorylation, and therefore activation of the receptor. This results in the inhibition of various downstream signaling cascades such as the extracellular signal-related kinase 1/2 (ERK1/2) and the phosphatidylinositol 3′-kinase (PI3K)/AKT pathway, both involved in cell proliferation and apoptosis (Okano et al. 2000; Nahta et al. 2003; Xia et al. 2005).

Lapatinib binds the inactive form of EGFR, and by doing so, it differs from other EGFR tyrosine kinase inhibitors like erlotinib or gefitinib, which bind the active EGFR conformation. Lapatinib also has a slower dissociation rate compared to other TKIs. Both could contribute to a greater duration of effect at the target site (Wood et al. 2004).

There are several theoretical advantages of small molecule inhibitors of both HER1 and HER2 compared with the monoclonal antibody cetuximab, which targets the extracellular domain of HER1, or trastuzumab, which targets the extracellular domain of HER2. In cancer, HER1 and HER2 receptors can be truncated. While still exhibiting tyrosine kinase activity, these truncated forms lack the extracellular domain of the receptors. They are necessarily resistant to the

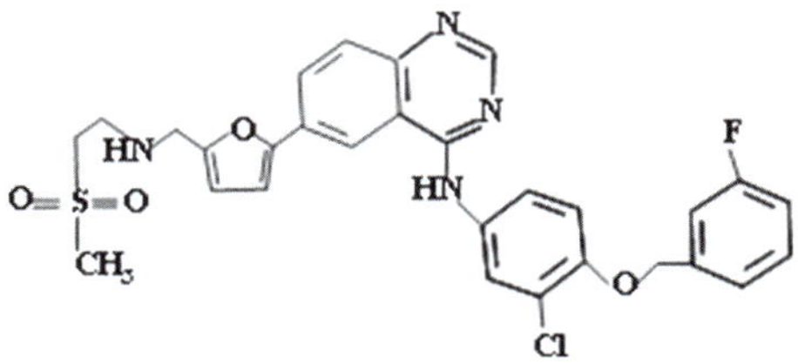

Fig. 2 Chemical structure of lapatinib. Lapatinib is a 4-anilinoquinazoline derivative, distinguishing it from the small head group quinazoline tyrosine kinase inhibitors such as erlotinib and gefitinib

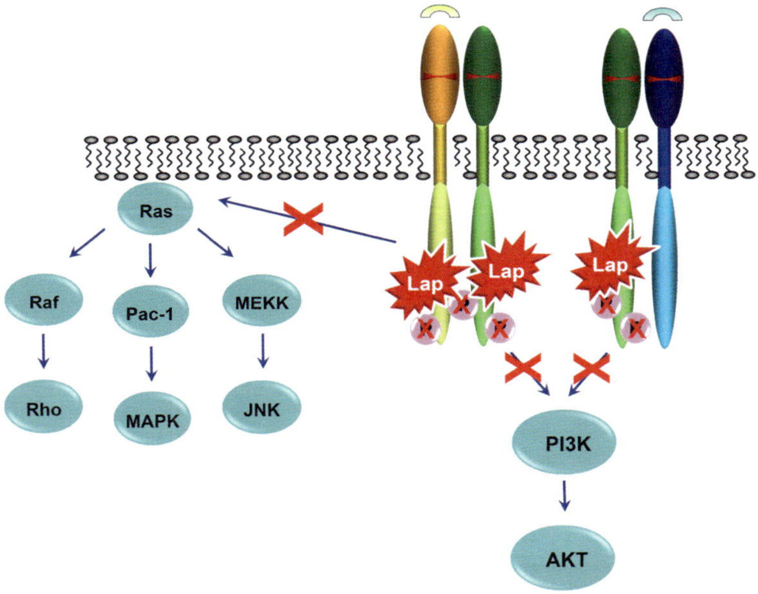

Fig. 3 Intracellular action of lapatinib. Lapatinib binds to the tyrosine kinase domain of HER1 and HER2 blocking the ATP-binding site and thus preventing (symbolized by "X") the activation of downstream cascades. HER1 is depicted in *yellow*, HER2 in *green*, and HER3 in *blue*. Ligands are shown as *semicircles* in corresponding color. Abbreviations: *Lap* lapatinib, *JNK* Jun N-terminal kinase, *MAPK* mitogen-activated protein kinase, *MEKK* MAPK/extracellular signal-related kinase (*ERK*) kinase, *PI3K* phosphatidyl-inositol-3-kinase

treatment with antibodies binding the extracellular HER domain. However, truncated HER2 is still sensitive to the TKI lapatinib (Xia et al. 2004). Another distinctive feature of lapatinib compared to antibody-based anti-HER strategies is its biodistribution. Lapatinib is the first approved small molecule inhibitor with the ability to cross the blood–brain barrier, making it suitable for targeting brain metastases, a common feature in patients with breast cancer, particularly the ones expressing HER2 (Gril et al. 2008; Lin et al. 2008).

3 Pharmacology

Lapatinib is administered orally and intestinal resorption rates vary. Food intake can increase bioavailability twofold to threefold (Singh and Malhotra 2004; Rahman et al. 2007; Ratain and Cohen 2007). To decrease variability, lapatinib intake is recommended no less than one hour before or at least one hour after food intake. In the blood, lapatinib is bound to 99 % to proteins, mainly albumin and acidic alpha-1 glycoprotein. The peak plasma level of lapatinib occurs 3–6 h after administration, and the half-life is approximately 17–24 h. Therefore, the drug is administered at a once-daily schedule. The drug accumulates upon repetitive administration, and equilibrium plasma levels are reached after 6–7 days of administration (Medina and Goodin 2008). Lapatinib is eliminated by hepatic metabolism, primarily through cytochrome P450(CYP)3A4 and biliary excretion. Hence, inducers or inhibitors of CYP3A4 may alter the metabolism of lapatinib, and in turn, lapatinib may increase the level of other CYP3A4 substrates (e.g., benzodiazepines and calcium channel blockers) as well as CYP2C8 substrates (e.g., amiodarone and pioglitazone) (Burris et al. 2005; GlaxoSmithKline 2007; Medina and Goodin 2008). Thus, administration of the drug in patients with impaired liver function, e.g., due to liver cirrhosis or diffuse hepatic metastases, has to be done—if at all—with particular care in a dose-reduced schedule, even though it has not been systemically investigated in this setting so far. The recommended single daily dose of lapatinib is 1,250 mg in combination with capecitabine as second-line therapy in patients with advanced HER2-positive breast cancer and 1,500 mg in combination with hormone therapy for postmenopausal patients with advanced hormone receptor and HER2-positive breast cancer, respectively (Geyer et al. 2006; Johnston et al. 2009).

4 Results from Clinical Trials

4.1 Efficacy in Breast Cancer

Several preclinical data provided the biological rationale to evaluate lapatinib in patients with HER2-positive breast cancer (Konecny et al. 2006; Nelson and Dolder 2006; Chu et al. 2008). A number of phase I–III clinical trials were conducted or are ongoing in breast cancer at different stages, evaluating lapatinib as a single agent or in combination with other therapeutics including chemotherapy, hormone therapy, or monoclonal anti-HER2 antibodies (Table 1). Phase I clinical trials suggested a favorable side effect profile of lapatinib, revealing good tolerability for the majority of volunteers or patients, respectively (Bence et al. 2005; Burris et al. 2005; Moy and Goss 2007). Phase II and III studies demonstrated partly substantial clinical activity of lapatinib in HER2-positive breast cancer patients, as discussed below.

Table 1 Lapatinib in phase I–III clinical trials

Indication	Treatment	Patients (n)	Phase	Response (%)			References
				CR	PR	SD	
Healthy volunteers	L[1a]	47	I	NA	NA	NA	Bence et al. (2005)
Various solid tumors	L[2b]	59	I	0	7	41	Burris et al. (2005)
Various solid tumors	X + L[4b]	45	I	2	7	49	Chu et al. 2007
Breast, ovarian, endometrial cancer	Let + L[3b]	39	I	0	6	59	Chu et al. (2008)
Metastatic breast cancer (second-line)	L[5b]	36	II	0	8	14	Blackwell et al. (2004)
	a: X + L[4b]	163	III	< 1	21		Geyer et al. (2006)
	b: X	161		0	14		
	L[7c]	237	II	0	6	37	Lin et al. (2009)
	a: X + L[4b]	13	II	0	38	46	Lin et al. (2011)
	b : Top + L[4b]	9		0	0	33	
	a: L[5b]	145	III	2	5	28	Blackwell et al. (2010)
	b: T + L[6b]	146		1	9	39	
Metastatic breast cancer (first-line)	*a*: L[5b]	69	II	0	22	58	Gomez et al. (2008)
	b: L[8c]	69		0	26	45	
	a: P + L[5b]	291	III	5	30	33	Di Leo et al. (2008)
	b: P	288		2	23	43	
	a: Let	642	III	4	27	25	Johnston et al. (2009)
	b: Let + L[5b]	644		5	28	26	
	a: P + T + L[6b]	29	III	3	76	10	Esteva et al. (2013)

(continued)

Table 1 (continued)

Indication	Treatment	Patients (n)		Phase	Response (%)			References
					CR	PR	SD	
	b: P + T + L[6b]	14			7	64	7	
	c: P + T + L[7b]	20			5	65	10	
	a: Tax + L[4b]	312		III	NA	NA	NA	Gelmon et al. (2012)
	b: Tax + T	317						
Breast cancer (adjuvant)	*a*: L[5b]	1571		III	NA	NA	NA	TEACH, Goss et al. (2012)
	b: Plac	1576						
	a: T	d.n.a.		III	d.n.a.	d.n.a.	d.n.a.	ALTTO, Tomasello et al. (2008)
	b: L[5b]							
	c: T followed by L[5b]							
	d: T + L[6b]							
Breast cancer (neoadjuvant)	*a*: P + L[5b]	154	III	25				NeoALTTO, Baselga et al. (2012)
	b: P + T	149		30				
	c: P + T + L[6b]	152		51				
	a: EC + D + T	307	III	30				GeparQuinto, Untch et al. (2012)
	b: EC + D + L[4b]	308		21				
	a: P + FEC + T	36	II	25				CHERLOB, Guarneri et al. (2012)
	b: P + FEC + L[4b]	38		26				
	c: P + FEC + T + L[7b]	45		46				
	a: Let + L[5b]	d.n.a.	II	d.n.a.	d.n.a.	d.n.a.		LETLOB, Frassoldati et al. (2008)

(continued)

Table 1 (continued)

Indication	Treatment	Patients (n)	Phase	Response (%)			References
				CR	PR	SD	
	b: Let + Plac						
	a: PAC + T	d.n.a.	III	52			NSABP (B-41), Robidoux et al. (2012)
	b: PAC + L[4b]			53			
	c: PAC + T + L[7b]			62			
Advanced gastroesophageal cancer	*a*: P + L[5c]	132	III	NA	NA	NA	TyTAN, Bang (2012)
(second-line)	*b*: P	129					
Advanced gastroesophageal cancer	*a*: XelOX + L[5b]	273	III	NA	NA	NA	Hecht et al. (2013)
(first-line)	*b*: XelOX + Plac	272	III	NA	NA	NA	
	L[4b]	47	II	0	12	L[4b]	Iqbal et al. (2007)

CR complete response, *PR* partial response, *SD* stable disease, *NA* not applicable, *d.n.a* data not available, *a* cohort A, *b* cohort B, *c* cohort C, *d* cohort D *A* doxorubicin, *C* cyclophosphamide, *D* docetaxel, *E* epirubicin, *F* fluorouracil; FOLFOX oxaliplatin; folinic acid; fluorouracil, *L* lapatinib; Let letrozole, *P* paclitaxel; Plac placebo, *T* trastuzumab; Tax taxane; Top topotecan, *X* capecitabine, *XelOX* capecitabine, oxaliplatin

[a]single and multiple doses, [b]once daily, [c]twice a day

[1]10–175 mg, [2]500–600 mg, [3]1,250–1,500 mg, [4]1,250 mg, [5]1,500 mg, [6]1,000 mg, [7]750 mg, [8]500 mg

4.1.1 Second-Line Treatment in Advanced Breast Cancer

Based on the results of the pivotal EGF100151 trial, lapatinib was first approved in 2007 by the FDA and in 2008 by the EMEA for its combined use with capecitabine in patients with advanced HER2-positive breast cancer after progression upon therapy with anthracyclines, taxanes, and trastuzumab (Geyer et al. 2006). In this open-label phase III trial, patients were randomized to receive either capecitabine alone (201 patients) or a reduced dose of capecitabine and lapatinib (198 patients). Time to disease progression (TTP) was the primary end point of this study. A planned interim analysis (Geyer et al. 2006) revealed 49 disease progression events in the lapatinib group versus 72 events in the control group, resulting in a 51 % risk reduction in time to progression. Due to these data, randomization within this trial was stopped and patients in the control arm could also receive lapatinib in addition to capecitabine. An update analysis of the trial confirmed the positive results of the interim analysis with TTP improvement from 4.3 to 6.2 months upon addition of lapatinib to capecitabine (HR = 0.57 (95 % CI 0.43–0.77), $p < 0.001$) (Cameron et al. 2008). Because premature enrollment termination and subsequent crossover resulted in an insufficient statistical power, exploratory analyses demonstrated only a trend toward a survival advantage with combination therapy (Cameron et al. 2010).

A pertinent question concerns the benefit of combining anti-HER-TKIs with monoclonal anti-HER2-antibodies as compared to either therapy alone. Among other recent studies, this issue was addressed in the EGF104900 phase III trial in the second-line setting in breast cancer (Blackwell et al. 2010). A total of 296 patients, with HER2-positive metastatic breast cancer being progressive on prior trastuzumab-containing regimens, were randomly assigned to receive either lapatinib alone or in combination with trastuzumab. Progression-free survival, as the primary end point of this study, was significantly longer in patients who received combination than in those with single-agent lapatinib therapy (median 12.0 weeks vs. 8.1 weeks, HR 0.73, 95 % CI 0.57–0.93, $p = 0.008$). These data support the idea that dual anti-HER2 therapy may result in a more complete blockade of HER2 signaling by synergistic interaction and their partly non-overlapping mechanisms of action, as it has been demonstrated in preclinical models (Konecny et al. 2006; Scaltriti et al. 2009).

Brain metastases are a major problem among patients treated with trastuzumab for metastatic HER2-positive breast cancer with incidence rates of 28–43 % (Clayton et al. 2004). The efficacy of lapatinib in breast cancer patients with brain metastases refractory to standard therapy was assessed in the EGF105084 phase II trial (Lin et al. 2009). Patients included in this trial had brain metastases and had previously received trastuzumab as well as brain irradiation. Thus, the study addressed a group of patients with particularly unfavorable prognosis. Patients received lapatinib monotherapy, and tumor response (>50 % size reduction) was the primary end point. Of 237 patients, 6 % achieved a partial response, and 37 % achieved stable disease. Although these clinical benefit rates appear moderate, they have to be seen in view of a group of patients with very little treatment options and an extremely high risk of disease progression. A direct comparison of lapatinib and trastuzumab, each in combination with capecitabine, in patients with brain metastases is currently evaluated in an ongoing randomized phase III trial (GlaxoSmithKline 2013). A total of 250 patients in each group have been analyzed so far, showing no significant difference in the number of patients with brain metastases as the site of first relapse (8 patients in lapatinib group, 12 patients in trastuzumab group, $p = 0.36$, OR 0.65, 95 % CI 0.26–1.63). Thus, lapatinib may be a valid alternative to trastuzumab as combination partner to chemotherapy in patients with brain metastases of breast cancer.

4.1.2 First-Line Treatment in Advanced Breast Cancer

In January 2010, lapatinib was approved for first-line treatment of postmenopausal women with hormone receptor-positive metastatic breast cancer that overexpresses the HER2 receptor and for whom hormonal therapy is indicated. This approval was based on the EGF30008 phase III trial, in which 1,286 postmenopausal women with hormone receptor-positive metastatic breast cancer, irrespective of HER2-expression status, were included (Johnston et al. 2009). Patients were randomized to receive either the aromatase inhibitor letrozole alone or in combination with lapatinib. In HER2-positive patients ($n = 219$), the addition of lapatinib increased progression-free survival from 3.0 to 8.2 months (HR 0.71, 95 % CI 0.53–0.96, $p = 0.019$), while HER2-negative patients ($n = 952$) showed no improvement in progression-free survival. It remains unclear which HER-inhibiting combination partner for hormone therapy is better and whether a combination of trastuzumab and lapatinib may have yielded even better results than either one drug alone as an addition to hormone therapy.

Lapatinib in combination with taxane-based chemotherapy has been proven to be effective as first-line treatment in HER2-positive metastatic breast cancer in several phase III studies (Di Leo et al. 2008; Guan et al. 2013). A direct comparison of lapatinib and trastuzumab has been done recently (Gelmon et al. 2012). In this phase III trial, 636 therapy-naïve patients with metastatic breast cancer were randomized to receive a taxane-based chemotherapy either with lapatinib or with trastuzumab, each for 24 weeks, following anti-HER2 monotherapy for 4 years or until progressive disease. After a median follow-up of 12.9 months in the lapatinib arm, and 14 months in the trastuzumab arm, respectively, patients receiving trastuzumab had a significantly longer progression-free survival (11.4 months) compared to patients receiving lapatinib (8.8 months; HR 1.33), with more adverse events, particularly diarrhea, in the lapatinib group. Hence, in patients with HER2-positive metastatic breast cancer, trastuzumab appears to be the preferred combination partner to chemotherapy for first-line therapy, at least if HER2-targeted therapy is confined to one agent.

The efficacy and safety of a dual anti-HER2 inhibition with lapatinib and trastuzumab combined with a taxane-based chemotherapy as first-line therapy in metastatic breast cancer is addressed in an ongoing randomized, double-blind, placebo-controlled phase III study. Irrespective of this trial, a safety study with three different dose regimens of paclitaxel, trastuzumab, and lapatinib was conducted in 63 patients with advanced breast cancer, revealing higher rates of severe diarrhea in patients receiving standard doses of lapatinib (Esteva et al. 2013). Therefore, it remains an open question whether this triple combination offers a manageable safety profile with superior efficacy in first-line setting of metastatic HER2-positive breast cancer compared to taxane-based chemotherapy with trastuzumab alone.

4.1.3 Neoadjuvant Treatment in Early Breast Cancer

A number of recent trails investigated the role of lapatinib in neoadjuvant therapy of breast cancer.

The randomized phase III GeparQuinto trial evaluated potential benefits of either lapatinib or trastuzumab, each combined with epirubicin and cyclophosphamide, followed by docetaxel as chemotherapy backbone prior to surgical removal of the primary tumor in the breast (Untch et al. 2012). Of 309 patients assigned to chemotherapy plus trastuzumab, 30.3 % showed pathological complete response (pCR), defined as absence of invasive tumor cells in the breast at the time of surgery. In contrast, only 22.7 % of 311 patients receiving chemotherapy with lapatinib showed pCR. Thus, neoadjuvant chemotherapy with trastuzumab resulted in a significantly higher pCR rate than did chemotherapy with lapatinib (OR 0.68).

The combination of the two drugs in the neoadjuvant setting was assessed in the lapatinib and/or trastuzumab treatment optimization (NeoALTTO) study. In this randomized, open-label, multicenter phase III trial, women with HER2-positive early breast cancer were randomized to receive either trastuzumab and lapatinib or each drug individually, both in combination with paclitaxel chemotherapy (Baselga et al. 2012). The rate of pCR was significantly higher in the cohort with combined anti-HER2 therapy with both lapatinib and trastuzumab (51.3 %) than in the group given trastuzumab alone (29.5 %; difference 21.1 %) with no significant difference between the trastuzumab and lapatinib groups (24.7). These results strongly support the combined use of the two HER2-targeted agents in combination with chemotherapy in this setting.

The recent phase III study NSABP B-41 also evaluated the dual HER2 inhibition in neoadjuvant treatment of breast cancer, and the results were comparable to the NeoALTTO results; however, the difference in favor of the dual HER2-inhibition was not statistically significant (Robidoux et al. 2012). All of the 529 included women received standard neoadjuvant chemotherapy with 4 cycles of doxorubicin plus cyclophosphamide, followed by weekly paclitaxel. In addition to paclixatel, women were randomly assigned to receive trastuzumab, lapatinib or both. The group of women receiving the combination of anti-HER2 therapy showed a (not statistically significantly) higher percentage of pCR than women receiving trastuzumab alone (62 % vs. 52.5 %; $p = 0.095$). Groups with either lapatinib or trastuzumab alone had similar percentages of pCR (53.2 % vs. 52.5 %).

Therefore, dual inhibition of HER2 might be a valid approach to the treatment of HER2-positive breast cancer in the neoadjuvant setting, but important aspects, such as best dose for optimum efficiency and tolerability of lapatinib, as well as detailed patient selection may need further evaluation.

4.1.4 Adjuvant Treatment in Early Breast Cancer

To address the role of lapatinib in the adjuvant setting, the Adjuvant Lapatinib and/or Trastuzumab Treatment Optimization (ALTTO) study has been initiated with 8,000 patients to be enrolled worldwide (Tomasello et al. 2008). This is an ongoing randomized trial evaluating the effectiveness of trastuzumab, lapatinib, and the combination of both drugs simultaneously as well as in sequential order, as adjuvant therapy in women with early-stage HER2-positive breast cancer. Based on a pre-planned interim analysis in 2011, the independent data monitoring committee recommended to discontinue the lapatinib monotherapy arm, because lapatinib did not appear to be as good as trastuzumab with respect to disease-free survival. Final results of the trial have not been presented so far.

Recently, the results of the Tykerb evaluation after chemotherapy (TEACH) trial, a large randomized phase III study, have been published (Goss et al. 2012). 3,147 women with HER2-positive early breast cancer who had completed trastuzumab-free adjuvant chemotherapy and had no evidence of disease were randomly assigned to receive daily lapatinib or placebo for up to 12 months. After a median follow-up of 4 years, disease-free survival (DFS) events occurred in 13 % in the lapatinib group and 17 % in the placebo group (HR 0.83; $p = 0.053$), thus not meeting the prespecified criteria for statistical significance. Exploratory analyses restricted to patients with confirmed HER2-positive status by central fluorescence in situ hybridization (FISH) review (78 % in the lapatinib group and 80 % in the placebo group) indicated a slight but significant benefit for patients receiving lapatinib. Subgroup analyses in terms of therapy onset showed significant improvement in DFS in patients starting lapatinib treatment within 1 year after surgery (HR 1.03; $p = 0.04$), while there was no significant benefit over placebo therapy for patients with initiation of lapatinib later than 1 year after surgery.

Considering these results, as well as the interim analyses of the ALTTO trial, as well as historical data from adjuvant trastuzumab trials, lapatinib as single anti-HER2 inhibitor in addition to standard chemotherapy, although not ineffective, is very unlikely to gain importance in the adjuvant therapy setting in breast cancer. Its value in combination with trastuzumab remains an open question so far. Single-agent HER2 inhibition with lapatinib in combination with chemotherapy might only be an option in the adjuvant setting in patients with HER2-positive breast cancer in whom trastuzumab is contraindicated, e.g., due to heart failure.

4.2 Efficacy in Gastroesophageal Cancer

Preclinical and early clinical evidence showed promising activity of lapatinib not only in breast cancer, but also in HER2-overexpressing gastroesophageal cancer cell lines (Kim et al. 2008; Wainberg et al. 2010).

In contrast, clinical trials revealed only limited efficacy of lapatinib in patients with gastric cancer so far. The Asian phase III clinical trial TyTAN evaluated the benefit of lapatinib in second-line therapy of advanced HER2-positive gastric cancer (Bang 2012). Patients were randomized to receive either paclitaxel plus lapatinib ($n = 132$) or paclitaxel alone ($n = 129$). In the intent-to-treat population, median overall survival was superior upon combined treatment compared with paclitaxel alone, but this was only statistically significant in the subgroup of patients with HER2 immunohistochemistry 3+ (14 months vs. 7.6 months, HR 0.59). This emphasizes the importance of the exact definition of HER2 positivity in gastric cancer (Boku 2013). In first-line therapy of advanced HER2-positive gastric cancer, lapatinib alone, as well as in combination with chemotherapy, demonstrated only limited activity; thus, lapatinib may not provide additional value over current standard treatment with chemotherapy and trastuzumab (Iqbal et al. 2007; Hecht et al. 2013). So far, there are no data on combined treatment with lapatinib and trastuzumab in gastroesophageal cancer.

4.3 Tolerability

In a phase I study, oral administration of lapatinib revealed good tolerability in healthy volunteers (Bence et al. 2005). Commonly reported side effects included diarrhea, nausea, vomiting, skin rash, and headache. In a dose escalation study of 67 heavily pretreated HER2-positive cancer patients, the main toxicity was diarrhea. This was linearly related to the dose of lapatinib (500–1,600 mg), but not to serum concentration, suggesting direct toxic effects on the intestinal epithelium (Rana and Sridhar 2012).

In the pivotal EGF100151 trial, diarrhea and skin rash, the most common adverse events, occurred more frequently in the combination arm with capecitabine and lapatinib (Geyer et al. 2006). The difference was due to an increase in grade 1 events. Toxicity-related interruption of therapy (43 %), the need for dose reduction (42–43 %), or complete stop of treatment due to intolerance (14 %) was approximately equal in both treatment arms.

In the approval study for postmenopausal women with hormone receptor-positive metastatic breast cancer, the combination of lapatinib and letrozole caused grade 3 and grade 4 diarrhea in 10 % of patients compared to 1 % of patients receiving letrozole alone, resulting in discontinuation (15 %), dose interruption (36 %), or supportive treatment without dose adjustments (31 %) (Johnston et al. 2009).

In all phase III trials evaluating lapatinib in the neoadjuvant setting, grade 3 adverse events, mainly diarrhea, were more common in patients receiving lapatinib with or without trastuzumab than in patients receiving trastuzumab alone (Baselga et al. 2012; Robidoux et al. 2012; Untch et al. 2012). There was no significant difference in frequency of adverse events between patients receiving lapatinib alone or in combination with trastuzumab. Hence, trastuzumab appears not to aggravate gastrointestinal toxicity of single-agent lapatinib.

Taken together, diarrhea is a frequent problem under therapy with lapatinib, but symptoms appear to be mostly manageable.

Treatment with lapatinib is less frequently associated with cardiac failure than treatment with trastuzumab, in which reduction in left ventricular output has been a significant concern, prevents simultaneous treatment with anthracyclines, and excludes patients with coexisting cardiac failure (Perez et al. 2008). Nevertheless, because cardiac events were slightly more common in patients receiving lapatinib than in patients in control arms, routine evaluation of cardiac function is usually recommended before initiating treatment with lapatinib (Geyer et al. 2006).

Additional, quite infrequently reported adverse events upon treatment with lapatinib were hepatotoxicity and interstitial pneumonitis (GlaxoSmithKline 2007). Therefore, routine laboratory evaluation of liver function and clinical observation of pulmonary function are recommended before and during treatment with lapatinib.

However, altogether, life-threatening events (grade 4) or death (grade 5) attributable to lapatinib treatment seems to be very rare (Moy and Goss 2007).

5 Conclusion and Future Perspectives

Patients with HER2-positive breast cancer have a high risk of disease progression upon treatment with conventional chemotherapeutic drugs but benefit enormously of the additional targeted treatment with trastuzumab. Failure to respond to trastuzumab-containing therapeutic regimens in advanced breast cancer as well as contraindications for trastuzumab therapy has posed a therapeutic dilemma to patients and clinicians. For these patients, lapatinib, in combination with capecitabine, is effective after progressive disease following standard therapy with anthracyclines, taxanes, and trastuzumab and as well as in postmenopausal women with advanced, triple-positive breast cancer in combination with hormonal therapy. However, there have also been drawbacks in the evaluation of its efficacy: In first-line therapy of breast cancer, therapy with lapatinib in combination with standard chemotherapy did not show superiority over trastuzumab and chemotherapy in both, early and advanced HER2-positive breast cancer, but resulted in higher toxicity with subsequent treatment interruption. Hence, in first-line therapy, the role of lapatinib may be limited to special settings such as for patients with cardiac failure or patients with brain metastases. But so far, the drug has not been approved for this line of indication.

Open questions remain regarding the future role of lapatinib in the treatment of HER2-positive cancer. Such questions include (1) what is the role of lapatinib in adjuvant therapy of early breast cancer, particularly in simultaneous and sequential combination with trastuzumab, since patients did not seem to benefit from lapatinib alone in this situation? (2) What is the best way of dual inhibition of HER2 with lapatinib and trastuzumab in the neoadjuvant situation? (3) Is lapatinib an equal or even more efficient alternative to trastuzumab in patients with HER2-

positive breast cancer and brain metastases and in combination with which concomitant chemotherapy? (4) Since trastuzumab may be effective in alternative combination regimens after disease progression upon previous trastuzumab treatment, what is the exact value of the combination of trastuzumab with lapatinib versus either drug alone in advanced breast cancer? (5) Is capecitabine or paclitaxel the ideal combination partner to lapatinib in advanced breast cancer or are there superior combination partners? (6) What is the role of dual HER2 inhibition with lapatinib and trastuzumab in strongly HER2-positive gastroesophageal cancer? (7) What is the role of a potential triple HER2-targeted therapy using lapatinib, trastuzumab, and pertuzumab with or without concomitant chemotherapy? Many of these topics will be addressed in ongoing or future clinical trials. The results are eagerly awaited, but may not be available for quite some time. Until then, the combination of lapatinib with capecitabine in HER2-positive, trastuzumab-resistant breast cancer as well as the combination of lapatinib with letrozole as first-line therapy in triple-positive breast cancer is the only approved, but not the only effective, applications of this agent.

References

Bang Y (2012) A randomized, open-label, phase III study of lapatinib in combination with weekly paclitaxel versus weekly paclitaxel alone in the second-line treatment of HER2 amplified advanced gastric cancer (AGC) in Asian population: Tytan study. J Clin Oncol 30(34):11

Bang YJ, Van Cutsem E et al (2010) Trastuzumab in combination with chemotherapy versus chemotherapy alone for treatment of HER2-positive advanced gastric or gastro-oesophageal junction cancer (ToGA): a phase 3, open-label, randomised controlled trial. Lancet 376 (9742):687–697

Baselga J, Bradbury I et al (2012) Lapatinib with trastuzumab for HER2-positive early breast cancer (NeoALTTO): a randomised, open-label, multicentre, phase 3 trial. Lancet 379(9816):633–640

Bence AK, Anderson EB et al (2005) Phase I pharmacokinetic studies evaluating single and multiple doses of oral GW572016, a dual EGFR-ErbB2 inhibitor, in healthy subjects. Invest New Drugs 23(1):39–49

Blackwell K, Kaplan E et al (2004) A phase II, open-label, multicenter study of GW572016 in patients with trastuzumab-refractory metastatic breast cancer. J Clin Oncol 22(3006)

Blackwell KL, Burstein HJ et al (2010) Randomized study of Lapatinib alone or in combination with trastuzumab in women with ErbB2-positive, trastuzumab-refractory metastatic breast cancer. J Clin Oncol 28(7):1124–1130

Boku N (2013) HER2-positive gastric cancer. Gastric Cancer (Epub ahead of print)

Burris HA 3rd (2004) Dual kinase inhibition in the treatment of breast cancer: initial experience with the EGFR/ErbB-2 inhibitor lapatinib. Oncologist 9(Suppl 3):10–15

Burris HA 3rd, Hurwitz HI et al (2005) Phase I safety, pharmacokinetics, and clinical activity study of lapatinib (GW572016), a reversible dual inhibitor of epidermal growth factor receptor tyrosine kinases, in heavily pretreated patients with metastatic carcinomas. J Clin Oncol 23(23):5305–5313

Cameron D, Casey M et al (2008) A phase III randomized comparison of lapatinib plus capecitabine versus capecitabine alone in women with advanced breast cancer that has progressed on trastuzumab: updated efficacy and biomarker analyses. Breast Cancer Res Treat 112(3):533–543

Cameron D, Casey M et al (2010) Lapatinib plus capecitabine in women with HER-2-positive advanced breast cancer: final survival analysis of a phase III randomized trial. Oncologist 15(9):924–934
Chen C, Yang JM et al (2013) Prognostic role of human epidermal growth factor receptor in gastric cancer: a systematic review and meta-analysis. Arch Med Res 44(5):380–389
Chu QS, Schwartz G et al (2007) Phase I and pharmacokinetic study of lapatinib in combination with capecitabine in patients with advanced solid malignancies. J Clin Oncol 25(24): 3753–3758
Chu QS, Cianfrocca ME et al (2008) A phase I and pharmacokinetic study of lapatinib in combination with letrozole in patients with advanced cancer. Clin Cancer Res 14(14): 4484–4490
Citri A, Yarden Y (2006) EGF-ERBB signalling: towards the systems level. Nat Rev Mol Cell Biol 7(7):505–516
Clayton AJ, Danson S et al (2004) Incidence of cerebral metastases in patients treated with trastuzumab for metastatic breast cancer. Br J Cancer 91(4):639–643
Danielsen AJ, Maihle NJ (2002) The EGF/ErbB receptor family and apoptosis. Growth Factors 20(1):1–15
Di Leo A, Gomez HL et al (2008) Phase III, double-blind, randomized study comparing lapatinib plus paclitaxel with placebo plus paclitaxel as first-line treatment for metastatic breast cancer. J Clin Oncol 26(34):5544–5552
Esteva FJ, Franco SX et al (2013) An open-label safety study of lapatinib plus trastuzumab plus paclitaxel in first-line HER2-positive metastatic breast cancer. Oncologist 18(6):661–666
Frassoldati A, Guarneri V et al (2008) Letrozole versus letrozole plus Lapatinib (GW572016) in hormone-sensitive, HER2-negative operable breast cancer: a double-blind, randomized, phase II study with biomarker evaluation (EGF109077-LAP107692/LETLOB). Clin Breast Cancer 8(1):97–100
Gelmon KA, Boyle F et al. (2012) Open-label phase III randomized controlled trial comparing taxane-based chemotherapy (Tax) with lapatinib (L) or trastuzumab (T) as first-line therapy for women with HER2+ metastatic breast cancer: interim analysis (IA) of NCIC CTG MA.31/ GSK EGF 108919. J Clin Oncol 30: 812. (ASCO Annual Meeting Abstracts) (LBA671)
Geyer CE, Forster J et al (2006) Lapatinib plus capecitabine for HER2-positive advanced breast cancer. N Engl J Med 355(26):2733–2743
GlaxoSmithKline (2007) Lapatinib (package insert)
GlaxoSmithKline (2013) Lapatinib plus capecitabine versus trastuzumab plus capecitabine in ErbB2 (HER2) positive metastatic breast cancer. From http://clinicaltrials.gov/show/NCT00820222
Gomez HL, Doval DC et al (2008) Efficacy and safety of lapatinib as first-line therapy for ErbB2-amplified locally advanced or metastatic breast cancer. J Clin Oncol 26(18):2999–3005
Goss PE, Smith IE et al (2012) Adjuvant lapatinib for women with early-stage HER2-positive breast cancer: a randomised, controlled, phase 3 trial. Lancet Oncol 14(1):88–96
Graus-Porta D, Beerli RR et al (1997) ErbB-2, the preferred heterodimerization partner of all ErbB receptors, is a mediator of lateral signaling. EMBO J 16(7):1647–1655
Gril B, Palmieri D et al (2008) Effect of lapatinib on the outgrowth of metastatic breast cancer cells to the brain. J Natl Cancer Inst 100(15):1092–1103
Guan Z, Xu B et al (2013) Randomized trial of lapatinib versus placebo added to paclitaxel in the treatment of human epidermal growth factor receptor 2-overexpressing metastatic breast cancer. J Clin Oncol 31(16):1947–1953
Guarneri V, Frassoldati A et al (2012) Preoperative chemotherapy plus trastuzumab, lapatinib, or both in human epidermal growth factor receptor 2-positive operable breast cancer: results of the randomized phase II CHER-LOB study. J Clin Oncol30(16):1989–1995

Hecht J R, Y J Bang et al (2013) Lapatinib in combination with capecitabine plus oxaliplatin (CapeOx) in HER2-positive advanced or metastatic gastric, esophageal, or gastroesophageal adenocarcinoma (AC): The TRIO-013/LOGiC Trial. J Clin Oncol **31**(18):abstract-LBA4001 [ASCO Annual Meeting Proceedings (Post-Meeting Edition)]
Hong L, Han Y et al (2013) Prognostic value of epidermal growth factor receptor in patients with gastric cancer: a meta-analysis. Gene 529(1):69–72
Horn L, Lovly C (2012) Update on HER1-3 in advanced non-small-cell lung cancer. J Thorac Oncol 7(16):S369–S371
Iqbal S, Goldman B et al. (2007). S0413: a phase II SWOG study of GW572016 (lapatinib) as first line therapy in patients with advanced or metastatic gastric cancer. J Clin Oncol 25(18):4621 (ASCO Annual Meeting Proceedings (Post-Meeting Edition))
Johnston S, Pippen J Jr et al (2009) Lapatinib combined with letrozole versus letrozole and placebo as first-line therapy for postmenopausal hormone receptor-positive metastatic breast cancer. J Clin Oncol 27(33):5538–5546
Kim JW, Kim HP et al (2008) The growth inhibitory effect of lapatinib, a dual inhibitor of EGFR and HER2 tyrosine kinase, in gastric cancer cell lines. Cancer Lett 272(2):296–306
Klapper LN, Kirschbaum MH et al (2000) Biochemical and clinical implications of the ErbB/HER signaling network of growth factor receptors. Adv Cancer Res 77:25–79
Kohler J, Schuler M (2013) Afatinib, Erlotinib and Gefitinib in the first-line therapy of EGFR mutation-positive lung adenocarcinoma: a review. Onkologie 36(9):510–518
Konecny GE, Pegram MD et al (2006) Activity of the dual kinase inhibitor lapatinib (GW572016) against HER-2-overexpressing and trastuzumab-treated breast cancer cells. Cancer Res 66(3):1630–1639
Lin NU, Winer EP (2004) New targets for therapy in breast cancer: small molecule tyrosine kinase inhibitors. Breast Cancer Res 6(5):204–210
Lin NU, Carey LA et al (2008) Phase II trial of lapatinib for brain metastases in patients with human epidermal growth factor receptor 2-positive breast cancer. J Clin Oncol 26(12): 1993–1999
Lin NU, Dieras V et al (2009) Multicenter phase II study of lapatinib in patients with brain metastases from HER2-positive breast cancer. Clin Cancer Res 15(4):1452–1459
Lin NU, Eierman W et al (2011) Randomized phase II study of lapatinib plus capecitabine or lapatinib plus topotecan for patients with HER2-positive breast cancer brain metastases. J Neurooncol 105(3):613–620
Medina PJ, Goodin S (2008) Lapatinib: a dual inhibitor of human epidermal growth factor receptor tyrosine kinases. Clin Ther 30(8):1426–1447
Mendelsohn J, Baselga J (2003) Status of epidermal growth factor receptor antagonists in the biology and treatment of cancer. J Clin Oncol 21(14):2787–2799
Moy B, Goss PE (2007) Lapatinib-associated toxicity and practical management recommendations. Oncologist 12(7):756–765
Nahleh ZA (2008) Molecularly targeted therapy in breast cancer: the new generation. Recent Patents Anticancer Drug Discov 3(2):100–104
Nahta R, Hortobagyi GN et al (2003) Growth factor receptors in breast cancer: potential for therapeutic intervention. Oncologist 8(1):5–17
Nelson MH, Dolder CR (2006) Lapatinib: a novel dual tyrosine kinase inhibitor with activity in solid tumors. Ann Pharmacother 40(2):261–269
Okano J, Gaslightwala I et al (2000) Akt/protein kinase B isoforms are differentially regulated by epidermal growth factor stimulation. J Biol Chem 275(40):30934–30942
Olayioye MA, Neve RM et al (2000) The ErbB signaling network: receptor heterodimerization in development and cancer. EMBO J 19(13):3159–3167
Perez EA, Koehler M et al (2008) Cardiac safety of lapatinib: pooled analysis of 3689 patients enrolled in clinical trials. Mayo Clin Proc 83(6):679–686
Piccart-Gebhart MJ, Procter M et al (2005) Trastuzumab after adjuvant chemotherapy in HER2-positive breast cancer. N Engl J Med 353(16):1659–1672

Prenzel N, Fischer OM et al (2001) The epidermal growth factor receptor family as a central element for cellular signal transduction and diversification. Endocr Relat Cancer 8(1):11–31
Rahman A, Pazdur R et al (2007) The value meal: effect of food on lapatinib bioavailability. J Clin Oncol 25(33):5333–5335
Rana P, Sridhar SS (2012) Efficacy and tolerability of lapatinib in the management of breast cancer. Breast Cancer (Auckl) 6:67–77
Rapidis AD, Vermorken JB et al (2008) Targeted therapies in head and neck cancer: past, present and future. Rev Recent Clin Trials 3(3):156–166
Ratain MJ, Cohen EE (2007) The value meal: how to save $1,700 per month or more on lapatinib. J Clin Oncol 25(23):3397–3398
Rivera F, Vega-Villegas ME et al (2008) Cetuximab, its clinical use and future perspectives. Anticancer Drugs 19(2):99–113
Robidoux A, Tang G et al (2012) Evaluation of lapatinib as a component of neoadjuvant therapy for HER2+ operable breast cancer: NSABP protocol B-41. J Clin Oncol 30:812 (ASCO Annual Meeting Abstract LBA506)
Romond EH, Perez EA et al (2005) Trastuzumab plus adjuvant chemotherapy for operable HER2-positive breast cancer. N Engl J Med 353(16):1673–1684
Scaltriti M, Verma C et al (2009) Lapatinib, a HER2 tyrosine kinase inhibitor, induces stabilization and accumulation of HER2 and potentiates trastuzumab-dependent cell cytotoxicity. Oncogene 28(6):803–814
Singh BN, Malhotra BK (2004) Effects of food on the clinical pharmacokinetics of anticancer agents: underlying mechanisms and implications for oral chemotherapy. Clin Pharmacokinet 43(15):1127–1156
Sliwkowski MX (2003) Ready to partner. Nat Struct Biol 10(3):158–159
Stebbing J, Copson E et al (2000) Herceptin (trastuzamab) in advanced breast cancer. Cancer Treat Rev 26(4):287–290
Stern DF (2000) Tyrosine kinase signalling in breast cancer: ErbB family receptor tyrosine kinases. Breast Cancer Res 2(3):176–183
Stern HM (2012) Improving treatment of HER2-positive cancers: opportunities and challenges. Sci Transl Med 4(127):127rv2
Tomasello G, de Azambuja E et al (2008) Jumping higher: is it still possible? The ALTTO trial challenge. Expert Rev Anticancer Ther 8(12):1883–1890
Untch M, Loibl S et al (2012) Lapatinib versus trastuzumab in combination with neoadjuvant anthracycline-taxane-based chemotherapy (GeparQuinto, GBG 44): a randomised phase 3 trial. Lancet Oncol 13(2):135–144
Wainberg ZA, Anghel A et al (2010) Lapatinib, a dual EGFR and HER2 kinase inhibitor, selectively inhibits HER2-amplified human gastric cancer cells and is synergistic with trastuzumab in vitro and in vivo. Clin Cancer Res 16(5):1509–1519
Witton CJ, Reeves JR et al (2003) Expression of the HER1-4 family of receptor tyrosine kinases in breast cancer. J Pathol 200(3):290–297
Wood ER, Truesdale AT et al (2004) A unique structure for epidermal growth factor receptor bound to GW572016 (Lapatinib): relationships among protein conformation, inhibitor off-rate, and receptor activity in tumor cells. Cancer Res 64(18):6652–6659
Xia W, Liu LH et al (2004) Truncated ErbB2 receptor (p95ErbB2) is regulated by heregulin through heterodimer formation with ErbB3 yet remains sensitive to the dual EGFR/ErbB2 kinase inhibitor GW572016. Oncogene 23(3):646–653
Xia W, Gerard CM et al (2005) Combining lapatinib (GW572016), a small molecule inhibitor of ErbB1 and ErbB2 tyrosine kinases, with therapeutic anti-ErbB2 antibodies enhances apoptosis of ErbB2-overexpressing breast cancer cells. Oncogene 24(41):6213–6221
Yarden Y, Sliwkowski MX (2001) Untangling the ErbB signalling network. Nat Rev Mol Cell Biol 2(2):127–137

Sorafenib: Targeting Multiple Tyrosine Kinases in Cancer

Jens Hasskarl

Abstract

Sorafenib (BAY 43-9006, Nexavar®) is an oral multiple tyrosine kinase inhibitor. Main targets are receptor tyrosine kinase pathways frequently deregulated in cancer such as the Raf–Ras pathway, vascular endothelial growth factor (VEGF) pathway, and FMS-like tyrosine kinase 3 (FLT3). Sorafenib was approved by the FDA in fast track for advanced renal cell cancer and hepatocellular cancer and shows good clinical activity in thyroid cancer. Multiple clinical trials are undertaken to further investigate the role of sorafenib alone or in combination for the treatment of various tumor entities.

Contents

J. Hasskarl (✉)
Department Innere Medizin, Klinik für Innere Medizin I, Schwerpunkt Hämatologie, Onkologie und Stammzelltransplantation, Hugstetter Str. 55, 79102 Freiburg, Germany
e-mail: jens.hasskarl@uniklinik-freiburg.de

U. M. Martens (ed.), *Small Molecules in Oncology*, Recent Results in Cancer Research 201, DOI: 10.1007/978-3-642-54490-3_8,

1 Introduction

Cancer cells exhibit multiple changes in cell cycle control, apoptosis, proliferation, and invasion. In many cases, excessive growth factors signaling leads to increased proliferation of cells. Growth factor receptors (GFRs) function as cell surface receptors for circulating growth factors, cytokines, and hormones. A majority of these receptors possess unique tyrosine kinase domains, so-called receptor tyrosine kinases (RTK). They consist of an extracellular ligand binding domain and an intracellular catalytic domain. Activating mutations within the RTK domains important for signal transduction result in constitutive activation of downstream signaling pathways found in many cancers (McInnes and Sykes 1997). These pathways include Raf kinase, platelet-derived growth factor (PDGF), vascular endothelial growth factor receptor (VEGFR) 2 and 3 kinases, and c-Kit, the receptor for stem cell factor. More than 15 different classes of RTK have been identified to date (Fig. 1). They function during normal growth and development but are also closely connected to tumorigenesis. Protein kinases are constitutively activated in many molecular pathways that contribute to malignant transformation and growth factor independent growth. Thus, GFRs and their RTKs have become attractive targets for tumor therapy.

There are three general approaches to target RTKs: (1) targeting the ligand before it binds to the receptor, (2) targeting the extracellular domain of the receptors, and (3) targeting the intracellular RTK domain. While (1) and (2) can be achieved by antibody technologies or decoys, small molecule inhibitors, so-called receptor tyrosine kinase inhibitors (RTKI), have been designed to target the intracellular RTK domains. The first RTKI approved for the treatment of chronic myelogenous leukemia (CML) was imatinib (STI-571, Glivec®) (Savage and Antman 2002). Sorafenib (BAY 43-9006, Nexavar®) is a small molecular inhibitor of multiple protein kinases. Sorafenib was approved by the US Food and Drug Administration (FDA) in 2005 for the treatment of advanced renal cell cancer (RCC) and shortly after received marketing authorization in the EU (Wilhelm et al. 2006). It was approved for treatment of hepatocellular carcinoma (HCC) in 2007. Based on recent trial results in thyroid cancer, approval for this indication is expected.

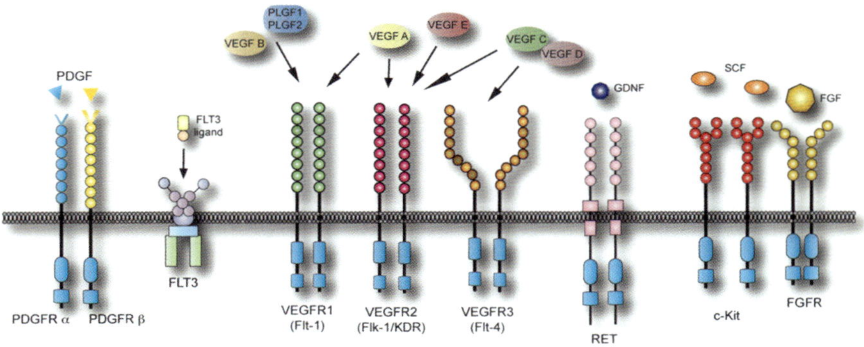

Fig. 1 Growth factor receptor and associated protein kinases targeted by sorafenib. Platelet-derived growth factor receptor (PDGFR), *FLT3*, vascular endothelial growth factor receptor (*VEGFR*), placental growth factor (*PLGF*), rearranged during transfection (*RET*), glial-derived neurotrophic factor (*GDNF*), stem cell factor (*SCF*), and fibroblast growth factor (*FGFR*). Modified from Hicklin and Ellis (2005), Sebolt-Leopold and Herrera (2004), Stirewalt and Radich (2003)

Fig. 2 Structure of sorafenib (4-[4-[[4-chloro-3-(trifluoromethyl)-phenyl]-carbamoyl-amino]-phenoxy]-N-methyl-pyridine-2-carboxamide) (Wishart et al. 2008)

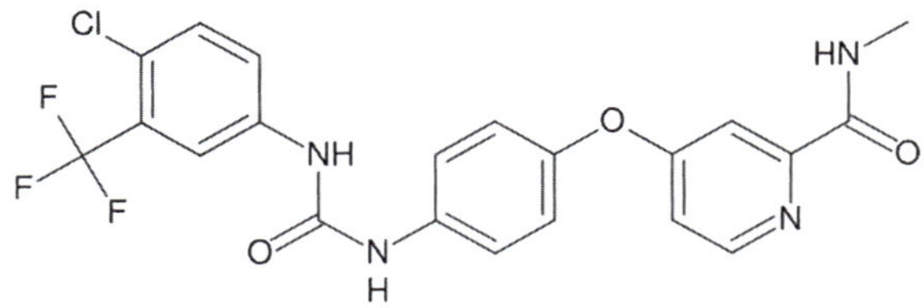

2 Structure and Mechanism of Action

Sorafenib (Fig. 2) is an inhibitor of multiple seronine/threonine and RTK including vascular endothelial growth factor (VEGF) receptor 2, FMS-like tyrosine kinase 3 (FLT3), platelet-derived growth factor (PDGF) receptor, and fibroblast growth factor receptor-1 (FGFR1). It was originally designed as inhibitor of the Raf kinases A-Raf, B-Raf, and C-Raf (Raf1) by chemical optimization (Wilhelm et al. 2006) and co-developed by Bayer Pharmaceuticals and Onyx Pharmaceutical.

Raf kinases are the initial kinases in the Ras/Raf/MEK pathway/mitogen-activated protein kinase (MAPK) pathway (Friday and Adjei 2008) and are frequently deregulated in human cancers, resulting in altered cellular growth and survival. Sorafenib inhibits wild-type and oncogenic Raf (b-Raf, c-Raf, V600E b-Raf), VEGFR 1–3, PDGFR-β, FGFR1, c-kit, Flt-3, and RET (Carlomagno et al. 2006; Gollob et al. 2006; Wilhelm et al. 2004) (Figs. 1 and 3). Sorafenib does not inhibit MEK1, ERK1, epithelial growth factor receptor 1 (EGFR1/HER1/ErbB-1), HER2/neu (ErbB-2), or insulin-like growth factor receptor 1 (IGFR1) (Wilhelm et al. 2006,

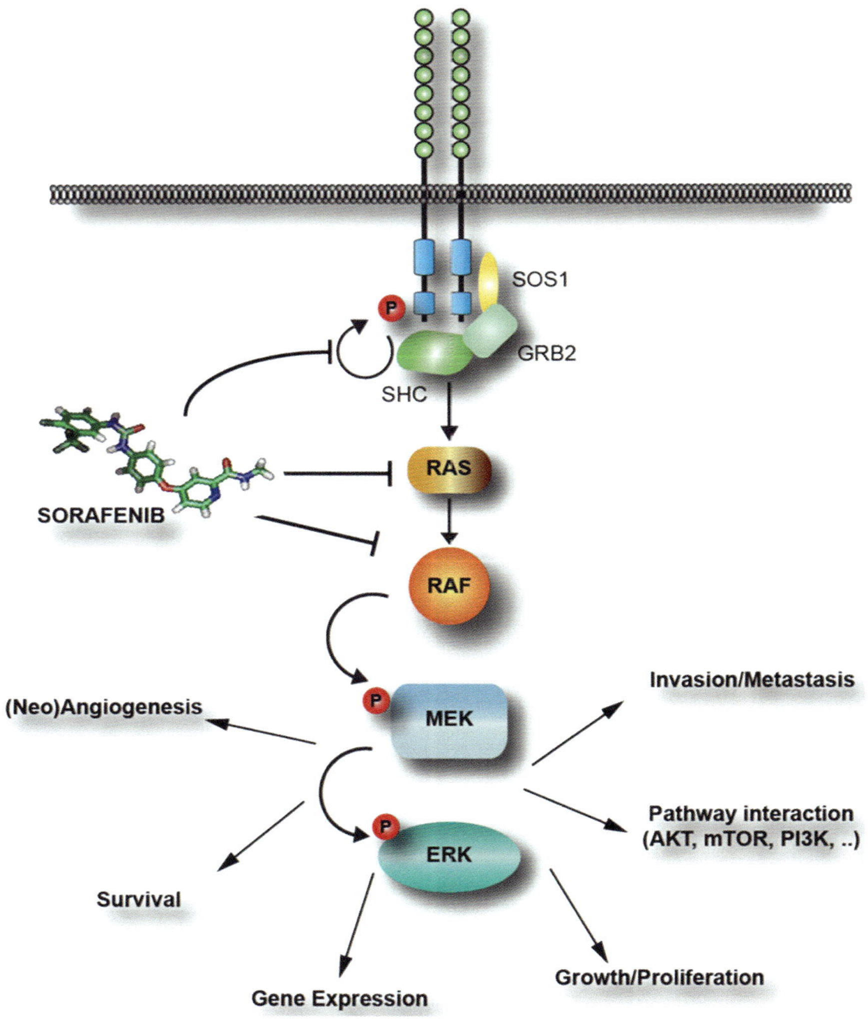

Fig. 3 Signaling pathways targeted by sorafenib. Sorafenib blocks signal transduction and (auto)phosphorylation of receptor tyrosine kinases and inhibits Raf kinases. Inhibition of Raf kinases results in decreased tumor angiogenesis and proliferation, reduced invasiveness, and facilitates apoptosis. Extracellular signal-regulated kinase (*ERK*), son of sevenless homolog (*SOS1*), growth factor receptor-bound protein 2 (*GRB2*), Src homology 2 domain containing (*SHC*), and MAPK/ERK kinase (*MEK*). Modified from Wilhelm et al. (2006). Structure of sorafenib modified from DrugBank (Wishart et al. 2008)

2004). In numerous xenograft tumor models, sorafenib alone or in combination with other agents showed broad-spectrum antitumor activity in colon, breast and non-small-cell lung cancer (NSCLC), melanoma, thyroid cancer, hepatocellular (HCC) and RCC, lymphoma, and Flt-3 mutant leukemia (Table 1).

Table 1 Xenograft tumor models

Tumor type	References
Colon cancer	Wilhelm et al. (2004)
Breast cancer	Valabrega et al. (2011), Wilhelm et al. (2004)
Non-small-cell lung cancer	Carter et al. (2007), Wilhelm et al. (2004)
Renal cell cancer	Chang et al. (2007)
Thyroid cancer	Carlomagno et al. (2006), Kim et al. (2007), Salvatore et al. (2006)
Melanoma	Karasarides et al. (2004), Smalley et al. (2008)
Hepatocellular carcinoma	Liu et al. (2006), Wang et al. (2008)
Leukemia	Auclair et al. (2007), Hu et al. (2011), Zhang et al. (2008)
Lymphoma	Carlo-Stella et al. (2013)
Cholangiocarcinoma	Sugiyama et al. (2011)

3 Clinical Data

3.1 Phase I

Various phase I studies in patients with solid or hematologic tumors of sorafenib alone or in combination with standard cytotoxic chemotherapy were launched (Table 2). These trials proved the safety and suggested clinical efficacy of sorafenib (Clark et al. 2005; Kupsch et al. 2005; Moore et al. 2005; Strumberg et al. 2005). Most frequent adverse events observed were hypertension, rash, diarrhea, hand–foot syndrome, and fatigue, whereas hematologic side effects were mild. Side effects improved promptly after stop of sorafenib medication. Form these trials, the standard dose of sorafenib was determined as 400 mg twice daily. Although resorption is influenced by concomitant food intake, bioavailability is not altered. Plasma half-life is approximately 36 h. Maximum plasma levels are reached three hours after ingestion, and steady-state levels are reached after one week. 99.5 % of sorafenib is protein bound. It is hardly metabolized and excreted in feces (ca. 80 %) and urine (ca. 20 %). Metabolism of sorafenib is independent of age and gender. Plasma levels in patients with reduced liver function (Child-Pugh A and B) or reduced kidney function (creatinin clearance >30 ml/min) do not differ from healthy subjects.

3.2 Experience in Special Patient Populations

There are no data about sorafenib in patients with severe liver disease (Child-Pugh C) or severely reduced kidney function (creatinin clearance <30 ml/min) or patients on hemodialysis.

Table 2 Phase I clinical trials with sorafenib

Indication	Sorafenib dose	Dose(s) combination partner(s)	References
Solid tumors	400 mg bid	Irinotecan 125 mg/m^2 or 140 mg^2	Mross et al. (2007)
Solid tumors	400 mg bid	Doxorubibin 60 mg/m^2	Richly et al. (2006)
Solid tumors	200 mg bid	Carboplatin (AUC 5) Pemetrexed 500 mg/m^2	Davies et al. (2011)
Solid tumors, colorectal cancer	400 mg bid	Oxaliplatin 130 mg/m^2	Kupsch et al. (2005)
Solid tumors, advanced leukemias (pediatric)	200 mg bid (solid tumors) 150 mg bid (leukemias)	–	Widemann et al. (2012)
Solid tumors, RCC, NSCLC	400 mg bid*	Vorinostat 300 mg qd*	Dasari et al. (2013)
Solid tumors Pancreatic cancer	400 mg bid	Gemcitabine 1000 mg/m^2	Siu et al. (2006)
Solid tumors, Melanoma	400 mg bid	Carboplatin AUC6 Paclitaxel 225 mg/m^2	Flaherty et al. (2008)
RCC, Melanoma	400 mg bid	Interferon α-2a 9 Mio IU	Escudier et al. (2007b)
NSCLC	400 mg bid	Carboplatin AUC 5 Paclitaxel 200 mg/m^2	Okamoto et al. (2010)
NSCLC	400 mg bid	Gefitinib 250 mg qd	(Adjei et al. 2007)
HCC (Japan)	400 mg bid	–	Furuse et al. (2008), Minami et al. (2008)
MDS/sAML	300 mg bid	–	Crump et al. (2010)
MDS/AML	600 mg qd	Cytarabine 10 mg bid	Macdonald et al. (2013)
Refractory AML	400 mg bid	–	Borthakur et al. (2011)
Refractory AML (pediatric)	150 mg bid	Cytarabine 1 g/m^2 Clofarabine 40 mg/m^2	Inaba et al. (2011)
Lymphoma	400 mg bid	Vorinostat 200 mg bid	Sayar et al. (2010)

*Doses not tolerated in expansion cohorts: *bid* twice daily, *qd* once daily, *RCC* renal cell carcinoma, *AML* acute myelogenous leukemia, *MDS* myelodysplastic syndrome, *HCC* hepatocellular carcinoma, *NSCLC* non-small-cell lung cancer, *AUC* area under the curve

3.3 Experience in Pediatric Patients

There are sparse data on sorafenib in children. Most published data are from phase I trials. Recommended dose for phase II trials for children with solid tumors was

Table 3 Registered active interventional clinical trials (phase I-III) with sorafenib

Indication	Phase I	Phase I/II	Phase II	Phase III
Advanced cancer/leukemia/lymphoma	8	–	1	–
AML/MDS	4	1	2	3
Brain tumors	1	1	1	–
Breast cancer	2	–	2	1
Childhood malignancies	1	–	1	–
CLL	–	–	1	–
Colorectal cancer	2	–	4	–
HCC	6	5	18	11
Melanoma	1	–	1	–
NSCLC	2	–	1	–
Ovarian cancer	–	–	1	–
RCC	1	1	5	1
Sarcoma	1	–	2	–
SCLC	–	–	1	–
Urothelial cancer	1	–	1	–

Reference www.clinicaltrials.gov

determined at 200 mg/m^2 bid and 150 mg/m^2 bid for leukemias. Adverse effects were similar to those observed in adult patients (Widemann et al. 2012). When administered in combination with bevacizumab (15 mg/kg qd 3 weeks) and cyclophosphamide (50 mg/m^2 qd), the recommended phase II dose of sorafenib was 90 mg/m^2 bid (Navid et al. 2013).

3.4 Active Clinical Trials

Up to June 2013, 574 trials using sorafenib for the treatment of solid tumors and hematologic malignancies have been registered (http://www.cinicaltrials.gov). The majority of these are phase I and II trials. Currently, 94 trials are listed as active, the greater part of which are phase II and III trials in RCC and HCC (Table 3).

3.5 Sorafenib in the Treatment of Renal Cell Cancer

Primary treatment of RCC is surgical resection. RCC had been regarded as chemotherapy-resistant tumor. With the introduction of TKIs, the prognosis of patients with metastatic or inoperable RCC improved tremendously. RCC is characterized by dense vascularization, most likely due to high activity of VEGF and VEGFR, resistance to conventional cytotoxic chemotherapy, and upregulation of Raf1 and

EGFR (Oka et al. 1995). Thus, a drug targeting the VEGF pathway and the Ras pathway such as sorafenib seemed perfect for treatment of RCC. In phase I trials, some patients with RCC showed significant and sustained disease stabilization (Clark et al. 2005; Strumberg et al. 2002). Based on these observations, sorafenib was tested as monotherapy for RCC in a phase II randomized discontinuation trial (Ratain et al. 2006). Of 202 patients, 36 % had an objective tumor response and 32 % showed disease stabilization. Median progression-free survival was increased from 6 to 24 weeks ($p = 0.0087$). These results were substantiated by the Treatment Approaches in Renal cancer Global Evaluation Trial (TARGET) phase III trial (Escudier et al. 2007a). Here, 903 patients with renal-cell carcinoma after treatment failure (mostly cytokine) were randomized to receive sorafenib (400 mg bid) or placebo. Primary study endpoint was overall survival. Because a planned interim analysis showed significantly prolonged progression-free survival in the sorafenib arm (5.5 vs. 2.8 months; HR 0.44; 95 % CI 0.35–0.55; $p < 0.01$), crossover was allowed. Patients receiving sorafenib had a 39 % reduced risk of death compared to placebo (HR 0.72; 95 % CI 0.54–0.94; $p = 0.02$), missing the predefined statistical boundary (Escudier et al. 2007a). Based on the above results, sorafenib was approved for treatment of advanced RCC. Currently, sorafenib is tested in various trials and combinations for treatment of RCC (Table 2). Three ongoing phase III trials (NCT01481870, NCT01613846, NCT00732914) are trying to define the optimal sequence of TKIs in RCC treatment.

The INTORSECT trial randomized 512 patients with advanced RCC who had failed first-line therapy with sunitinib to receive either sorafenib or temsirolimus. While PFS tended to be increased in the temsirolimus arm, the effect did not reach statistical significance (PFS 4.28 vs. 3.91 months; HR 0.87, 95 % CI 0.71–1.07; $p = 0.1933$). Furthermore, OS was significantly longer in the sorafenib arm (OS 16.64 vs. 12.27 months; HR 1.31, 95 % CI 1.05–1.63; $p = 0.014$), clearly favoring sorafenib (Hutson et al. 2012). The randomized phase III AXIS trial compared the VEGFR-TKI axitinib with sorafenib as second-line therapy in patients with advanced RCC. Seven hundred and twenty-three patients were randomized to receive axitinib (5 mg bid) or sorafenib (400 mg bid). The median PFS was 6.7 months with axitinib compared to 4.7 months with sorafenib (HR 0.67; 95 % CI 0.54–0.81; $p < 0.0001$) (Rini et al. 2011). Median overall survival was 20.1 months with axitinib and 19.2 months with sorafenib (HR 0.97; 95 % CI 0.80–1.17; $p = 0.3744$) (Motzer et al. 2013b). Another phase III trial, TIVO-1, randomized 517 patients with RCC to receive sorafenib (400 mg bid) or tivozanib (1.5 mg qd), a pan VEGFR-TKI until progression. Median PFS was 11.9 months for tivozanib compared with 9.1 months for sorafenib (HR 0.797; 95 % CI 0.64–0.99; $p = 0.042$) (Motzer et al. 2012). OS tended to be reversed in favor of the sorafenib arm. At time of final OS analysis, mortality rates were 45.4 % in the tivozanib group compared to 39.3 % in the sorafenib group (HR 1.25; 95 % CI 0.95–1.62; $p = 0.105$), with a median OS of 28.8 months for tivozanib and 29.3 months for sorafenib (Motzer et al. 2013a). This difference in OS, which might have been influenced by the study design, led the FDA to not grant approval of tivozanib for RCC based on TIVO-1.

3.6 Sorafenib in the Treatment of Hepatocellular Cancer

Like in RCC, preclinical and early clinical studies had suggested activity in RCC. In a phase II study, 137 patients with chemo-naive advanced HCC were treated with 400 mg sorafenib bid Median TTP was 4.2 months, and median OS was 9.2 months. Side effects were generally tolerable and comparable with other trials (Abou-Alfa et al. 2006). This led to a multicenter randomized, double-blind, placebo-controlled phase III trial testing efficacy of 400 mg sorafenib bid in patients with advanced chemo-naive HCC, the SHARP trial (Llovet et al. 2008). In this trial, 602 HCC patients with good liver function (>95 % Child-Pugh Class A) were randomized to receive either sorafenib 400 mg or matching placebo orally bid until progression (Llovet et al. 2008). The primary endpoint was overall survival, which showed an improvement from 7.9 to 10.7 months in patients receiving sorafenib compared to placebo (HR 0.69; 95 % CI, 0.55–0.87; $p = 0.0001$) in all subgroups analyzed (Bruix et al. 2012). Likewise, time to radiologic progression increased from 2.8 months to 5.5 ($p < 0.001$). Because of this trial, sorafenib was approved for the treatment of advanced HCC. Similar results were reported for another randomized phase III trial, the Sorafenib Asia Pacific (AP) trial: 226 patients (>95 % Child-Pugh A) were randomized 2:1 to sorafenib 400 mg bid or matching placebo. Patients treated with sorafenib had longer median OS (6.5 vs. 4.2 months; HR 0.68; 95 % CI 0.50–0.93; $p = 0.014$) and TTP (2.8 vs. 1.4 months; $p = 0.0005$) (Cheng et al. 2009, 2012). Sorafenib is tested in various settings and combinations worldwide (Table 3).

3.7 Sorafenib in the Treatment of Lung Cancer

At time of writing, 32 phase I and II trials of sorafenib monotherapy or in combination with various other agents have been or are being conducted in patients with advanced non-small-cell lung cancer (NSCLC) (www.clinicaltrials.gov; Table 2). Sorafenib has been evaluated in three phase III trials in combination with paclitaxel and carboplatin, and gemcitabine and cisplatin. The first trial to report was stopped prematurely after interim analysis showed futility of success and a higher mortality in patients with squamous cell carcinoma treated with sorafenib (HR = 1.85; 95 % CI, 1.22–2.81) (Scagliotti et al. 2010) and led to termination of a very similar trial in Asia. Another phase III trial of sorafenib in combination with gemcitabine and cisplatin also missed its primary endpoint (Paz-Ares et al. 2012). Sorafenib has demonstrated some clinical activity in pretreated NSCLC patients in a randomized discontinuation trial (Wakelee et al. 2012) and in k-Ras mutated patients (Dingemans et al. 2013). Molecular screening might further help to identify patients to whom sorafenib might be of greater benefit (Ellis and Al-Saleh 2012; Kuiper et al. 2012).

Sorafenib has also been investigated in small-cell lung cancer (SCLC) as maintenance therapy or in combination with topotecan for refractory SCLC. While clinical activity was noted, the therapy was felt to be too toxic in comparison with other available therapies (Gitlitz et al. 2008; Leach et al. 2010; Sharma et al. 2012).

3.8 Sorafenib in the Treatment of Breast Cancer

Clinicaltrials.gov lists currently 4 active phase I-III trials with sorafenib alone or in combination in breast cancer. Most prior trials had shown a high degree of toxicity when combined with other agents (Gradishar 2012). Single-agent activity was negligible (Bianchi et al. 2009; Moreno-Aspitia et al. 2009). Combination of sorafenib with anastrozole in aromatase inhibitor (AI)-resistant breast cancer was primarily toxic (Isaacs et al. 2011). Combination with paclitaxel in a neoadjuvant setting was quite toxic (Spigel et al. 2011) and did not exert clinical benefit in first-line setting (Gradishar et al. 2013). Combination of sorafenib with gemcitabine or capecitabine led to a modest but statistically significant PFS-benefit in patients with advanced HER2-negative breast cancer (median PFS 3.4 vs. 2.7 months; HR 0.65; 95 % CI 0.45–0.95; $p = 0.02$) (Schwartzberg et al. 2013). Another randomized, double-blind, placebo-controlled phase II trial evaluated sorafenib in combination with capecitabine in 229 patients with advanced HER2-negative breast cancer (Baselga et al. 2012). Patients receiving the combination had longer PFS compared to patients receiving capecitabine and placebo (median PFS, 6.4 vs. 4.1 months; HR 0.58; 95 % CI 0.41–0.81; $p = 0.001$). Of note, toxicity was significant, and no difference in OS was noted. A phase III confirmatory trial using a reduced sorafenib dose is currently recruiting patients.

3.9 Sorafenib in the Treatment of Malignant Melanoma

B-Raf is a target of sorafenib and has been identified as therapeutic target in melanoma (Karasarides et al. 2004). Unfortunately, sorafenib as single agent failed to show clinical efficacy in a phase II trial (Egberts et al. 2011; Eisen et al. 2006). Nevertheless, when tested in combination with carboplatin and paclitaxel or dacarbacin, objective responses were noted (Flaherty et al. 2008; McDermott et al. 2008). In contrast, the SWOG S0512 phase II trial evaluating sorafenib (400 mg bid) in combination with carboplatin (AUC 6) and paclitaxel (225 mg/m^2) in 25 patients with metastatic uveal melanoma failed to show objective tumor responses (Bhatia et al. 2012). Combination of sorafenib with tipifarnib or temsirolimus in a phase III trial did not show enough efficacy to pursuit this strategy (Margolin et al. 2012). Two phase III trials failed to show relevant clinical activity of sorafenib in combination with carboplatin (AUC 6) and paclitaxel (225 mg/m^2) in metastatic melanoma. No clinical benefit was observed in first-line or in second-line treatment (Flaherty et al. 2013; Hauschild et al. 2009).

3.10 Sorafenib in the Treatment of Prostate Cancer

Several phase II studies of sorafenib in hormone-independent prostate cancer (Aragon-Ching et al. 2009; Beardsley et al. 2012; Chi et al. 2008; Dahut et al.

2008; Safarinejad 2008; Steinbild et al. 2007) failed to show convincing activity of sorafenib in prostate cancer.

3.11 Sorafenib in the Treatment of Head and Neck Cancer

Like in prostate cancer, single-agent sorafenib reached only show modest results in patients with squamous cell carcinoma of the head and neck (Elser et al. 2007; Williamson et al. 2010).

3.12 Sorafenib in the Treatment of Ovarian Cancer

Dual inhibition of the VEGF pathway with sorafenib (200 mg bid) and bevacizumab (5 mg/m^2 or 10 mg/m^2) showed promising tumor response in a phase I dose-escalation trial (Azad et al. 2008). Objective responses were seen in 6 (43 %) of 13 patients with ovarian cancer. Unfortunately, 74 % required sorafenib dose reduction, indicating that the combination of sorafenib with bevacizumab might be too toxic for routine use. Combination of sorafenib with carboplatin (AUC 5) and paclitaxel (175 mg/m^2) was highly toxic, so that a trial with planned 102 patients was prematurely stopped after 4 patients had been enrolled (Polcher et al. 2010). Combination of sorafenib with other agents resulted in very limited antitumor activity but substantial toxicity (Bodnar et al. 2011; Matei et al. 2011; Ramasubbaiah et al. 2011; Welch et al. 2010).

3.13 Sorafenib in the Treatment of Brain Tumors

Two case reports described good response of cerebral metastases of RCC (Ranze et al. 2007; Valcamonico et al. 2008), demonstrating efficacy of sorafenib in the brain. A retrospective subgroup analysis of the TARGET trial in RCC reported a lower incidence of brain metastases in patients treated with sorafenib compared to placebo (Massard et al. 2010). Treatment of patients with glioblastoma with temozolomide and sorafenib (Hainsworth et al. 2010; Reardon et al. 2011), or sorafenib and temsirolimus did not improve PFS (Lee et al. 2012).

3.14 Sorafenib in the Treatment of Thyroid Cancer

Various phase II trials in metastatic, iodine-refractory thyroid carcinoma, showed very promising clinical activity of sorafenib (Ahmed et al. 2011; Gupta-Abramson et al. 2008; Schneider et al. 2012) with the exception of anaplastic thyroid carcinoma, where the activity was quite low (Savvides et al. 2013). Impressive clinical activity of sorafenib in differentiated thyroid carcinoma was confirmed in the phase III DECISION trial, reported at ASCO 2013. A total of 417 patients with progressive locally advanced or metastatic radio iodine-refractory differentiated thyroid cancer were randomized to receive sorafenib 400 mg bid or placebo. Tumor response was assessed every 8 weeks by independent radiologic review using modified RECIST 1.0. In this trial, sorafenib almost doubled median PFS from 5.8 to 10.8 months (HR 0.58, 95 % CI 0.45–0.75, $p < 0.0001$). Median OS had not been reached at time of presentation but is likely to be confounded by crossover to sorafenib: 70 % of patients progressing on placebo started open-label sorafenib. OR was 12.2 % versus 0.5 % ($p < 0.0001$) (Brose et al. 2011, 2013).

3.15 Sorafenib in the Treatment of Hematologic Diseases

Mutations of the FLT3 gene have been identified in approximately one-third of acute myelogenous leukemia (AML) patients. FLT3-mutations are associated with a poor prognosis in these patients. The most frequent mutation of FLT3 in AML is internal tandem duplications (FLT3-ITD). In this setting, sorafenib might be a new compound to improve therapeutic options of FLT3-mutant AML. In a mouse model, sorafenib reduced the tumor burden of FLT3-mutated blasts, and a phase I study showed clinical activity of sorafenib in FLT3-mutant patients (Zhang et al. 2008). A total of 13 phase I and II trials are using sorafenib in combination with other agents for treatment of leukemia and lymphomas (Table 2). Most clinical data suggesting antileukemic activity of sorafenib come from case reports or retrospective case series (Metzelder et al. 2009, 2010, 2012; Rollig et al. 2012; Safaian et al. 2009; Schroeder et al. 2010). In a case series of 16 patients with advanced FLT3-ITD-mutated AML relapsed after HSCT, activity of sorafenib was negligible (Sharma et al. 2011).

In phase I trials, response to sorafenib given as single agent was sometimes impressive but transient arguing for its use in combination with chemotherapy (Borthakur et al. 2011; Crump et al. 2010; Man et al. 2012). A phase I trial in 12 pediatric patients with acute leukemia sorafenib was tested in combination with cytarabine and clofarabine. Six patients (3 FLT3-ITD and 3 FLT3-wt AML) achieved CR (Inaba et al. 2011). A phase I/II trial of sorafenib in combination with cytarabine and idarubicin in 61 patients with AML (<65 years) reported interesting activity of this combination especially in FLT3-ITD-mutated patients. Patients in phase II were treatment naive at study entry. Complete response was observed in 18 (75 %) patients (14 (93 %) FLT3-ITD mutated, 24 (66 %) with FLT3 wild type (WT) ($p = 0.033$) (Ravandi et al. 2010). Another phase I/II study in 21 elderly patients with AML ($n = 17$) and high-risk AML ($n = 4$) unsuitable for standard chemotherapy performed by the NCIC Clinical Trials Group showed only very limited activity of the combination of sorafenib with cytarabine (Macdonald et al. 2013). A German multicenter phase II trial (NCT00373373) presented at ASH 2010 evaluated the efficacy of sorafenib versus placebo (each in combination with standard chemotherapy) in 197 elderly patients with AML. Arms were well balanced. No benefit of adding sorafenib to chemotherapy was observed in this trial. A subgroup analysis in FLT-ITD-mutated patients (14.2 %) also failed to show differences in EFS or OS (Serve et al. 2010). Combination of sorafenib with 5-azacytidine could be an active treatment for FLT3-ITD-mutated AML (Ravandi et al 2013). An ongoing phase III trial is evaluating the activity of bortezomib and sorafenib with chemotherapy in patients with newly diagnosed AML (NCT01371981). Thus, activity of sorafenib in AML needs to be confirmed in larger prospective randomized controlled and adequately powered studies with molecular stratification.

Sorafenib alone or in combination is also under investigation in CML, CLL, multiple myeloma, and other lymphoma types.

4 Clinical Safety Profile of Sorafenib

Sorafenib has a predictable safety profile that has been established in various phase III trials and in clinical routine. Side effects are hemorrhage, rash and hand-foot syndrome, diarrhea, hypertension, cardiac ischemia/infarction, and QT-prolongation.[1] For full safety profile, refer to summary of product characteristics.

5 Conclusion and Future Perspectives

Identification of tumor-specific pathways led to the development of sorafenib as a rationally designed pathway-specific drug. Positive trials in RCC and HCC led to the rapid approval of sorafenib for the treatment of RCC and HCC by the FDA and EMA. Approval for treatment of differentiated thyroid carcinoma is expected in the near future. Results of several clinical trials (e.g., in NSCLC) have not stood up to the high expectation. Multiple clinical trials in various tumor entities are still on their way and will hopefully show efficacy in patent populations with a high unmet medical need, such as FLT3-positive AML.

References

Abou-Alfa GK, Schwartz L, Ricci S, Amadori D, Santoro A, Figer A et al (2006) Phase II study of sorafenib in patients with advanced hepatocellular carcinoma. J Clin Oncol 24:4293–4300

Adjei AA, Molina JR, Mandrekar SJ, Marks R, Reid JR, Croghan G et al (2007) Phase I trial of sorafenib in combination with gefitinib in patients with refractory or recurrent non-small cell lung cancer. Clin Cancer Res 13:2684–2691

Ahmed M, Barbachano Y, Riddell A, Hickey J, Newbold KL, Viros A et al (2011) Analysis of the efficacy and toxicity of sorafenib in thyroid cancer: a phase II study in a UK based population. Eur J Endocrinol 165:315–322

[1] *Source* Fachinfo Nexavar® February 2013.

Aragon-Ching JB, Jain L, Gulley JL, Arlen PM, Wright JJ, Steinberg SM et al (2009) Final analysis of a phase II trial using sorafenib for metastatic castration-resistant prostate cancer. BJU Int 103:1636–1640
Auclair D, Miller D, Yatsula V, Pickett W, Carter C, Chang Y et al (2007) Antitumor activity of sorafenib in FLT3-driven leukemic cells. Leukemia 21:439–445
Azad NS, Posadas EM, Kwitkowski VE, Steinberg SM, Jain L, Annunziata CM et al (2008) Combination targeted therapy with sorafenib and bevacizumab results in enhanced toxicity and antitumor activity. J Clin Oncol 26:3709–3714
Baselga J, Segalla JG, Roche H, Del Giglio A, Pinczowski H, Ciruelos EM et al (2012) Sorafenib in combination with capecitabine: an oral regimen for patients with HER2-negative locally advanced or metastatic breast cancer. J Clin Oncol 30:1484–1491
Beardsley EK, Hotte SJ, North S, Ellard SL, Winquist E, Kollmannsberger C et al (2012) A phase II study of sorafenib in combination with bicalutamide in patients with chemotherapy-naive castration resistant prostate cancer. Invest New Drugs 30:1652–1659
Bhatia S, Moon J, Margolin KA, Weber JS, Lao CD, Othus M et al (2012) Phase II Trial of Sorafenib in Combination with Carboplatin and Paclitaxel in Patients with Metastatic Uveal Melanoma: SWOG S0512. PLoS One 7:e48787
Bianchi G, Loibl S, Zamagni C, Salvagni S, Raab G, Siena S et al (2009) Phase II multicenter, uncontrolled trial of sorafenib in patients with metastatic breast cancer. Anticancer Drugs 20:616–624
Bodnar L, Gornas M, Szczylik C (2011) Sorafenib as a third line therapy in patients with epithelial ovarian cancer or primary peritoneal cancer: a phase II study. Gynecol Oncol 123:33–36
Borthakur G, Kantarjian H, Ravandi F, Zhang W, Konopleva M, Wright JJ et al (2011) Phase I study of sorafenib in patients with refractory or relapsed acute leukemias. Haematologica 96:62–68
Brose MS, Nutting CM, Sherman SI, Shong YK, Smit JW, Reike G et al (2011) Rationale and design of decision: a double-blind, randomized, placebo-controlled phase III trial evaluating the efficacy and safety of sorafenib in patients with locally advanced or metastatic radioactive iodine (RAI)-refractory, differentiated thyroid cancer. BMC Cancer 11:349
Brose MS, Nutting C, Jarzab B, Elisei R, Siena S, Bastholt L et al (2013) Sorafenib in locally advanced or metastatic patients with radioactive iodine-refractory differentiated thyroid cancer: the phase III DECISION trial. J Clin Oncol 31:4
Bruix J, Raoul JL, Sherman M, Mazzaferro V, Bolondi L, Craxi A et al (2012) Efficacy and safety of sorafenib in patients with advanced hepatocellular carcinoma: subanalyses of a phase III trial. J Hepatol 57:821–829
Carlomagno F, Anaganti S, Guida T, Salvatore G, Troncone G, Wilhelm SM et al (2006) BAY 43-9006 inhibition of oncogenic RET mutants. J Natl Cancer Inst 98:326–334
Carlo-Stella C, Locatelli SL, Giacomini A, Cleris L, Saba E, Righi M et al (2013) Sorafenib inhibits lymphoma xenografts by targeting MAPK/ERK and AKT pathways in tumor and vascular cells. PLoS One 8:e61603
Carter CA, Chen C, Brink C, Vincent P, Maxuitenko YY, Gilbert KS et al (2007) Sorafenib is efficacious and tolerated in combination with cytotoxic or cytostatic agents in preclinical models of human non-small cell lung carcinoma. Cancer Chemother Pharmacol 59:183–195
Chang YS, Adnane J, Trail PA, Levy J, Henderson A, Xue D et al (2007) Sorafenib (BAY 43-9006) inhibits tumor growth and vascularization and induces tumor apoptosis and hypoxia in RCC xenograft models. Cancer Chemother Pharmacol 59:561–574
Cheng AL, Kang YK, Chen Z, Tsao CJ, Qin S, Kim JS et al (2009) Efficacy and safety of sorafenib in patients in the Asia-Pacific region with advanced hepatocellular carcinoma: a phase III randomised, double-blind, placebo-controlled trial. Lancet Oncol 10:25–34
Cheng AL, Guan Z, Chen Z, Tsao CJ, Qin S, Kim JS et al (2012) Efficacy and safety of sorafenib in patients with advanced hepatocellular carcinoma according to baseline status: subset analyses of the phase III Sorafenib Asia-Pacific trial. Eur J Cancer 48:1452–1465

Chi KN, Ellard SL, Hotte SJ, Czaykowski P, Moore M, Ruether JD et al (2008) A phase II study of sorafenib in patients with chemo-naive castration-resistant prostate cancer. Ann Oncol 19:746–751

Clark JW, Eder JP, Ryan D, Lathia C, Lenz HJ (2005) Safety and pharmacokinetics of the dual action Raf kinase and vascular endothelial growth factor receptor inhibitor, BAY 43-9006, in patients with advanced, refractory solid tumors. Clin Cancer Res 11:5472–5480

Crump M, Hedley D, Kamel-Reid S, Leber B, Wells R, Brandwein J et al (2010) A randomized phase I clinical and biologic study of two schedules of sorafenib in patients with myelodysplastic syndrome or acute myeloid leukemia: a NCIC (National Cancer Institute of Canada) clinical trials group study. Leuk Lymphoma 51:252–260

Dahut WL, Scripture C, Posadas E, Jain L, Gulley JL, Arlen PM et al (2008) A phase II clinical trial of sorafenib in androgen-independent prostate cancer. Clin Cancer Res 14:209–214

Dasari A, Gore L, Messersmith WA, Diab S, Jimeno A, Weekes CD et al (2013) A phase I study of sorafenib and vorinostat in patients with advanced solid tumors with expanded cohorts in renal cell carcinoma and non-small cell lung cancer. Invest New Drugs 31:115–125

Davies JM, Dhruva NS, Walko CM, Socinski MA, Bernard S, Hayes DN et al (2011) A phase I trial of sorafenib combined with cisplatin/etoposide or carboplatin/pemetrexed in refractory solid tumor patients. Lung Cancer 71:151–155

Dingemans AM, Mellema WW, Groen HJ, van Wijk A, Burgers SA, Kunst PW et al (2013) A phase II study of sorafenib in patients with platinum-pretreated, advanced (Stage IIIb or IV) non-small cell lung cancer with a KRAS mutation. Clin Cancer Res 19:743–751

Egberts F, Gutzmer R, Ugurel S, Becker JC, Trefzer U, Degen A et al (2011) Sorafenib and pegylated interferon-alpha2b in advanced metastatic melanoma: a multicenter phase II DeCOG trial. Ann Oncol 22:1667–1674

Eisen T, Ahmad T, Flaherty KT, Gore M, Kaye S, Marais R et al (2006) Sorafenib in advanced melanoma: a Phase II randomised discontinuation trial analysis. Br J Cancer 95:581–586

Ellis PM, Al-Saleh K (2012) Multitargeted anti-angiogenic agents and NSCLC: clinical update and future directions. Crit Rev Oncol Hematol 84:47–58

Elser C, Siu LL, Winquist E, Agulnik M, Pond GR, Chin SF et al (2007) Phase II trial of sorafenib in patients with recurrent or metastatic squamous cell carcinoma of the head and neck or nasopharyngeal carcinoma. J Clin Oncol 25:3766–3773

Escudier B, Eisen T, Stadler WM, Szczylik C, Oudard S, Siebels M et al (2007a) Sorafenib in advanced clear-cell renal-cell carcinoma. N Engl J Med 356:125–134

Escudier B, Lassau N, Angevin E, Soria JC, Chami L, Lamuraglia M et al (2007b) Phase I trial of sorafenib in combination with IFN alpha-2a in patients with unresectable and/or metastatic renal cell carcinoma or malignant melanoma. Clin Cancer Res 13:1801–1809

Flaherty KT, Schiller J, Schuchter LM, Liu G, Tuveson DA, Redlinger M et al (2008) A phase I trial of the oral, multikinase inhibitor sorafenib in combination with carboplatin and paclitaxel. Clin Cancer Res 14:4836–4842

Flaherty KT, Lee SJ, Zhao F, Schuchter LM, Flaherty L, Kefford R et al (2013) Phase III trial of carboplatin and paclitaxel with or without sorafenib in metastatic melanoma. J Clin Oncol 31:373–379

Friday BB, Adjei AA (2008) Advances in targeting the Ras/Raf/MEK/Erk mitogen-activated protein kinase cascade with MEK inhibitors for cancer therapy. Clin Cancer Res 14:342–346

Furuse J, Ishii H, Nakachi K, Suzuki E, Shimizu S, Nakajima K (2008) Phase I study of sorafenib in Japanese patients with hepatocellular carcinoma. Cancer Sci 99:159–165

Gitlitz BJ, Glisson BS, Moon J, Reimers H, Gandara DR (2008) Sorafenib in patients with platinum (plat) treated extensive stage small cell lung cancer (E-SCLC): A SWOG (S0435) phase II trial. J Clin Oncol 26:8039

Gollob JA, Wilhelm S, Carter C, Kelley SL (2006) Role of Raf kinase in cancer: therapeutic potential of targeting the Raf/MEK/ERK signal transduction pathway. Semin Oncol 33:392–406

Gradishar WJ (2012) Sorafenib in locally advanced or metastatic breast cancer. Expert Opin Investig Drugs 21:1177–1191

Gradishar WJ, Kaklamani V, Sahoo TP, Lokanatha D, Raina V, Bondarde S et al (2013) A double-blind, randomised, placebo-controlled, phase 2b study evaluating sorafenib in combination with paclitaxel as a first-line therapy in patients with HER2-negative advanced breast cancer. Eur J Cancer 49:312–322

Gupta-Abramson V, Troxel AB, Nellore A, Puttaswamy K, Redlinger M, Ransone K et al (2008) Phase II trial of sorafenib in advanced thyroid cancer. J Clin Oncol 26:4714–4719

Hainsworth JD, Ervin T, Friedman E, Priego V, Murphy PB, Clark BL et al (2010) Concurrent radiotherapy and temozolomide followed by temozolomide and sorafenib in the first-line treatment of patients with glioblastoma multiforme. Cancer 116:3663–3669

Hauschild A, Agarwala SS, Trefzer U, Hogg D, Robert C, Hersey P et al (2009) Results of a phase III, randomized, placebo-controlled study of sorafenib in combination with carboplatin and paclitaxel as second-line treatment in patients with unresectable stage III or stage IV melanoma. J Clin Oncol 27:2823–2830

Hicklin DJ, Ellis LM (2005) Role of the vascular endothelial growth factor pathway in tumor growth and angiogenesis. J Clin Oncol 23:1011–1027

Hu S, Niu H, Inaba H, Orwick S, Rose C, Panetta JC et al (2011) Activity of the multikinase inhibitor sorafenib in combination with cytarabine in acute myeloid leukemia. J Natl Cancer Inst 103:893–905

Hutson T, Escudier B, Esteban E, Bjarnason GA, Lim HY, Pittman K et al (2012) Temsirolimus vs sorafenib as second line therapy in metastatic renal cell carcinoma: results from the intorsect trial. Ann Oncol 23:LBA22 PR

Inaba H, Rubnitz JE, Coustan-Smith E, Li L, Furmanski BD, Mascara GP et al (2011) Phase I pharmacokinetic and pharmacodynamic study of the multikinase inhibitor sorafenib in combination with clofarabine and cytarabine in pediatric relapsed/refractory leukemia. J Clin Oncol 29:3293–3300

Isaacs C, Herbolsheimer P, Liu MC, Wilkinson M, Ottaviano Y, Chung GG et al (2011) Phase I/II study of sorafenib with anastrozole in patients with hormone receptor positive aromatase inhibitor resistant metastatic breast cancer. Breast Cancer Res Treat 125:137–143

Karasarides M, Chiloeches A, Hayward R, Niculescu-Duvaz D, Scanlon I, Friedlos F et al (2004) B-RAF is a therapeutic target in melanoma. Oncogene 23:6292–6298

Kim S, Yazici YD, Calzada G, Wang ZY, Younes MN, Jasser SA et al (2007) Sorafenib inhibits the angiogenesis and growth of orthotopic anaplastic thyroid carcinoma xenografts in nude mice. Mol Cancer Ther 6:1785–1792

Kuiper JL, Lind JS, Groen HJ, Roder J, Grigorieva J, Roder H et al (2012) VeriStrat((R)) has prognostic value in advanced stage NSCLC patients treated with erlotinib and sorafenib. Br J Cancer 107:1820–1825

Kupsch P, Henning BF, Passarge K, Richly H, Wiesemann K, Hilger RA et al (2005) Results of a phase I trial of sorafenib (BAY 43-9006) in combination with oxaliplatin in patients with refractory solid tumors, including colorectal cancer. Clin Colorectal Cancer 5:188–196

Leach JW, Swenson K, Anderson E, Menge MR, Tsai ML (2010) A phase I study of weekly topotecan (T) in combination with sorafenib (S) for treatment of relapsed or refractory small cell lung cancer (SCLC). J Clin Oncol 28:e18086

Lee EQ, Kuhn J, Lamborn KR, Abrey L, DeAngelis LM, Lieberman F et al (2012) Phase I/II study of sorafenib in combination with temsirolimus for recurrent glioblastoma or gliosarcoma: North American brain tumor consortium study 05-02. Neuro Oncol 14:1511–1518

Liu L, Cao Y, Chen C, Zhang X, McNabola A, Wilkie D et al (2006) Sorafenib blocks the RAF/MEK/ERK pathway, inhibits tumor angiogenesis, and induces tumor cell apoptosis in hepatocellular carcinoma model PLC/PRF/5. Cancer Res 66:11851–11858

Llovet JM, Ricci S, Mazzaferro V, Hilgard P, Gane E, Blanc JF et al (2008) Sorafenib in advanced hepatocellular carcinoma. N Engl J Med 359:378–390

Macdonald DA, Assouline SE, Brandwein J, Kamel-Reid S, Eisenhauer EA, Couban S et al (2013) A phase I/II study of sorafenib in combination with low dose cytarabine in elderly patients with acute myeloid leukemia or high-risk myelodysplastic syndrome from the National Cancer Institute of Canada Clinical Trials Group: trial IND.186. Leuk Lymphoma 54:760–766

Man CH, Fung TK, Ho C, Han HH, Chow HC, Ma AC et al (2012) Sorafenib treatment of FLT3-ITD(+) acute myeloid leukemia: favorable initial outcome and mechanisms of subsequent nonresponsiveness associated with the emergence of a D835 mutation. Blood 119:5133–5143

Margolin KA, Moon J, Flaherty LE, Lao CD, Akerley WL 3rd, Othus M et al (2012) Randomized phase II trial of sorafenib with temsirolimus or tipifarnib in untreated metastatic melanoma (S0438). Clin Cancer Res 18:1129–1137

Massard C, Zonierek J, Gross-Goupil M, Fizazi K, Szczylik C, Escudier B (2010) Incidence of brain metastases in renal cell carcinoma treated with sorafenib. Ann Oncol 21:1027–1031

Matei D, Sill MW, Lankes HA, DeGeest K, Bristow RE, Mutch D et al (2011) Activity of sorafenib in recurrent ovarian cancer and primary peritoneal carcinomatosis: a gynecologic oncology group trial. J Clin Oncol 29:69–75

McDermott DF, Sosman JA, Gonzalez R, Hodi FS, Linette GP, Richards J et al (2008) Double-blind randomized phase II study of the combination of sorafenib and dacarbazine in patients with advanced melanoma: a report from the 11715 Study Group. J Clin Oncol 26:2178–2185

McInnes C, Sykes BD (1997) Growth factor receptors: structure, mechanism, and drug discovery. Biopolymers 43:339–366

Metzelder S, Wang Y, Wollmer E, Wanzel M, Teichler S, Chaturvedi A et al (2009) Compassionate use of sorafenib in FLT3-ITD-positive acute myeloid leukemia: sustained regression before and after allogeneic stem cell transplantation. Blood 113:6567–6571

Metzelder S, Finck A, Fey M, Scholl S, Kroger M, Reiter A et al (2010) Sorafenib monotherapy is effective in relapsed and refractory Flt3-ITD positive acute myeloid leukemia, particularly after allogenic stem cell transplantation. ASH Annual Meeting Abstracts 116:3314

Metzelder SK, Schroeder T, Finck A, Scholl S, Fey M, Gotze K et al (2012) High activity of sorafenib in FLT3-ITD-positive acute myeloid leukemia synergizes with allo-immune effects to induce sustained responses. Leukemia 26:2353–2359

Minami H, Kawada K, Ebi H, Kitagawa K, Kim YI, Araki K et al (2008) Phase I and pharmacokinetic study of sorafenib, an oral multikinase inhibitor, in Japanese patients with advanced refractory solid tumors. Cancer Sci 99:1492–1498

Moore M, Hirte HW, Siu L, Oza A, Hotte SJ, Petrenciuc O et al (2005) Phase I study to determine the safety and pharmacokinetics of the novel Raf kinase and VEGFR inhibitor BAY 43-9006, administered for 28 days on/7 days off in patients with advanced, refractory solid tumors. Ann Oncol 16:1688–1694

Moreno-Aspitia A, Morton RF, Hillman DW, Lingle WL, Rowland KM Jr, Wiesenfeld M et al (2009) Phase II trial of sorafenib in patients with metastatic breast cancer previously exposed to anthracyclines or taxanes: North Central Cancer Treatment Group and Mayo Clinic Trial N0336. J Clin Oncol 27:11–15

Motzer RJ, Nosov D, Eisen T, Bondarenko IN, Lesovoy V, Lipatov ON et al (2012) Tivozanib versus sorafenib as initial targeted therapy for patients with advanced renal cell carcinoma: Results from a phase III randomized, open-label, multicenter trial. J Clin Oncol 30:4501

Motzer RJ, Eisen T, Hutson TE, Szczylik C, Krygowski M, Strahs AL et al (2013a) Overall survival results from a phase III study of tivozanib hydrochloride versus sorafenib in patients with renal cell carcinoma. J Clin Oncol 31:350

Motzer RJ, Escudier B, Tomczak P, Hutson TE, Michaelson MD, Negrier S et al (2013b) Axitinib versus sorafenib as second-line treatment for advanced renal cell carcinoma: overall survival analysis and updated results from a randomised phase III trial. Lancet Oncol 14:552–562

Mross K, Steinbild S, Baas F, Gmehling D, Radtke M, Voliotis D et al (2007) Results from an in vitro and a clinical/pharmacological phase I study with the combination irinotecan and sorafenib. Eur J Cancer 43:55–63

Navid F, Baker SD, McCarville MB, Stewart CF, Billups CA, Wu J et al (2013) Phase I and clinical pharmacology study of bevacizumab, sorafenib, and low-dose cyclophosphamide in children and young adults with refractory/recurrent solid tumors. Clin Cancer Res 19:236–246

Oka H, Chatani Y, Hoshino R, Ogawa O, Kakehi Y, Terachi T et al (1995) Constitutive activation of mitogen-activated protein (MAP) kinases in human renal cell carcinoma. Cancer Res 55:4182–4187

Okamoto I, Miyazaki M, Morinaga R, Kaneda H, Ueda S, Hasegawa Y et al (2010) Phase I clinical and pharmacokinetic study of sorafenib in combination with carboplatin and paclitaxel in patients with advanced non-small cell lung cancer. Invest New Drugs 28:844–853

Paz-Ares LG, Biesma B, Heigener D, von Pawel J, Eisen T, Bennouna J et al (2012) Phase III, randomized, double-blind, placebo-controlled trial of gemcitabine/cisplatin alone or with sorafenib for the first-line treatment of advanced, nonsquamous non-small-cell lung cancer. J Clin Oncol 30:3084–3092

Polcher M, Eckhardt M, Coch C, Wolfgarten M, Kubler K, Hartmann G et al (2010) Sorafenib in combination with carboplatin and paclitaxel as neoadjuvant chemotherapy in patients with advanced ovarian cancer. Cancer Chemother Pharmacol 66:203–207

Ramasubbaiah R, Perkins SM, Schilder J, Whalen C, Johnson CS, Callahan M et al (2011) Sorafenib in combination with weekly topotecan in recurrent ovarian cancer, a phase I/II study of the Hoosier Oncology Group. Gynecol Oncol 123:499–504

Ranze O, Hofmann E, Distelrath A, Hoeffkes HG (2007) Renal cell cancer presented with leptomeningeal carcinomatosis effectively treated with sorafenib. Onkologie 30:450–451

Ratain MJ, Eisen T, Stadler WM, Flaherty KT, Kaye SB, Rosner GL et al (2006) Phase II placebo-controlled randomized discontinuation trial of sorafenib in patients with metastatic renal cell carcinoma. J Clin Oncol 24:2505–2512

Ravandi F, Cortes JE, Jones D, Faderl S, Garcia-Manero G, Konopleva MY et al (2010) Phase I/II study of combination therapy with sorafenib, idarubicin, and cytarabine in younger patients with acute myeloid leukemia. J Clin Oncol 28:1856–1862

Ravandi F, Alattar ML, Grunwald MR, Rudek MA, Rajkhowa T, Richie MA et al (2013) Phase II study of azacytidine plus sorafenib in patients with acute myeloid leukemia and FLT-3 internal tandem duplication mutation. Blood 121(23):4655–4662

Reardon DA, Vredenburgh JJ, Desjardins A, Peters K, Gururangan S, Sampson JH et al (2011) Effect of CYP3A-inducing anti-epileptics on sorafenib exposure: results of a phase II study of sorafenib plus daily temozolomide in adults with recurrent glioblastoma. J Neurooncol 101:57–66

Richly H, Henning BF, Kupsch P, Passarge K, Grubert M, Hilger RA et al (2006) Results of a Phase I trial of sorafenib (BAY 43-9006) in combination with doxorubicin in patients with refractory solid tumors. Ann Oncol 17:866–873

Rini BI, Escudier B, Tomczak P, Kaprin A, Szczylik C, Hutson TE et al (2011) Comparative effectiveness of axitinib versus sorafenib in advanced renal cell carcinoma (AXIS): a randomised phase III trial. Lancet 378:1931–1939

Rollig C, Brandts C, Shaid S, Hentrich M, Kramer A, Junghanss C et al (2012) Survey and analysis of the efficacy and prescription pattern of sorafenib in patients with acute myeloid leukemia. Leuk Lymphoma 53:1062–1067

Safaian NN, Czibere A, Bruns I, Fenk R, Reinecke P, Dienst A et al (2009) Sorafenib (Nexavar) induces molecular remission and regression of extramedullary disease in a patient with FLT3-ITD$^+$ acute myeloid leukemia. Leuk Res 33:348–350

Safarinejad MR (2008) Safety and efficacy of sorafenib in patients with castrate resistant prostate cancer: a phase II study. Urol Oncol 28:21–27

Salvatore G, De Falco V, Salerno P, Nappi TC, Pepe S, Troncone G et al (2006) BRAF is a therapeutic target in aggressive thyroid carcinoma. Clin Cancer Res 12:1623–1629

Savage DG, Antman KH (2002) Imatinib mesylate—a new oral targeted therapy. N Engl J Med 346:683–693

Savvides P, Nagaiah G, Lavertu P, Fu P, Wright JJ, Chapman R et al (2013) Phase II trial of sorafenib in patients with advanced anaplastic carcinoma of the thyroid. Thyroid 23:600–604

Sayar H, Cripe L, Cangany M, Weisenbach J, Sargent KJ, Goswami C et al (2010) Cyclic administration of combination of sorafenib and vorinostat in poor-risk AML: a pharmacodynamically-oriented extended phase I trial. ASH Annu Meet Abs 116:3272

Scagliotti G, Novello S, von Pawel J, Reck M, Pereira JR, Thomas M et al (2010) Phase III study of carboplatin and paclitaxel alone or with sorafenib in advanced non-small-cell lung cancer. J Clin Oncol 28:1835–1842

Schneider TC, Abdulrahman RM, Corssmit EP, Morreau H, Smit JW, Kapiteijn E (2012) Long-term analysis of the efficacy and tolerability of sorafenib in advanced radio-iodine refractory differentiated thyroid carcinoma: final results of a phase II trial. Eur J Endocrinol 167:643–650

Schroeder T, Zohren F, Saure C, Bruns I, Czibere A, Safaian NN et al (2010) Sorafenib treatment in 13 patients with acute myeloid leukemia and activating FLT3 mutations in combination with chemotherapy or as monotherapy. Acta Haematol 124:153–159

Schwartzberg LS, Tauer KW, Hermann RC, Makari-Judson G, Isaacs C, Beck JT et al (2013) Sorafenib or Placebo with Either Gemcitabine or Capecitabine in Patients with HER-2-Negative Advanced Breast Cancer That Progressed during or after Bevacizumab. Clin Cancer Res 19:2745–2754

Sebolt-Leopold JS, Herrera R (2004) Targeting the mitogen-activated protein kinase cascade to treat cancer. Nat Rev Cancer 4:937–947

Serve H, Wagner R, Sauerland C, Brunnberg U, Krug U, Schaich M et al (2010) Sorafenib in combination with standard induction and consolidation therapy in elderly AML patients: results from a randomized, placebo-controlled phase II trial. ASH Ann Meet Abs 116:333

Sharma M, Ravandi F, Bayraktar UD, Chiattone A, Bashir Q, Giralt S et al (2011) Treatment of FLT3-ITD-positive acute myeloid leukemia relapsing after allogeneic stem cell transplantation with sorafenib. Biol Blood Marrow Transplant 17:1874–1877

Sharma N, Pennell NA, Halmos B, Ma PM, Dowlati A (2012) Phase II trial of sorafenib in conjunction with chemotherapy and as maintenance therapy in extensive-stage small cell lung cancer (SCLC): Final results. J Clin Oncol 30:e17563

Siu LL, Awada A, Takimoto CH, Piccart M, Schwartz B, Giannaris T et al (2006) Phase I trial of sorafenib and gemcitabine in advanced solid tumors with an expanded cohort in advanced pancreatic cancer. Clin Cancer Res 12:144–151

Smalley KS, Xiao M, Villanueva J, Nguyen TK, Flaherty KT, Letrero R et al (2008) CRAF inhibition induces apoptosis in melanoma cells with non-V600E BRAF mutations. Oncogene 28(1):85–94

Spigel DR, Hainsworth JD, Burris HA 3rd, Molthrop DC, Peacock N, Kommor M et al (2011) A pilot study of adjuvant doxorubicin and cyclophosphamide followed by paclitaxel and sorafenib in women with node-positive or high-risk early-stage breast cancer. Clin Adv Hematol Oncol 9:280–286

Steinbild S, Mross K, Frost A, Morant R, Gillessen S, Dittrich C et al (2007) A clinical phase II study with sorafenib in patients with progressive hormone-refractory prostate cancer: a study of the CESAR Central European Society for Anticancer Drug Research-EWIV. Br J Cancer 97:1480–1485

Stirewalt DL, Radich JP (2003) The role of FLT3 in haematopoietic malignancies. Nat Rev Cancer 3:650–665

Strumberg D, Voliotis D, Moeller JG, Hilger RA, Richly H, Kredtke S et al (2002) Results of phase I pharmacokinetic and pharmacodynamic studies of the Raf kinase inhibitor BAY 43-9006 in patients with solid tumors. Int J Clin Pharmacol Ther 40:580–581

Strumberg D, Richly H, Hilger RA, Schleucher N, Korfee S, Tewes M et al (2005) Phase I clinical and pharmacokinetic study of the Novel Raf kinase and vascular endothelial growth factor receptor inhibitor BAY 43-9006 in patients with advanced refractory solid tumors. J Clin Oncol 23:965–972

Sugiyama H, Onuki K, Ishige K, Baba N, Ueda T, Matsuda S et al (2011) Potent in vitro and in vivo antitumor activity of sorafenib against human intrahepatic cholangiocarcinoma cells. J Gastroenterol 46:779–789

Valabrega G, Capellero S, Cavalloni G, Zaccarello G, Petrelli A, Migliardi G et al (2011) HER2-positive breast cancer cells resistant to trastuzumab and lapatinib lose reliance upon HER2 and are sensitive to the multitargeted kinase inhibitor sorafenib. Breast Cancer Res Treat 130:29–40

Valcamonico F, Ferrari V, Amoroso V, Rangoni G, Simoncini E, Marpicati P et al (2008). Long-lasting successful cerebral response with sorafenib in advanced renal cell carcinoma. J Neurooncol 91:47–50

Wakelee HA, Lee JW, Hanna NH, Traynor AM, Carbone DP, Schiller JH (2012) A double-blind randomized discontinuation phase-II study of sorafenib (BAY 43-9006) in previously treated non-small-cell lung cancer patients: eastern cooperative oncology group study E2501. J Thorac Oncol 7:1574–1582

Wang Z, Zhou J, Fan J, Qiu SJ, Yu Y, Huang XW et al (2008) Effect of rapamycin alone and in combination with sorafenib in an orthotopic model of human hepatocellular carcinoma. Clin Cancer Res 14:5124–5130

Welch SA, Hirte HW, Elit L, Schilder RJ, Wang L, Macalpine K et al (2010) Sorafenib in combination with gemcitabine in recurrent epithelial ovarian cancer: a study of the Princess Margaret Hospital Phase II Consortium. Int J Gynecol Cancer 20:787–793

Widemann BC, Kim A, Fox E, Baruchel S, Adamson PC, Ingle AM et al (2012) A phase I trial and pharmacokinetic study of sorafenib in children with refractory solid tumors or leukemias: a Children's Oncology Group Phase I Consortium report. Clin Cancer Res 18:6011–6022

Wilhelm SM, Carter C, Tang L, Wilkie D, McNabola A, Rong H et al (2004) BAY 43-9006 exhibits broad spectrum oral antitumor activity and targets the RAF/MEK/ERK pathway and receptor tyrosine kinases involved in tumor progression and angiogenesis. Cancer Res 64:7099–7109

Wilhelm S, Carter C, Lynch M, Lowinger T, Dumas J, Smith RA et al (2006) Discovery and development of sorafenib: a multikinase inhibitor for treating cancer. Nat Rev Drug Discov 5:835–844

Williamson SK, Moon J, Huang CH, Guaglianone PP, LeBlanc M, Wolf GT et al (2010) Phase II evaluation of sorafenib in advanced and metastatic squamous cell carcinoma of the head and neck: Southwest Oncology Group Study S0420. J Clin Oncol 28:3330–3335

Wishart DS, Knox C, Guo AC, Cheng D, Shrivastava S, Tzur D et al (2008) DrugBank: a knowledgebase for drugs, drug actions and drug targets. Nucleic Acids Res 36:D901–D906

Zhang W, Konopleva M, Shi YX, McQueen T, Harris D, Ling X et al (2008) Mutant FLT3: a direct target of sorafenib in acute myelogenous leukemia. J Natl Cancer Inst 100:184–198

Sunitinib in the Treatment of Advanced Solid Tumors

Amal Imbulgoda, Daniel Y. C. Heng and Christian Kollmannsberger

Abstract

Sunitinib is an oral multikinase inhibitor that blocks the vascular endothelial growth factor receptor (VEGFR), platelet-derived growth factor receptor (PDGFR) alpha and beta, c-kit, and other receptors. These attributes have proven to be efficacious in the treatment of metastatic renal cell carcinoma (RCC), unresectable gastrointestinal stromal tumors (GIST), and well-differentiated advanced pancreatic neuroendocrine tumors (PNET). Though activity has been reported in other tumor types, phase III trials have not yet demonstrated improved survival outcomes in these cancers. Most side effects including hypertension, hand-foot syndrome, and diarrhea are generally well manageable. This review will detail the preclinical data leading up to the results of the pivotal phase III clinical trials that have led to the widespread use of sunitinib in advanced RCC, GIST, and PNET.

Contents

A. Imbulgoda · D. Y. C. Heng
Medical Oncology, Tom Baker Cancer Center, Calgary, Canada

C. Kollmannsberger (✉)
Medical Oncology, British Columbia Cancer Agency, 600 West 10th Avenue, Vancouver, BC V5Z 4E6, Canada
e-mail: ckollmannsberger@bccancer.bc.ca

U. M. Martens (ed.), *Small Molecules in Oncology*, Recent Results in Cancer Research 201, DOI: 10.1007/978-3-642-54490-3_9,

1 Structure and Mechanism of Action

Sunitinib is an oral multikinase inhibitor that blocks VEGFR-1, VEGFR-2 (IC_{50} 4 nM), VEGFR-3, PDGFR-alpha (IC_{50} 69 nM) and beta (IC_{50} 39 nM), c-kit (IC_{50} 1–10 nM), FLT-3 (IC_{50} 250 nM), RET (IC_{50} 50 nM), fibroblast growth factor receptor-1 (FGFR-1) (IC_{50} 880 nM), and colony-stimulating factor 1 (CSF-1) (IC_{50} 50–100 nM) (Christensen 2007; Mendel et al. 2003; Chow and Eckhardt 2007). Note that IC_{50} values must be interpreted with caution as there is great variation between laboratories using different cell lines and in vitro activity may not reflect the same magnitude as in vivo activity. The molecular formula of sunitinib is $C_{22}H_{27}FN_4O_2$, and its structure is represented in Fig. 1 (Sun et al. 2003).

Sunitinib attaches to the adenosine triphosphate (ATP)-binding pocket of these receptor tyrosine kinases. By acting as a competitive inhibitor of ATP, sunitinib prevents activation and downstream cellular signaling (Christensen 2007). Receptor tyrosine kinases play an integral role in the signaling cascade of VEGF and PDGF. Each receptor has an extracellular domain that binds their respective ligand. The transmembrane region spans the membrane into the cytoplasm, and the intracellular domain holds the tyrosine kinase responsible for downstream signal activation. Upon ligand binding, the receptor tyrosine kinases dimerize or multimerize to induce a conformational change that allows ATP binding, resulting in autophosphorylation and transphosphorylation. These phosphorylated tyrosine domains are then able to activate downstream signal transduction by phosphorylation of various other proteins.

2 Preclinical Data

Mouse xenograft studies have demonstrated that sunitinib can cause tumor regression, growth arrest, and reduced tumor growth in a dose-dependent manner. Videomicroscopy has shown evidence of tumor vessel density reduction compared with controls (Laird et al. 2000). These studies suggest that sunitinib has antiangiogenic properties that may explain at least in part its antitumor activity.

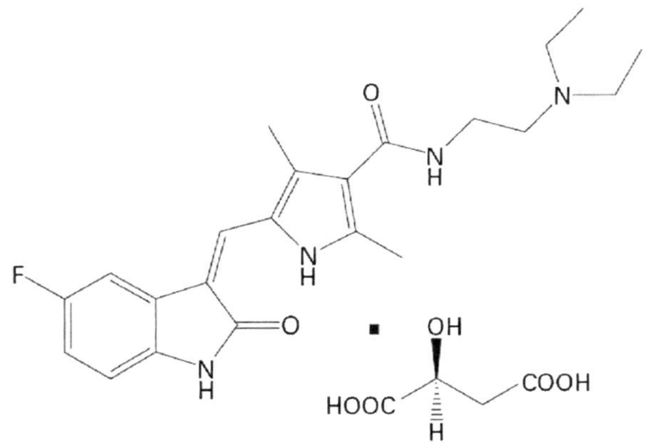

Fig. 1 Molecular structure of sunitinib malate

3 Clinical Data

Phase I dose-finding studies were performed in healthy individuals and those with solid malignancies. A single dose of 50 mg given to healthy individuals was shown to be well tolerated and safe. The time to maximal concentration was 8 h, and the estimated half-life was 60 h (Houk et al. 2005).

Phase I repeat dosing studies (Houk et al. 2005; Faivre et al. 2006) have been performed investigating daily or every 2-day schedules of sunitinib administered in 3 week cycles (2 weeks on, 1 week off), 4 week cycles (2 weeks on, 2 weeks off), and 6 week cycles (4 weeks on, 2 weeks off). Daily dosing of 50 mg produced target plasma concentrations above the 50 ng/mL required to inhibit platelet-derived growth factor receptor (PDGFR) and vascular endothelial growth factor receptor (VEGFR). Plasma concentrations declined to pre-dose levels during the 14 day rest period. Dose-limiting toxicities of fatigue, asthenia, and thrombocytopenia were observed, and thus, the final dose of 50 mg, 4 weeks on and 2 weeks off, was adopted as the standard for future clinical trials.

3.1 Renal Cell Carcinoma

Metastatic renal cell carcinoma (RCC) portends a poor prognosis and will cause an estimated 13,680 deaths in the USA in 2013 (Siegel et al. 2013). Previously, immunotherapy agents such as interleukin-2 and interferon (IFN) alpha were the only treatments available and demonstrated low response rates of approximately 15 % (McDermott et al. 2005; Yang et al. 2003; Negrier et al. 1998, 2007; Coppin et al. 2005, 2008). Based on the increasing knowledge of the biology underlying RCC, agents targeting relevant biologic pathways have been investigated (Cohen and McGovern 2005). This initially developed from the understanding of patients with von Hippel–Lindau (VHL) syndrome that is an inherited, autosomal dominant genetic disorder that commonly manifests by the development of clear cell RCC in most affected patients.

Clear cell RCCs, which account for 85 % of all RCCs, commonly demonstrate aberrations of the VHL gene (Kovacs et al. 1997; Rini and Small 2005) in both hereditary and non-hereditary forms. A single VHL allele deletion occurs in approximately 78.4–98 % of sporadic tumors (Banks et al. 2006; Gnarra et al. 1994; Shuin et al. 1994; Kondo et al. 2002; Brauch et al. 2000; Kenck et al. 1996). For the remaining allele, VHL gene mutations are seen in 34–57 %, while gene inactivation via hypermethylation of CpG-rich DNA islands occurs in about 5–20.4 % of clear cell RCC (Banks et al. 2006; Kondo et al. 2002; Brauch et al. 2000; Clifford et al. 1998; Foster et al. 1994). Thus, it is clear that in both hereditary and sporadic cases of clear cell RCC, VHL abnormalities are a key factor in pathogenesis.

When the VHL gene is mutated or inactivated, the VHL gene product can no longer regulate the degradation of the hypoxia inducible factor (HIF) alpha, which is a transcription factor (Fig. 2). Normally, low oxygen conditions cause HIF alpha to accumulate and bind to HIF beta thereby creating a complex that transcriptionally activates genes related to glucose metabolism, apoptosis, angiogenesis, and endothelial stabilization. In patients with aberrant VHL, HIF alpha is not destroyed and thus is left to freely accumulate without degradation even under normal oxygen conditions. There are over 100 HIF-responsive genes, which include growth factors and their receptors such as VEGF and PDGF (Cohen and McGovern 2005; Rini and Small 2005). These pathways are targeted by sunitinib and have been studied in phase II/III studies to determine efficacy.

3.1.1 Phase II/III Studies in Metastatic RCC

Two multicenter phase II trials treated cytokine-refractory metastatic clear cell RCC patients with sunitinib (Motzer et al. 2006a, b). They demonstrated that 34–40 % of patients receiving oral sunitinib at 50 mg daily for 4 weeks out of a 6 week cycle achieved a partial response (PR) while 27–29 % maintained stable disease (SD) according to the response evaluation criteria in solid tumors (RECIST) guidelines. The median time to progression in the combined analysis of these two studies was 8.2 months. These data led the Food and Drug Administration (FDA) to provisionally approve sunitinib in the treatment of advanced RCC pending confirmation in a randomized controlled trial.

The resulting pivotal phase III trial (Motzer et al. 2007) enrolled 750 patients to compare first-line sunitinib with first-line interferon. This demonstrated a statistically significant difference in progression-free survival (PFS) (11 vs. 5 months) with a hazard ratio of 0.42 ($P < 0.001$). Overall survival data for sunitinib was presented recently showing an impressive difference when compared with interferon (26.4 vs. 21.8 months) (Figlin et al. 2008). Due to the crossover of patients from the interferon group to sunitinib or another VEGF-targeted agent after preliminary results were presented, a dilution of the overall survival benefit may have

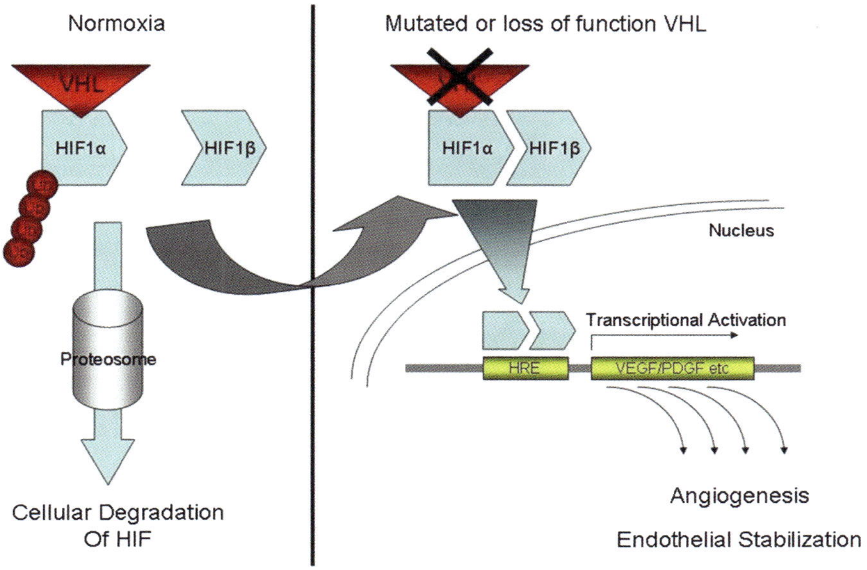

Fig. 2 Normal function of VHL in the normoxic state compared to the aberrant VHL state. Under normal conditions, VHL binds to HIFα and polyubiquinates it to mark it for destruction in the cellular proteosome. When VHL function is lost, HIFα binds HIFβ and then translocates into the nucleus to activate HIF-responsive elements (*HRE*). This results in transcriptional activation of genes important in angiogenesis and endothelial stabilization

occurred. It is important to note that this is the first-randomized study in which the median overall survival of patients with metastatic RCC exceeded 2 years. Based on this data, this agent has become a standard of care for the first-line treatment of metastatic RCC.

It is important to note that the vast majority patients enrolled in this trial (94 %) had favorable or intermediate risk Memorial Sloan Kettering Cancer Center (MSKCC) prognostic criteria (Motzer et al. 2002) and only patients with clear cell histology were enrolled. Thus, the generalizability of this data to patients with poor prognostic profiles or non-clear cell histologies is uncertain. Retrospective studies and population-based experiences have demonstrated that indeed sunitinib has activity in poor risk groups and non-clear cell histologies albeit response rates and overall survival were shorter in these subgroups compared with other patients with mRCC (Kollmannsberger et al. 2007a; Choueiri et al. 2008).

Because papillary (10–15 %), chromophobe (5–10 %), and collecting duct (<1 %) histologies account for a minority of metastatic RCCs, clinical trials investigating sunitinib have excluded these patients with non-clear cell histologies (Heng and Bukowski 2007). A retrospective analysis of 20 patients with non-clear cell mRCC treated with sunitinib demonstrated a response rate of 16 % and a PFS of 11.9 months (Choueiri et al. 2008). In an expanded access trial of sunitinib

(Gore et al. 2007), 2,341 patients were enrolled for which 87.8 % had clear cell histology, 11.8 % had non-clear cell histology, and 0.4 % had missing data about their subtype. Of the 276 patients with non-clear cell histology, the overall response rate was 5.4, 41.6 % had SD, and the PFS for this subgroup was 6.7 months. This is compared with the entire cohort of 2,341 patients in whom the overall response rate was 9.3, 43 % had SD and the PFS for the entire cohort was 8.9 months. Although the quality of data obtained from expanded access trials may not be as precise or accurate as randomized controlled trials, this study demonstrates that patients with non-clear cell histology appear to have a clinically meaningful response to sunitinib.

Sunitinib is being investigated in the adjuvant setting where high-risk localized disease has been resected. The Adjuvant Sorafenib or Sunitinib for Unfavorable Renal Carcinoma intergroup trial (ASSURE, NCT00326898) randomizes high-risk nephrectomized patients to 1 year of sorafenib, sunitinib, or placebo (ASSURE).

Studies combining targeted therapies are being performed with the known caveat that combination therapies are associated with high financial cost and possibly increased toxicity. A phase I trial of bevacizumab and sunitinib in a variety of solid tumors led by the Cleveland Clinic reported 1 unconfirmed PR in a patient with papillary RCC out of 9 evaluable patients (Cooney et al. 2007). Another phase I trial of this combination given exclusively to patients with metastatic RCC reported 4/13 patients with PRs (Feldman et al. 2007). Using a different combination, a randomized phase II trial studying bevacizumab and erlotinib [an inhibitor of the epidermal growth factor receptor (EGFR) pathway] versus bevacizumab and placebo revealed no benefit to the combination in terms of overall response rate or PFS (Bukowski et al. 2007). Currently, combinations of targeted therapy remain experimental, and they should only be employed in the context of a clinical trial.

3.2 Gastrointestinal Stromal Tumors

Gastrointestinal stromal tumors (GIST) are the most common mesenchymal malignancies of the gastrointestinal tract. GISTs are thought to arise from the interstitial cells of Cajal, or a common precursor, and are most commonly found in the stomach and small intestine with metastases most commonly to the liver and peritoneum (Nowain et al. 2005). Although surgery remains the mainstay curative treatment for GIST, half of all patients already have metastatic disease at the time of diagnosis. Additionally, 45–90 % of patients will relapse following even a complete resection (Dematteo et al. 2008). Approximately 85 % of GISTs manifest a mutation in the KIT receptor tyrosine kinase: 67 % in the intracellular domain in exon 11, 18 % in the extramembrane domain in exon 9, and a smaller proportion in exons 13 and 17 (Corless et al. 2004; Heinrich et al. 2003a). The constitutive activation of this receptor affects downstream cellular signaling cascades that promote cellular proliferation and prevent apoptosis. An additional

5–7 % of patients with GIST have an activating mutation of PDGFR-alpha (Corless et al. 2004; Heinrich et al. 2003a). Largely, because of these two types of mutations, imatinib mesylate, which is both a c-kit and PDGFR-alpha inhibitor has become the first-line standard of care in patients with metastatic GIST as demonstrated in a series of randomized trials (Verweij et al. 2004; Demetri et al. 2002; Blanke et al. 2008).

Imatinib was the first-targeted therapy used in the treatment of metastatic GIST, and one of the first to be used in any solid tumor. However, 12–14 % of patients with GIST have primary resistance to imatinib, and 40 % of patients who had initial responses to imatinib develop secondary resistance to the drug after a median of 18–26 months (Verweij et al. 2004). Secondary resistance may develop as a result of secondary mutations in the KIT or PDGFR-alpha kinases, gene amplification, or loss of target expression (Weisberg and Griffin 2003; Van Glabbeke et al. 2005). Thus, second-line therapy for metastatic GIST was greatly needed, and sunitinib has assumed this role.

3.2.1 GIST Clinical Trials

The efficacy and safety of sunitinib was initially evaluated in an open-label phase I/II study where the optimum dosing was determined to be 50 mg daily for 4 weeks followed by a 2-week break (6 week cycle). Ninety-seven imatinib-resistant or intolerant patients were enrolled in this trial. Of these, 7 % had RECIST-defined PRs, and 27 % had SD for 6 months or longer. The time to tumor progression (TTP) was 34 weeks (Maki et al. 2005).

Subsequently, a phase III double-blinded randomized placebo-controlled trial was performed with a 2:1 randomization scheme. Three hundred and twelve patients with imatinib-refractory or resistant unresectable GIST were accrued (Demetri et al. 2006). Eight percent of patients exhibited a PR in the sunitinib group versus 0 % in the placebo group. The median TTP was 27.3 weeks in those treated with sunitinib versus 6.4 weeks in those treated placebo (HR 0.33, $p < 0.0001$). The hazard ratio for overall survival was 0.49 in favor of the sunitinib group ($p = 0.007$) though median survivals had not yet been reached for this analysis. This pivotal study formed the basis for the FDA to approve sunitinib in patients with unresectable GIST with disease progression or intolerance to imatinib (Goodman et al. 2007).

Upon the presentation of these results, patients in the trial were unblinded so that all could receive open-label sunitinib (Demetri et al. 2006). Despite this crossover, improvements in TTP were maintained (28.4 vs. 8.2 weeks $p < 0.0001$). The crossover also allowed for a comparison of overall survival in patients who were treated immediately with sunitinib versus those that were initially treated with placebo and then crossed over to sunitinib (delayed administration). The overall survival of the delayed (24.3 weeks) versus the immediate (28.9 weeks) administration groups was comparable. Although this result is interesting, one must be cautious in its interpretation because the delayed administration group is selected in that patients survived long enough to eventually crossover.

Response to sunitinib appears to be affected by pre-imatinib tumor genotypes. It appears that those patients with wild-type genotypes or a primary KIT exon 9 mutation have a significantly longer PFS and overall survival than patients with exon 11 mutations (Heinrich et al. 2008). This is contrary to the pattern seen with imatinib wherein exon 11 mutations are associated with greater response rates and improved survival compared with wild type or exon 9-mutated KIT (Heinrich et al. 2003b).

Investigations into the appropriate dosing schedule of sunitinib were made after anecdotal experience demonstrated tumor growth while on the 2-week sunitinib break (George et al. 2008). A phase II open-label, multicenter trial randomized 60 imatinib-refractory patients to either morning or evening sunitinib dosing at 37.5 mg daily continuously without the 2-week break. Twelve percent of patients had a PR, and the median PFS was 32 weeks. Although cross-trial comparisons should be interpreted with caution, these outcomes appeared comparable to those seen in the aforementioned phase III trial of sunitinib dosed at 50 mg daily for 4 weeks followed by a 2-week break (Demetri et al. 2006). The continuous dosing trial included the analysis of VEGF, soluble (s)VEGFR-2, sVEGFR-3, and sKIT concentrations in these patients, which confirmed the persistent pharmacologic effect of sunitinib with continuous dosing. There was no rebound in these concentrations, which are otherwise observed during off-treatment periods with continuous dosing. Finally, a decrease in plasma sKIT after the first 3 cycles and particularly after cycle 5 ($p = 0.007$) was associated with a longer overall survival compared with those without a decrease in plasma sKIT (George et al. 2008). These preliminary results will require further prospective evaluation as to whether continuous dosing is just as efficacious as intermittent dosing and whether biomarkers such as sKIT can be used to predict prognosis or response.

3.3 Pancreatic Neuroendocrine Tumors

Pancreatic neuroendocrine tumors (PNET) are characterized by the expression of neuroendocrine markers such as synaptophysin and chromogranin A (Ehehalt et al. 2009). These neoplasms are rare, with an incidence of approximately two cases per million in the USA; however, this number has been increasing over time (Halfdanarson et al. 2008). Most cases are sporadic (Modlin et al. 2008), but may associated with the familial genetic syndromes VHL, multiple endocrine neoplasia type 1, neurofibromatosis type 1, and tuberous sclerosis (Ehehalt et al. 2009).

PNET are heterogeneous with respect to clinical presentation, biology, propensity to metastasize, and prognosis (Mansour and Chen 2004). The 2010 WHO scheme for digestive system neuroendocrine tumors attempts to classify PNET by histology, i.e., well-differentiated (low or intermediate grade) and poorly differentiated, based on mitotic counts and Ki-67 indices (Klimstra et al. 2010). Also, some PNET can be separated into functioning, i.e., causing symptoms by secretion of excess hormones, or non-functioning.

A variety of treatment modalities exist for the treatment of PNET. In those tumors that are localized, surgery can be curative. Unfortunately, over 60 % of PNET are metastatic at diagnosis (Halfdanarson et al. 2008). Surgery also has a palliative role in these patients, particularly in the setting of liver metastases. Hepatic artery embolisation, somatostatin analogs, interferons, and cytotoxic chemotherapy have been used in unresectable disease as well (Mansour and Chen 2004). In the period from 1973 to 2000, the median overall survival for metastatic disease was a dismal 17 months, but has improved over time (Halfdanarson et al. 2008). Since then, a better understanding of the molecular biology of PNET has stimulated the development of more effective targeted therapies, which have now become standard of care treatment.

Molecular signaling pathways implicated in the pathogenesis of PNET include VEGF, PDGF, mTOR, EGFR, and c-kit (Casanovas et al. 2005; Hansel et al. 2003; Inoue et al. 2002; La Rosa et al. 2003; Terris et al. 1998; Chaudhry et al. 1992; Fjällskog et al. 2003, 2007; Yao et al. 2011; Wulbrand et al. 1998). As an inhibitor of VEGF and PDGF, sunitinib was considered a promising candidate for clinical study. Faivre et al. (2006) in their phase I dose-escalation trial, enrolled four patients with unspecified neuroendocrine tumors, one of whom had an objective response. This finding prompted a phase II trial.

3.3.1 PNET Clinical Trials

A phase II, multicenter, open-label trial treated 107 patients with advanced neuroendocrine tumors (66 with PNET, 41 with carcinoid tumors) with 6 week cycles of sunitinib (50 mg daily for 4 weeks, then 2-weeks off) (Kulke et al. 2008). In the PNET cohort, the overall objective response rate (ORR) was 16.7 %, with all of those patients experiencing PRs. An additional 56.1 % had SD lasting at least 6 months. Median TTP was 4.0 months. Efficacy in the carcinoid group was modest—only one patient had a response to treatment.

The promising findings in the PNET cohort led to the opening of a multinational, double-blind phase III trial (Raymond et al. 2011). In this study, 171 patients were randomly assigned 1:1 to sunitinib 37.5 mg continuous daily administration or placebo. Only patients with pathologically confirmed, well-differentiated tumors were eligible to participate. The trial was stopped early because an interim safety analysis revealed a clear difference in terms of deaths (10 vs. 25 %), PFS, and severe adverse events favoring the sunitinib arm. Subsequently, 59 patients in the placebo arm crossed over to sunitinib in a new clinical trial. In the intent-to-treat population, the estimated median PFS was 11.4 months for sunitinib versus 5.5 for placebo, with a hazard ratio for progression or death of 0.42 ($p < 0.001$). ORR was 9.3 % for the treatment arm versus 0 % ($p = 0.007$). Median overall survival was not reached at the time of trial closure. The most recent data, at 2 years following closure, report a median PFS of 12.6 versus 5.8 months still favoring sunitinib (HR 0.32, $P = 0.00001$) (Vinik et al. 2012). Median OS was estimated at 33.0 versus 26.7 months (HR 0.71, $P = 0.11$). The authors reported that 69 % of patients had crossed over from placebo upon disease progression.

3.4 Other Solid Tumors

Preliminary evidence has suggested promising activity of sunitinib in other tumor groups. Dose-finding studies of sunitinib in addition to standard chemotherapy and preliminary efficacy analyses have also been reported in prostate, bladder, testicular, and colorectal cancers among other solid malignancies. Recently, phase III-randomized trials comparing sunitinib to standard of care therapy in metastatic breast, lung, and colorectal cancers have been completed.

3.4.1 Breast

In a phase II trial of 64 patients with refractory, metastatic breast cancer, sunitinib treatment resulted in an 11 % ORR mostly seen in patients with triple negative (ER-, PR-, HER2-) breast cancers or HER2 positive cancers previously treated with trastuzumab (Burstein et al. 2008). This led to the opening of two randomized, open-label phase III trials comparing sunitinib 37.5 mg daily (2-weeks on/1-week off) with the standard of care in patients with advanced triple negative breast cancers. Both were negative studies (Barrios et al. 2010; Bergh et al. 2012). The comparator treatments were capecitabine 1,250 mg/m^2 (1,000 mg/m^2 in patients >65 years) twice daily on days 1–14 every 3 weeks and docetaxel (100 mg/m^2 every 3 weeks), respectively. The combination of sunitinib (25 mg continuous daily dosing) with paclitaxel (90 mg/m^2) was compared with bevacizumab (another VEGF inhibitor, 10 mg/kg) plus paclitaxel in patients with unresectable or advanced HER-2 negative breast cancer (Robert et al. 2011). This trial was terminated due to futility in reaching the primary endpoint of improved median PFS.

3.4.2 Non-small Cell Lung Cancer (NSCLC)

A phase III study of erlotinib combined with sunitinib 37.5 mg daily or placebo in previously treated advanced NSCLC showed no improvement in the primary endpoint of median OS (Scagliotti et al. 2012). The currently active phase III CALBG 30607 trial is assigning patients with advanced NSCLC who have achieved a response or SD with four cycles of platinum-based chemotherapy to sunitinib or placebo as maintenance therapy (Sunitinib Malate).

3.4.3 Colorectal

In metastatic colorectal cancer, a phase III study comparing FOLFIRI plus sunitinib (37.5 mg daily; 4 weeks on/2 weeks off) with FOLFIRI plus placebo was stopped prematurely because of potential futility and clearly more toxicity in the sunitinib arm (Carrato et al. 2013). The mFOLFOX6 regimen in combination with sunitinib was compared to mFOLFOX6 plus bevacizumab in a phase II study. This trial was recently terminated early, and the results have yet to be reported (FOLFOX).

3.4.4 Non-GIST Sarcomas

A phase II trial has looked at the efficacy of sunitinib in metastatic and locally advanced incurable soft tissue neoplasms (George et al. 2009). Fifty-three patients with a variety of sarcomas were treated with sunitinib 37.5 mg daily continuously,

48 of whom were assessable for response. One patient with desmoplastic round cell tumor had a PR by RECIST criteria. This individual stayed on treatment for 56 weeks before experiencing progression of disease. Another six patients (12 %) had SD at 24 weeks. Twenty-one participants in the trial also had FDG-PET imaging done at baseline and after 2 weeks of therapy. An impressive 48 % experienced a PR, and 52 % had SD based on European Organisation for Research and Treatment of Cancer (EORTC) criteria.

3.4.5 Thyroid

Sunitinib has shown evidence of efficacy in phase II trials involving patients with some forms of metastatic thyroid cancer refractory to other treatments. Cohen et al. (2008) reported on a study that enrolled 37 patients with differentiated thyroid cancer (DTC) and six patients with medullary thyroid cancer (MTC).

They were treated with 50 mg daily on a 4-weeks on/2-weeks off schedule. In the 31 evaluable DTC patients completing two cycles, a PR was seen in 13 % and SD in 68 %. In the MTC group, 83 % had SD. Interim results of the THYSU trial showed that in 15 patients with MTC, five (33.3 %) had a PR and four (26.7 %) had SD on the 50 mg daily, 4 weeks on/2 weeks off schedule (Ravaud et al. 2010). On the 37.5 mg continuous daily dosing schedule, another study of 35 patients (28 DTC, 7 MTC) found a response rate of 31 % and median time to progression of 12.8 months (Carr et al. 2010).

3.4.6 Ovarian/Fallopian/Primary Peritoneal

Interim results of a phase II study of sunitinib in previously treated patients with recurrent ovarian, fallopian tube, or primary peritoneal carcinomas have exhibited two PRs and 10 patients with SD out of the 17 patients enrolled (Biagi et al. 2008).

4 Toxicity

Most side effects increase in intensity as the cycle progresses but then decrease during the 2-week break. Side effects can be managed with preventative and symptomatic measures, dose reductions or delays and schedule changes. Patients usually start at a dose of 50 mg orally for 4 weeks and take a 2-week break. If toxicities become an issue, sunitinib can be dose-reduced to 37.5 mg for 4 weeks followed by a 2-week break. If another dose reduction is required, 25 mg for 4 weeks followed by a 2-week break can be considered; however, a number of patients will be underdosed with 25 mg daily and may show progression of their disease. Recently published data suggest that a dose-response relationship exists for sunitinib, particularly in renal cell carcinoma (Houk et al. 2007). Therefore, grade 1/2 toxicities should be managed symptomatically, while dose reductions should be reserved for those patients with otherwise intolerable side effects. If side effects become intolerable in the third or fourth week, a schedule change to 50 mg/day for 2 weeks followed by a 1-week break rather than a dose reduction may be helpful and allow to maintain a high dose intensity.

Table 1 Precautions and side effects of sunitinib

Precautions	Common and major side effects
• Caution in preexisting uncontrolled hypertension, left ventricular dysfunction, or arrhythmias	• Fatigue
	• Hand-foot syndrome
	• Diarrhea
• Avoid pregnancy and breastfeeding	• Hypertension
	• Mucositis/Stomatitis
	• Hypothyroidism
	• Yellow discoloration of skin (not jaundice)
	• Bleeding
	• Cardiotoxicity

The most common side effects of sunitinib include generalized fatigue and anorexia. It is important to rule out other underlying causes of these symptoms. More characteristic side effects include hand-foot syndrome, diarrhea, hypertension, mucositis, and stomatitis (Table 1) (Kollmannsberger et al. 2007b).

The hand-foot syndrome is a blistering and potentially ulcerating condition of pressure points that can be quite painful. Patients should use moisturizing lotions for their hands and feet and avoid injuries or overuse, which may exacerbate the pressure points. Tight jewelery and shoes, shaving of the blisters, and exposure to extremes of temperature should be avoided as these may exacerbate the symptoms.

Diarrhea can be managed with agents including loperamide and diphenoxylate, and patients should refrain from taking laxatives. The diarrhea usually resolves once the 2-week break commences. Hypertension should be regularly monitored and treated with standard antihypertensives according to existing hypertension guidelines; however, those drugs that interact with CYP3A4 (see Drug Interactions) should be avoided. Mucositis and stomatitis can be treated with good oral hygiene, non-alcoholic mouthwashes (e.g., with baking soda), viscous lidocaine, non-peroxide toothpastes, and lip creams or balms.

Skin and hair manifestations are also common. A generalized yellow discoloration of the skin due to sunitinib and its active metabolite and can often be confused for jaundice. Occasionally, a maculopapular or seborrheic dermatitis-like rash can appear with sunitinib therapy. Additionally, depigmentation of the hair can occur 5–6 weeks into treatment. All these manifestations are reversible upon discontinuation of the drug.

Sunitinib-induced hypothyroidism is a phenomenon with greater incidence upon progressive cycles of sunitinib. Although the mechanism is not completely understood, there may be some similarities to propylthiouracil in the way it inhibits thyroid peroxidise (Wong et al. 2007). In preclinical models, thyroid capillary regression and an increase in thyroid-stimulating hormone (TSH) have been demonstrated. Patients on sunitinib therapy should have their TSH measured on day 1 and 28 of the first 4 cycles and if normal, monitored every 2–3 months (Wolter et al. 2008). When patients develop hypothyroidism, hormone replacement should be initiated to treat the associated symptoms and to achieve biochemical normalization (Rini et al. 2007).

Cardiotoxicity is a rare but well-recognized adverse effect of sunitinib. A meta-analysis including 6,935 patients in phase II/III trials treated with this drug reported an overall incidence of congestive heart failure (CHF) of 4.1 % (Richards et al. 2011). Severe CHF (grade 3 or higher) was found in 1.5 %. Subgroup analysis revealed no significant differences in rates of CHF between RCC and non-RCC trials, studies with and without cardiac monitoring, and trials with an observed PFS less than that of the median PFS of all trials and those with a longer PFS. In a retrospective analysis from a single institution, 48 patients treated with sunitinib were assessable (Witteles et al. 2008). Eighty-five percent had a diagnosis of renal cell carcinoma. Seven (14.6 %) patients experienced symptomatic grade 3/4 left ventricular dysfunction 22–435 days after initiation of sunitinib. Three out of five patients with subsequent cardiac evaluations had persistent left ventricular dysfunction after discontinuation of sunitinib and initiation of standard heart failure therapy. The mean age of patients experiencing cardiotoxicity was 67 years. A history of CHF ($p = 0.002$), coronary artery disease ($p = 0.05$), and lower body mass index ($p = 0.03$) were factors associated with increased risk. Of note, in contrast to anthracycline-induced cardiotoxicity, sunitinib-induced cardiotoxicity appears reversible and can be treated according to heart failure recommendations. As more evidence is emerging on cardiotoxicity, clinicians should consider performing baseline cardiac imaging and monitor for symptoms of CHF in patients with predisposing risk factors or a prior history of heart disease.

Sunitinib-induced hypertension has been reported in 11–26 % (2–10 % grade 3/4) of patients in phase III trials (Motzer et al. 2007; Demetri et al. 2006; Barrios et al. 2010; Bergh et al. 2012; Robert et al. 2011; Carrato et al. 2013). A small study of 14 patients with advanced RCC after unilateral nephrectomy demonstrated substantial increases in blood pressure within the first 4 weeks of treatment. These changes were detected by home blood pressure monitoring (HBPM) and were not as evident on office measurements. The authors propose that HBPM may have a role in the earlier detection of antiangiogenic agent-related hypertension (Azizi et al. 2008).

Bleeding occurred in 19.3 % of patients in a meta-analysis that included 3,445 patients in phase II/III trials of sunitinib (Je et al. 2009). High grade bleeding, including cases of fatal pulmonary and cerebral hemorrhage, was seen in 3.0 %. This study also found similar results for sorafenib, another VEGF inhibitor. Caution is advised in prescribing these agents to patients who are already on antiplatelet or anticoagulant therapy.

Macrocytosis has also been documented in patients receiving sunitinib. In a retrospective analysis, the macrocytosis resolves when the drug is stopped for other reasons. In the limited number of bone marrow examinations in these patients, no evidence of metastases were found. Although the long-term clinical implications are unknown, macrocytosis does not appear to cause any deleterious effects (Rini et al. 2008). Other well-recognized hematologic side effects include thrombocytopenia and neutropenia which occur in approximately 20 % of patients, which may require dose delays or reductions (Motzer et al. 2006a, b, 2007).

5 Drug Interactions

It is important to note that the active metabolite of sunitinib, SU012662, is produced by the cytochrome P450-3A4 system (CYP3A4). Drugs that are inhibitors of the CYP3A4 system such as ketoconazole, aprepitant, diltiazem, fluoxetine, glyburide, grapefruit juice, propranolol, and verapamil could reduce the amount of active metabolite produced. CPY3A4 inducer drugs such as rifampin, carbamazepine, phenytoin, St. John's wort, and troglitazone could potentially increase the active metabolite and associated side effects. Thus, concurrent administration of sunitinib with these drugs, especially those requiring a narrow therapeutic window, should be avoided (Kollmannsberger et al. 2007b). When given together, close observation of toxicity and response with appropriate dose adjustments is mandatory.

6 Biomarkers

Several candidate biomarkers have emerged, particularly with respect to metastatic renal cell carcinoma, which may help identify those patients who are more likely to benefit from sunitinib and those at higher risk for toxicity. These include several genetic and circulating markers. Clinically, certain toxicities may be indicative of treatment efficacy (Yuasa et al. 2011). Further validation in clinical studies is required, however, before these biomarkers are incorporated into routine clinical care.

Single nucleotide polymorphisms with potential prognostic value in sunitinib-treated renal cell carcinoma have been identified. These include variants of genes encoding for ATP-binding cassette proteins (involved in gastrointestinal tract absorption of sunitinib), CYP3A5 and NR1I3 (both involved in drug metabolism), PDGFR-alpha, and VEGFR2 (Yuasa et al. 2011). One prospective study enrolled 101 patients receiving first-line sunitinib in RCC, and tested for 16 single nucleotide polymorphisms that were identified as potentially relevant to sunitinib efficacy and toxicity, based on the findings of previous research (Garcia-Donas et al. 2011). Identified were two missense mutations in VEGFR3 associated with reduced PFS, and one high-metabolizing allele of CYP3A5*1 which had a statistically significant hazard ratio (HR 3.75, $p = 0.022$) for toxicity-related dose reduction.

In patients treated with sunitinib, levels of some circulating biomarkers rise or fall. These responses appear to have prognostic value. In mRCC, markers of interest include VEGF/soluble VEGF receptor, placental growth factor, circulating endothelial progenitors, and circulating endothelial cells (Yuasa et al. 2011). In GIST, lower levels of soluble KIT following treatment were predictive of improved TTP in one study (DePrimo et al. 2009).

Retrospective analyses of trials of sunitinib in mRCC have suggested that the development of hypertension, hand-foot syndrome, asthenia, hypothyroidism, neutropenia, and thrombocytopenia may be associated with improved survival (Rini et al. 2011; Donskov et al. 2011a, 2012; Schmidinger et al. 2011). Similarly, in GIST patients, hypertension, neutropenia, and asthenia were again identified as potential biomarkers of efficacy (George et al. 2012; Donskov et al. 2011b; Davis et al. 2011).

7 Summary and Perspectives

Sunitinib and other VEGF-targeted therapies have revolutionized the treatment of advanced RCC, GIST, and PNET. Through the identification of relevant pathways associated with tumor growth and angiogenesis, we now have effective tools to treat these patients more effectively. Sunitinib has become a first-line standard of care for patients with metastatic RCC and well-differentiated PNET, and it is a standard of care for patients with GIST after progressing on or being intolerant to imatinib. Research is underway to determine if sunitinib will have efficacy in other tumor types.

References

ASSURE: Adjuvant Sorafenib or Sunitinib for Unfavorable Renal Carcinoma. http://clinicaltrials.gov/ct2/show/NCT00326898

Azizi M, Chedid A, Oudard S (2008) Home blood-pressure monitoring in patients receiving sunitinib. N Engl J Med 358:95–97

Banks RE, Tirukonda P, Taylor C et al (2006) Genetic and epigenetic analysis of von Hippel–Lindau (VHL) gene alterations and relationship with clinical variables in sporadic renal cancer. Cancer Res 66:2000–2011

Barrios CH, Liu MC, Lee SC et al (2010) Phase III randomized trial of sunitinib versus capecitabine in patients with previously treated HER2-negative advanced breast cancer. Breast Cancer Res Treat 121:121–131

Bergh J, Bondarenko IM, Lichinitser MR et al (2012) First-line treatment of advanced breast cancer with sunitinib in combination with docetaxel versus docetaxel alone: results of a prospective, randomized phase III study. J Clin Oncol 30:921–929

Biagi JJ, Oza AM, Grimshaw R et al (2008) A phase II study of sunitinib (SU11248) in patients (pts) with recurrent epithelial ovarian, fallopian tube or primary peritoneal carcinoma—NCIC CTG IND 185. J Clin Oncol 26:5522

Blanke CD, Rankin C, Demetri GD et al (2008) Phase III randomized, intergroup trial assessing imatinib mesylate at two dose levels in patients with unresectable or metastatic gastrointestinal stromal tumors expressing the kit receptor tyrosine kinase: S0033. J Clin Oncol 26:626–632

Brauch H, Weirich G, Brieger J et al (2000) VHL alterations in human clear cell renal cell carcinoma: association with advanced tumor stage and a novel hot spot mutation. Cancer Res 60:1942–1948

Bukowski RM, Kabbinavar FF, Figlin RA et al (2007) Randomized phase II study of erlotinib combined with bevacizumab compared with bevacizumab alone in metastatic renal cell cancer. J Clin Oncol 25:4536–4541
Burstein HJ, Elias AD, Rugo HS et al (2008) Phase II study of sunitinib malate, an oral multitargeted tyrosine kinase inhibitor, in patients with metastatic breast cancer previously treated with an anthracycline and a taxane. J Clin Oncol 26:1810–1816
Carr LL, Mankoff DA, Goulart BH et al (2010) Phase II study of daily sunitinib in FDG-PET-positive, iodine-refractory differentiated thyroid cancer and metastatic medullary carcinoma of the thyroid with functional imaging correlation. Clin Cancer Res 16:5260–5268
Carrato A, Swieboda-Sadlej A, Staszewska-Skurczynska M et al (2013) Fluorouracil, leucovorin, and irinotecan plus either sunitinib or placebo in metastatic colorectal cancer: a randomized, phase III trial. J Clin Oncol 31:1341–1347
Casanovas O, Hicklin DJ, Bergers G et al (2005) Drug resistance by evasion of antiangiogenic targeting of VEGF signaling in late-stage pancreatic islet tumors. Cancer Cell 8:299–309
Chaudhry A, Papanicolaou V, Oberg K et al (1992) Expression of platelet-derived growth factor and its receptors in neuroendocrine tumors of the digestive system. Cancer Res 52:1006–1012
Choueiri TK, Plantade A, Elson P et al (2008) Efficacy of sunitinib and sorafenib in metastatic papillary and chromophobe renal cell carcinoma. J Clin Oncol 26:127–131
Chow LQ, Eckhardt SG (2007) Sunitinib: from rational design to clinical efficacy. J Clin Oncol 25:884–896
Christensen JG (2007) A preclinical review of sunitinib, a multitargeted receptor tyrosine kinase inhibitor with anti-angiogenic and antitumour activities. Ann Oncol 18(Suppl 10):x3–x10
Clifford SC, Prowse AH, Affara NA et al (1998) Inactivation of the von Hippel–Lindau (VHL) tumour suppressor gene and allelic losses at chromosome arm 3p in primary renal cell carcinoma: evidence for a VHL-independent pathway in clear cell renal tumourigenesis. Genes Chromosomes Cancer 22:200–209
Cohen HT, McGovern FJ (2005) Renal-cell carcinoma. N Engl J Med 353:2477–2490
Cohen EE, Needles BM, Cullen KJ et al (2008) Phase 2 study of sunitinib in refractory thyroid cancer. J Clin Oncol 26(suppl; abstract 6025)
Cooney MM, Garcia J, Brell J et al (2007) A phase I study of bevacizumab in combination with sunitinib in advanced solid tumors. J Clin Oncol 25:15532
Coppin C, Porzsolt F, Awa A et al (2005) Immunotherapy for advanced renal cell cancer. Cochrane Database Syst Rev (1):CD001425
Coppin C, Le L, Porzsolt F et al (2008) Targeted therapy for advanced renal cell carcinoma. Cochrane Database Syst Rev (2):CD006017
Corless CL, Fletcher JA, Heinrich MC (2004) Biology of gastrointestinal stromal tumors. J Clin Oncol 22:3813–3825
Davis MP, Goldstein D, George S et al (2011) Asthenia and fatigue as predictors of sunitinib efficacy in gastrointestinal stromal tumour (GIST). Eur J Cancer 47(suppl; abstract 1140)
Dematteo RP, Gold JS, Saran L et al (2008) Tumor mitotic rate, size, and location independently predict recurrence after resection of primary gastrointestinal stromal tumor (GIST). Cancer 112:608–615
Demetri GD, von Mehren M, Blanke CD et al (2002) Efficacy and safety of imatinib mesylate in advanced gastrointestinal stromal tumors. N Engl J Med 347:472–480
Demetri GD, van Oosterom AT, Garrett CR et al (2006) Efficacy and safety of sunitinib in patients with advanced gastrointestinal stromal tumour after failure of imatinib: a randomised controlled trial. Lancet 368:1329–1338
DePrimo SE, Huang X, Blackstein ME et al (2009) Circulating levels of soluble KIT serve as a biomarker for clinical outcome in gastrointestinal stromal tumor patients receiving sunitinib following imatinib failure. Clin Cancer Res 15:5869–5877
Donskov F, Cams A, Barrios CH et al (2011a) Neutropenia and thrombocytopenia during treatment as biomarkers of sunitinib efficacy in patients with metastatic renal cell carcinoma (mRCC). Eur J Cancer 47(suppl; abstract 1141)

Donskov F, von Mehren M, Cams A et al (2011b) Neutropenia as a biomarker of sunitinib efficacy in patients (Pts) with gastrointestinal stromal tumour (GIST). Eur J Cancer 47(suppl; abstract 1138)

Donskov F, Michaelson MD, Puzanov I et al (2012) Comparative assessment of sunitinib-associated adverse events as potential biomarkers of efficacy in metastatic renal cell carcinoma (mRCC). Ann Oncol 23(suppl; abstract 785O)

Ehehalt F, Saeger HD, Schmidt CM et al (2009) Neuroendocrine tumors of the pancreas. Oncologist 14:456–467

Faivre S, Delbaldo C, Vera K et al (2006) Safety, pharmacokinetic, and antitumor activity of SU11248, a novel oral multitarget tyrosine kinase inhibitor, in patients with cancer. J Clin Oncol 24:25–35

Feldman DR, Kondagunta GV, Ronnen EA et al (2007) Phase I trial of bevacizumab plus sunitinib in patients (pts) with metastatic renal cell carcinoma (mRCC). J Clin Oncol 25:5099

Figlin RA, Hutson TE, Tomczak P et al (2008) Overall survival with sunitinib versus interferon (IFN)-alfa as first-line treatment of metastatic renal cell carcinoma (mRCC). J Clin Oncol 26:5024

Fjällskog ML, Lejonklou MH, Oberg KE et al (2003) Expression of molecular targets for tyrosine kinase receptor antagonists in malignant endocrine pancreatic tumors. Clin Cancer Res 9:1469–1473

Fjällskog ML, Hessman O, Eriksson B et al (2007) Upregulated expression of PDGF receptor beta in endocrine pancreatic tumors and metastases compared to normal endocrine pancreas. Acta Oncol 46:741–746

Foster K, Prowse A, van den Berg A et al (1994) Somatic mutations of the von Hippel–Lindau disease tumour suppressor gene in non-familial clear cell renal carcinoma. Hum Mol Genet 3:2169–2173

Garcia-Donas J, Esteban E, Leandro-García LJ et al (2011) Single nucleotide polymorphism associations with response and toxic effects in patients with advanced renal-cell carcinoma treated with first-line sunitinib: a multicentre, observational, prospective study. Lancet Oncol 12:1143–1150

George S, Blay JY, Casali PG et al (2008) Continuous daily dosing (CDD) of sunitinib (SU) in pts with advanced GIST: updated efficacy, safety, PK and pharmacodynamic analysis. J Clin Oncol 26:10554

George S, Merriam P, Maki RG et al (2009) Multicenter phase II trial of sunitinib in the treatment of nongastrointestinal stromal tumor sarcomas. J Clin Oncol 27:3154–3160

George S, Reichardt P, Lechner T et al (2012) Hypertension as a potential biomarker of efficacy in patients with gastrointestinal stromal tumor treated with sunitinib. Ann Oncol 23:3180–3187

Gnarra JR, Tory K, Weng Y et al (1994) Mutations of the VHL tumour suppressor gene in renal carcinoma. Nat Genet 7:85–90

Goodman VL, Rock EP, Dagher R et al (2007) Approval summary: sunitinib for the treatment of imatinib refractory or intolerant gastrointestinal stromal tumors and advanced renal cell carcinoma. Clin Cancer Res 13:1367–1373

Gore ME, Porta C, Oudard S et al (2007) Sunitinib in metastatic renal cell carcinoma (mRCC): preliminary assessment of toxicity in an expanded access trial with subpopulation analysis. J Clin Oncol 25:5010

Halfdanarson TR, Rabe KG, Rubin J et al (2008) Pancreatic neuroendocrine tumors (PNETs): incidence, prognosis and recent trend toward improved survival. Ann Oncol 19:1727–1733

Hansel DE, Rahman A, Hermans J et al (2003) Liver metastases arising from well-differentiated pancreatic endocrine neoplasms demonstrate increased VEGF-C expression. Mod Pathol 16:652–659

Heinrich MC, Corless CL, Demetri GD et al (2003) Kinase mutations and imatinib response in patients with metastatic gastrointestinal stromal tumor. J Clin Oncol 21:4342–4349

Heinrich MC, Maki RG, Corless CL et al (2008) Primary and secondary kinase genotypes correlate with the biological and clinical activity of sunitinib in imatinib-resistant gastrointestinal stromal tumor. J Clin Oncol 26:5352–5359
Heng DY, Bukowski RM (2007) Renal cell carcinoma: evolving approaches to advanced non-clear cell carcinoma. Oncol Rev 1:170–176
Houk B, Garrett M, Bello C (2005) Population pharmacokinetics of SU011248 and its primary metabolite SU12662 in oncology patients and healthy volunteers. In: Presented at the EORTC/AACR/NCI molecular targets meeting, Philadelphia, PA, 14–18 Nov 2005
Houk BE, Bello CL, Michaelson MD et al (2007) Exposure-response of sunitinib in metastatic renal cell carcinoma (mRCC): a population pharmacokinetic/pharmacodynamic (PKPD) approach. J Clin Oncol 25:5027
Inoue M, Hager JH, Ferrara N et al (2002) VEGF-A has a critical, nonredundant role in angiogenic switching and pancreatic beta cell carcinogenesis. Cancer Cell 1:193–202
Je Y, Schutz FA, Choueiri TK (2009) Risk of bleeding with vascular endothelial growth factor receptor tyrosine-kinase inhibitors sunitinib and sorafenib: a systematic review and meta-analysis of clinical trials. Lancet Oncol 10:967–974
Kenck C, Wilhelm M, Bugert P et al (1996) Mutation of the VHL gene is associated exclusively with the development of non-papillary renal cell carcinomas. J Pathol 179:157–161
Klimstra DS, Arnold R, Capella C et al (2010) Neuroendocrine neoplasms of the pancreas. WHO classification of tumours of the digestive system, pp 322–326
Kollmannsberger C, Heng DY, Murray N et al (2007a) A population-based study evaluating metastatic renal cell cancer (mRCC) patients treated with interferon (IFN) alone, first-line IFN then second-line sunitinib, or sunitinib alone. J Clin Oncol 25:15572
Kollmannsberger C, Soulieres D, Wong R et al (2007b) Sunitinib therapy for metastatic renal cell carcinoma: recommendations for management of side effects. Can Urol Assoc J 1:S41–S54
Kondo K, Yao M, Yoshida M et al (2002) Comprehensive mutational analysis of the VHL gene in sporadic renal cell carcinoma: relationship to clinicopathological parameters. Genes Chromosomes Cancer 34:58–68
Kovacs G, Akhtar M, Beckwith BJ et al (1997) The Heidelberg classification of renal cell tumours. J Pathol 183:131–133
Kulke MH, Lenz HJ, Meropol NJ et al (2008) Activity of sunitinib in patients with advanced neuroendocrine tumors. J Clin Oncol 26:3403–3410
La Rosa S, Uccella S, Finzi G et al (2003) Localization of vascular endothelial growth factor and its receptors in digestive endocrine tumors: correlation with microvessel density and clinicopathologic features. Hum Pathol 34:18–27
Laird AD, Vajkoczy P, Shawver LK et al (2000) SU6668 is a potent antiangiogenic and antitumor agent that induces regression of established tumors. Cancer Res 60:4152–4160
Maki RG, Fletcher JA, Heinrich MC et al (2005) Results from a continuation trial of SU11248 in patients (pts) with imatinib (IM)-resistant gastrointestinal stromal tumor (GIST). J Clin Oncol 23:9011
Mansour JC, Chen H (2004) Pancreatic endocrine tumors. J Surg Res 120:139–161
McDermott DF, Regan MM, Clark JI et al (2005) Randomized phase III trial of high-dose interleukin-2 versus subcutaneous interleukin-2 and interferon in patients with metastatic renal cell carcinoma. J Clin Oncol 23:133–141
Mendel DB, Laird AD, Xin X et al (2003) In vivo antitumor activity of SU11248, a novel tyrosine kinase inhibitor targeting vascular endothelial growth factor and platelet-derived growth factor receptors: determination of a pharmacokinetic/pharmacodynamic relationship. Clin Cancer Res 9:327–337
Modlin IM, Oberg K, Chung DC et al (2008) Gastroenteropancreatic neuroendocrine tumours. Lancet Oncol 9:61–72
Motzer RJ, Bacik J, Murphy BA et al (2002) Interferon-alfa as a comparative treatment for clinical trials of new therapies against advanced renal cell carcinoma. J Clin Oncol 20:289–296

Motzer RJ, Michaelson MD, Redman BG et al (2006a) Activity of SU11248, a multitargeted inhibitor of vascular endothelial growth factor receptor and platelet-derived growth factor receptor, in patients with metastatic renal cell carcinoma. J Clin Oncol 24:16–24

Motzer RJ, Rini BI, Bukowski RM et al (2006b) Sunitinib in patients with metastatic renal cell carcinoma. JAMA 295:2516–2524

Motzer RJ, Hutson TE, Tomczak P et al (2007) Sunitinib versus interferon alfa in metastatic renal-cell carcinoma. N Engl J Med 356:115–124

Negrier S, Escudier B, Lasset C et al (1998) Recombinant human interleukin-2, recombinant human interferon alfa-2a, or both in metastatic renal-cell carcinoma. Groupe francais d'immunotherapie. N Engl J Med 338:1272–1278

Negrier S, Perol D, Ravaud A et al (2007) Medroxyprogesterone, interferon alfa-2a, interleukin 2, or combination of both cytokines in patients with metastatic renal carcinoma of intermediate prognosis: results of a randomized controlled trial. Cancer 110:2468–2477

Nowain A, Bhakta H, Pais S et al (2005) Gastrointestinal stromal tumors: clinical profile, pathogenesis, treatment strategies and prognosis. J Gastroenterol Hepatol 20:818–824

Randomized study of sunitinib plus FOLFOX versus bevacizumab plus FOLFOX in metastatic colorectal cancer. http://clinicaltrials.gov/show/NCT00609622

Ravaud A, de la Fouchardière C, Asselineau J et al (2010) Efficacy of sunitinib in advanced medullary thyroid carcinoma: intermediate results of phase II THYSU. Oncologist 15:212–213

Raymond E, Dahan L, Raoul JL et al (2011) Sunitinib malate for the treatment of pancreatic neuroendocrine tumors. N Engl J Med 364:501–513

Richards CJ, Je Y, Schutz FA et al (2011) Incidence and risk of congestive heart failure in patients with renal and nonrenal cell carcinoma treated with sunitinib. J Clin Oncol 29:3450–3456

Rini BI, Small EJ (2005) Biology and clinical development of vascular endothelial growth factor-targeted therapy in renal cell carcinoma. J Clin Oncol 23:1028–1043

Rini BI, Tamaskar I, Shaheen P et al (2007) Hypothyroidism in patients with metastatic renal cell carcinoma treated with sunitinib. J Natl Cancer Inst 99:81–83

Rini BI, Choueiri TK, Elson P et al (2008) Sunitinib-induced macrocytosis in patients with metastatic renal cell carcinoma. Cancer 113:1309–1314

Rini BI, Cohen DP, Lu DR et al (2011) Hypertension as a biomarker of efficacy in patients with metastatic renal cell carcinoma treated with sunitinib. J Natl Cancer Inst 103:763–773

Robert NJ, Saleh MN, Paul D et al (2011) Sunitinib plus paclitaxel versus bevacizumab plus paclitaxel for first-line treatment of patients with advanced breast cancer: a phase III, randomized, open-label trial. Clin Breast Cancer 11:82–92

Scagliotti GV, Krzakowski M, Szczesna A et al (2012) Sunitinib plus erlotinib versus placebo plus erlotinib in patients with previously treated advanced non-small-cell lung cancer: a phase III trial. J Clin Oncol 30:2070–2078

Schmidinger M, Vogl UM, Bojic M et al (2011) Hypothyroidism in patients with renal cell carcinoma: blessing or curse? Cancer 117:534–544

Shuin T, Kondo K, Torigoe S et al (1994) Frequent somatic mutations and loss of heterozygosity of the von Hippel–Lindau tumor suppressor gene in primary human renal cell carcinomas. Cancer Res 54:2852–2855

Siegel R, Naishadham D, Jemal A (2013) Cancer statistics, 2013. CA Cancer J Clin 63:11–30

Sun L, Liang C, Shirazian S et al (2003) Discovery of 5-[5-fluoro-2-oxo-1,2- dihydroindol-(3Z)-ylidenemethyl]-2,4- dimethyl-1H-pyrrole-3-carboxylic acid (2-diethylaminoethyl)amide, a novel tyrosine kinase inhibitor targeting vascular endothelial and platelet-derived growth factor receptor tyrosine kinase. J Med Chem 46:1116–1119

Sunitinib malate as maintenance therapy in treating patients with Stage III or Stage IV non-small cell lung cancer previously treated with combination chemotherapy. http://clinicaltrials.gov/show/NCT00693992

Terris B, Scoazec JY, Rubbia L et al (1998) Expression of vascular endothelial growth factor in digestive neuroendocrine tumours. Histopathology 32:133–138
Van Glabbeke M, Verweij J, Casali PG et al (2005) Initial and late resistance to imatinib in advanced gastrointestinal stromal tumors are predicted by different prognostic factors: a European Organisation for Research and Treatment of Cancer–Italian Sarcoma Group–Australasian Gastrointestinal Trials Group study. J Clin Oncol 23:5795–5804
Verweij J, Casali PG, Zalcberg J et al (2004) Progression-free survival in gastrointestinal stromal tumours with high-dose imatinib: randomised trial. Lancet 364:1127–1134
Vinik A, Van Cutsem E, Niccoli P et al (2012) Updated results from a phase III trial of sunitinib versus placebo in patients with progressive, unresectable, well-differentiated pancreatic neuroendocrine tumor (NET). J Clin Oncol 30(suppl; abstract 4118)
Weisberg E, Griffin JD (2003) Resistance to imatinib (Glivec): update on clinical mechanisms. Drug Resist Updat 6:231–238
Witteles RM, Telli ML, Fisher GA et al (2008) Cardiotoxicity associated with the cancer therapeutic agent sunitinib malate. J Clin Oncol 26:9597
Wolter P, Stefan C, Decallonne B et al (2008) The clinical implications of sunitinib-induced hypothyroidism: a prospective evaluation. Br J Cancer 99:448–454
Wong E, Rosen LS, Mulay M et al (2007) Sunitinib induces hypothyroidism in advanced cancer patients and may inhibit thyroid peroxidase activity. Thyroid 17:351–355
Wulbrand U, Wied M, Zöfel P et al (1998) Growth factor receptor expression in human gastroenteropancreatic neuroendocrine tumours. Eur J Clin Invest 28:1038–1049
Yang JC, Sherry RM, Steinberg SM et al (2003) Randomized study of high-dose and low-dose interleukin-2 in patients with metastatic renal cancer. J Clin Oncol 21:3127–3132
Yao JC, Shah MH, Ito T et al (2011) Everolimus for advanced pancreatic neuroendocrine tumors. N Engl J Med 364:514–523
Yuasa T, Takahashi S, Hatake K et al (2011) Biomarkers to predict response to sunitinib therapy and prognosis in metastatic renal cell cancer. Cancer Sci 102:1949–1957

Regorafenib

Thomas J. Ettrich and Thomas Seufferlein

Abstract

Regorafenib (BAY 73-4506, Stivarga®) is an oral diphenylurea multikinase inhibitor that targets angiogenic (VEGFR1-3, TIE2), stromal (PDGFR-β, FGFR), and oncogenic receptor tyrosine kinases (KIT, RET, and RAF). Regorafenib is the first small-molecule multikinase inhibitor to achieve survival benefits in metastatic colorectal cancer that has progressed after all standard therapies. Consequently, regorafenib was FDA approved for this indication. In addition, regorafenib treatment resulted in a significant improvement in progression-free survival (PFS) compared with placebo in patients with metastatic gastrointestinal stromal tumors (GIST) after progression on standard treatments and is also an FDA approved indication. Currently, regorafenib is examined in several clinical trials (mostly phase II) in different tumor entities, including renal cell carcinoma (RCC), hepatocellular carcinoma (HCC), and soft tissue sarcoma (STS).

Contents

T. J. Ettrich (✉) · T. Seufferlein
Department of Internal Medicine I, University of Ulm, Albert-Einstein-Allee 23, 89081 Ulm, Germany
e-mail: thomas.seufferlein@uniklinik-ulm.de

U. M. Martens (ed.), *Small Molecules in Oncology*, Recent Results in Cancer Research 201, DOI: 10.1007/978-3-642-54490-3_10,

1 Structure, Mechanism of Action, and Pharmacokinetics

See (Fig. 1)

1.1 Mechanism of Action

Regorafenib is a small-molecule inhibitor of various membrane bound and intracellular kinases involved in normal cellular functions as well as pathologic processes such as oncogenesis, tumor angiogenesis, and maintenance of the tumor microenvironment. In biochemical in vitro or cell-based assays, regorafenib or its major human active metabolites M-2 and M-5 inhibited the activity of RET, VEGFR 1-3, KIT, PDGFR-alpha, PDGFR-beta, FGFR1, FGFR2, TIE2, DDR2, TrkA, Eph2A, RAF-1, BRAF, BRAFV600E, SAPK2, PTK5, and Abl at concentrations that can be achieved clinically.

1.2 Pharmacokinetics and Elimination

The standard dose of regorafenib is 160 mg taken orally once daily as tablets. The mean relative bioavailability of orally taken regorafenib is 69 %. Regorafenib undergoes enterohepatic circulation with multiple plasma concentration peaks observed across the 24-h dosing interval. Regorafenib is highly bound (99.5 %) to human plasma proteins and metabolized by CYP3A4 and UGT1A9. The main circulating metabolites of regorafenib in human plasma are M-2 (N-oxide) and M-5 (N-oxide and N-desmethyl). Both metabolites have similar in vitro pharmacological activity and are highly protein bound (>99.0 %). The elimination

Fig. 1 Chemical structure of regorafenib

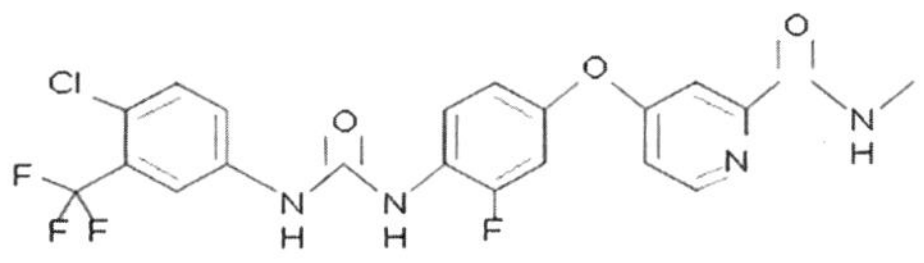

half-lives for regorafenib and its M-2 metabolite in plasma are 28 h and 25 h, respectively. M-5 has a longer elimination half life of 51 h. Approximately 71 % of a radiolabeled dose of regorafenib was excreted via feces, and 19 % of the dose was excreted via urine. Based on a population pharmacokinetic analysis, there is no clinically relevant effect of age, gender, or weight on the pharmacokinetics of regorafenib.

1.3 Regorafenib in Renal or Hepatic Impairment

Because of its major elimination via feces, no differences in the mean steady-state exposure to regorafenib, its M-2 or M-5 metabolite were observed in patients with mild renal impairment compared to patients with normal renal function. There is no clinical data for patients with severe renal impairment or end-stage renal disease. There were no clinically important differences observed in the mean exposure to regorafenib, M-2, or M-5 in patients with mild or moderate hepatic impairment (Child-Pugh A and B) compared to the patients with normal hepatic function. There are no clinical data for patients with severe hepatic impairment (Child-Pugh C).

2 Preclinical Data

Regorafenib is a multitarget small-molecule compound with potent activity against a number of angiogenic and stromal TKs (tyrosine kinases), including VEGFR-2, TIE-2, FGFR-1, and the PDGFR. Regorafenib also blocks KIT, RET, wild type, and V600 mutant BRAF. An antiangiogenic effect of regorafenib was demonstrated in vivo by dynamic contrast-enhanced magnetic resonance imaging. Regorafenib administered once orally at 10 mg/kg significantly decreased the extravasation of Gadomer, an intravascular macromolecular MRI contrast agent, in the vasculature of rat GS9L glioblastoma tumor xenografts (Wilhelm et al. 2011). In a daily dosing study, the pharmacodynamic effects persisted for 48 h after the last dosing and correlated with tumor growth inhibition (TGI). A significant reduction in the tumor microvessel area was observed in a human colorectal xenograft after daily dosing at 10 and 30 mg/kg.

Regorafenib exhibited potent dose-dependent TGI in various preclinical human xenograft models in mice with tumor shrinkage observed in breast MDA-MB-231 and renal 786-O carcinoma models (Wilhelm et al. 2011). Pharmacodynamic analyses of the breast cancer model revealed a strong reduction in Ki-67 immunoreactivity (a proliferation marker) and phosphorylation/activation of ERK 1/2.

Various low concentrations of regorafenib were examined in vitro in two human HCC cell lines with respect to its effects on alpha-fetoprotein (AFP) levels, cell growth, migration, and invasion (Carr et al. 2013). AFP secretion was inhibited at 0.1–1 μM regorafenib. Cell migration and invasion were inhibited at similar drug concentrations. Interestingly, a ten-fold higher drug concentration was required to inhibit cell growth in both AFP positive and negative cell lines (Carr et al. 2013). These data demonstrate that regorafenib is an active multikinase inhibitor with a distinct target profile.

3 Clinical Data

3.1 Regorafenib in Metastatic Colorectal Cancer

There are only limited treatment options available for patients with metastatic colorectal cancer progressing after all approved standard therapies. However, many patients maintain a good performance status and are eligible for further therapy. An international phase III trial, the CORRECT-trial (Grothey et al. 2013) was performed to assess regorafenib in patients with metastatic colorectal cancer (mCRC) progressing after all approved standard therapies. Seven hundred and sixty patients with a good performance status (ECOG 0 and 1) were randomized in a 2:1 ratio to receive regorafenib ($n = 505$) or placebo ($n = 255$), respectively. The primary endpoint of overall survival was met at a preplanned interim analysis. Median overall survival was 6.4 months in the regorafenib group versus 5.0 months in the placebo group (hazard ratio 0.77; 95 % CI 0.64–0.94; one-sided $p = 0.0052$). Treatment-related adverse events occurred in 465 (93 %) patients assigned to regorafenib and in 154 (61 %) of those assigned to placebo. The most common adverse events of grade 3 or higher related to regorafenib were hand-foot skin reaction (HFSR) (83 patients, 17 %), fatigue (48, 10 %), diarrhea (36, 7 %), hypertension (36, 7 %), and rash or desquamation (29, 6 %). Thus, regorafenib is the first small-molecule multikinase inhibitor with survival benefits in mCRC progressing after all standard therapies. The FDA approved the use of regorafenib for this indication on September 27th, 2012 (Table 1).

The combination of regorafenib with FOLFOX or FOLFIRI as first- or second-line treatment of mCRC was tested in a multicenter, phase Ib study (Schultheis et al. 2013) with forty-five patients. Safety and pharmacokinetics were the primary objectives, tumor response was the secondary objective. Patients were treated every 2 weeks with mFOLFOX 6 or FOLFIRI. On days 4–10, patients received regorafenib 160 mg orally once daily. The median duration of treatment was 108 days (range 2–345 days). Treatment was stopped for adverse events or death (17 patients), disease progression (11 patients), and withdrawal of consent or by investigators decision (11 patients). Drug-related adverse events occurred in 44 patients (≥grade 3 in 32 patients: mostly neutropenia and leukopenia, HFSR, and hypophosphatemia). Thirty-three patients

Table 1 Results from the CORRECT-trial (Grothey et al. 2013) in patients with colorectal cancer

	Regorafenib ($n = 500$)	Placebo ($n = 253$)	
mOS (month)	6.4	5.0	HR 0.77; 95 % CI 0.64–0.94; $p = 0.0052$
mPFS (month)	1.9	1.7	HR 0.49, 95 % CI 0.42–0.58, $p < 0.0001$
CR	0	0	
PR	4 %	1 %	($p = 0.19$)
DCR	41 %	15 %	($p < 0.0001$), 6 weeks after randomization

mOS median overall survival, *mPFS* progression-free survival, *HR* hazard ratio, *CI* confidence interval, *CR* complete remission, *PR* partial remission, *DCR* disease control rate

achieved disease control (partial response or stable disease) for a median of 126 days (range 42–281 days). With 71 % ≥grade 3 toxicity in this small study, regorafenib exhibited a not ideal tolerability in this setting. Currently (2013), two phase II trials, examining regorafenib in the first-line or second-line situation are under way (regorafenib + FOLFIRI vs. Placebo + FOLFIRI as second-line therapy in mCRC—NCT01298570 and mFOLFOX6 in combination with regorafenib as first-line treatment of mCRC—NCT01289821). No results of these trials are as yet available (Table 2).

3.2 Regorafenib in Metastatic Gastrointestinal Stromal Tumors

Metastatic gastrointestinal stromal tumors (mGIST) is a life-threatening disease with no therapy of proven efficacy after failure of imatinib and sunitinib. Mutant KIT and PDGFR-alpha, both regorafenib targets, remain dominant oncogenic drivers in GIST refractory to imatinib and sunitinib. Efficacy and safety of regorafenib were evaluated in a multicenter, single-arm phase II trial ($n = 34$) of regorafenib in patients with advanced GIST after failure of imatinib and sunitinib (George et al. 2012). This trial revealed positive results for regorafenib with respect to tumor control. Consequently, the GRID-trial, an international, multicenter, randomized, double-blind, placebo-controlled phase III trial in unresectable, locally advanced or metastatic GIST, who had been previously treated with imatinib and sunitinib, was initiated (Demetri et al. 2013).

The primary outcome measure in this trial was progression-free survival (PFS) based on disease assessment by independent radiological review using the modified RECIST 1.1 criteria. In modified RECIST, lymph nodes and bone lesions are not counted as target lesions and a progressively growing new tumor nodule within a preexisting tumor mass is classified as progression. The key secondary outcome measure was overall survival.

One hundred and ninety-nine patients were randomized 2:1 to receive regorafenib ($n = 133$) or placebo ($n = 66$), respectively. Median PFS per independent-blinded central review was 4.8 months (IQR 1.4–9.2) for regorafenib and

Table 2 Toxicity data (adverse events: CTC Grade 3 and 4) taken from the CORRECT-trial (Grothey et al. 2013)

Event	Regorafenib (n = 500)		Placebo (n = 253)	
	Grade 3 (%)	Grade 4	Grade 3	Grade 4
Any event	51	3 %	12 %	2 %
Fatigue	9	<1 %	5 %	<1 %
Hand-foot-skin reaction	17	0	<1 %	0
Diarrhea	7	<1 %	1 %	0
Anorexia	3	0	3 %	0
Voice changes	<1	0	0	0
Hypertension	7	0	1 %	0
Oral mucositis	3	0	0	0
Rash or desquamation	6	0	0	0
Nausea	<1	0	0	0
Fever	1	0	0	0
Vomiting	1	0	0	0
Sensory neuropathy	<1	0	0	0
Muscle pain	<1	0	<1 %	0
Headache	1	0	0	0
Pain, abdomen	<1	0	0	0
Laboratory event				
Thrombocytopenia	3	<1 %	<1 %	0
Hyperbilirubinemia	2	0	1 %	0
Proteinuria	1	0	<1 %	0
Anemia	2	<1 %	0	0
Hypophosphatemia	4	0	<1 %	0

0.9 months (0.9–1.8) for placebo [hazard ratio (HR) 0.27, 95 % CI 0.19–0.39; $p < 0.0001$]. Upon progression, 56 patients (85 %) assigned to placebo crossed over to regorafenib. Drug-related adverse events were reported in 130 (98 %) patients assigned to regorafenib and 45 (68 %) patients assigned to placebo. The most common regorafenib-related adverse events of grade 3 or higher were hypertension (31 of 132, 23 %), HFSR (26 of 132, 20 %), and diarrhea (seven of 132, 5 %).

Thus, oral regorafenib significantly improves PFS compared with placebo in patients with metastatic GIST after progression on standard treatments. These results led to the approval of regorafenib for this indication by the FDA on February 25, 2013.

3.3 Regorafenib in Hepatocellular Carcinoma

For hepatocellular carcinoma (HCC), there is currently only one published open-label, phase II safety study as second-line therapy of intermediate or advanced HCC (Bruix et al 2013). Thirty-six patients with stage B or C HCC according to the Barcelona Clinic Liver Cancer (BCLC) classification and only mildly impaired liver function (Class A according to the Child-Pugh classification) received regorafenib 160 mg once daily in cycles of 3 weeks on/1 week off treatment until disease progression, unacceptable toxicity, death or patient/physician decision to discontinue. The primary objective of this trial was safety, secondary objectives included efficacy (including time to progression and overall survival). The median treatment duration was 19.5 weeks (range 2–103 weeks). At data cutoff, three patients remained on treatment. Reasons for discontinuation were adverse events ($n = 20$), disease progression ($n = 10$), withdrawal of consent ($n = 2$), and death ($n = 1$). The most frequent treatment-related adverse events were HFSR (any grade $n = 19$; $\geq$grade 3 $n = 5$), diarrhea ($n = 19$; $\geq$grade 3 $n = 2$), fatigue ($n = 19$; $\geq$grade 3 $n = 6$), hypothyroidism ($n = 15$; $\geq$grade 3 $n = 0$), anorexia ($n = 13$; $\geq$grade 3 $n = 0$), hypertension ($n = 13$; $\geq$grade 3 $n = 1$), nausea ($n = 12$; $\geq$grade 3 $n = 0$), and voice changes ($n = 10$; $\geq$grade 3 $n = 0$). Disease control was achieved in 26 patients (partial response $n = 1$; stable disease $n = 25$). Median time to progression was 4.3 months. Median overall survival was 13.8 months. These data show that regorafenib has an acceptable tolerability and evidence of antitumour activity as single agent in patients with intermediate or advanced HCC that progressed following first-line sorafenib.

To provide further evidence for the use of regorafenib in HCC, the RESOURCE-trial (NCT01774344), a randomized, double-blind, placebo-controlled, multicenter phase III study of regorafenib in patients with advanced HCC, who progressed on sorafenib treatment, is recruiting since May 2013. Primary endpoint of the study is overall survival. Approximately 530 patients will be randomly assigned in a 2:1 ratio to regorafenib or placebo.

3.4 Regorafenib in Metastatic Renal Cell Carcinoma

Regorafenib inhibits VEGF receptors 1, -2, and -3 and PDGF receptors like other antiangiogenic tyrosine-kinase inhibitors approved for treatment of advanced renal cell cancer. Regorafenib also inhibits other potentially important angiogenic kinases like TIE2, activation of which is thought to be important in tumor escape mechanisms.

A phase II, open-label, non-randomized study assessed the safety and efficacy of the multikinase inhibitor regorafenib for the treatment of renal cell carcinoma (RCC) (Eisen et al. 2012). Patients with previously untreated metastatic or unresectable clear cell renal-cell carcinoma received oral regorafenib (160 mg per day) in cycles of 3 weeks on, 1 week off until disease progression. The primary efficacy endpoint was the proportion of patients who achieved an objective overall response. Forty-nine patients received regorafenib. Median duration of treatment was 7.1 months (range 0.7–34.4), and at the time of data cutoff, six patients (12 %) were still on treatment. Forty-eight patients were assessable for tumor response. Nineteen patients (39.6 %, 90 % CI 27.7–52.5) had an objective response, all of which were partial responses. Grade 3 drug-related adverse events were common, most frequently hand and foot skin reaction (16 patients, 33 %), diarrhea (5 patients, 10 %), renal failure (5 patients, 10 %), fatigue (4 patients, 8 %), and hypertension (3 patients, 6 %). Two patients had grade 4 treatment-related adverse events: two cardiac ischemia or infarction, one hypomagnesaemia, and one chest or thorax pain. Four patients died during study treatment or within 30 days of last dose. Two of these deaths were regarded likely to be related to the study drug. In summary, based on this phase II trial, the efficacy of regorafenib in the first-line setting of unresectable RCC appears comparable with that of other targeted first-line drugs. However, testing regorafenib in standard phase III trials seems inappropriate in view of its toxic effects.

3.5 Regorafenib in Soft Tissue Sarcoma

There is no clinical data for the treatment of advanced or metastatic soft tissue sarcoma (STS) with regorafenib. Currently, a multinational, randomized, placebo-controlled phase II trial of regorafenib in metastatic soft tissue sarcoma (REGOSARC, NCT01900743) has been initiated. The study recruits patients with metastatic STS having received at least doxorubicin (or another anthracyclin) as a previous treatment. One hundred and ninety-two patients will be randomly assigned in a 1:1 ratio. Primary endpoint of the study is PFS. No results are as yet available.

4 Detailed Analysis of Toxicity

4.1 Dermatological Toxicity

In the CORRECT-trial (Grothey et al. 2013) (mCRC, 760 patients), regorafenib caused adverse reactions involving the skin and subcutaneous tissues (72 % vs. 24 %), including HFSR and severe rash requiring dose modification. Serious adverse skin reactions including erythema multiforme (0.2 % vs. 0 %) and Stevens–Johnson syndrome (0.2 % vs. 0 %) were more frequent in regorafenib-treated patients. Toxic epidermal necrolysis occurred in 0.17 % of 1,200 regorafenib-treated patients across all clinical trials.

In a meta-analysis (Belum et al. 2013), 1,078 patients treated with regorafenib for mCRC, GIST, RCC, and HCC were included. The overall incidence of all-grade and high-grade HFSR were 60.5 and 20.4 %, respectively. The relative risk (RR) of all-grade and high-grade HFSR with regorafenib compared to controls was increased for all-grade ($RR = 5.4$) and high-grade ($RR = 41.99$) HFSR. Interestingly, the incidence of HFSR varied significantly with tumor type ($p = 0.007$) and was 71.4 % in RCC, 60.2 % in GIST, 50.0 % in HCC, and 46.6 % in mCRC, respectively.

4.2 Hypertension, Cardiac Ischemia, and Infarction

In the CORRECT-trial (Grothey et al. 2013) (mCRC, 760 patients), regorafenib increased the incidence of hypertension (30 % vs. 8 %), myocardial ischemia, and infarction (1.2 % vs. 0.4 %).

4.3 Hepatotoxicity

In the CORRECT-trial (Grothey et al. 2013) (mCRC, 760 patients), fatal hepatic failure occurred in 1.6 % of patients in the regorafenib arm and in 0.4 % of patients in the placebo arm; all of the patients with hepatic failure had metastatic liver disease.

4.4 Gastrointestinal Perforation or Fistula

In the GRID-trial (George et al. 2012) (GIST, 199 patients), 2.1 % of regorafenib-treated patients who were treated during the blinded or open-label portion of the study developed gastrointestinal fistula or perforation; two cases were fatal.

4.5 Hemorrhage

Regorafenib increased the incidence of hemorrhage in the CORRECT-trial (Grothey et al. 2013) (mCRC, 760 patients). The overall incidence (CTC Grades 1–5) was 21 % in regorafenib-treated group compared with 8 % in placebo group. Fatal hemorrhage occurred in 0.6 % of regorafenib-treated patients and involved the respiratory, gastrointestinal, or genitourinary tract.

4.6 Embryo–Fetal Toxicity

Regorafenib was found to be embryonic lethal and teratogenic in rats and rabbits at concentrations lower than those achieved in man at the recommended dose. Thus, the drug is likely to cause harm when administered during pregnancy.

5 Drug Interactions

5.1 Effect of Strong CYP3A4 Inducers

Co-administration of a strong CYP3A4 inducer (e.g., rifampicin, phenytoin, carbamazepine, phenobarbital, and St. John's Wort) together with regorafenib decreased the mean exposure of regorafenib, increased the mean exposure of the active metabolite M-5, and resulted in no change in the mean exposure of the active metabolite M-2. Concomitant use should be avoided.

5.2 Effect of Strong CYP3A4 Inhibitors

Co-administration of a strong CYP3A4 inhibitor (e.g., clarithromycin, grapefruit juice, itraconazole, ketoconazole, posaconazole, telithromycin, and voriconazole) with regorafenib increased the mean exposure to regorafenib and decreased the mean exposure to the active metabolites M-2 and M-5. Thus, concomitant use should be avoided.

5.3 Effect of Regorafenib on UGT1A1 Substrates

Regorafenib and its metabolites (M-2 and M-5) competitively inhibit UGT1A9 and UGT1A1 at therapeutically relevant concentrations. Eleven patients received irinotecan-containing combination chemotherapy together with regorafenib at a dose of 160 mg (Schultheis et al. 2013). The mean AUC of irinotecan increased by 28 % when irinotecan was administered 5 days after the final of 7 doses of regorafenib.

6 Biomarkers

There are (negative) predictive biomarkers for antiEGFR agents. In contrast, there are so far no biomarkers for antiangiogenic agents including regorafenib. An analysis of plasma biomarkers and KRAS mutations in patients with mCRC treated with regorafenib (Strumberg et al. 2012) (phase I study, 38 patients) revealed that during regorafenib treatment VEGF plasma levels increased by

62.4 % (change in arithmetic mean), and 95.6 % at days 21 and 49, respectively. sVEGFR decreased by 35.8 % (day 21) and 42.8 % (day 49), respectively. KRAS mutations were detected in 53 % of patients. Changes in VEGF and sVEGFR-2 did not correlate with PFS. Patients with mutated or wild-type KRAS were equally distributed among those who benefitted clinically (PFS $\geq$ 100 days). The observed changes in angiogenic plasma cytokines are supportive of the antiangiogenic activity of regorafenib in patients with advanced CRC. The KRAS status was not predictive for a clinical benefit as determined by PFS.

7 Summary and Perspectives

Regorafenib is a novel, orally active multikinase inhibitor that is fairly well tolerated as single agent in the clinical setting as judged by the available data from phase I, II, and III trials. The toxicity profile is comparable to other oral multikinase inhibitors with similar targets. Regorafenib has promising antineoplastic activity in several tumor entities. Two large, randomized phase III studies in patients with "difficult to treat" clinical settings, advanced mGIST and advanced mCRC, have shown a benefit for regorafenib treatment regarding overall survival (CRC) and progression-free survival (GIST). Consequently, regorafenib as single agent treatment has been approved by the FDA for the palliative last-line situation in mCRC and mGIST. Further extensive clinical development as a single agent or in combination with standard chemotherapeutic agents in various malignant tumors is warranted and ongoing.

References

Belum VR, Wu S, Lacouture ME (2013) Risk of hand-foot skin reaction with the novel multikinase inhibitor regorafenib: a meta-analysis. Invest New Drugs 31(4):1078–1086

Bruix J, Tak WY, Gasbarrini A, Santoro A, Colombo M, Lim HY, Mazzaferro V, Wiest R, Reig M, Wagner A et al (2013) Regorafenib as second-line therapy for intermediate or advanced hepatocellular carcinoma: multicentre, open-label, phase II safety study. Eur j cancer 49:3412–3419

Carr BI, D'Alessandro R, Refolo MG, Iacovazzi PA, Lippolis C, Messa C, Cavallini A, Correale M, Di Carlo A (2013) Effects of low concentrations of regorafenib and sorafenib on human HCC cell AFP, migration, invasion, and growth in vitro. J Cell Physiol 228(6):1344–1350

Demetri GD, Reichardt P, Kang YK, Blay JY, Rutkowski P, Gelderblom H, Hohenberger P, Leahy M, von Mehren M, Joensuu H et al (2013) Efficacy and safety of regorafenib for advanced gastrointestinal stromal tumours after failure of imatinib and sunitinib (GRID): an international, multicentre, randomised, placebo-controlled, phase 3 trial. Lancet 381(9863):295–302

Eisen T, Joensuu H, Nathan PD, Harper PG, Wojtukiewicz MZ, Nicholson S, Bahl A, Tomczak P, Pyrhonen S, Fife K et al (2012) Regorafenib for patients with previously untreated metastatic or unresectable renal-cell carcinoma: a single-group phase 2 trial. Lancet Oncol 13(10):1055–1062

George S, Wang Q, Heinrich MC, Corless CL, Zhu M, Butrynski JE, Morgan JA, Wagner AJ, Choy E, Tap WD et al (2012) Efficacy and safety of regorafenib in patients with metastatic and/or unresectable GI stromal tumor after failure of imatinib and sunitinib: a multicenter phase II trial. J Clin Oncol Off j Am Soc Clin Oncol 30(19):2401–2407

Grothey A, Van Cutsem E, Sobrero A, Siena S, Falcone A, Ychou M, Humblet Y, Bouche O, Mineur L, Barone C et al (2013) Regorafenib monotherapy for previously treated metastatic colorectal cancer (CORRECT): an international, multicentre, randomised, placebo-controlled, phase 3 trial. Lancet 381(9863):303–312

Schultheis B, Folprecht G, Kuhlmann J, Ehrenberg R, Hacker UT, Kohne CH, Kornacker M, Boix O, Lettieri J, Krauss J et al (2013) Regorafenib in combination with FOLFOX or FOLFIRI as first- or second-line treatment of colorectal cancer: results of a multicenter, phase Ib study. Ann Oncol Off j Eur Soc Med Oncol 24(6):1560–1567

Strumberg D, Scheulen ME, Schultheis B, Richly H, Frost A, Buchert M, Christensen O, Jeffers M, Heinig R, Boix O et al (2012) Regorafenib (BAY 73-4506) in advanced colorectal cancer: a phase I study. Br J Cancer 106(11):1722–1727

Wilhelm SM, Dumas J, Adnane L, Lynch M, Carter CA, Schutz G, Thierauch KH, Zopf D (2011) Regorafenib (BAY 73-4506): a new oral multikinase inhibitor of angiogenic, stromal and oncogenic receptor tyrosine kinases with potent preclinical antitumor activity. Int j cancer J int du cancer 129(1):245–255

Crizotinib

David F. Heigener and Martin Reck

Abstract

Crizotinib is an ATP-competitive small-molecule inhibitor of the receptor tyrosine kinases (RTK) c-Met, anaplastic lymphoma kinase (ALK), and ROS1. There is convincing clinical evidence for the effectiveness in non-small-cell lung cancer (NSCLC) harboring EML4-ALK rearrangements resulting in constitutional activation of the ALK-RTK. The drug is approved for this entity, which represents no more than 3–5 % of all NSCLC. However, in this population, impressive response rates are generated. The same seems to be true for ROS-1 rearrangements; however, these only occur in approximately 1 % of all NSCLC. The role in c-Met altered cancers needs to be determined. Toxicities include visual impairment, nausea, peripheral edema, QT-prolongation, and liver enzyme elevation. Also, the occurrence of renal cysts is reported. Fluorescence in situ hybridization (FISH) detecting the ALK rearrangement has to be performed on tumor tissue to predict crizotinib efficacy. The role of immunohistochemistry in this setting needs to be determined. It has high concordance with FISH results when strongly positive or completely negative. The high efficacy of crizotinib in ALK- and ROS-positive lung cancer as new molecular targets beside the epidermal growth factor receptor (EGFR) underscores the importance of molecular typing in NSCLC.

D. F. Heigener (✉) · M. Reck
Department of Thoracic Oncology, LungenClinic Grosshansdorf, Grosshansdorf, Germany
e-mail: D.heigener@lungenclinic.de

U. M. Martens (ed.), *Small Molecules in Oncology*, Recent Results in Cancer Research 201, DOI: 10.1007/978-3-642-54490-3_11,

Contents

1 Structure and Mechanism of Action

Crizotinib (R)-3-[1-(2,6-dichloro-3-flourophenyl)ethoxyl]-5-(1-piperidin-4-yl-1H-pyrazol-4-yl)pyridine-2-ylamine (Fig. 1) was initially developed as a second-generation, selective c-Met (mesenchymal to epidermal transition) inhibitor developed from a compound named PHA-665752 by Pfizer. This first-generation compound was modulated to become a potent small-molecule inhibitor of c-Met (Cui et al. 2011). It is an adenosine triphosphate (ATP) inhibitor of receptor tyrosine kinases. Besides c-Met, it inhibits anaplastic lymphoma kinase (ALK), ROS-1, and possibly other targets (Table 1) (Curran 2012).

Crizotinib in combination with its target, i.e., ALK, creates an inactive conformation of this oncogenic protein by inhibiting its phosphorylation as shown by crystalline structure analysis (Sasaki et al. 2010).

2 Preclinical Data

Much preclinical data were obtained on its property of inhibiting c-Met. The IC_{50} inhibiting the phosphorylation of wild-type c-Met in vitro in several human tumor cell lines has a mean of 4–8 nM. It inhibited cell growth and induced apoptosis in human GTL16 gastric carcinoma cell lines and supressed migration of tumor cells in vitro (Rodig and Shapiro 2010).

In ALK-translocated cell lines, crizotinib inhibited downstream effector functions and induced apoptosis (Christensen et al. 2007). Moreover, the compound has antiangiogenic properties in preclinical studies (Zou et al. 2007).

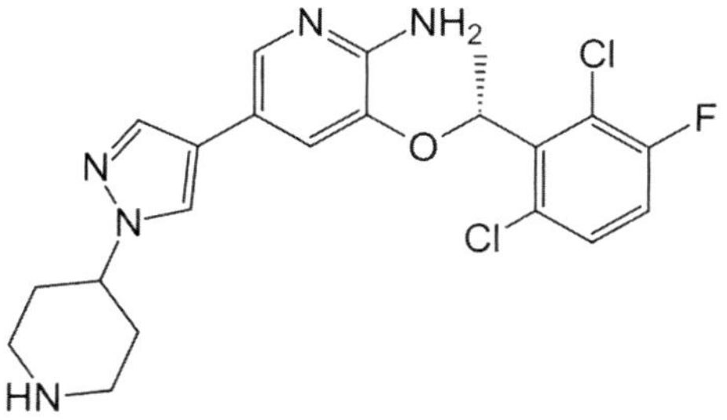

Fig. 1 Molecular structure of crizotinib

Table 1 Targets of crizotinib, reported entities harboring this target and relative frequency in NSCLC

Targets of Crizotinib	Types of cancer	Frequency of alteration in NSCLC
ALK rearrangement	NSCLC, lymphoma	4 %
ROS-1 rearrangement	NSCLC, chronic myelomonocytic leukemia, gastric carcinoma	1 %
c-Met amplification	NSCLC, breast cancer, bladder, ovarian cancer, brain tumors, skin tumors, kidney tumors, sarcomas	2–4 % in previously untreated patients, up to 20 % in patients treated with EGFR-TKI

For sources and abbreviations, see text. c-Met frequency is reported on www.mycancergenome.org/content/disease/lung-cancer/met/59

3 Clinical Data

3.1 NSCLC

In a phase 1 trial, patients with any solid tumor and no further approved treatment option were treated with increasing doses of crizotinib. Two hundred and fifty milligrams bid was the maximum tolerated dose. In this cohort, two patients with non-small-cell lung cancer had improvements in tumor-symptoms. Thus, an expansion cohort was created consisting of patients with NSCLC harboring an EML4/ALK rearrangement. They received the maximum tolerated dose (250 mg bid) in continuous 28-day cycles (2010). Median progression-free survival was 9.7 months (95 % CI 7.7–12.8). Estimated overall survival (OS) at 6 and 12 months was 87.9 % (95 % CI 81.3–92.3) and 74.8 % (66.4–81.5), respectively; however, the median was not reached by time of the publication. Thirty-nine patients continued to receive crizotinib for more than 2 weeks after progression because of perceived ongoing clinical benefit from the drug (12 for at least 6 months from the time of their initial investigator-defined disease progression)

Table 2 Efficacy of crizotinib compared to chemotherapies. The hazard ratios are for the comparison to crizotinib in all instances

Arm	PFS (months)	Hazard ratio	*P*-value
Crizotinib	7.7	0.49	<0.001
Chemotherapy	3.0		
Pemetrexed	4.2	0.59	<0.001
Docetaxel	2.6	0.3	<0.001

(Camidge et al. 2012). These data were considered sufficient for accelerated approval of crizotinib in the United States. However, the European Medical Agency (EMA) demanded further trials to prove superiority of crizotinib compared to standard chemotherapy. This trial compared crizotinib to either pemetrexed or docetaxel (by investigators' decision) in ALK-positive patients as second-line therapy (PROFILE 1007).Three hundred and eighteen patients were randomized to either crizotinib or chemotherapy. Primary endpoint was PFS. OS was not feasible, because crossover of chemotherapy patients into a single-arm crizotinib trial (PROFILE 1005) was pre-planned. A median of eleven cycles of crizotinib and four cycles of chemotherapy were administered, respectively. Chemotherapy consisted of docetaxel in 41 % of patients and pemetrexed in 57 % of patients, respectively. Median PFS was 7.7 versus 3.0 months favoring crizotinib [HR 0.49; confidence interval (CI) 0.37–0.64; $p < 0.0001$]. Interestingly, there was also a different PFS regarding to chemotherapy: Patients receiving pemetrexed had a median of 4.3 months compared to docetaxel with 2.6 months ($p < 0.0001$) with the difference between pemetrexed and crizotinib remaining significant ($p = 0.0004$, Table 2). Response rates to crizotinib, pemetrexed, and docetaxel were 65.7, 29.3, and 6.9 %, respectively. The preliminary data on OS showed no significant difference between crizotinib (20.3 months) and chemotherapy (22.8 months, $p = 0.5394$) because 111 out of 174 patients in the chemotherapy arm subsequently received crizotinib (Shaw et al. 2013a) and thus benefitted from the drug as well. These results are in line with all phase III trials of epidermal growth factor receptor (EGFR) tyrosine kinase inhibitors in patients harboring EGFR-activating mutations: Despite impressive advantages in PFS compared to chemotherapy, no OS difference could be detected due to crossover to EGFR-TKI in subsequent lines of therapy (Hirsch et al. 2013).

There is indirect evidence that crizotinib prolongs OS in patients harboring an ALK rearrangement: In a retrospective comparison of 82 patients with ALK rearrangement receiving crizotinib, 36 patients with ALK rearrangement not receiving crizotinib, 67 patients with an activating EGFR mutation, and 253 patients with wild-type EGFR and ALK survival was compared. ALK-positive patients treated second or third line with crizotinib had a one-year survival of 70 % (95 % CI 50–83 %). ALK-positive patients treated with any other second- or third-line therapy had a one-year survival of 44 % (95 CI 23–64 %; HR 0.36; 95 % CI 0.17–0.75; $p = 0.004$). Survival of ALK-positive patients receiving crizotinib was comparable to those who harbor an activating EGFR mutation receiving an EGFR-TKI [one-year survival % (95 % CI 58–81) vs. 74 % (61–83)]. ALK-positive patients not treated with crizotinib had similar survival as "double-wild-type" patients [median OS 20 months (95 % CI 13–26) vs. 15 months (13–17)]; $p = 0.244$ (Shaw et al. 2011).

A frequent site of treatment failure is the central nervous system, possibly due to the fact that crizotinib concentration in cerebrospinal fluid is much lower than in blood plasma [cerebrospinal fluid-to-plasma ratio 0.0026 (Costa et al. 2011)] and many patients develop brain metastases in their relatively long course of crizotinib treatment. As suspected by the results of the PROFILE 1007 trial, continuation of crizotinib paired with local treatment (i.e., radiation) seems to be beneficial. In 21 ALK-positive patients who developed central nervous system progression and radiation to these lesions, seven continued crizotinib without further progression for more than 4 months (Takeda et al. 2013).

Some of the resistance mechanisms leading to crizotinib failure are already discovered. In fact, the first report on crizotinib resistance was published "back to back" with the first clinical efficacy results described above (Choi et al. 2010). Drugs which might overcome this resistance are in clinical development.

ROS-1 rearrangements occur in about 1 % of patients with NSCLC. ROS1 and ALK are "kissing cousins," i.e., closely akin within the human kinome. In vitro essays with crizotinib showed that the drug was capable of inhibiting growth of ROS-1-positive NSCLC cell lines (Yasuda et al. 2012). So it was straightforward to test crizotinib in patients with a ROS-1 rearrangement. Patients were recruited in the dose escalation trial mentioned above (Kwak et al. 2010) as an own cohort. Forty patients harboring such a rearrangement could be identified. Thirty-five could be evaluated for response, and 32 were still receiving the drug at the time of data analysis. Overall response rate was 60 % with two complete and 19 partial responses. Disease control rate was 66 % at 16 weeks of treatment, and thus, median PFS is not reached at the time of first publication (Ou et al. 2013).

Data reporting the activity of crizotinib in c-MET-positive NSCLC cell lines suggest that its efficacy seems to be restricted to c-MET amplification rather than mutations in the corresponding gene (Tanizaki et al. 2011). A case report by Ou and colleagues reports on a patient with NSCLC harboring a c-MET amplification but no ALK rearrangement. Crizotinib resulted in a durable response in this patient (Ou et al. 2011). Because c-MET amplification is a known mechanism of EGFR resistance, a current trial investigates the safety and feasibility of combining crizotinib with a potent EGFR and HER-2 inhibitor [PF-00299804 (dacomitinib); NCT01121575].

3.2 Other Entities

In gastric carcinomas, ROS-1 rearrangements and c-MET amplifications are described (Lee et al. 2013; Okamoto et al. 2012) suggesting a possible benefit of crizotinib in these subsets.

Targets drugable with crizotinib are also found in Ewing sarcomas (Fleuren et al. 2013), anaplastic large-cell lymphoma (Ordemann et al. 2013), inflammatory myofibroblastic tumors (Tothova and Wagner 2012), chronic myelomonocytic leukemia (Cilloni et al. 2013), and neuroblastoma (Matthay et al. 2012) (Table 1). However, the clinical evidence is preliminary at best.

4 Toxicity

Crizotinib is comparably well tolerable. According to an analysis of phase I/II trials, most adverse events were mild to moderate with only 3–6 % of treatment interruption due to adverse events. In the order of frequency, the adverse events are the following:

- Visual disturbances (in 62 % of patients) including light flashes or perception of overlying shadows or after images (Salgia et al. 2011). However, the disturbances were all short in duration and had minimal influence on quality of life or activities of daily living.
- Nausea occurred in approximately 50 % of patients, diarrhea and vomiting occurred too. Again, these disturbances were mild and of short duration.
- Further frequent side effects were peripheral edema, constipation, fatigue, decreased appetite, and dizziness (Xalkori 2012).
- In 1.3 % of cases, administration of crizotinib can result in prolongation of the QT interval in the electrocardiogram (ECG) (Xalkori 2012). Patients already showing a prolonged QT interval or taking drugs known to prolong it should be monitored periodically with an ECG (Curran 2012).

5 Drug Interactions

Crizotinib is primarily metabolized in the liver by CYP3A which can result in drug interactions with CYP3A inducers like rifampicin, resulting in decreased plasma levels of crizotinib. CYP3A inhibitors like ketoconazole can lead to increased plasma levels of crizotinib. Finally, crizotinib itself may act as a CYP3A inhibitor, raising plasma levels of other substrates like midazolam (Curran 2012).

6 Biomarkers

The efficacy of crizotinib was tested in small subsets of patients with NSCLC, who are clearly defined on a molecular basis.

By now, three targets for crizotinib are identified: rearrangements in ALK and ROS as well as c-Met mutations. The gold standard for detection of ALK or ROS rearrangements is fluorescence in situ hybridization (FISH). For ALK, 15 % of cells must show this rearrangement for being classified as "ALK positive." This number is not chosen arbitrary but represents the double standard deviation from the number of ALK rearrangements found in normal tissue. FISH is a time-consuming procedure and can only be done by specially trained personnel. A valid screening test is thus needed. Overexpression of ALK measured by immunohistochemistry (IHC) is a promising candidate tool as shown by Park and colleagues: In a series of 262 patients representing an enriched cohort (no EGFR mutation) of patients, IHC and ALK FISH were performed on formalin-fixed, paraffin-embedded tissue. ALK protein was expressed in 28 (10.7 %) tumors in 262 patients. ALK FISH was positive in 25 (9.5 %) cases. All patients with IHC score of 3 ($n = 9$) were FISH positive, and all patients with score of 0 ($n = 234$) were FISH negative. Among patients with IHC scores of 1 and 2, five (83.3 %, 5/6) and eleven (84.6 %, 11/13) were FISH positive, respectively. The sensitivity and specificity of ALK IHC with intensity score of 1 or more were 100 and 98.7 %, respectively. So maybe in the future, people with an IHC score of 3 do not need a FISH for confirmation (and can be classified as "ALK positive") as do patients with a score of 0 ("ALK negative"), preserving the method for patients with an indeterminate IHC score of 1 or 2 (Park et al. 2012).

7 Summary and Perspectives

Crizotinib revealed to be a potent drug for a very small subset of patients with NSCLC, i.e., those with an ALK or ROS rearrangement. Its role in patients with a c-MET amplification remains to be clarified. The major challenge is the management of crizotinib resistance which will inevitably occur in almost every patient. Interestingly, many patients developing clinical progression under treatment with crizotinib do not show a resistance mutation on rebiopsy and are successfully treated with another ALK inhibitor with an even higher affinity to its target, LDK-378 (Shaw et al. 2013b).

Hopefully, in the future, we will be able to treat the majority of patients suffering from NSCLC on a molecular targeted base with similar success as those with ALK and ROS rearrangements (Table 2).

References

Camidge DR, Bang YJ, Kwak EL, Iafrate AJ, Varella-Garcia M, Fox SB et al (2012) Activity and safety of crizotinib in patients with ALK-positive non-small-cell lung cancer: updated results from a phase 1 study. Lancet Oncol 13(10):1011–1019

Choi YL, Soda M, Yamashita Y, Ueno T, Takashima J, Nakajima T et al (2010) EML4-ALK mutations in lung cancer that confer resistance to ALK inhibitors. N Engl J Med 363(18):1734–1739

Christensen JG, Zou HY, Arango ME, Li Q, Lee JH, McDonnell SR et al (2007) Cytoreductive antitumor activity of PF-2341066, a novel inhibitor of anaplastic lymphoma kinase and c-Met, in experimental models of anaplastic large-cell lymphoma. Mol Cancer Ther 6(12):3314–3322

Cilloni D, Carturan S, Bracco E, Campia V, Rosso V, Torti D et al (2013) Aberrant activation of ROS1 represents a new molecular defect in chronic myelomonocytic leukemia. Leuk Res 37(5):520–530

Costa DB, Kobayashi S, Pandya SS, Yeo WL, Shen Z, Tan W et al (2011) CSF concentration of the anaplastic lymphoma kinase inhibitor crizotinib. J Clin Oncol 29(15):e443–e445

Cui JJ, Tran-Dube M, Shen H, Nambu M, Kung PP, Pairish M et al (2011) Structure based drug design of crizotinib (PF-02341066), a potent and selective dual inhibitor of mesenchymal-epithelial transition factor (c-MET) kinase and anaplastic lymphoma kinase (ALK). J Med Chem 54(18):6342–6363

Curran MP (2012) Crizotinib: in locally advanced or metastatic non-small cell lung cancer. Drugs 72(1):99–107

Fleuren ED, Roeffen MH, Leenders WP, Flucke UE, Vlenterie M, Schreuder HW et al (2013) Expression and clinical relevance of MET and ALK in Ewing sarcomas. Int J Cancer 133(2):427–436

Hirsch FR, Janne PA, Eberhardt WE, Cappuzzo F, Thatcher N, Pirker R et al (2013) Epidermal growth factor receptor inhibition in lung cancer: status 2012. J Thorac Oncol 8(3):373–384

Kwak EL, Bang YJ, Camidge DR, Shaw AT, Solomon B, Maki RG et al (2010) Anaplastic lymphoma kinase inhibition in non-small-cell lung cancer. N Engl J Med 363(18):1693–1703

Lee J, Lee SE, Kang SY, Do IG, Lee S, Ha SY et al (2013) Identification of ROS1 rearrangement in gastric adenocarcinoma. Cancer 119(9):1627–1635

Matthay KK, George RE, Yu AL (2012) Promising therapeutic targets in neuroblastoma. Clin Cancer Res 18(10):2740–2753

Okamoto W, Okamoto I, Arao T, Kuwata K, Hatashita E, Yamaguchi H et al (2012) Antitumor action of the MET tyrosine kinase inhibitor crizotinib (PF-02341066) in gastric cancer positive for MET amplification. Mol Cancer Ther 11(7):1557–1564

Ordemann R, Stohlmacher J, Beuthien-Baumann B, Platzek I, van den Hoff J, Kroschinsky F et al (2013) Use of targeted therapy for refractory ALK-positive anaplastic large cell lymphoma as a bridging strategy prior to allogeneic transplantation. Ann Hematol 92(1):125–127

Ou SH, Kwak EL, Siwak-Tapp C, Dy J, Bergethon K, Clark JW et al (2011) Activity of crizotinib (PF02341066), a dual mesenchymal-epithelial transition (MET) and anaplastic lymphoma kinase (ALK) inhibitor, in a non-small cell lung cancer patient with de novo MET amplification. J Thorac Oncol 6(5):942–946

Ou SH, Bang YJ, Camidge DR, Riely G (2013) Efficacy and safety of crizotinib in patients with advanced ROS1-rearranged non-small cll lung cancer (NSCLC). J Clin Oncol 31:8032

Park HS, Lee JK, Kim DW, Kulig K, Kim TM, Lee SH et al (2012) Immunohistochemical screening for anaplastic lymphoma kinase (ALK) rearrangement in advanced non-small cell lung cancer patients. Lung Cancer 77(2):288–292

Rodig SJ, Shapiro GI (2010) Crizotinib, a small-molecule dual inhibitor of the c-Met and ALK receptor tyrosine kinases. Curr Opin Invest Drugs 11(12):1477–1490

Salgia R, Solomon B, Shaw AT, Camidge DR (2011) Visual effects in anaplastic lymphoma kinase (ALK)-positive advanced non-small cell lung cancer (NSCLC) treated with crizotinib. J Clin Oncol 30:7596

Sasaki T, Okuda K, Zheng W, Butrynski J, Capelletti M, Wang L et al (2010) The neuroblastoma-associated F1174L ALK mutation causes resistance to an ALK kinase inhibitor in ALK-translocated cancers. Cancer Res 70(24):10038–10043

Shaw AT, Yeap BY, Solomon BJ, Riely GJ, Gainor J, Engelman JA et al (2011) Effect of crizotinib on overall survival in patients with advanced non-small-cell lung cancer harbouring ALK gene rearrangement: a retrospective analysis. Lancet Oncol 12(11):1004–1012

Shaw AT, Kim DW, Nakagawa K, Seto T, Crino L, Ahn MJ et al (2013a) Crizotinib versus Chemotherapy in advanced ALK-positive lung cancer. N Engl J Med 368:2385–2394

Shaw AT, Mehra R, Kim DW, Felip E (2013b) Clinical activity of the ALK inhibitor LDK378 in advanced, ALK-positive NSCLC. J Clin Oncol 31(suppl), abstr 8010. 2013

Takeda M, Okamoto I, Nakagawa K (2013) Clinical impact of continued Crizotinib administration after isolated central nervous system progression in patients with lung cancer positive for ALK rearrangement. J Thorac Oncol 8(5):654–657

Tanizaki J, Okamoto I, Okamoto K, Takezawa K, Kuwata K, Yamaguchi H et al (2011) MET tyrosine kinase inhibitor crizotinib (PF-02341066) shows differential antitumor effects in non-small cell lung cancer according to MET alterations. J Thorac Oncol 6(10):1624–1631

Tothova Z, Wagner AJ (2012) Anaplastic lymphoma kinase-directed therapy in inflammatory myofibroblastic tumors. Curr Opin Oncol 24(4):409–413

Xalkori (crizotinib) prescribing information. Pfizer Inc. 2012

Yasuda H, de Figueiredo-Pontes LL, Kobayashi S, Costa DB (2012) Preclinical rationale for use of the clinically available multitargeted tyrosine kinase inhibitor crizotinib in ROS1-translocated lung cancer. J Thorac Oncol 7(7):1086–1090

Zou HY, Li Q, Lee JH, Arango ME, McDonnell SR, Yamazaki S et al (2007) An orally available small-molecule inhibitor of c-Met, PF-2341066, exhibits cytoreductive antitumor efficacy through antiproliferative and antiangiogenic mechanisms. Cancer Res 67(9):4408–4417

Cabozantinib: A MET, RET, and VEGFR2 Tyrosine Kinase Inhibitor

Carsten Grüllich

Abstract

Cabozantinib is a receptor tyrosine kinase inhibitor with activity against MET, VEGFR2, FLT3, c-KIT, and RET. Activity of cabozantinib toward a broad range of tumor models could be detected in several preclinical studies. Of note, cabozantinib decreases metastasis potential and tumor invasiveness when compared with placebo or agents that target VEGFR and have no activity against MET. Clinical phase I and II studies with cabozantinib have been conducted in various malignancies including medullary thyroid cancer (MTC), NSCLC, breast, ovarian, pancreatic, and prostate cancer. In MTC, gain of function mutations of RET are central for tumorigenesis. Hereditary forms of MTC (MEN II) are caused by germline mutations of RET, in sporadic MTC in up to 50 % of cases RET mutations occur. Additionally, activating molecular changes in VEGFR and MET pathways have also been implicated in MTC progression. Clinical responses with cabozantinib in MTC could be observed in early clinical trials, and following confirmation of clinical benefit in a randomized phase III trial, cabozantinib gained FDA approval for first-line treatment of advanced MTC in 2012. In prostate cancer models, MET expression increases with androgen ablation and clinical progression of bone and lymph node metastasis. A phase II trial with cabozantinib also showed very promising response rates in patients with metastatic prostate cancer. Therefore, randomized phase III studies are currently ongoing to validate the efficacy of cabozantinib in heavily pretreated prostate cancer patients.

C. Grüllich (✉)
Department of Medical Oncology, National Center for Tumor Diseases, Heidelberg University Medical Center, Im Neuenheimer Feld 460, 69120 Heidelberg, Germany
e-mail: carsten.gruellich@med.uni-heidelberg.de

U. M. Martens (ed.), *Small Molecules in Oncology*, Recent Results in Cancer Research 201, DOI: 10.1007/978-3-642-54490-3_12,

Contents

1 Introduction

The tyrosine kinase MET is the receptor for hepatocyte growth factor (HGF), a cytokine with anti-apoptotic, pro-migratory, and mitogenic activity. Multiple signaling cascades can be recruited to the intracellular domain of MET (MEK, PI3K, and Jak/Stat) leading to their activation. Activation of MET can disrupt cell–cell contacts and facilitates cell migration (Trusolino and Comoglio 2002). These promigratory effects mediated by MET play an important role during embryogenesis and are also active in adults during tissue damage repair (Takayama et al. 1996). It has also been demonstrated that the HGF/MET pathway has protective activity in several degenerative diseases, including liver cirrhosis, nephropathies, and lung fibrosis (Matsumoto and Nakamura 2001; Michalopoulos and DeFrances 1997; Mizuno et al. 2001). Further, MET is expressed in endothelial cells and plays a role in pro-angiogeneic signaling (Bussolino et al. 1992).

Taken together, these properties make MET a typical candidate for oncogenic aberration and cancerous transformation by MET has been demonstrated early. Since its discovery, activating changes in MET have been described in numerous cancers consisting either of activating mutations, gene duplications or transcriptional activation, that result in overexpression of wild-type MET (Table 1). The activating events in MET can either occur during primary tumorigenesis or as secondary events that drive further progression of the malignant phenotype (Trusolino and Comoglio 2002). Activating mutations have been identified in hereditary and sporadic papillary renal carcinoma (Soman et al. 1991; Schmidt et al. 1997); overexpression of MET has been detected in many tumors, including pancreatic cancer, prostate cancer, NSCLC, and gastric cancer (Soman et al. 1991; Schmidt et al. 1997; Houldsworth et al. 1990; Direnzo et al. 1995). In NSCLC, MET overexpression has been shown to be a mechanism of secondary resistance during treatment with EGFR antagonists (Bean et al. 2007), and in prostate cancer MET is upregulated during hormonal ablation and higher expression levels are also associated with progression of bone and lymph node metastasis (Sirotnak et al. 2004; Verras et al. 2007).

Different strategies to target MET for anticancer therapy are being followed, blockade of ligand binding by HGF antagonists or monoclonal antibodies against MET and HGF and cell permeable tyrosine kinase inhibitors. Several substances are currently being developed by different pharmaceutical companies and tested in clinical trials. Cabozantinib, developed by Exelexis, is a fairly broad-spectrum tyrosine kinase inhibitor with activity not only against MET but also against VEGFR2, FLT3, c-KIT and RET. It was the first orally available MET inhibitor to enter clinical trials in 2005 (Yakes et al. 2011). Phase I and II clinical trials have been completed in gastric, renal cell, pancreatic, and prostate cancer (Kurzrock et al. 2011; Smith et al. 2013; Schoffski et al. 2012). A successful phase III trial in medullary thyroid cancer (MTC) has been completed and met its primary endpoint showing a median PFS of 11.2 months for the cabozantinib arm over 4.0 months for the placebo arm (Schoffski et al. 2012). Besides activating changes in MET activating mutations of the proto-oncogene RET are also found in hereditary and in sporadic cases of MTC. Dual kinase inhibition by cabozantinib may contribute to its clinical activity in MTC. Based on this positive trial, cabozantinib was granted FDA approval for the first-line treatment of metastatic MTC in 2012. In prostate cancer, a positive randomized, placebo-controlled phase II study with cabozantinib has been completed and currently a phase III trial is recruiting patients.

Cabozantinib has shown clinical activity in a couple of clinical trials in different tumor entities. The importance of MET activation for tumor progression has been confirmed in numerous cancers. Multiple tyrosine kinase might be especially beneficial in certain tumors. This review will summarize the preclinical and clinical data for cabozantinib in cancer treatment.

2 Preclinical Properties and Pharmakokinetics

Cabozantinib, initially coded XL 184, was developed by Exelexis (South San Francisco, CA). It was shown to have inhibitory activity at pharmacological doses against MET, VEGFR2, RET, KIT, FLT-3, AXL, and TIE-2 (tunica interna endothelial cell kinase 2), kinases that all play a role in the development and progression of different tumor diseases. Preclinically, MET phosphorylation was shown to be reduced in peripheral nerve sheath tumor cells by cabozantinib at low concentrations. Studies with xenografts in nude mice demonstrated reduced cell proliferation, reduced vascular density and increased apoptosis. Tumor size was decreasing in a dose-dependent manner upon treatment with cabozantinib (Yakes et al. 2011). Penetration of the blood–brain barrier was shown to be at 20 % of plasma levels. In a phase I trial, the pharmakokinetics of cabozantinib were established. Oral bioavailability was demonstrated, and the maximum tolerated dose was determined at 175 mg once daily (equals 140 mg free base). Peak plasma concentrations were reached after 5 h following oral administration. The half-life was shown to be 91 $\pm$ 33 h (Kurzrock et al. 2011).

3 Clinical Trials

3.1 Phase I

The phase I trial of cabozantinib was carried out to determine the maximum tolerated dose (MTD). Included were various solid tumor entities (Kurzrock et al. 2011). The MTD was determined at 175 mg per day. Following early reports of activity in medullary thyroid cancer (MTC) an expansion cohort for patients with MTC was added to the trial. A total of 85 patients were treated within the trial; 37 of these had MTC. 35 of 37 MTC patients had measurable disease by RECIST. Of these, in 10 a partial response was confirmed and 25 had tumor shrinkage less than 30 % or disease stabilization for at least 6 months. Interestingly, three patients with a confirmed response had been pretreated with vandetanib or sorafenib that also target RET and VEGFR. This supports the hypothesis of MET being an escape mechanism to VEGFR inhibition. Tumor genotyping was performed in 31 patients with MTC; activating mutation of RET were detected in 25 of 31 patients. However, there was no correlation between mutations and clinical response. The tumor of one patient that was rapidly progressing harbored no RET mutation but an activating B-RAF mutation, which is downstream of RET and MET. In a subset of MTC patients ($n = 15$) analyzed for MET mutations in the tumor DNA, no mutations were detected and copy number gain was only assessed in a few samples and in three patients found to be increased.

Toxicity was similar to other VEGFR tyrosine kinase inhibitors. Treatment-related adverse events (AE) were reported in 77 of 85 patients (90 %). Of these, 43 % reported grade one or two AEs. The most frequent AEs were diarrhea, rash, hand–foot syndrome, liver enzyme elevation, fatigue, hypertension, nausea, and mucositis. One grade four AE was pulmonary embolism attributed to cabozantinib. Further, dose-limiting toxicities (DLT) were hand–foot syndrome and liver enzyme elevations.

3.2 Phase III EXAM Trial

A large phase III trial in medullary thyroid cancer was directly initiated following the responses seen in phase I. The "Efficacy of XL184 in Advanced Medullary Thyroid Cancer (EXAM)" trial was a randomized, double-blind, placebo-controlled trial (Schoffski et al. 2012). A total of 330 patients with MTC were randomized in a 2:1 ratio to cabozantinib versus placebo. The primary endpoint was progression-free survival (PFS), and crossing over was not allowed. Secondary endpoints included overall survival (OS) and response rate. Interim results were presented at the 2012 American Society of Clinical Oncology Annual Meeting. The primary endpoint had been met with a median PFS of 7.2 months in the treatment arm versus 4.0 months in the placebo arm. The difference reached statistical significance with a hazard ratio of 0.28. One-year progression-free survival was reported as 47.3 % in the treatment arm versus 7.2 % in the placebo arm. All subgroups showed an increased PFS in the treatment arm, including prior treatment with TKI and RET mutations. Overall response rate was 28 % in the cabozantinib group versus 0 % in the placebo group ($P \leq 0.0001$); duration of response was 14.6 months, that was similar in both RET mutation-positive and RET mutation-negative patients. Overall survival data had not yet reached the required number of events for analysis, but there was no difference between the two arms at this early stage. At interim analysis 45 % of patients in the cabozantinib arm remained on treatment versus 13 % in the placebo group. The primary reason for treatment discontinuation was progression of disease (20 % in the treatment arm versus 60 % in the placebo arm). Adverse events were reason for discontinuation in 16 % and 8 % of cases, respectively. Adverse events were more common in the treatment arm with diarrhea and hand–foot syndrome of all grades in over 50 % of patients. Further, fatigue, hypertension, and mucositis was also reported more often in the treatment arm. Assessment of calcitonin after 12 weeks of treatment showed a strong correlation with response. Calcitonin fell by a mean of 45 % in the treatment arm and increased by a mean of 57 % in the placebo arm.

3.3 Phase II Trial in Prostate Cancer

Based on responses observed in the phase I Trial, a phase II discontinuation trial was conducted in patients with castrate refractory prostate cancer (CRPC) (Smith et al. 2013). Patients received cabozantinib at 100 mg daily for 12 weeks. Then, patients with stable disease were randomized to cabozantinib versus placebo in a 1:1 ratio. Primary endpoints were objective response at 12 weeks and PFS after randomization. The randomized part was stopped early because of the observed cabozantinib activity. Enrolled were 171 men with CRPC. Improvement on bone scan was observed in 68 % of patients including complete resolution in 12 %. 31 patients with stable disease at week 12 were randomized. Median PFS was 23.9 weeks (95 % CI, 10.7–62.4 weeks) with cabozantinib and 5.9 weeks (95 % CI, 5.4–6.6 weeks) with placebo (hazard ratio, 0.12; $P < 001$). Bone pain improved in 67 % of evaluable patients, with a decrease in narcotics use in 56 %. The most common grade three adverse events were fatigue (16 %), hypertension (12 %), and hand–foot syndromes (8 %). PSA changes did not correlate with radiographic changes in this trial. Biomarker analysis on MET mutational and expression status has not been performed in this trial. Based on the positive clinical results, two phase III trials (COMET-1 and COMET-2) are currently enrolling patients with CRPC who progressed after taxane-based chemotherapy. The control arm consists of placebo in the COMET-1 trial and mitoxantron plus prednisone in the COMET-2 trial.

4 Discussion

Cabozantinib is a multikinase inhibitor with significant activity against MET, RET, and VEGFR among others. This combination of target specificity might prove especially useful in tumors where multiple target inhibition might prevent tumor escape mechanisms to one target from getting activated. In MTC, the dual kinase inhibition of RET and MET seems to be particularly active. Both kinases have been implicated in tumorigenesis in this cancer. RET mutation is found as many as 50 % of MTC tumor samples, while MET seems to be active mainly by overexpression. The influence of RET and MET was supported in a phase I trial, where activity of cabozantinib against MTC was observed in RET-mutated and RET-unmutated tumors, alike (Kurzrock et al. 2011). The phase III EXAM trial confirmed a clinical benefit for the treatment of MTC patients with cabozantinib. Progression-free survival was improved to 7.2 months over 4.0 months with placebo, and cabozantinib was FDA approved in 2012 (Schoffski et al. 2012). The final analysis of overall survival will further help defining the role of cabozantinib in this disease. In 2011, vadetanib, an inhibitor of RET and VEGFR but not MET, was already approved for MTC by also showing a PFS benefit over placebo. Head-to-head comparisons are needed in the future to define the roles of both substances.

Cabozantinib also showed promising activity in a phase II trial for castrate-resistant prostate cancer (CRPC) (Smith et al. 2013). The trial was conducted in a discontinuation design, where patients were randomized after 12 weeks of cabozantinib to treatment versus placebo. The trial was stopped early because of the rapid clinical benefit with cabozantinib and the high rate of progression in patients receiving placebo after randomization. Improvement of bone scans was seen in 67 % and reduction in pain in 57 % of patients. Two phase III trials in CRPC are currently recruiting patients. COMET-1 is comparing cabozantinib to placebo and COMET-2 to mitoxantrone plus prednisone. Both trials will help defining the clinical benefit of cabozantinib in CRPC.

The toxicities of cabozantinib are similar to those seen with other TKIs. Diarrhea, hand–foot syndrome, liver enzyme elevation, fatigue, and hypertension have been reported as the most common side effects. In general, side effects are mostly mild to moderate with the MTD determined by phase I and should be manageable by supportive means in clinical practice.

MET inhibition or multikinase inhibition as offered by substances like cabozantinib is a promising approach for various other tumors, where MET has been shown to play a role, including renal cell cancer, gastric cancer, and pancreatic cancer. Recently, MET activation has been shown to act as an escape mechanism in EGFR-mutated non-small-cell lung cancer during EGFR targeting therapy (Bean et al. 2007). Therefore, combinations of EGFR and MET inhibitors, which

Table 1 Types of molecular lesion of MET found in human cancers

Molecular lesion	Tumor entity
TPR-MET translocation	Gastric cancer
MET gene amplification	EGFR targeting therapy-resistant non-small-cell lung cancer
	Esophageal cancer
	Gastric cancer
	Liver metastasis from colon cancer
	Medulloblastoma
Germline MET mutations	Papillary renal cell cancer
	Gastric cancer
Somatic MET mutations	Papillary renal cell carcinoma
	Childhood hepatocellular carcinoma
	Lymph node metastases of head and neck squamous cell carcinomas
MET transcriptional activation	Thyroid carcinoma
	Ovarian carcinoma
	Pancreatic carcinoma
	Prostatic carcinoma
	Renal cell carcinoma
	Hepatocellular carcinoma
	Breast carcinoma
	Colorectal carcinoma
	Oral squamous cell carcinoma

have been shown to be active in vitro (Sennino et al. 2012; Nakagawa et al. 2012), are attractive approaches for clinical trials. However, excessive toxicities could be a limiting factor for clinical use.

In conclusion, cabozantinib is a tyrosine kinase that has shown clinical activity in a variety of cancers and is approved for treatment of advanced medullary thyroid cancer. A clinical benefit for prostate cancer is currently being evaluated in phase III trials. Hence, cabozantinib is the first clinically approved MET inhibitor. Further indications remain to be elucidated. The exploratory biomarker analyses within the trials show the need for a better understanding of the pathways involved, especially of resistance and escape mechanism. And finally, for certain tumor entities, tyrosine kinase inhibitors with activity against multiple targets appear to be superior over substances that are specific only to a single target.

References

Bean J et al (2007) MET amplification occurs with or without T790 M mutations in EGFR mutant lung tumors with acquired resistance to gefitinib or erlotinib. Proc Natl Acad Sci USA 104(52):20932–20937

Bussolino F et al (1992) Hepatocyte growth-factor is a potent angiogenic factor which stimulates endothelial-cell motility and growth. J Cell Biol 119(3):629–641

Direnzo MF et al (1995) Overexpression and amplification of the Met/Hgf receptor gene during the progression of colorectal-cancer. Clin Cancer Res 1(2):147–154

Houldsworth J et al (1990) Gene amplification in gastric and esophageal adenocarcinomas. Cancer Res 50(19):6417–6422

Kurzrock R et al (2011) Activity of XL184 (Cabozantinib), an oral tyrosine kinase inhibitor, in patients with medullary thyroid cancer. J Clin Oncol 29(19):2660–2666

Matsumoto K, Nakamura T (2001) Hepatocyte growth factor: renotropic role and potential therapeutics for renal diseases. Kidney Int 59(6):2023–2038

Michalopoulos GK, DeFrances MC (1997) Liver regeneration. Science 276(5309):60–66

Mizuno S, Matsumoto K, Nakamura T (2001) Hepatocyte growth factor suppresses interstitial fibrosis in a mouse model of obstructive nephropathy. Kidney Int 59(4):1304–1314

Nakagawa T et al (2012) Combined therapy with mutant-selective EGFR inhibitor and met kinase inhibitor for overcoming erlotinib resistance in EGFR-mutant lung cancer. Mol Cancer Ther 11(10):2149–2157

Schmidt L et al (1997) Germline and somatic mutations in the tyrosine kinase domain of the MET proto-oncogene in papillary renal carcinomas. Nat Genet 16(1):68–73

Schoffski P et al (2012) An international, double-blind, randomized, placebo-controlled phase III trial (EXAM) of cabozantinib (XL184) in medullary thyroid carcinoma (MTC) patients (pts) with documented RECIST progression at baseline. J Clin Oncol 30(15)

Sennino B et al (2012) Suppression of tumor invasion and metastasis by concurrent inhibition of c-Met and VEGF signaling in pancreatic neuroendocrine tumors. Cancer Discov 2(3):270–287

Sirotnak FM et al (2004) Microarray analysis of progression to reduced prostate cancer androgen dependence: studies in unique models contrasts early and late molecular events. Mol Carcinog 41(3):150–163

Smith DC et al (2013) Cabozantinib in patients with advanced prostate cancer: results of a phase II randomized discontinuation trial. J Clin Oncol 31(4):412–419

Soman NR et al (1991) The Tpr-Met oncogenic rearrangement is present and expressed in human gastric-carcinoma and precursor lesions. Proc Natl Acad Sci USA 88(11):4892–4896

Takayama H et al (1996) Scatter factor/hepatocyte growth factor as a regulator of skeletal muscle and neural crest development. Proc Natl Acad Sci USA 93(12):5866–5871

Trusolino L, Comoglio PM (2002) Scatter-factor and semaphorin receptors: cell signalling for invasive growth. Nat Rev Cancer 2(4):289–300

Verras M et al (2007) The androgen receptor negatively regulates the expression of c-Met: implications for a novel mechanism of prostate cancer progression. Cancer Res 67(3):967–975

Yakes FM et al (2011) Cabozantinib (XL184), a Novel MET and VEGFR2 inhibitor, simultaneously suppresses metastasis, angiogenesis, and tumor growth. Mol Cancer Ther 10(12):2298–2308

Vemurafenib

Claus Garbe, Sail Abusaif and Thomas K. Eigentler

Abstract

The activating BRAF mutation V600E and related mutations in this codon are most important for the activation of the RAS/RAF/MEK/ERK mitogen-activated protein kinase (MAPK) signalling pathway in melanoma. BRAF V600E mutations have been detected in ~40 % of melanoma patients and BRAF V600K mutations in ~5 % of melanoma patients. Activation of the MAPK pathway results in continuous stimulation of cell proliferation and inhibits programmed cell death. Vemurafenib (PLX4032) was developed as a low molecular weight molecule for the inhibition of the mutated serine threonine kinase BRAF, and it selectively binds to the ATP-binding site of BRAF-V600E kinase and inhibits its activity. The biochemical affinity of vemurafenib for mutated BRAF translates to potent inhibition of ERK phosphorylation and of cell proliferation exclusively in BRAF-mutant cell lines. In animal model experiments, it was demonstrated that vemurafenib achieved tumour regressions in cells harbouring the BRAF V600E mutation. The clinical trials with vemurafenib in unresectable metastatic melanoma in phase I, II, and III for patients harbouring BRAF V600E mutations demonstrated all unexpected high objective response rates ranging between 50 and 80 %. Median progression-free survival was prolonged from two months with dacarbazine to seven months with vemurafenib, and median overall survival was respectively prolonged from 9 to 14 months. A major problem that remains is the development of resistance to vemurafenib treatment after several months in the majority of patients, and multiple resistance mechanisms have already

C. Garbe (✉) · S. Abusaif · T. K. Eigentler
Department of Dermatology, University Medical Centre, Liebermeisterstr 25, 72074, Tuebingen, Germany
e-mail: claus.garbe@med.uni-tuebingen.de

U. M. Martens (ed.), *Small Molecules in Oncology*, Recent Results in Cancer Research 201, DOI: 10.1007/978-3-642-54490-3_13,

been described. Under vemurafenib treatment, about 25 % of patients developed cutaneous squamous cell carcinomas of the keratoacanthoma type with low invasive potential and without occurrence of metastasis. The overall tolerability of the drug was quite good, and a number of patients remained on treatment for long times. As other solid tumours like papillary thyroid cancer, colorectal cancer, non-small-cell lung cancer, and ovarian cancer likewise harbour BRAF mutation, vemurafenib is also tested in these entities. In future, combinations of vemurafenib with other kinase inhibitors and with immunotherapies will improve its therapeutic potential.

Keywords
Vemurafenib • BRAF mutation • Melanoma • BRAF inhibitor

Contents

1 Introduction

The prognosis for patient with distant melanoma metastasis (AJCC stage IV melanoma) is generally poor with a median survival ranging from 8 to 10 months after diagnosis depending on the number and the sites of metastatic spread and serum LDH (Chapman et al. 2011). The 5 year survival rate is 5–10 % in patients with metastatic melanoma (Eigentler and Garbe 2006). Treatment with single-agent chemotherapy or with combined schedules can produce palliative clinical response in a minority of patients (Pflugfelder et al. 2011). The discovery of activating BRAF mutations in approximately 50 % of patients with melanoma led to the development of a first targeted therapy of an activated oncogene in cutaneous melanoma, and clinical trials in other tumour entities are under way.

Mutations in the BRAF gene which substitute the valine at amino acid position 600 with glutamic acid (V600E) represent over 80 % of the BRAF mutations. Other variants of BRAF mutation are V600K with ~10 %, and less common V600R and V600D. Vemurafenib is also active in these less common BRAF V600 mutations, probably to a lower degree. BRAF mutations were mainly found in melanoma, colorectal cancer, papillary thyroid cancer, non-small-cell lung cancer, and ovarian cancer. Additionally, nearly all patients with hairy cell leukaemia carry the BRAF V600E mutation.

Targeted therapy represents nowadays a promising therapy for metastatic melanoma harbouring a drug-sensitive mutation. Vemurafenib was licensed for the treatment of non-resectable metastasised melanoma by the Food and Drug Administration Agency in the USA in August 2011 and by the European Medicines Agency in Europe in February 2012 on the basis of a phase III study for the treatment of patients carrying a BRAF V600 mutation (USFDA 2011; Hoffmann-La Roche Ltd 2012). With evaluated response rates ranging between 60 and 88 %, vemurafenib represents a therapeutic milestone in melanoma patients since decades (Flaherty et al. 2010; Schreck and Rapp 2006; Chapman et al. 2012). Additionally, an increase in overall survival up to 14 months compared to 9 months with standard chemotherapy treatment was reported, whereas some patients are still under treatment after 2 years (Chapman et al. 2012). Before treating patients with vemurafenib, patients must have a positive result from a BRAF mutational testing.

2 Structure and Mechanism of Action

BRAF is a member of the RAF family of serine threonine kinases (ARAF, BRAF, and CRAF) which are part of the RAS/RAF/MEK/ERK mitogen-activated protein kinase (MAPK) signalling pathway (Schreck and Rapp 2006).

Therapy targeting the MAPK pathway through inhibition of oncogenic mutations in the BRAF kinase has become a standard treatment for patients who have metastatic melanoma with activating BRAF mutations. Mitogen-activated protein kinase cascades are key signalling pathways involved in the regulation of normal cell proliferation, survival, and differentiation. The RAF/MEK/ERK signalling has implications in a wide variety of cellular functions. This pathway is central for cell proliferation, cell cycle arrest, terminal differentiation, and cell death. RAF activates the MAPK kinase MEK1/2 which subsequently phosphorylates ERK1/2 (Peyssonnaux and Eychene 2001). Mutated BRAF V600E has a critical role for the proliferation and survival of melanoma cells through activation of the MAPK pathway. The mutation in the V600 codon changes the molecular confirmation of BRAF to the activated (phosphorylated) status. In June 2002, Davies and colleagues reported mutations of the BRAF gene in human cancers. BRAF mutation-induced oncogenes are present in approximately 5–10 % of all human malignancies (Davies et al. 2002). BRAF is the most frequently mutated protein kinase in melanoma (Greenman et al. 2007) and was identified in ~50 % of malignant melanomas, in 15 % of thyroid tumours, in 8 % of colon carcinomas, in 4 % of all solid tumours, and up to 100 % in hairy cell leukaemia (Davies et al. 2002; Tiacci et al. 2011).

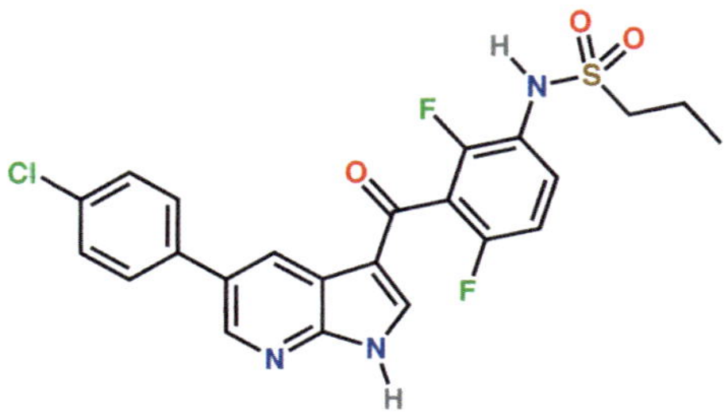

Fig. 1 Structure of vemurafenib: propane-1-sulphonic acid {3-[5-(4-chlorophenyl)-1H-pyrolo[2,3-b]pyridine-3-carbonyl]-2,4-difluoro-phenyl}-amide

Vemurafenib is a low molecular weight molecule, an orally available, selective inhibitor of BRAF with the V600E mutation but does not inhibit BRAF wild type; it selectively binds to the ATP-binding site of BRAF-V600E kinase and inhibits its activity (Fig. 1).

3 Preclinical Data

The discovery of the mutations in the BRAF gene, which represent approximately two-thirds of activating mutations in the oncogene protein kinases, was an important step in understanding the aetiology of metastatic melanoma.

The biochemical affinity of vemurafenib for mutated BRAF translates to cellular potent inhibition of ERK phosphorylation and of cell proliferation exclusively in BRAF-mutant cell lines. In preclinical cell line experiments, it was demonstrated that vemurafenib inhibited proliferation in cells harbouring the BRAF V600E mutation. Vemurafenib likewise caused tumour regressions of BRAF-mutant xenografts (Bollag et al. 2010).

4 Pharmacokinetics and Drug Interactions

After oral administration of a single 960 mg dose of vemurafenib, the substance was absorbed with a time needed to reach maximum concentration (tmax) of approximately 4 h. Mean maximum concentration achieved in the blood (Cmax) at the 960 mg dose level was approximately 4.8 ± 3.3 µg/ml. Clearance is approximately 30 L/day. The mean half-life time (t1/2) is 50 h, resulting in sixfold–ninefold accumulation between day 1 and day 15. Vemurafenib is excreted via faeces (94 %) and urine (1 %) (Shah et al. 2013; European Medicines Agency 2013).

Vemurafenib is metabolised by CYP3A4, and the metabolites make up 5 % of the components in plasma. The parent compound makes up for the remaining 95 %. Results from an in vivo drug–drug interaction study in patients with cancer demonstrated that vemurafenib is a moderate CYP1A2 inhibitor, a weak CYP2D6 inhibitor and a CYP3A4 inducer. Ketoconazole, itraconazole, clarithromycin, atazanavir, nefazodone, saquinavir, telithromycin, ritonavir, indinavir, nelfinavir, and voriconazole are potent CYP3A4 inhibitors; concomitant administration of strong CYP3A4 inhibitors increases plasma concentration of vemurafenib (Shah et al. 2013; European Medicines Agency 2013).

Phenytoin, carbamazepine, rifampicin, rifabutin, rifapentine, and phenobarbital are CYP3A4 inhibitors; concomitant administration of strong CYP3A4 inhibitors decreases plasma concentration of vemurafenib. Co-administration of vemurafenib increased the AUC of caffeine (CYP1A2 substrate) 2.6-fold and increased the AUC of dextromethorphan (CYP2D6 substrate) by 47 %, while it decreased the AUC of midazolam (CYP3A4 substrate) by 39 %. Co-administration of vemurafenib resulted in an 18 % increase in AUC of S-warfarin (CYP2C9 substrate) (Shah et al. 2013; European Medicines Agency 2013).

5 Vemurafenib in Melanoma

The clinical trials with vemurafenib in phase I, II, and III for patients harbouring BRAF V600E mutations demonstrated all unexpected high objective response rates and improvement in progression-free and overall survival. The tolerability of the drug was quite good, and many patients remained on treatment for long times (Chapman et al. 2011; Flaherty et al. 2010; Sosman et al. 2012).

The results from a phase I study for the first time reported a high objective response rate in patients with metastatic melanoma harbouring BRAF mutations. Data of the phase I trial (BRIM1) were published In August 2010 (Flaherty et al. 2010). This trial had a two-phase design (dose escalation phase and an extension phase). Complete or partial tumour responses occurred in 26 of 32 patients within the extension phase (81 %). The response duration for the patients in dose escalation phase ranged from 2 to more than 18 months. The median progression-free survival among all patients was more than 7 months. In the dose escalation phase, 11 of 16 patients (69 %) with BRAF-V600E mutant melanoma had a complete or partial response, who were treated with doses of 240 mg twice daily or higher. Forty percentage of the extension cohort had dose reduction from 960 mg twice daily to 720, 600 or 480 mg twice daily due to the side effects which were demonstrated to be proportional to the dose of the drug. Predominantly cutaneous side effects have been observed as rash, photosensitivity, cutaneous squamous cell carcinoma, and palmar–plantar dysaesthesia. Furthermore, fatigue and arthralgia were reported in nearly one-third of patient in the extension phase. Well-differentiated cutaneous squamous cell carcinoma was diagnosed in more than 20 % of patients with low invasive potential and no metastatic course. The maximum tolerated dose was found to be 960 mg orally twice daily (Flaherty et al. 2010).

A multicentre, open-label phase II trial was conducted in patients with metastatic melanoma who had previously been treated with one or more prior systemic therapy (BRIM2) (Sosman et al. 2012). In this trial, 132 patients with melanoma harbouring a BRAF V600 mutation were treated with vemurafenib at a dose of 960 mg until the development of unacceptable toxic effects or disease progression. The median duration of response was 6.8 months (95 % CI: 5.6—not reached). The confirmed overall response rate was 53 %. Adverse events (AEs) were generally reversible (with dose modification or interruption). The most common adverse events (all grades) were arthralgia (seen in 59 % of patients), rash (52 %), and photosensitivity reactions (52 %). The most common grade 3 adverse event was cutaneous squamous cell carcinoma (seen in 26 % of patients), the majority of which were centrally reviewed as keratoacanthoma type. Forty-five percentage of patients required dose reductions, most commonly for rash, arthralgia, and liver function test abnormalities (Sosman et al. 2012).

In June 2011, the results from an open-label phase III study with a total of 672 patients with previously untreated melanoma with the BRAF V600E mutation were reported (Chapman et al. 2011). This study has been performed in order to evaluate the efficacy of vemurafenib as a monotherapy in comparison with dacarbazine chemotherapy. Vemurafenib treatment showed remarkable tumour responses in approximately 48 % of patients with vemurafenib treatment compared with 55 % for those on dacarbazine chemotherapy. Vemurafenib was associated with a relative reduction of 63 % in the risk of death and of 74 % in the risk of tumour progression (Chapman et al. 2011).

Vemurafenib is associated with a significant improved overall survival and progression-free survival in comparison with dacarbazine chemotherapy in patients with previously untreated, V600E BRAF-mutated metastatic melanoma.

6 Toxicity

Vemurafenib is generally well tolerated with manageable side effects. The adverse events reported in vemurafenib clinical studies were demonstrated to be proportional to the dose and exposure to the drug. The toxic effects were largely related to the skin, joints, liver, and CNS.

Only few patients needed to discontinue treatment permanently in the clinical studies due to adverse events. The frequency of adverse events leading to permanent discontinuation of treatment in phase I and phase II trials was 7 % and 3 %. Most common adverse reactions (in $\geq$30 % treated patients) were the following: arthralgia, rash, alopecia, fatigue, photosensitivity reactions, nausea, pruritus, and skin papillomas including squamous cell cancer. Prolongation of the QT interval was also reported. Thirty-one percentage of patients in the extension phase developed well-differentiated SCC with low invasive potential and without development of metastases (Flaherty et al. 2010).

In the phase II study, the most common adverse events reported were arthralgia, rash, mild to moderate photosensitivity reactions, fatigue, and alopecia (Sosman et al. 2012). Transient elevations of liver-enzyme levels were likewise reported. Three patients had transient palsies of the seventh cranial nerve, one patient had retinal-vein occlusion, and another patient had acute renal failure. Twenty-six percentage of patients developed SCC or keratoaconthoma; the median time to development of the first cutaneous squamous cell carcinoma or keratoacanthoma lesion was 8 weeks. The most common grade 3 adverse reactions were cutaneous SCC and rash. The possible mechanisms of developing SCC appears to be paradoxically increasing signalling of the MAPK pathway in cancer cells with wild-type BRAF that carry upstream RAS mutations, through signalling via CRAF (Oberholzer et al. 2012).

7 Vemurafenib in Colorectal Cancer

Approximately 10 % of all patients with colorectal cancer have BRAF(V600E) mutation (Tanaka et al. 2006). Patients with metastatic colorectal BRAF V600E mutation had poorer survival as compared with BRAF wild-type patients (Tie et al. 2011). The clinical responses to the vemurafenib in clinical trials were only 5 % in BRAF-mutant colorectal cancer (Kopetz et al. 2010). The low response rate for vemurafenib treatment in patients harbouring BRAF mutation is possibly explained by resistance to the kinase therapy. Therefore, the parallel blockade of the epidermal growth factor receptor (EGFR) may be a successful strategy in colon cancers, as this showed a strong synergy with BRAF(V600E) blockade. Inhibition of the activity of EGFR with cetuximab, erlotinib, or gefitinib and combination with BRAF inhibitor may be more effective in those patients (Prahallad et al. 2012). Another resistance mechanism to BRAF inhibitors has been reported in BRAF-mutant colon cancer which is the activation of the PI3K/AKT pathway. Therefore, inhibiting the PI3K pathway in combination with vemurafenib in BRAF-mutant CRC cell lines provided an improved anti-tumour action (Mao et al. 2013).

8 Vemurafenib in Papillary Thyroid Cancer

Forty-five to fifty percentage of patients with papillary thyroid cancers were reported to have activating BRAF mutations (Xing 2007). The incidence rate of BRAF mutation in recurrent or metastatic PTCs was approximately 80 %. A phase I study with vemurafenib showed a partial response and prolonged stabilization of disease in all patients with PTC treated with vemurafenib (Kim et al. 2013).

9 Vemurafenib in Non-Small-Cell Lung Cancer

BRAF mutations are reported in approximately 1–5 % of NSCLCs. The majority of the mutations were non-V600E (Naoki et al. 2002). Gautschi et al. (2012) reported one case with V600E mutation in NSCLC that responded to vemurafenib.

10 Vemurafenib in Hairy Cell Leukaemia

In 2011, Tiacci and colleagues reported of a 100 % detection rate of the BRAF V600E mutation in patients suffering from hairy cell leukaemia (Tiacci et al. 2011). Meanwhile, case reports were published indicating partial and complete remissions even for low doses of vemurafenib (Dietrich et al. 2012; Peyrade et al. 2013).

11 Biomarkers and Monitoring of Vemurafenib Treatment

Biomarkers in metastatic melanoma are used to assess the progression of disease, predict the response of treatment, and are part of staging examinations. In 2009, the American Joint Committee on Cancer (AJCC) included the serum lactate dehydrogenase (LDH) to classify stage IV into the M categories, M1a (soft tissue metastasis), M1b (pulmonary involvement), and M1c (involvement of other visceral organs or elevated LDH) (Balch et al. 2009). LDH is expressed ubiquitously in different healthy tissues. Elevated serum concentrations of the intracellular enzyme are mainly a result of cell lysis. Moreover, increased serum LDH levels occur in different tumour entities and indicate a high turnover of tumour cells as well as necrosis in fast-growing tumours. Increased LDH values are associated with high tumour burden and seem to be particularly elevated in liver metastases (Finck et al. 1983; Sirott et al. 1993).

Another prognostic factor for stage VI metastatic melanoma is serum S100B. In immunohistochemistry, routine staining with S100 polyclonal antibody is able to detect macrophages, monocytes, interdigitating reticulum cells, Langerhans cells, and cells from the neural crest including glia, Schwann cells, and melanocytes (Gogas et al. 2009; Hauschild et al. 1999). Serum S100B has been shown to be elevated at stage I/II in 0–12.0 %, at stage III in 8.7–31 %, and at stage IV in 48–100 % (Carlson et al. 2005). Weide et al. assessed the use of biomarker in melanoma patients with distant metastases. Serum markers LDH and S100B were found to be independent prognostic factors in melanoma patients with distant metastases, and both factors were associated with similar hazard ratios (Weide et al. 2012).

A retrospective study in 44 patients with stage IV melanoma who were treated with vemurafenib evaluated the potential of the tumour marker S100B as response and progression markers during vemurafenib treatment. Computed tomography scans and measurement of LDH and S100B levels were performed every

6–8 weeks. The correlation between response or progression and LDH and S100B levels was analysed. A good correlation between S100B and LDH decline and a RECIST-confirmed response was observed, especially when S100B and/or LDH were elevated at baseline. However, the correlation in case of tumour progression and S100B/LDH levels was low. Therefore, monitoring the course of the disease with tumour markers is thus not an alternative to monitoring with imaging examinations (Abusaif et al. 2013).

12 Summary and Perspectives

Vemurafenib is a very active drug in unresectable metastatic melanoma. Eighty-five percentage of patients develop tumour regressions up to objective responses in about 50 % of patients. The median progression-free survival time is 7 months; up to this duration, half of the patients have developed resistance to vemurafenib. A small percentage of patients of 10–15 % are now for 18–36 months on treatment and may develop late or no resistance. A major clinical challenge in vemurafenib treatment is the development of acquired vemurafenib resistance and the subsequent often rapid tumour progression. Several mechanisms of resistance to vemurafenib have been reported. The remarkable advances in the direct oncogene therapy in melanoma and the understanding of the mechanisms of vemurafenib resistance has led to the development of novel agents; particularly, the combination of BRAF and MEK inhibitors showed initial promising results. Several clinical trials are in progress using this combination with the different compounds of at least three international drug companies. Other kinase inhibitors probably of the PI3K-AKT signalling pathway will likewise be tested in combination with vemurafenib. Furthermore, these concepts of molecular targeted therapies will be combined with the new immunotherapies in melanoma, and it remains an open question whether simultaneous or sequential schedules will be used in future.

References

Abusaif S, Jradi Z, Held L et al (2013) S100B and lactate dehydrogenase as response and progression markers during treatment with vemurafenib in patients with advanced melanoma. Melanoma Res 2013, Epub ahead of print

Balch CM, Gershenwald JE, Soong SJ et al (2009) Final version of 2009 AJCC melanoma staging and classification. J Clin Oncol 27:6199–6206

Bollag G, Hirth P, Tsai J et al (2010) Clinical efficacy of a RAF inhibitor needs broad target blockade in BRAF-mutant melanoma. Nature 467:596–599

Carlson JA, Ross JS, Slominski A et al (2005) Molecular diagnostics in melanoma. J Am Acad Dermatol 52:743–775

Chapman PB, Hauschild A, Robert C et al (2011) Improved survival with vemurafenib in melanoma with BRAF V600E mutation. N Engl J Med 364:2507–2516

Chapman PB, Hauschild A, Robert C et al (2012) Updated overall survival (OS) results for BRIM-3, a phase III randomized, open-label, multicenter trial comparing BRAF inhibitor

vemurafenib (vem) with dacarbazine (DTIC) in previously untreated patients with BRAFV600E-mutated melanoma. J Clin Oncol 30:8502
Davies H, Bignell GR, Cox C et al (2002) Mutations of the BRAF gene in human cancer. Nature 417:949–954
Dietrich S, Glimm H, Andrulis M, von Kalle C, Ho AD, Zenz T (2012) BRAF inhibition in refractory hairy-cell leukemia. N Engl J Med 366:2038–2040
Eigentler TK, Garbe C (2006) Malignant melanoma: classification and staging of malignant melanoma. Front Radiat Ther Oncol 39:149–158
European Medicines Agency (2013) Zelboraf—Annex I—Summary of product characteristics. 19 June 2013
Finck SJ, Giuliano AE, Morton DL (1983) LDH and melanoma. Cancer 51:840–843
Flaherty KT, Puzanov I, Kim KB et al (2010) Inhibition of mutated, activated BRAF in metastatic melanoma. N Engl J Med 363:809–819
Gautschi O, Pauli C, Strobel K et al (2012) A patient with BRAF V600E lung adenocarcinoma responding to vemurafenib. J Thorac Oncol 7:e23–e24
Gogas H, Eggermont AM, Hauschild A et al (2009) Biomarkers in melanoma. Ann Oncol 20(6):vi8–vi13
Greenman C, Stephens P, Smith R et al (2007) Patterns of somatic mutation in human cancer genomes. Nature 446:153–158
Hauschild A, Engel G, Brenner W et al (1999) S100B protein detection in serum is a significant prognostic factor in metastatic melanoma. Oncology 56:338–344
Hoffmann-La Roche Ltd (2012) Roche's Zelboraf receives EU approval for the treatment of people with deadly form of skin cancer. http://www.roche.com/media/media_releases/med-cor-2012-02-20.htm
Kim KB, Cabanillas ME, Lazar AJ et al (2013) Clinical responses to vemurafenib in patients with metastatic papillary thyroid cancer harboring BRAF(V600E) mutation. Thyroid 23:1277–1283
Kopetz S, Desai J, Chan E et al (2010) PLX4032 in metastatic colorectal cancer patients with mutant BRAF tumours. J Clin Oncol 28:3534
Mao M, Tian F, Mariadason JM et al (2013) Resistance to BRAF inhibition in BRAF-mutant colon cancer can be overcome with PI3K inhibition or demethylating agents. Clin Cancer Res 19:657–667
Naoki K, Chen TH, Richards WG, Sugarbaker DJ, Meyerson M et al (2002) Missense mutations of the BRAF gene in human lung adenocarcinoma. Cancer Res 62:7001–7003
Oberholzer PA, Kee D, Dziunycz P et al (2012) RAS mutations are associated with the development of cutaneous squamous cell tumours in patients treated with RAF inhibitors. J Clin Oncol 30:316–321
Peyrade F, Re D, Ginet C et al (2013) Low-dose vemurafenib induces complete remission in a case of hairy-cell leukaemia with a V600E mutation. Haematologica 98:e20–e22
Peyssonnaux C, Eychene A (2001) The Raf/MEK/ERK pathway: new concepts of activation. Biol Cell 93:53–62
Pflugfelder A, Eigentler TK, Keim U et al (2011) Effectiveness of carboplatin and paclitaxel as first- and second-line treatment in 61 patients with metastatic melanoma. PLoS One 6:e16882
Prahallad A, Sun C, Huang S et al (2012) Unresponsiveness of colon cancer to BRAF(V600E) inhibition through feedback activation of EGFR. Nature 483:100–103
Schreck R, Rapp UR (2006) Raf kinases: oncogenesis and drug discovery. Int J Cancer 119:2261–2271
Shah N, Iyer RM, Mair HJ et al (2013) Improved human bioavailability of vemurafenib, a practically insoluble drug, using an amorphous polymer-stabilized solid dispersion prepared by a solvent-controlled coprecipitation process. J Pharm Sci 102:967–981
Sirott MN, Bajorin DF, Wong GY et al (1993) Prognostic factors in patients with metastatic malignant melanoma: a multivariate analysis. Cancer 72:3091–3098

Sosman JA, Kim KB, Schuchter L et al (2012) Survival in BRAF V600-mutant advanced melanoma treated with vemurafenib. N Engl J Med 366:707–714

Tanaka H, Deng G, Matsuzaki K et al (2006) BRAF mutation, CpG island methylator phenotype and microsatellite instability occur more frequently and concordantly in mucinous than non-mucinous colorectal cancer. Int J Cancer 118:2765–2771

Tiacci E, Trifonov V, Schiavoni G et al (2011) BRAF mutations in hairy-cell leukemia. N Engl J Med 364:2305–2315

Tie J, Gibbs P, Lipton L et al (2011) Optimizing targeted therapeutic development: analysis of a colorectal cancer patient population with the BRAF(V600E) mutation. Int J Cancer 128:2075–2084

U.S. Food and Drug Administration (2011) FDA approves Zelboraf and companion diagnostic test for late-stage skin cancer. http://www.roche.com/media/media_releases/med-cor-2012-02-20.htm

Weide B, Elsasser M, Buttner P et al (2012) Serum markers lactate dehydrogenase and S100B predict independently disease outcome in melanoma patients with distant metastasis. Br J Cancer 107:422–428

Xing M (2007) BRAF mutation in papillary thyroid cancer: pathogenic role, molecular bases, and clinical implications. Endocr Rev 28:742–762

Dabrafenib

Radhika Kainthla, Kevin B. Kim and Gerald S. Falchook

Abstract

Dabrafenib was developed as a highly specific reversible inhibitor of V600-mutant BRAF kinase, an oncogenic mutation driving proliferation in many different types of aggressive tumors. Metastatic melanoma has a high prevalence of V600-mutant BRAF, and clinical trials showed that dabrafenib improved response rates and median progression-free survival in patients with V600E BRAF mutations, including those with brain metastasis. Preliminary results suggest that dabrafenib may also have some role in non-melanoma V600-mutant solid tumors; however, more studies are needed. With a well-tolerated toxicity profile and few drug interactions, dabrafenib is effective as a monotherapy; however, resistance eventually develops in most patients after persistent exposure to the drug. Current research focuses on combination strategies with dabrafenib to not only improve response rates but also overcome resistance.

R. Kainthla (✉)
Department of Internal Medicine, Baylor College of Medicine, Houston, TX, USA
e-mail: kainthla@bcm.edu

K. B. Kim
Department of Melanoma Medical Oncology, The University of Texas
MD Anderson Cancer Center, Houston, TX, USA

G. S. Falchook
Department of Investigational Cancer Therapeutics, The University of Texas
MD Anderson Cancer Center, Houston, TX, USA
e-mail: gfalchoo@mdanderson.org

U. M. Martens (ed.), *Small Molecules in Oncology*, Recent Results in Cancer Research 201, DOI: 10.1007/978-3-642-54490-3_14,

Contents

1 Introduction

The prevalence of specific mutations driving oncogenesis in many tumors has led to increased interest in the development of targeted therapies. Activating mutations in the mitogen-activated protein kinase (MAPK) pathway are well-known for their contribution to uncontrolled proliferation (Fig. 1) (Dhillon et al. 2007; Fang and Richardson 2005; Seger and Krebs 1995). Substitution of glutamine for valine at amino acid 600 (V600E) in the serine/threonine protein kinase BRAF locks the enzyme into a 500-fold more active conformation compared to the wild type and has been identified in a variety of cancers, including cutaneous melanoma, papillary thyroid carcinoma, and colorectal cancer (Davies et al. 2002; Frasca et al. 2008; Kalady et al. 2012; Long et al. 2011; Wan et al. 2004). Associated with more aggressive disease courses and worse overall prognoses, V600E BRAF mutations are ideal for targeted therapy (Frasca et al. 2008; Kalady et al. 2012; Long et al. 2011).

2 Mechanism of Action

Dabrafenib (Tafinlar, GSK2118436) was systematically developed from a thiazole core after the addition of a sulfonamide demonstrated potent inhibition of V600E BRAF (Fig. 2) (Rheault et al. 2013). As an ATP-competitive, reversible inhibitor, dabrafenib binds to the active formation of BRAF kinase and prevents downstream propagation of pro-growth signals, leading to cell cycle arrest (Laquerre et al. 2009).

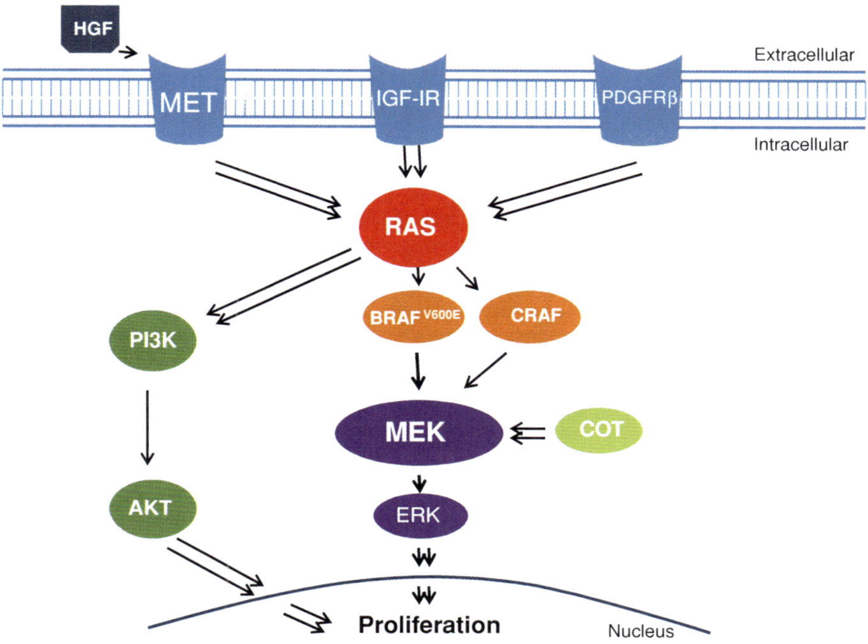

Fig. 1 MAPK signaling cascade and the redundancy leading to oncogenesis. *Single arrows* signify directpathways. *Double arrows* reflect a culmination of multiple steps in the signaling cascade. (Adapted from Kainthla et al. 2013)

Fig. 2 Structure of dabrafenib

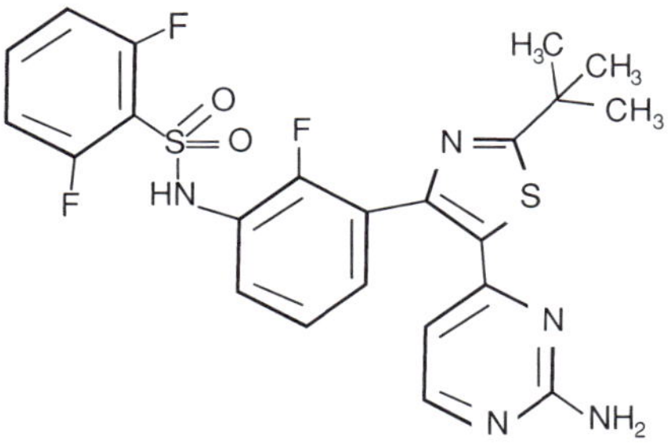

3 Preclinical Data

3.1 Dabrafenib Activity in V600 BRAF-Mutant Cell Lines

Preclinical studies demonstrated that dabrafenib decreases the expression of downstream-phosphorylated ERK in V600E BRAF-mutant cells. Dabrafenib is almost 20 times more specific for V600E BRAF mutants than wild-type BRAF in multiple cancer cell lines with an IC_{50} of 0.6 and 12 nM, respectively. Dabrafenib also displays inhibition in cell lines containing alternative oncogenic BRAF mutations including substitution at amino acid 600 of valine with lysine (V600K) and aspartate (V600D) with an IC_{50} of 0.5 and 1.9 nM, respectively (Laquerre et al. 2009).

3.2 Dabrafenib and Immune Modulation

The activated BRAF kinase leads to the increased production of immunosuppressive cytokines that prevent the body's ability to contribute to antitumor activity (Sumimoto et al. 2006). Dabrafenib-induced inhibition of BRAF could allow the immune system to attack tumor cells and decrease the likelihood of reoccurrence; however, many immune cells rely on the MAPK pathway to function, and previous non-specific inhibitors of the cascade have led to immune dysfunction (Hong et al. 2012; Weichsel et al. 2008; Zhao et al. 2008). Hong et al. 2012 demonstrated that dabrafenib treatment does not negatively impact systemic immunity or the production of de novo tumor-specific T cells . Additionally, tumor biopsies from patients before and after dabrafenib treatment showed post-treatment tumors usually had higher concentrations of intratumoral and peritumoral $CD4^+$ and $CD8^+$ cells compared to pre-treated biopsies. Increased intratumoral $CD8^+$ cells are correlated with decreased tumor size and increased tumor necrosis. Progressing tumors had fewer $CD8^+$ cells present (Wilmott et al. 2012). These findings suggest that dabrafenib may work synergistically with an immune stimulator, such as interleukin-2, to improve antitumor activity.

3.3 Mechanisms of Dabrafenib Resistance

Sustained exposure to dabrafenib induces resistance in cell lines and tumor lesions that were once sensitive (Greger et al. 2012; Nazarian et al. 2010; Villanueva et al. 2010). The acquired mechanism of resistance has been extensively studied, and many have been identified (Fig. 1). Previously sensitive cells that developed resistance after continued exposure to dabrafenib did not demonstrate the development of new secondary mutations in V600E BRAF. Persistent downstream phosphorylation of MEK and ERK in the presence of dabrafenib in some tumor lesions suggests alternative resistance pathways that are still dependent on the MAPK cascade for oncogenesis (Greger et al. 2012; Johnnessen et al. 2010; Nazarian et al. 2010; Villanueva et al. 2010). For example, utilization of different isoforms of RAF, such as CRAF, via an acquired new activating mutation in N-RAS, continues the unregulated MAPK signaling (Dumaz et al. 2006; Greger et al. 2012; Nazarian et al. 2010). Alternatively, an increase in the expression of COT-1, another serine/threonine kinase, leads to increased downstream phosphorylation of MEK independent of RAF (Johnnessen et al. 2010). Similarly, upregulation of different receptor tyrosine kinases, such as PDGFRβ and IGF-1R, has also been identified in BRAF inhibitor-resistant cells (Nazarian et al. 2010; Villanueva et al. 2010). Another mechanism of resistance involves alternative splicing of V600E BRAF (p61 BRAF) that leads to dimerization of the variant RAF proteins independent of RAS and continues downstream ERK phosphorylation in the presence of RAF inhibitors (Poulikakos et al. 2011).

Resistance to dabrafenib has been demonstrated in previously sensitive cell lines with evidence of persistent downstream MEK phosphorylation even after continued exposure to dabrafenib. When trametinib, a MEK inhibitor, was subsequently administered with dabrafenib to these cell lines with acquired resistance, restoration of sensitivity was observed, suggesting a role of dual inhibition with dabrafenib and trametinib to combat acquired dabrafenib resistance (Greger et al. 2012).

In addition, resistance can also develop through activating mutations in other proliferative pathways. Both MAPK and PI3K/mTOR cascades share S6 ribosomal protein (S6P) (Greger et al. 2012). In the setting of BRAF inhibition, studies have identified an increase in AKT and mTOR phosphorylation in the PI3K/mTOR pathway (Mendoza et al. 2011; Sanchez-Hernandez et al. 2012). Even with dual dabrafenib and trametinib therapy, S6P continued to be phosphorylated downstream. The addition of a dual PI3K/mTOR inhibitor to either dabrafenib or trametinib led to decreased S6P activation when compared to combination dabrafenib and trametinib therapy. Dual dabrafenib and PI3K/mTOR inhibitor treatment decreased proliferation in parental and resistant cell lines and offers an alternative strategy in overcoming dabrafenib resistance (Greger et al. 2012).

Although dabrafenib has high selectivity for V600E BRAF, the tumor microenvironment can also confer resistance to BRAF inhibition. In in vitro studies, cells initially sensitive to RAF inhibition became resistant when cultured with stromal cells that replicate the tumor microenvironment. Using antibody array-based analysis, hepatocyte growth factor (HGF) was identified as the factor inducing resistance. In the presence of RAF inhibitors, recombinant HGF was able to induce resistance when added to media containing initially sensitive cells (Straussman et al. 2012). Increased expression of MET kinase, which is a membrane receptor for HGF, was detected in melanoma cells with newly acquired resistance, but MET levels were undetectable in patients that remained sensitive to RAF inhibition (Straussman et al. 2012; Wilson et al. 2012). Activated MET kinase can contribute to oncogenesis through activation of either the MAPK pathways via utilization of CRAF to bypass BRAF inhibition or the PI3K-AKT pathway (Puri et al. 2007; Straussman et al. 2012). The role of HGF/MET signaling was further established when inhibitors to each were able to eliminate resistance in some V600E BRAF-mutant cells (Straussman et al. 2012). All these preliminary results suggest that adding HGF/MET inhibitors to dabrafenib therapy may increase response rates and possibly delay the emergence of resistance.

4 Metastatic Melanoma

4.1 Monotherapy

Melanoma has the highest mortality rate among all the skin cancer subtypes (American Cancer Society 2013). Standard chemotherapy options have modest response rates of less than 20 % as single agents and significant toxicities when administered in combination regimens (Agarwala et al. 2004; Atkins et al. 1999; Guirguis et al. 2002). BRAF mutations have been identified in about 50–60 % of metastatic melanoma with V600E BRAF mutants comprising about 80–90 % of these mutations (Davies et al. 2002; Long et al. 2011; Shinozaki et al. 2004). V600K BRAF is another common mutation observed in about 20 % of BRAF-mutant melanomas (Long et al. 2011). Given the prevalence of V600 BRAF mutations and their impact on the activation of the MAPK pathway, metastatic melanoma containing this oncogenic protein is an ideal target for dabrafenib treatment.

The first-in-human phase I clinical trial of dabrafenib in patients with metastatic melanoma yielded encouraging results. The drug was well-tolerated, and dose escalation failed to identify the maximum tolerated dose despite reaching concentrations sufficient for inhibition. The recommended phase II dose (RP2D) selected was 150 mg by mouth twice daily. At the RP2D, patients with V600E BRAF had a confirmed response rate of 57 % compared to 37 % observed in those with V600K BRAF (Table 1). Median progression-free survival was similar in patients with V600E or V600K at 5.5 and 5.6 months, respectively. No therapy was stopped secondary to side effects, and no deaths occurred directly from the treatment (Falchook et al. 2012).

With these promising results, a phase III trial compared dabrafenib to standard dacarbazine treatment in patients with V600E BRAF-mutant metastatic melanoma. Patients had no prior treatment other than high-dose IL-2. Participants had a good Eastern Cooperative Oncology Group (ECOG) performance status of 0 or 1 and no active central nervous system metastasis. The confirmed response rate in patients receiving dabrafenib treatment was 50 % compared to only 6 % in those on dacarbazine therapy per the study's independent review committee (Table 1). In the dabrafenib group, the partial response rate was 47 % while 3 % had a complete response (Hauschild et al. 2012). The median progression-free survival with dabrafenib was 6.9 months while patients receiving dacarbazine had a median progression-free survival of 2.7 months (Hauschild et al. 2013). Overall, dabrafenib proved to have significantly better response rates and median progression-free survival compared to dacarbazine in patients with V600E BRAF-mutant metastatic melanoma.

Table 1 Comparison of endpoints in dabrafenib clinical trials treating patients with metastatic melanoma

	# of patients enrolled[1]	Response rate (confirmed CR and PR)	Stable disease	Progression-free survival
Dabrafenib: phase I/II (Falchook et al. 2012)				
All patients	36	19 (53 %)	Not reported	5.5 months
V600E	28	16 (57 %)		5.5 months
V600K	8	3 (37 %)		5.6 months
Dabrafenib versus Dacarbazine: phase III (Hauschild et al. 2012)				
Dabrafenib	187	93 (50 %)	78 (42 %)	6.9 months[2]
Dacarbazine	63	4 (6 %)	30 (48 %)	2.7 months
Dabrafenib for brain metastasis: phase II (Long et al. 2012)				
Initial treatment				
V600E	74	29 (39 %)	31 (42 %)	16.1 weeks
V600K	15	1 (7 %)	4 (27 %)	8.1 weeks
Previously treated				
V600E	65	20 (31 %)	38 (58 %)	16.6 weeks
V600K	18	4 (22 %)	5 (28 %)	15.9 weeks
Dabrafenib with trametinib: phase I/II (Flaherty et al. 2012)				
Dabrafenib monotherapy	54	29 (54 %)	22 (41 %)	5.8 months
Dabrafenib+trametinib	54	41 (76 %)	13 (24 %)	9.4 months

CR complete response, *PR* partial response
[1]At the recommended phase 2 dose
[2]Hauschild et al. (2013)
Adapted from Kainthla et al. (2013)

4.2 Monotherapy in Brain Metastasis

In addition to the high response rate observed in metastatic melanoma, dabrafenib also demonstrated activity at the RP2D in a subset of ten patients with untreated brain metastases in the first-in-human phase I trial. Nine of these patients responded to treatment with four having a complete resolution of the brain lesions and a median progression-free survival of 4.2 months (Falchook et al. 2012). Based on these preliminary results, a phase II trial compared dabrafenib treatment in V600E and V600K BRAF-mutant melanoma in patients with untreated or locally treated brain metastases (Table 1) (Long et al. 2012). Local treatment included craniotomy with tumor resection, whole-brain radiation, or stereotactic radiosurgery. Participants with V600E BRAF mutations and no prior treatment had a 39 % intracranial response rate with a 3 % complete response rate and a median progression-free survival of 16.1 weeks. Those with prior local brain treatment and V600E BRAF-mutant melanoma had a partial response rate of 31 % and a median progression-free survival of 16.6 weeks. In comparison, V600K BRAF mutants were less responsive to dabrafenib treatment. The intracranial response rates in the untreated and previously treated cohort were 7 and 22 %, respectively, with none having a complete response. The median progression-free survival was 8.1 weeks in those with no prior treatment and 15.9 weeks in patients with prior local treatment (Long et al. 2012). Although V600E BRAF mutants had better response rates and median progression-free survival than V600K BRAF mutants, the overall results demonstrate that dabrafenib can be a reasonable first-line treatment option in both V600E and V600K BRAF-mutant metastatic melanoma with active brain metastasis, especially if patients have multiple intracranial metastasis.

4.3 Combination Therapy with Trametinib

Unfortunately, the effectiveness of dabrafenib in those with V600 BRAF mutations is limited as almost half the responders with metastatic melanoma have disease progression after 6 months, and eventually, nearly all develop resistance (Falchook et al. 2012; Hauschild et al. 2012; Long et al. 2012).

In a phase I and randomized phase II trial, dabrafenib was combined with trametinib, a MEK inhibitor, to evaluate the response rate and median progression-free survival as well as the development of cutaneous squamous cell carcinoma compared to dabrafenib monotherapy. Eligible patients had confirmed V600E or V600K BRAF-mutant metastatic melanoma with no prior treatment. The phase I portion of the study identified the RP2D to be dabrafenib 150 mg oral twice daily with trametinib 2 mg oral daily (Flaherty et al. 2012).

The combination regimen at the RP2D of each drug met the primary endpoints when compared to dabrafenib alone (Table 1). The response rate for dabrafenib with trametinib was 76 % (67 % partial response rate and 9 % complete response rate) compared to 54 % with dabrafenib monotherapy. Consistent with previous trials, the partial response rate for monotherapy was 50 % with a complete response rate of 4 %. The median progression-free survival duration with the combination treatment was also significantly improved at 9.4 months compared to 5.8 months with only dabrafenib treatment (Flaherty et al. 2012). Overall, combining dabrafenib with trametinib improved response rates and median progression-free survival compared to dabrafenib monotherapy.

Table 2 The response in different non-melanoma V600 BRAF-mutant solid tumors to dabrafenib treatment from the first-time-in-human clinical trial (Falchook et al. 2012)

Cancer type	No. of patients	Partial response	Stable disease
Papillary thyroid cancer	9	2	0
Colorectal cancer	9	1	7
Non-small cell lung cancer	1	1	0
GIST	1	0	1
Ovarian cancer	1	0	1

5 Other Cancers With V600E BRAF Mutations

5.1 Dabrafenib Monotherapy

In addition to metastatic melanoma, V600E BRAF mutations drive oncogenesis in many different types of cancers (Davies et al. 2011; Frasca et al. 2008; Kalady et al. 2012). The first-in-human phase I trial had a small subset of patients with non-melanoma, V600E BRAF-mutant solid tumors, which showed response to dabrafenib treatment (Table 2) (Falchook et al. 2012). Two out of nine patients with papillary thyroid cancer demonstrated a partial response as did the only patient with non-small-cell lung cancer. Of the nine participants with colorectal cancer, one had a partial response while seven had stable disease. One patient with gastrointestinal stromal tumor (GIST) and one person with ovarian cancer achieved stable disease with measurable decreases in tumor size (Falchook et al. 2012). The patient with V600E BRAF-mutant GIST, who had failed previous standard treatment, demonstrated a 20 % decrease in tumor size. The tumor decreased in size until 24 weeks and then plateaued before progressing at 8 months (Falchook et al. 2013). Ultimately, these preliminary results suggest a beneficial role of dabrafenib in non-melanoma cancers with V600E BRAF mutations; however, larger studies are needed to further investigate the potential use of dabrafenib in other cancers.

5.2 Combination Therapy with Trametinib in Colorectal Cancer (CRC)

Dabrafenib as a monotherapy in V600E BRAF-mutant CRC had modest response rates when compared to metastatic melanoma in the first-in-human phase I trial (Falchook et al. 2012). In metastatic melanoma, dabrafenib and trametinib combination therapy demonstrated improved response rates and median progression-free survival compared to dabrafenib monotherapy, so a small expansion cohort with V600 BRAF-mutant CRC was included in the phase I/II clinical trial of dabrafenib with trametinib (Corcoran et al. 2012; Flaherty et al. 2012). Almost all had failed prior therapy. Patients received 150 mg of dabrafenib twice daily and 2 mg of trametinib daily. Among the thirty-six participants available for evaluation, four (11 %) had at least a 30 % reduction in tumor size while eight (22 %) had minor responses, defined as a decrease in tumor size by 10–29 %. Median progression-free survival for the entire cohort was 3.4 months (Corcoran et al. 2013). About one-third of patients experienced a decrease in tumor size with combination therapy. Further investigation is needed to determine the role of dabrafenib and possible addition of trametinib in patients with V600 BRAF-mutant CRC.

6 Toxicity

Dabrafenib is well-tolerated overall. The most common side effects observed included hyperkeratosis of the skin (39 %), headache (35 %), arthralgia (35 %), and pyrexia (32 %). The most serious adverse effect was the development of cutaneous squamous cell carcinoma (10 %) (Hauschild et al. 2013). Grades 3 and 4 adverse effects were rare and included pyrexia (3 %), palmar-plantar erythrodysaesthesia (2 %), and fatigue (1 %) (Hauschild et al. 2012).

When dabrafenib was combined with trametinib, the most common adverse effect was pyrexia, which was more frequent in combination therapy (71 %) than monotherapy (26 %). Neutropenia (11 %) was the most common grade 3 or 4 adverse effect. The incidence of cutaneous squamous cell carcinoma decreased from 19 to 7 % when dabrafenib was combined with trametinib compared to dabrafenib alone. However, patients receiving the combination therapy experienced MEK inhibitor-associated adverse effects not seen in those taking monotherapy, including decreased ejection fraction (9 %) and chorioretinopathy (2 %), but none of these events were grade 3 or higher (Flaherty et al. 2012). Overall, dabrafenib combined with trametinib was well-tolerated.

7 Drug Interactions

Dabrafenib induces cytochrome P450 (CYP) 3A4 activity; therefore, dabrafenib should not be given with other substances that affect or are substrates of CYP3A4, CYP2C8, CYP2C9, CYP2C19, or CYP2B6 (Dabrafenib 2013). Additionally, increased gastric pH or concomitant ingestion of certain foods when taking dabrafenib decreases the drug's bioavailability (Ouellet et al. 2013). Therefore, dabrafenib should not be administered in patients taking medications that increase gastric pH and should be taken either 1 h before or 2 h after a meal (Dabrafenib 2013; Ouellet et al. 2013).

8 Biomarkers

8.1 Predictors of Response

Activating V600 BRAF mutations correlate with response to dabrafenib. No responses have been observed in patients without V600 BRAF mutations so far. In the first-in-human phase I trial, 6 patients without BRAF mutations were treated, and no antitumor activity was observed (Falchook et al. 2012). Subsequent studies have excluded those without V600 BRAF mutations. Therefore, V600 BRAF mutations are necessary but not always sufficient to achieve response to dabrafenib treatment. Additionally, the presence of a higher copy number of cyclin D1, lower copy number of cyclin-dependent kinase inhibitor 2A, or PTEN loss/mutation in patients with V600 BRAF mutations are associated with shorter median progression-free survival duration with dabrafenib treatment (Nathanson et al. 2013).

8.2 Pharmacodynamic Markers

A decrease in phosphorylated ERK (pERK), an enzyme downstream to BRAF, was detected in serial tumor biopsies in the phase I trial following dabrafenib treatment (Falchook et al. 2012). Monitoring pERK levels provides not only evidence of efficacy but also insight into whether mechanisms of resistance rely on MAPK-dependent pathways to propagate oncogenesis.

9 Summary and Perspectives

Dabrafenib was developed as a specific inhibitor of V600E BRAF, a common oncogenic protein present in different types of cancers. With a high prevalence of V600E BRAF mutations, metastatic melanoma is an ideal tumor type for BRAF-targeted therapy. Clinical trials in those with metastatic melanoma demonstrated improved response rates and median progression-free survival in patients with V600E BRAF mutations receiving dabrafenib compared to standard therapy. Based on the positive clinical trial results, in May 2013, the Food and Drug Administration (FDA) approved the use of dabrafenib in the treatment of unresectable or metastatic melanoma with V600E BRAF mutations (USFDA 2013). With a well-tolerated toxicity profile, few drug interactions, and taken orally twice daily, dabrafenib can conveniently be administered as an outpatient treatment.

Although the use of dabrafenib as a monotherapy in metastatic melanoma has been established, more studies are needed to determine the full potential of dabrafenib in cancer therapy. Preliminary studies suggest the drug has antitumor activity in other types of cancers with V600 BRAF mutations, but further investigation is still ongoing. Additionally, continued exposure to dabrafenib induces resistance in both preclinical studies and clinical trials. Combining dabrafenib with other inhibitors that target pathways conferring redundancy to the MAPK cascade may not only delay resistance but also increase overall response rates. Future studies will focus on taking advantage of the interplay among the tumor microenvironment, immune system, and intracellular signaling causing tumor progression to determine effective dabrafenib combination treatment strategies.

References

Agarwala SS, Kirkwood JM, Gore M et al (2004) Temozolomide for the treatment of brain metastases associated with metastatic melanoma: a phase II study. J Clin Oncol 22:2101–2107

American Cancer Society (2013) Cancer facts and figures 2013. American Cancer Society, Atlanta

Atkins MB, Lotze MT, Dutcher JP et al (1999) High-dose recombinant interleukin 2 therapy for patients with metastatic melanoma: analysis of 270 patients treated between 1985 and 1993. J Clin Oncol 17:2105–2116

Corcoran RB, Falchook GS, Infante JR et al (2012) BRAF V600 mutant colorectal cancer (CRC) expansion cohort from the phase I/II clinical trial of BRAF inhibitor dabrafenib (GSK2118436) plus MEK inhibitor trametinib (GSK1120212). J Clin Oncol (ASCO Meeting Abstract)

Corcoran RB, Falchook GS, Infante JR et al (2013) Pharmacodynamic and efficacy analysis of the BRAF inhibitor dabrafenib (GSK436) in combination with the MEK inhibitor trametinib (GSK212) in patients with BRAFV600 mutant colorectal cancer (CRC). J Clin Oncol (Meeting Abstract)

Dabrafenib (2013) Research Triangle Park. NC, GlaxoSmithKline, (package insert)

Davies H, Bignell GR, Cox C et al (2002) Mutations of the BRAF gene in human cancer. Nature 417:949–954

Dhillon AS, Hagan S, Rath O et al (2007) MAP kinase signaling pathways in cancer. Oncogene 26:3279–3290

Dumaz N, Hayward R, Martin J et al (2006) In melanoma, RAS mutations are accompanied by switching signaling from BRAF to CRAF and disrupted cyclic AMP signaling. Cancer Res 66:9483–9491

Falchook GS, Long GV, Kurzrock R et al (2012) Dabrafenib in patients with melanoma, untreated brain metastases, and other solid tumors: a phase 1 dose-escalation trial. The Lancet 379:1893–1901

Falchook GS, Trent JC, Heinrich MC et al (2013) BRAF mutant gastrointestinal stromal tumor: First report of regression with BRAF inhibitor dabrafenib (GSK2118436) and whole exomic sequencing for analysis of acquired resistance. Oncotarget 4:310–315

Fang JY, Richardson BC (2005) The MAPK signaling pathways and colorectal cancer. Lancet Oncol 6:322–327

Flaherty KT, Infante JR, Daud A et al (2012) Combined BRAF and MEK inhibition in melanoma with BRAF V600 mutations. N Engl J Med 367:1694–1703

Frasca F, Nucera C, Pellegriti G et al (2008) BRAF (V600E) mutation and the biology of papillary thyroid cancer. Endocr Relat Cancer 15:191–205

Greger JG, Eastman SD, Zhang V et al (2012) Combinations of BRAF, MEK, and PI3K/mTOR inhibitors overcome acquired resistance to the BRAF inhibitor GSK2118436 dabrafenib, mediated by NRAS or MEK mutations. Mol Cancer Ther 11:909–920

Guirguis LM, Yang JC, White DE et al (2002) Safety and efficacy of high-dose interleukin-2 therapy in patients with brain metastases. J Immunother 25:82–87

Hauschild A, Grob J, Dimidov LV et al (2012) Dabrafenib in BRAF-mutated metastatic melanoma: a multicentre, open-label, phase 3 randomised controlled trial. The Lancet 380:358–365
Hauschild A, Grob J, Dimidov LV et al (2013) An update on BREAK-3, a phase III, randomized trial: Dabrafenib (DAB) versus dacarbazine (DTIC) in patients with BRAF V600E-positive mutation metastatic melanoma (MM). J Clin Oncol (ASCO Meeting Abstract)
Hong DS, Vence L, Falchook GS et al (2012) BRAF(V600) inhibitor GSK2118436 targeted inhibition of mutant BRAF in cancer patients does not impair overall immune competency. Clin Cancer Res 8:2326–3715
Johnnessen CM, Boehm JS, Kim SY (2010) COT/MAP3K8 drives resistance to RAF inhibition through MAP kinase pathway reactivation. Nature 468:968–972
Kainthla R, Kim KB, Falchook GS (2013) Dabrafenib for treatment of BRAF-mutant melanoma. Pharm Pers Med 7:21–29
Kalady MF, Dejulius KL, Sanchez JA et al (2012) BRAF mutations in colorectal cancer are associated with distinct clinical characteristics and worse prognosis. Dis Colon Rectum 55:128–133
Laquerre S, Arnone M, Moss K et al (2009) Abstract B88: a selective Raf kinase inhibitor induces cell death and tumor regression of human cancer cell lines encoding B-Raf V600E mutation. Mol Ca Ther (Meeting Abstract 8)
Long GV, Menzies AM, Nagrial AM et al (2011) Prognostic and clinicopathologic associations of oncogenic BRAF in metastatic melanoma. J Clin Oncol 29:1239–1246
Long GV, Trefzer U, Davies MA et al (2012) Dabrafenib in patients with Val600Glu or Val600Lys BRAF-mutant melanoma metastatic to the brain (BREAK-MB): A multicentre, open-label, phase 2 trial. The Lancet 13:1087–1095
Mendoza MC, Er Emrah E, Blenis J (2011) The RAS-ERK and PI3K-mTOR pathways: cross-talk and compensation. Biochem Sci 36:320–328
Nathanson KL, Martin AM, Wubbenhorst B et al (2013) Tumor genetic analyses of patients with metastatic melanoma treated with the BRAF inhibitor dabrafenib (GSK2118436). Clin Cancer Res 19:4868–4878
Nazarian R, Shi H, Wang Q et al (2010) Melanomas acquire resistance to B-RAF (V600E) inhibition by RTK or N-RAS upregulation. Nature 468:973–977
Ouellet D, Grossmann KF, Limentani G et al (2013) Effects of particle size, food, and capsule shell composition on the oral bioavailability of dabrafenib, a BRAF inhibitor, in patients with BRAF mutation-positive tumors. J of Pharm Sci 102:3100–3109
Poulikakos PI, Persaud Y, Janakirman M et al (2011) RAF inhibitor resistance is mediated by dimerization of aberrantly spliced BRAF(V600E). Nature 480:387–390
Puri N, Ahmed S, Janamanchi V et al (2007) c-Met is a potentially new therapeutic target for treatment of human melanoma. Clin Cancer Res 13:2246–2253
Rheault TR, Stellwagen JC, Adjabeng GM et al (2013) Discovery of dabrafenib: A selective inhibitor of Raf kinases with antitumor activity against B-Raf-driven tumors. ACS Med Chem Lett 4:358–362
Sanchez-Hernandez I, Baquero P, Calleros L et al (2012) Dual inhibition of (V600E) BRAF and the PI3K/AKT/mTOR pathway cooperates to induce apoptosis in melanoma cells through a MEK-independent mechanism. Cancer Lett 314:244–255
Seger R, Krebs EG (1995) The MAPK signaling cascade. FASEB J 9:726–735
Shinozaki M, Fujimoto A, Morton DL et al (2004) Incidence of BRAF oncogene mutation and clinical relevance for primary cutaneous melanomas. Clin Cancer Res 10:1753–1757
Straussman R, Morikawa T, Shee K et al (2012) Tumor micro-environment elicits innate resistance to RAF inhibitors through HGF secretion. Nature 487:500–504
Sumimoto H, Imabayashi F, Iwata T et al (2006) The BRAF-MAPK signaling pathway is essential for cancer-immune evasion in human melanoma cells. J Exp Med 203:1651–1656
U.S. Food and Drug Administration (2013) Dabrafenib. Retrieved from http://www.fda.gov/Drugs/InformationOnDrugs/ApprovedDrugs/ucm354477.htm, 29 May 2013

Villanueva J, Vultur A, Lee JT et al (2010) Acquired resistance to BRAF inhibitors mediated by a RAF kinase switch in melanoma can be overcome by cotargeting MEK and IGF-1R/PI3K. Cancer Cell 18:683–695

Wan PT, Garnett MJ, Roe SM et al (2004) Mechanism of activation of the RAF-ERK signaling pathway by oncogenic mutations of B-RAF. Cell 116:855–867

Weichsel R, Dix C, Woolridge L et al (2008) Profound inhibition of antigen-specific T-cell effector functions by dasatinib. Clin Cancer Res 14:2484–2491

Wilmott JS, Long GV, Howie JR et al (2012) Selective BRAF inhibitors induce marked T-cell infiltration into human metastatic melanoma. Clin Cancer Res 18:1386–1394

Wilson TR, Fridlyand J, Yan Y et al (2012) Widespread potential for growth-factor-driven resistance to anticancer kinase inhibitors. Nature 487:505–509

Zhao W, Gu YH, Song R et al (2008) Sorafenib inhibits activation of human peripheral blood T cells by targeting LCK phosphorylation. Leukemia 22:1226–1233

Trametinib

Robert Zeiser

Abstract

The mitogen-activated protein kinase (MEK MAPK/ERK kinase) signaling pathways play a critical role in regulation of diverse cellular activities, including survival, differentiation, proliferation, motility, and angiogenesis. Therefore, MEK inhibition was recognized as a promising target for antineoplastic therapy. While multiple MEK inhibitors have been tested clinically only trametinib (GSK1120212), an oral MEK inhibitor which is selective for MEK1 and MEK2 has shown promising activity in several clinical trials on melanoma and colorectal cancer and it is being evaluated by the FDA for the treatment of metastatic melanoma. Mechanistically it was shown that trametinib induces cell cycle arrest in vitro. In this overview, important preclinical and clinical data for trametinib are presented including mechanism-based in vitro studies as well as findings from different clinical studies. Future clinical trial in different solid tumor entities will define the therapeutic role of this targeted therapy approach, possibly as a combination with other targeted therapies such as BRAF inhibitors.

Contents

R. Zeiser (✉)
Department of Hematology and Oncology, Freiburg University Medical Center, Albert Ludwigs University, Hugstetterstr. 55, 79106 Freiburg, Germany
e-mail: robert.zeiser@uniklinik-freiburg.de

U. M. Martens (ed.), *Small Molecules in Oncology*, Recent Results in Cancer Research 201, DOI: 10.1007/978-3-642-54490-3_15,

1 Structure and Mechanism of Action

The mitogen-activated protein kinase (MAPK) signaling pathways involve a family of protein kinases that play critical roles in regulation of diverse cellular activities, including cell proliferation, survival, differentiation, motility, and angiogenesis (Thompson and Lyons 2005). The MAPK pathways transduce signals from various extracellular stimuli (growth factors, hormones, mitogens, cytokines, and environmental stress), leading to distinct intracellular responses (Chang and Karin 2001) as shown in Fig. 1. Mitogen-activated protein kinase or MAP2K or MAPKK are commonly known as MEK proteins. These MEK enzymes selectively phosphorylate serine/threonine and tyrosine residues within the activation loop of their specific MAP kinase substrates.

Trametinib (GSK1120212, JTP-74057) is a second-generation small molecule inhibitor of MEK kinase. It functions as allosteric, ATP non-competitive inhibitor with nanomolar activity against both MEK 1 and MEK 2 kinases with a half-maximal inhibitory concentration of 0.7–14.9 nmol/L for MEK1/MEK2 (Gilmartin et al. 2011; Yamaguchi et al. 2011). Inhibitors of MEK1/2 had been previously investigated as targeted therapies for tumors dependent on activating mutations in the MAPK pathway, but prior to trametinib, the success of MEK inhibitors with respect to clinical activity was limited due to the dependence of non-malignant cells on the MAPK pathway which precluded adequate dosing of the inhibitor (LoRusso et al. 2005; Yeh et al. 2007). When compared to other published MEK inhibitors, trametinib has a different pharmacokinetic profile, with a prolonged half-life, and small peak-to-trough ratios, which made it possible to overcome the narrow therapeutic index associated with MEK inhibition. Specificity of trametinib for MEK1/2 was confirmed against a panel of more than 180 kinases, including B-Raf, C-Raf, and MEK5 the closest kinase homolog (Yamaguchi et al. 2011), adjacent to the active site and defined on one side by the activation loop. The inhibitory effect of trametinib on cell growth was shown to be through inhibition of p-ERK 1/2. Therefore, most significant inhibition was achieved in tumor cell lines with mutant B-Raf or Ras (Yamaguchi et al. 2011). In vitro studies have demonstrated that trametinib decreases cell proliferation, causes G1 cell cycle arrest, and induces apoptosis. The structure and chemical characteristics of trametinib are shown in Fig. 2.

2 Preclinical Data

In the initial studies on trametinib, the proliferation across 94 cancer cell lines was evaluated systematically in vitro (Gilmartin et al. 2011; Yamaguchi et al. 2011). Among the different cell lines evaluated in the study, those with either $BRAF^{V600E}$

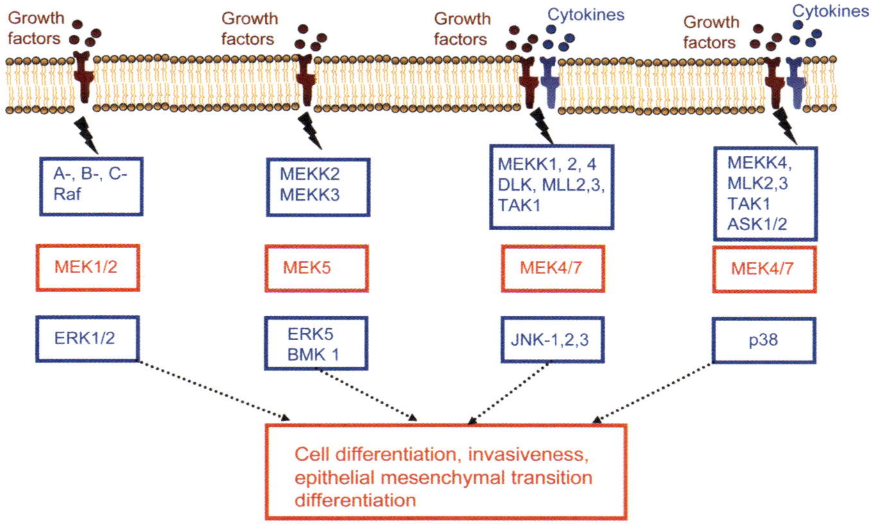

Fig. 1 The known MEK enzymes and their four signaling pathways. *Brown color* growth factor receptors, *blue color* cytokine receptors

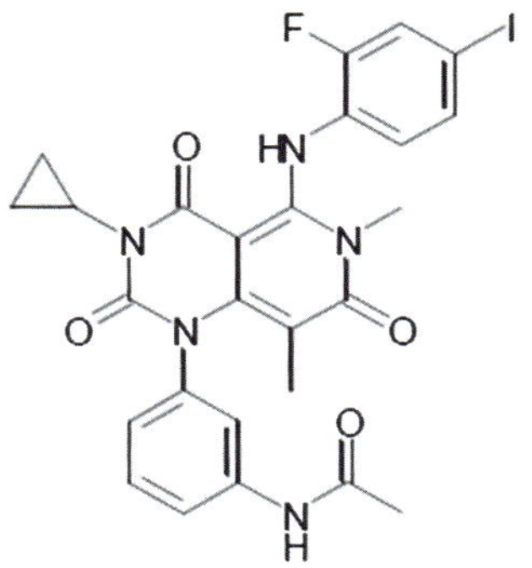

Fig. 2 The structure and chemical characteristics of trametinib. Mol. mass: 615.39 g/mol. Molecular formula: C26H23FIN5O4, chemical name: *N*-(3-{3-Cyclopropyl-5-[(2-fluoro-4-iodo-phenyl)amino]-6,8-dimethyl-2,4,7-trioxo-3,4,6,7-tetrahydropyrido[4,3-d]pyrimidin-1(2*H*)-yl} phenyl)acetamide

mutation or activating mutations in KRAS or NRAS were the most sensitive. In all cancer cell lines evaluated in this study, trametinib inhibited the MEK1/2-dependent activating dual phosphorylation of ERK1/2 on both T202 and Y204 (Gilmartin et al. 2011). The observation that trametinib did not directly inhibit either C-Raf or B-Raf activity in enzymatic assays led to the conclusion that the drug must bind to MEK such that it specifically blocks the accessibility of S217 to Raf kinases. Tumor cell proliferation assay curves for 94 cancer cell lines evaluating sensitivity to trametinib demonstrated that among cell lines with activating KRAS mutation, 16 of 25 (64 %) had a partial response to the drug and 19 of 25 (76 %) cell lines had cytotoxic or cytostatic responses (Gilmartin et al. 2011). These findings were then further studied in vivo in nude mice in which the tumor cells were implanted and grown as tumor xenografts (Gilmartin et al. 2011). The treatment with trametinib was initiated when the tumors had reached a volume of 150 mm^3 to mimic the clinical situation. Trametinib or vehicle was administered by oral garvage, and the maximum tolerated dose was defined as the highest dose that produced less than 20 % mortality and less than 20 % weight loss. The activity of trametinib against the tumor was defined according to clinical criteria including growth inhibition, partial remission (PR), or complete remission (CR). The preclinical studies showed efficient inhibition of p-ERK 1/2 which correlated with potent cell growth inhibition in tumor lines with mutant B-Raf or Ras (Gilmartin et al. 2011; Yamaguchi et al. 2011). In xenograft models of HT-29 and COLO205 colorectal tumor cell lines, trametinib demonstrated robust anticancer activity when administered daily for 14 days (Gilmartin et al. 2011; Yamaguchi et al. 2011). Pharmacokinetic profiling in mice indicated a mean effective half-life ($t_{1/2}$) of 33 h, with a low peak/trough ratio of around 1.6:2.8 after single or repeat dosing of trametinib (Gilmartin et al. 2011). This is compatible with other studies showing that pharmacological MEK inhibition completely abrogated tumor growth in BRAF mutant xenografts, whereas RAS mutant tumors were only partially inhibited (Solit et al. 2006). These preclinical findings provided robust evidence that MEK inhibition has in vivo antitumor activity and led to clinical trials.

3 Clinical Data

The rationale for clinical studies was build on the strong in vitro and mouse model data and on the finding in humans that mutated oncogenic forms of RAS are found in approximately 15 % of all cancers (Davies et al. 2002) with a variable prevalence of RAS mutations depending on the tumor types. KRAS mutations which predispose for sensitivity to trametinib responsiveness are frequently found in colorectal, lung, pancreatic, and cervical cancer (Schubbert et al. 2007), and activating BRAF mutations have been reported in approximately 60 % of cutaneous melanoma, approximately 50 % of papillary thyroid, 5–20 % of colorectal, approximately 30 % of ovarian, and approximately 26 % of germ cell tumors (Wellbrock et al. 2004; Honecker et al. 2009). Based on these findings, an early phase I dose increase trial of trametinib was performed, which enrolled 206 patients with different advanced solid tumors. This clinical trial determined that dose-limiting toxic effects of trametinib were rash, diarrhea, and central serous retinopathy (Infante et al. 2012). While these dose-limiting toxic effects grade 3–4 were infrequent (<8 %), common treatment-related adverse events were dermatitis acneiform (80 %) and diarrhea (42 %). The authors described the effective half-life of trametinib with about 4 days. Based on the results of this study, the recommended dose for the following phase II study was 2 mg per day. While the overall objective response rate in the different solid tumor types was 10 %, B-Raf mutant melanoma had a higher response rate of 33 % (Infante et al. 2012). These encouraging results led to several phase II/III clinical trials of trametinib alone or in combination with other agents including NCT01553851, NCT01682083, NCT01362296, NCT01619774, and NCT01245062 (details are available on clinicaltrials.gov). In the first published phase III trial of trametinib (METRIC trial), 322 patients with advanced melanoma previously treated with interferon or chemotherapy with a proven V600E or V600K B-Raf mutation were randomly assigned in a 2:1 ratio to receive oral trametinib or intravenous chemotherapy consisting of either dacarbazine or paclitaxel, every 3 weeks (Flaherty et al. 2012a, b). The median progression-free survival (PFS) of patients who received trametinib was significantly longer than that of patients who received chemotherapy (4.8 vs. 1.5 months, respectively) and at 6 months, the rate of overall survival (OS) was 81 % in the trametinib group versus 67 % in the chemotherapy group. These findings indicated that trametinib, as compared to chemotherapy, improved rates of PFS and OS among patients who had metastatic melanoma. The response rate was higher in trametinib-treated patients when compared with other MEK inhibitors such as selumetinib which had an response rate of 10 % in BRAF mutant melanoma (Kirkwood et al. 2012), and PD0325901 was poorly tolerated (Haura et al. 2010; LoRusso et al. 2010). Since in vitro studies and analyses of predose and postprogression tumor biopsies in clinical trials have shown both MEK-dependent and MEK-independent resistance following exposure to a BRAF inhibitor (Montagut et al. 2008; Johannessen et al. 2010; Nazarian et al. 2010; Villanueva et al. 2010; Fedorenko et al. 2011) a combination of trametinib with a BRAF inhibitor was a logical next step. In a more recent study dabrafenib and trametinib were combined and compared with trametinib monotherapy. The rate of pyrexia was increased with combination therapy, whereas the rate of proliferative skin lesions was nonsignificantly reduced. Progression-free survival was significantly improved in the combination therapy compared to monotherapy (Flaherty et al. 2012a, b). Based on the data from the clinical trials, the FDA has approved Mekinist (trametinib) as a single-agent oral treatment for unresectable or metastatic melanoma in adult patients with BRAF V600E or V600K mutations. This result was confirmed by a later study in which significant clinical activity was observed in BRAF inhibitor-naive melanoma patients while almost no clinical activity was observed as sequential therapy in patients previously treated with a BRAF inhibitor (Kim et al. 2013). These data lead to the conclusion that BRAF inhibitor resistance mechanisms likely confer resistance to MEK inhibitor monotherapy. Consequently, tramtinib was not approved for the indication melanoma in patients who have received a prior BRAF inhibitor therapy.

4 Toxicity

In individuals with advanced solid tumors, a dose increase study was performed to define the maximum tolerated dose (Infante et al. 2012). The most common treatment-related adverse events were rash or dermatitis acneiform (80 %) and diarrhea (42 %), most of which were grade 1 and 2. Dose-limiting toxicities included rash, central retinopathy, and diarrhea (Infante et al. 2012). Based on this study, the dose of 2 mg/day was chosen for further studies. In patients treated with trametinib for malignant melanoma, most common adverse events observed were rash, diarrhea, peripheral edema, fatigue, and dermatitis acneiform (Flaherty et al. 2012a, b). Among the patients with rash, less than 8 % had grade 3 or 4 rash. A decreased ejection fraction or ventricular dysfunction was observed in 14 patients (7 %) in the trametinib group; of these, patients 11 had a decreased ejection fraction and 3 had left ventricular dysfunction (Flaherty et al. 2012a, b). In the light of the reported toxicity data, the dose of 2 mg trametinib once a day was shown to be tolerable and the side effects were manageable. Administration of trametinib in combination with standard gemcitabine dosing (1,000 mg/m2 IV Days 1, 8, and 15 every 28 days) was shown to be feasible (Infante et al. 2013). Though most toxicities were manageable, the addition of trametinib was shown to lead to slightly higher gemcitabine-associated myelosuppression.

5 Drug Interactions

The low C_{max} in plasma with the 2 mg a day dose suggests that trametinib is low risk for drug interactions [unpublished data, mentioned in (Infante et al. 2012)]. In vitro and in vivo data suggest that GSK1120212 is unlikely to affect the PK of other drugs.

6 Biomarkers

Biomarkers are essential to identify patients with a better chance to respond to targeted therapies. In order to find predictive biomarkers for the sensitivity to trametinib, a recent study had profiled 218 solid tumor cell lines and 81 hematologic malignancy cell lines (Jing et al. 2012). The authors found that *RAF* and *RAS* mutations were a strong predictor of sensitivity to MEK inhibition by trametinib in solid tumor cells. By using transcriptomics analysis in *KRAS* mutant cell lines, the authors identified cell lines with a gene signature indicative of epithelial-to-mesenchymal transition (EMT) to be less sensitive to trametinib (Jing et al. 2012). Also, the gene *DUSP6* was identified to predict for trametinib sensitivity while a lack of expression was associated with resistance to the drug irrelevant of the *RAF/RAS* mutation status. When colon cancer cells had both *RAF/RAS* mutations and *PIK3CA/PTEN* mutations, this was predictive for a cytostatic response instead of a cytotoxic response (Jing et al. 2012). The evaluation of trametinib sensitivity within hematological malignancies demonstrated that acute myeloid leukemia and chronic myeloid leukemia cell lines were more sensitive than other entities (Jing et al. 2012). Overall, the different studies for trametinib sensitivity identified multiple biomarkers including mutant *RAF*, *RAS*, *PIK3CA/PTEN*, and *DUSP6* in solid tumors and thereby will help in the future to identify patients who could benefit from trametinib treatment.

7 Summary and Perspectives

Targeted therapies with small molecular inhibitors for solid tumors and hematological malignancies are moving rapidly from bench to bedside. The MEK inhibitor a trametinib has shown promising clinical efficacy and is being evaluated by the FDA for the treatment of metastatic melanoma. Since targeted therapies attempt to inactivate a mutated oncogenic pathway, critical to survival of cancer cells while sparing normal cells, which do not carry the mutation and are not similarly addicted to the pathway, informative biomarkers for trametinib have been identified including *RAF*, *RAS*, *PIK3CA/PTEN*, and *DUSP6*. Trametinib holds promise to overcome paradoxical MEK activation seen in different solid tumors such as melanoma that become resistant to BRAF inhibition and thereby contribute to the solution of a major clinical problem. This concept will not only apply to BRAF and MEK inhibitors, and combination of targeting agents against different signaling pathways may provide additional benefits and warrant further clinical studies.

References

Chang L, Karin M (2001) Mammalian MAP kinase signalling cascades. Nature 6:37–40

Davies H, Bignell GR, Cox C et al (2002) Mutations of the BRAF gene in human cancer. Nature 417:949–954

Fedorenko IV, Paraiso KH, Smalley KS (2011) Acquired and intrinsic BRAF inhibitor resistance in BRAF V600E mutant melanoma. Biochem Pharmacol 82:201–209

Flaherty KT, Infante JR, Daud A, Gonzalez R, Kefford RF, Sosman J et al (2012a) Combined BRAF and MEK inhibition in melanoma with BRAF V600 mutations. N Engl J Med 367:1694–1703

Flaherty KT, Robert C, Hersey P, Nathan P, Garbe C, Milhem M et al (2012b) Improved survival with MEK inhibition in BRAF-mutated melanoma. N Engl J Med 367:107–114

Gilmartin AG, Bleam MR, Groy A, Moss KG, Minthorn EA, Kulkarni SG et al (2011) GSK1120212 (JTP-74057) is an inhibitor of MEK activity and activation with favorable pharmacokinetic properties for sustained in vivo pathway inhibition. Clin Cancer Res 6:989–1000

Haura EB, Ricart AD, Larson TG, Stella PJ, Bazhenova L, Miller VA et al (2010) A phase II study of PD-0325901, an oral MEK inhibitor, in previously treated patients with advanced non-small cell lung cancer. Clin Cancer Res 16:2450–2457

Honecker F, Wermann H, Mayer F, Gillis AJM et al (2009) Microsatellite instability, mismatch repair deficiency, and BRAF mutation in treatment-resistant germ cell tumours. J Clin Oncol 27:2129–2136

Infante JR, Fecher LA, Falchook GS, Nallapareddy S, Gordon MS, Becerra C et al (2012) Safety, pharmacokinetic, pharmacodynamic, and efficacy data for the oral MEK inhibitor trametinib: a phase 1 dose-escalation trial. J Clin Oncol 6:773–781

Infante JR, Papadopoulos KP, Bendell JC, Patnaik A, Burris HA, Rasco D et al (2013) A phase 1b study of trametinib, an oral Mitogen-activated protein kinase kinase (MEK) inhibitor, in combination with gemcitabine in advanced solid tumours. Eur J Cancer (Epub ahead of print)

Jing J, Greshock J, Holbrook JD, Gilmartin A, Zhang X, McNeil E et al (2012) Comprehensive predictive biomarker analysis for MEK inhibitor GSK1120212. Mol Cancer Ther 11:720–729

Johannessen CM, Boehm JS, Kim SY, Thomas SR, Wardwell L, Johnson LA et al (2010) COT drives resistance to RAF inhibition through MAP kinase pathway reactivation. Nature 468:968–972

Kim KB, Kefford R, Pavlick AC, Infante JR, Ribas A, Sosman JA et al (2013) Phase II study of the MEK1/MEK2 inhibitor trametinib in patients with metastatic BRAF-mutant cutaneous melanoma previously treated with or without a BRAF inhibitor. J Clin Oncol 31:482–489

Kirkwood JM, Bastholt L, Robert C, Sosman J, Larkin J, Hersey P et al (2012) Phase II, open-label, randomized trial of the MEK1/2 inhibitor selumetinib as monotherapy versus temozolomide in patients with advanced melanoma. Clin Cancer Res 18:555–567

LoRusso PM, Adjei AA, Varterasian M, Gadgeel S, Reid J, Mitchell DY et al (2005) Phase I and pharmacodynamic study of the oral MEK inhibitor CI-1040 in patients with advanced malignancies. J Clin Oncol 23:5281–5293

LoRusso PM, Krishnamurthi SS, Rinehart JJ, Nabell LM, Malburg L, Chapman PB et al (2010) Phase I pharmacokinetic and pharmacodynamic study of the oral MAPK/ERK kinase inhibitor PD-0325901 in patients with advanced cancers. Clin Cancer Res 16:1924–1937

Montagut C, Sharma SV, Shioda T, McDermott U, Ulman M, Ulkus LE et al (2008) Elevated CRAF as a potential mechanism of acquired resistance to BRAF inhibition in melanoma. Cancer Res 68:4853–4861

Nazarian R, Shi H, Wang Q, Kong X, Koya RC, Lee H et al (2010) Melanomas acquire resistance to B-RAF(V600E) inhibition by RTK or N-RAS upregulation. Nature 468:973–977

Schubbert S, Shannon K, Bollag G (2007) Hyperactive Ras in developmental disorders and cancer. Nat Rev Cancer 7:295–308

Solit DB, Garraway LA, Pratilas CA, Sawai A, Getz G, Basso A et al (2006) BRAF mutation predicts sensitivity to MEK inhibition. Nature 439:358–362

Thompson N, Lyons J (2005) Recent progress in targeting the Raf/MEK/ERK pathway with inhibitors in cancer drug discovery. Curr Opin Pharmacol 6:350–356

Villanueva J, Vultur A, Lee JT, Somasundaram R, Fukunaga-Kalabis M, Cipolla AK et al (2010) Acquired resistance to BRAF inhibitors mediated by a RAF kinase switch in melanoma can be overcome by cotargeting MEK and IGF-1R/PI3K. Cancer Cell 18:683–695

Wellbrock C, Karasarides M, Marais R (2004) The RAF proteins take centre stage. Nature Rev Mol Cell Biol 5:875–885

Yamaguchi T, Kakefuda R, Tajima N, Sowa Y, Sakai T (2011) Antitumor activities of JTP-74057 (GSK1120212), a novel MEK1/2 inhibitor, on colorectal cancer cell lines in vitro and in vivo. Int J Oncol 39:23–31

Yeh TC, Marsh V, Bernat BA, Ballard J, Colwell H, Evans RJ et al (2007) Biological characterization of ARRY-142886 (AZD6244), a potent, highly selective mitogen-activated protein kinase kinase 1/2 inhibitor. Clin Cancer Res 13:1576–1583

Ruxolitinib

Heiko Becker, Monika Engelhardt, Nikolas von Bubnoff and Ralph Wäsch

Abstract

Ruxolitinib, formerly known as INCB018424 or INC424, is a potent and selective oral inhibitor of JAK1 and JAK2. Ruxolitinib has been approved for the treatment of myelofibrosis, which is characterized, biologically, by the activation of the JAK-STAT pathway and, clinically, by bone marrow fibrosis, splenomegaly, abnormal blood counts, and poor quality-of-life through associated symptoms. Ruxolitinib treatment results in a meaningful reduction in spleen size and symptom burden in the majority of myelofibrosis patients, and it may also have a favorable effect on survival. Treatment response apparently does not depend on the presence of a JAK2 V617F mutation. The predominant toxicities are thrombocytopenia and anemia. The metabolization of ruxolitinib through CYP3A4 needs to be considered particularly if co-administered with potent CYP3A4 inhibitors. Several further JAK inhibitors are currently studied in myelofibrosis or other immuno-inflammatory diseases.

Contents

H. Becker · M. Engelhardt · N. von Bubnoff · R. Wäsch (✉)
University Freiburg—Medical Center, Hugstetterstrasse 55, 79106, Freiburg, Germany
e-mail: ralph.waesch@uniklinik-freiburg.de

U. M. Martens (ed.), *Small Molecules in Oncology*, Recent Results in Cancer Research 201, DOI: 10.1007/978-3-642-54490-3_16,

1 Structure and Mechanism of Action

The Janus kinase (JAK) family consists of four intracellular, nonreceptor tyrosine kinases: JAK1, JAK2, JAK3, and TYK2. JAKs are constitutively bound to cytokine receptors. Upon binding of ligand, JAKs are activated and thereby phosphorylate and activate downstream targets such as signal transducers and activators of transcription (STAT) (Mertens and Darnell 2007). Thus, JAKs have a crucial role in regulation and homeostasis in hematopoiesis and immunity. In 2005, an activating mutation in the JAK2 pseudokinase, i.e., V617F, was identified in a high proportion of patients with myeloproliferative neoplasms (MPNs), and expression of the mutant JAK2 in a murine model resulted in an MPN-like disease (James et al. 2005; Quintás-Cardama et al. 2010). These findings drove the development of drugs to target wild-type and/or mutant JAK2. Ruxolitinib is the first of these drugs that has been approved for treatment.

Ruxolitinib was formerly known as INCB018424 or INC424. The chemical name is (*R*)-3-(4-(7*H*-pyrrolo[2,3-*d*]pyrimidin-4-yl)-1*H*-pyrazol-1-yl)-3-cyclopentylpropanenitrile phosphate, and its molecular weight is 404.36. The chemical structure is available in the PubChem Compound database through the identifier CID 25127112.

Ruxolitinib is an oral, reversible class I inhibitor and competes with ATP in the catalytic site of the JAK tyrosine kinases. Accordingly, ruxolitinib is not specific for the JAK2 V617F mutation. Its efficacy in myelofibrosis has been primarily attributed to attenuation of the inflammatory state caused by constitutive JAK-STAT activation and a nonspecific myelosuppression. Peak plasma concentrations of ruxolitinib are achieved within one hour after administration and decline in a monophasic or biphasic manner with a mean terminal half-life of 2.3 h (Shilling et al. 2010).

2 Preclinical Data

Ruxolitinib selectively inhibited JAK1 and JAK2 with IC_{50} values of 3.3 and 2.8 nM, respectively. The IC_{50} was approximately sixfold higher for TYK2 and 140-fold higher for JAK3 (Quintás-Cardama et al. 2010). Ruxolitinib also suppressed the proliferation of JAK2 V617-positive Ba/F3 cells with an IC_{50} of 127 nM as well as the cytokine-independent colony formation of erythroid progenitors from patients with JAK2 V617F-positive polycythemia vera with an IC_{50} of 67 nM (Quintás-Cardama et al. 2010). In Balb/c mice injected with JAK2 V617F-positive Ba/F3 cells, ruxolitinib reduced splenomegaly, decreased levels of circulating interleukin 6 and tumor necrosis factor alpha, and prolonged survival (Quintás-Cardama et al. 2010).

3 Clinical Data

The Food and Drug Administration (FDA) in the United States approved ruxolitinib for the treatment of myelofibrosis in 2011 and the European Medicines Agency (EMA) in 2012. Myelofibrosis can occur as primary myelofibrosis (PMF), post-essential thrombocythemia myelofibrosis (PETMF), or post-polycythemia vera myelofibrosis (PPVMF). It is characterized by progressive bone marrow fibrosis, splenomegaly, abnormal blood counts as well as constitutional symptoms (fever, weight loss, and night sweats) and other debilitating symptoms, such as fatigue, bone pain, early satiety, abdominal pain, and pruritus. Abnormal levels of pro-inflammatory cytokines and the activation of the JAK-STAT pathway are characteristic for myelofibrosis. JAK2 V617F mutations are found in approximately half of the patients. The median survival of patients with myelofibrosis depends on the presence of risk factors and varies according to the International Prognostic Scoring System (IPSS) between 2 years for patients with high risk and 11 years for those with low risk (Cervantes et al. 2009). Major causes of death are leukemic transformation and progressive disease (Cervantes et al. 2009). Except for allogeneic hematopoietic stem cell transplantation, the current therapeutic approaches are palliative and confer limited benefit.

In a phase 1/2 trial, which included 153 adult patients with myelofibrosis (93 % intermediate-2 and high risk), thrombocytopenia was found to be the dose-limiting toxic effect, and 25 mg twice daily was defined as the maximum tolerated dose (Verstovsek et al. 2010). Sixty-one (44 %) of 140 patients with splenomegaly had a ≥50 % reduction in palpable splenomegaly in the first 3 months of treatment. Response rates were highest among patients who received 15 mg twice daily (response rate 52 %) or 25 mg twice daily (response rate 49 %). Considering also those with a less pronounced effect on splenomegaly, ≥70 % of patients with 10, 15, or 25 mg twice daily had ≥25 % reduction in palpable spleen size in the first 2 months of treatment. Response rates were similar among patients with or without JAK2 V617F mutation. In accordance, the suppression of STAT3 phosphorylation was observed regardless of the presence of JAK2 V617F. In addition to the reduction in the spleen size, the majority of patients with 10, 15, or 25 mg twice daily had a ≥50 % improvement of myelofibrosis-related symptoms. With regard to the blood counts, the mean white blood cell count decreased from 29.8×10^9 to 16.0×10^9/L, and patients with elevated platelet counts at baseline (mean 728×10^9/L) had reduced platelet counts (336×10^9/L) at 3 months of treatment. In the long-term follow-up of 107 patients included in the phase 1/2 trial, the median duration of a meaningful spleen size reduction was approximately 2 years from the onset of the response (Verstovsek et al. 2012a).

Subsequent to the phase 1/2 trial, two phase 3 studies (COMFORT-I and COMFORT-II) were initiated. In both trials, patients had PMF, PETMF, or PPVMF with palpable splenomegaly of at least 5 cm below the costal margin and an IPSS intermediate-2 or high risk. The starting dose depended on the baseline platelet count and was 15 mg twice daily for platelets of 100×10^9/L–200×10^9/

L and 20 mg twice daily for platelets of more than 200 × 10^9/L. During the study, the dosing was reduced based on neutropenia or thrombocytopenia or escalated (to a maximum of 25 mg twice daily) to increase efficacy. While COMFORT-I was a double-blind, placebo-controlled trial including 155 patients in the ruxolitinib group and 154 in the placebo group, COMFORT-II was an open-label trial testing ruxolitinib in 146 patients against best available therapy (BAT, mostly hydroxyurea or glucocorticoids) in 73 patients.

The primary efficacy end point was the proportion of patients achieving a ≥35 % reduction in spleen volume at 24 weeks (COMFORT-I) or 48 weeks (COMFORT-II), as assessed by MRI or CT. The respective end point was reached by 42 % in the ruxolitinib and 1 % in the placebo group in COMFORT-I (Verstovsek et al. 2012b) and by 28 % in the ruxolitinib group compared with 0 % in the BAT group in COMFORT-II (Harrison et al. 2012a) (Fig. 1a, b). The median time to the first observation of ≥35 % reduction in spleen volume was 12 weeks in the ruxolitinib group in COMFORT-II. Overall, almost every patient who received ruxolitinib had some degree of spleen size reduction.

A secondary end point in COMFORT-I was the proportion of patients with a ≥50 % reduction in the total symptom score at 24 weeks measured by the modified Myelofibrosis Symptom Assessment Form. This end point was reached by 46 % of the ruxolitinib-treated patients and 5 % of the patients receiving placebo in COMFORT-I (Verstovsek et al. 2012b) (Fig. 1c). In contrast, only 4 % of the ruxolitinib group had significant worsening of symptoms (>50 % increase in total symptom score), compared with 33 % in the placebo group (Mesa et al. 2013). Comparable results regarding quality-of-life and symptoms were obtained in COMFORT-II (Harrison et al. 2012a).

Notably, ruxolitinib was effective in reducing spleen size and symptom burden regardless of age group (≤65 and >65 years), myelofibrosis subtype, IPSS risk group, pretreatment spleen size, pretreatment platelet count, and JAK2 V617F status (Verstovsek et al. 2013). Although there were no significant differences according to the JAK2 V617F status, JAK2 V617F-positive patients had a mean reduction in the spleen volume of 35 % and in the symptom burden of 53 %, whereas those negative for JAK2 V617F had reductions of 24 and 28 %, respectively (Verstovsek et al. 2012b).

Ruxolitinib-treated patients also had a survival benefit compared with those receiving placebo in COMFORT-I (HR 0.5, 95 %-CI 0.25–0.98, $P = 0.04$). In COMFORT-II, overall survival was similar between the ruxolitinib and BAT group after 48 weeks. Long-term outcome of COMFORT-I and COMFORT-II has been hitherto reported only in abstract form, but a survival advantage conferred by ruxolitinib in comparison with placebo appears to persist and, with the longer follow-up, may also become apparent in comparison with BAT (Verstovsek et al. 2012c; Vanucchi et al. 2013). In a sponsor-independent report on the long-term follow-up of 51 patients of the phase 1/2 trial, the overall survival of the ruxolitinib-treated patients was similar to that of 410 PMF patients treated with

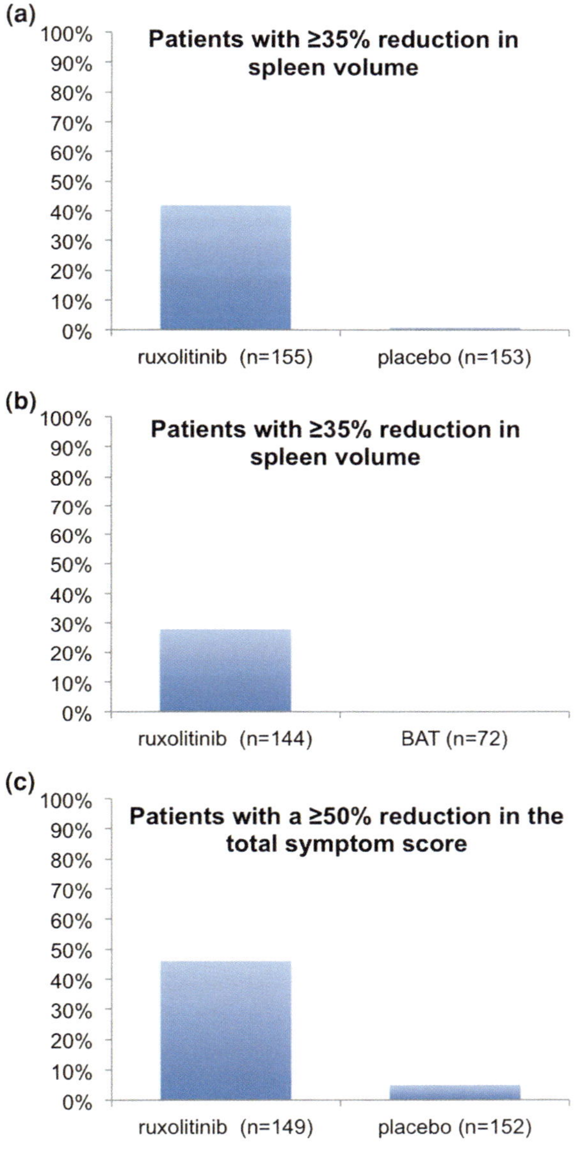

Fig. 1 Effects on spleen volume and symptoms. **a** Proportion of patients achieving a $\geq$35 % reduction in spleen volume at 24 weeks in COMFORT-I (Verstovsek et al. 2012b). **b** Proportion of patients achieving a $\geq$35 % reduction in spleen volume at 48 weeks in COMFORT-II (Harrison et al. 2012a). **c** Proportion of patients achieving a $\geq$50 % reduction in the total symptom score at 24 weeks in COMFORT-I, which was measured using the modified Myelofibrosis Symptom Assessment Form (Verstovsek et al. 2012b). *BAT* best available therapy

standard therapy ($P = 0.43$) (Tefferi et al. 2011). A second study reported on a different cohort of 107 patients who also received ruxolitinib in the phase 1/2 trial (Verstovsek et al. 2012a). After a median follow-up of 32 months, the overall survival rate among the ruxolitinib-treated patients was 69 %. In comparison with 310 matched historical control patients, ruxolitinib was associated with a longer overall survival among patients with high risk ($P = 0.006$), but not those with

Fig. 2 Discontinuation rates among the patients of the phase 1/2 trial. The *dark blue bars* indicate the rates among the 51 patients reported by Tefferi et al. (2011), and the *light blue bars* those among the 107 patients studied by Verstovsek et al. (2012a)

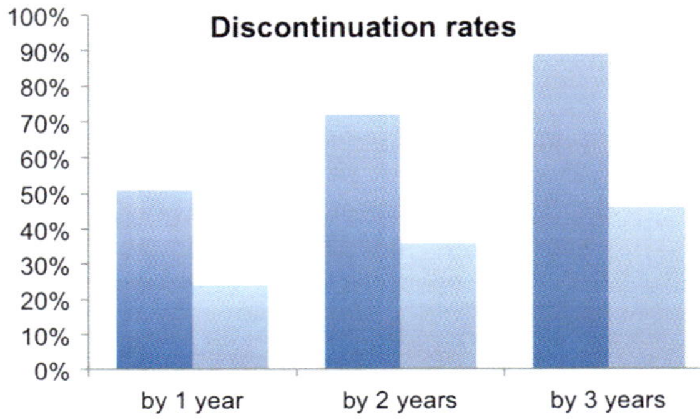

intermediate-2 risk myelofibrosis ($P = 0.71$). Since these findings are based on comparisons with historical controls, they have to be interpreted with caution. However, in accordance with these results, no survival difference was observed between intermediate-2 and high risk patients when treated with ruxolitinib (Verstovsek et al. 2012a). The finding of a survival benefit in one cohort of the phase 1/2 trial (Verstovsek et al. 2012a), but not another (Tefferi et al. 2011) was reasoned to be due to the lower discontinuation rates and a higher mean ruxolitinib dose in the cohort with the survival advantage by ruxolitinib (Verstovsek et al. 2012a) (Fig. 2). Disease progression or loss or lack of response was the reason for treatment discontinuation in 40 % of the patients in the report by Tefferi et al. (2011), whereas progressive disease was the cause for discontinuation in 11 % in the cohort studied by Verstovsek et al. (2012a).

Overall, ruxolitinib may have a favorable impact on survival, but the long-term follow-up data are yet premature, and moreover, the high crossover rate in the two phase 3 trials makes it difficult to determine the effect of ruxolitinib on survival. A possible favorable impact on survival by ruxolitinib has been hypothesized to be linked with the improvements of symptoms and, thus, performance status (Mascarenhas and Hoffmann 2013).

4 Toxicity

In the phase 3 clinical trials, the nonhematologic toxic effects were largely similar between the ruxolitinib and the placebo or BAT group (Verstovsek et al. 2012b; Harrison et al. 2012a). More frequently associated with ruxolitinib than with placebo in COMFORT-I were bruising, dizziness, and headache (mostly grade 1 or 2). In COMFORT-II, diarrhea (predominantly grade 1 or 2) was the only adverse event the rate of which was $\geq$10 % higher in the ruxolitinib than in the BAT group.

With regard to hematologic effects, thrombocytopenia and anemia occurred more frequently in patients receiving ruxolitinib than in those receiving placebo or BAT (Verstovsek et al. 2012b; Harrison et al. 2012a). Although anemia and thrombocytopenia were the most common adverse events, they rarely led to discontinuation of ruxolitinib. They were usually manageable with dose modifications, treatment interruption, or transfusion. In COMFORT-II, mandated dose reductions due to thrombocytopenia were required in 41 % of patients receiving ruxolitinib. Overall, dose reductions or treatment interruptions due to adverse events were more frequent in the ruxolitinib (63 %) than in the BAT group (15 %) in COMFORT-II. It was already observed in the antecedent phase 1/2 trial that patients with 25 mg twice daily more often had thrombocytopenia and new onset of anemia than those with 15 mg twice daily. The safety and efficacy of ruxolitinib in myelofibrosis patients with low platelet counts (50–99 $\times$ 10^9/L) have been addressed in recent phase 1/2 studies, final results of which are yet to be reported (Talpaz et al. 2012a, b; Harrison et al. 2012b). Moreover, after initiating ruxolitinib at 15 or 20 mg BID, patients titrated to 10 mg BID after nadir hemoglobin showed faster and more complete return to baseline hemoglobin levels without affecting efficacy (Verstovsek et al. 2012c).

Following interruption or discontinuation of ruxolitinib, symptoms of myelofibrosis returned to pretreatment levels within approximately 1 week (Verstovsek et al. 2012b). Among the adverse events that occurred after discontinuation, no pattern was observed that would suggest a withdrawal syndrome (Verstovsek et al. 2012b). However, as acknowledged in the FDA prescribing information, a patient's clinical course may worsen after discontinuation of ruxolitinib during acute illness (Tefferi et al. 2011, Tefferi and Pardanani 2011). Although such a ruxolitinib withdrawal syndrome due to a cytokine rebound remains to be established, the FDA recommends that a gradual tapering of ruxolitinib (e.g., by 5 mg twice daily each week) may be considered, when therapy is discontinued for reasons other than thrombocytopenia.

5 Drug Interactions

Ruxolitinib is primarily metabolized by cytochrome P450 3A4 (CYP3A4). Co-administration of ruxolitinib with the strong CYP3A4 inhibitor ketoconazole or the moderate CYP3A4 inhibitor erythromycin increased ruxolitinib plasma exposure by 91 and 27 %, respectively, which was consistent with the level of inhibition of interleukin 6-stimulated STAT3 phosphorylation (Shi et al. 2012). Co-administration of the CYP3A4 inducer rifampicin decreased the plasma levels of ruxolitinib by 71 %, but reduced the inhibition of STAT3 phosphorylation by only 10 %. This discrepancy may be explained by the presence of active ruxolitinib metabolites (Shi et al. 2012). Hence, adjustments in ruxolitinib doses may not be needed when co-administered with inducers or moderate inhibitors of CYP3A4, but ruxolitinib doses should be reduced by 50 % if co-administered with strong CYP3A4 inhibitors.

6 Biomarkers

Patients receiving ruxolitinib had increased plasma levels of leptin and erythropoietin and reduced plasma levels of proinflammatory tumor necrosis factor alpha and interleukin 6 (Verstovsek et al. 2010, 2012b; Harrison et al. 2012a). The decrease in proinflammatory cytokines was associated with symptomatic improvements by ruxolitinib in the phase 1/2 trial (Verstovsek et al. 2010).

7 Summary and Perspectives

Ruxolitinib is a potent and selective oral inhibitor of JAK1 and JAK2, which induces clinically meaningful responses in terms of reducing splenomegaly and debilitating symptoms in the majority of patients with myelofibrosis. Ruxolitinib may also have a favorable impact on survival. Ruxolitinib has not been shown to induce histopathologic or molecular remissions. Thus, ruxolitinib is a precious addition to the palliative substances currently used in the treatment of patients with myelofibrosis and splenomegaly and/or symptoms, primarily those who are not candidates for allogeneic stem cell transplantation or for clinical trials with newer JAK inhibitors. Based on the key role of JAKs in cytokine signaling, JAK inhibitors are also being studied in the treatment of other MPNs, such as polycythemia vera, as well as other immuno-inflammatory diseases, such as rheumatoid arthritis, inflammatory bowel disease, and psoriasis. Tofacitinib, which mainly inhibits JAK3, has been recently approved for the treatment of rheumatoid arthritis in the USA.

References

Cervantes F, Dupriez B, Pereira A et al (2009) New prognostic scoring system for primary myelofibrosis based on a study of the International Working Group for Myelofibrosis Research and Treatment. Blood 113(13):2895–2901

Harrison C, Kiladjian JJ, Al-Ali HK et al (2012a) JAK inhibition with ruxolitinib versus best available therapy for myelofibrosis. N Engl J Med 366(9):787–798

Harrison CN, Gisslinger H, Miller CB et al (2012b) Expand: a phase 1b, open-label, dose-finding study of ruxolitinib in patients with myelofibrosis and baseline platelet counts between 50 × 109/L and 99 × 109/L. Blood 120 (abstract 177) (ASH Annual Meeting Abstracts)

James C, Ugo V, Le Couédic JP et al (2005) A unique clonal JAK2 mutation leading to constitutive signalling causes polycythaemia vera. Nature 434(7037):1144–1148

Mascarenhas J, Hoffman R (2013) A comprehensive review and analysis of the effect of ruxolitinib therapy on the survival of patients with myelofibrosis. Blood 121(24):4832–4837

Mertens C, Darnell JE Jr (2007) SnapShot: JAK-STAT signaling. Cell 131(3):612

Mesa RA, Yasothan U, Kirkpatrick P (2012) Ruxolitinib. Nat Rev Drug Discov 11(2):103–104

Mesa RA, Gotlib J, Gupta V et al (2013) Effect of ruxolitinib therapy on myelofibrosis-related symptoms and other patient-reported outcomes in COMFORT-I: a randomized, double-blind, placebo-controlled trial. J Clin Oncol 31(10):1285–1292

Quintás-Cardama A, Vaddi K, Liu P et al (2010) Preclinical characterization of the selective JAK1/2 inhibitor INCB018424: therapeutic implications for the treatment of myeloproliferative neoplasms. Blood 115(15):3109–3117
Shi JG, Chen X, Emm T et al (2012) The effect of CYP3A4 inhibition or induction on the pharmacokinetics and pharmacodynamics of orally administered ruxolitinib (INCB018424 phosphate) in healthy volunteers. J Clin Pharmacol 52(6):809–818
Shilling AD, Nedza FM, Emm T et al (2010) Metabolism, excretion, and pharmacokinetics of [14C] INCB018424, a selective Janus tyrosine kinase 1/2 inhibitor, in humans. Drug Metab Dispos 38(11):2023–2031
Talpaz M, Hamburg SI, Jamieson K et al (2012a) Preliminary safety and efficacy from a phase II stud of ruxolitinib in patients with primary and secondary myelofibrosis with platelet counts of 50–100 × 109/L. Haematologica 97(s1):245 (abstract 0597)
Talpaz M, Paquette R, Afrin L et al (2012b) Efficacy, hematologic effects, and dose of ruxolitinib in myelofibrosis patients with low starting platelet counts (50–100 × 109/L): a comparison to patients with normal or high starting platelet counts. Blood 120 (abstract 176) (ASH Annual Meeting Abstracts)
Tefferi A, Pardanani A (2011) Serious adverse events during ruxolitinib treatment discontinuation in patients with myelofibrosis. Mayo Clin Proc 86(12):1188–1191
Tefferi A, Litzow MR, Pardanani A (2011) Long-term outcome of treatment with ruxolitinib in myelofibrosis. N Engl J Med 365(15):1455–1457
Vannucchi A, Cervantes F, Niederwieser D et al (2013) Long-term outcomes from a phase 3 study comparing ruxolitinib with best available therapy (BAT) for the treatment of myelofibrosis (MF): a 3-year update of COMFORT-II. Haematologica 98(s1):456 (abstract S1111)
Verstovsek S, Kantarjian H, Mesa RA et al (2010) Safety and efficacy of INCB018424, a JAK1 and JAK2 inhibitor, in myelofibrosis. N Engl J Med 363(12):1117–1127
Verstovsek S, Kantarjian HM, Estrov Z et al (2012a) Long-term outcomes of 107 patients with myelofibrosis receiving JAK1/JAK2 inhibitor ruxolitinib: survival advantage in comparison to matched historical controls. Blood 120(6):1202–1209
Verstovsek S, Mesa RA, Gotlib J et al (2012b) A double-blind, placebo-controlled trial of ruxolitinib for myelofibrosis. N Engl J Med 366(9):799–807
Verstovsek S, Mesa RA, Gotlib J, et al (2012c) Long-term outcome of ruxolitinib treatment in patients with myelofibrosis: durable reductions in spleen volume, improvements in quality of life, and overall survival advantage in COMFORT-I. Blood 120 (abstract 800) (ASH Annual Meeting Abstracts)
Verstovsek S, Mesa RA, Gotlib J et al (2013) The clinical benefit of ruxolitinib across patient subgroups: analysis of a placebo-controlled, Phase III study in patients with myelofibrosis. Br J Haematol 161(4):508–516

Ibrutinib

Mark-Alexander Schwarzbich and Matthias Witzens-Harig

Abstract

Abnormal B-cell receptor (BCR) signaling is a key mechanism of disease progression in B-cell malignancy. Bruton's tyrosine kinase (BTK) has a pivotal role in BCR signaling. Ibrutinib (PCI-32765) is a novel agent which serves as a covalent irreversible inhibitor of BTK. It is characterized by high selectivity for BTK and high potency. Preliminary data from phase I and ongoing phase II trials have proven very promising so far. It suggests the substance has high efficacy in B-cell malignancies such as chronic lymphocytic leukemia (CLL); diffuse large B-cell lymphoma (DLBCL), follicular lymphoma (FL), mantel cell lymphoma (MCL), and multiple myeloma (MM) and is very well tolerable. Most notably, the substance does not cause myelosuppression. This chapter discusses structure, mechanism of action, and toxicities of ibrutinib and also presents important preclinical and clinical data. Phase III trials will have to determine the definite role of ibrutinib in clinical practice but the data available so far suggests it may be a powerful new weapon in the battle against B-cell malignancies.

Contents

M.-A. Schwarzbich · M. Witzens-Harig (✉)
Universität Heidelberg, Heidelberg, Germany
e-mail: mathias.witzens-harig@med.uni-heidelberg.de

U. M. Martens (ed.), *Small Molecules in Oncology*, Recent Results in Cancer Research 201, DOI: 10.1007/978-3-642-54490-3_17,

1 Structure and Mechanism of Action

PCI-32765, better known as ibrutinib, is a small molecule first designed by Celera Genomics as a selective inhibitor of Bruton's tyrosine kinase (BTK) and is currently under development by Pharmacyclics, Inc and Johnson & Johnson's Janssen Pharmaceutica as a novel compound for treatment of B-cell malignancies such as chronic lymphocytic leukemia (CLL), follicular lymphoma (FL), mantle cell lymphoma, diffuse large B-cell lymphoma (DLBCL), and multiple myeloma (MM).

Ibrutinib works by covalent irreversible binding of Cystein residue 481 in the kinase domain of BTK. It is characterized by a high potency ($IC_{50} = 0.5$ nM) and selectivity for BTK. Only about 10 other kinases contain a homologous cystein residue and thus are prone to irreversible inhibition by ibrutinib. These include BMX, EGFR, HER2 and nHer4, BLK and JAK3. In addition, ibrutinib has some reversible inhibitory activity against a number of other kinases. The effect derived from this is probably of little significance clinically since the half-life in vivo is only about 2–3 h. The extent to which these off target effects contribute to the efficacy and toxicity of the substance are unknown (Pan et al. 2007; Honigberg et al. 2010).

For structure, chemical characteristics, and mode of action, please refer to Fig. 1.

In B-cell malignancies, antigen-dependent and independent B-cell receptor (BCR) signaling is widely appreciated as one of the main mechanism to promote disease progression (Stevenson et al. 2011; Woyach et al. 2012; Davis et al. 2010; Chiorazzi et al. 2005; Dühren-von Minden et al. 2012).

The BCR is a complex consisting of a membrane bound immunoglobulin (Ig) coupled with heterodimers of the transmembrane proteins CD79a (Igalpha) and CD79b (Igbeta). The cytoplasmatic residue of this heterodimer associates with Src-family kinases like LYN, Fyn, or BLK. Antigen recognition by the Ig results in clustering of BCRs. The associated Src-family kinases now start to phosphorylate each other and the immunoreceptor-based activation motifs (ITAM) in the cytoplasmatic tail of CD79a/b. The fully phosphorylated BCR now binds the protein tyrosine kinase Syk, which is phosphorylated and in turn activates downstream signaling cascades via molecules such as PI3K, Tec kinases, and GEFs. BLNK serves as a linker protein to enable the formation of the activation complex. Colligation with a co-receptor complex consisting of CD19/CD21/CD81 further increases the signal (Janeway et al. 2005).

BTK is a non-receptor tyrosine kinase of the Tec-kinase family. It is primarily expressed in B cells and is of central importance in BCR signaling. After being activated by Syk, it is using PLC gamma to activate transcription factors necessary for B-cell proliferation and differentiation like NFkappaB or NFAT and also protein kinases like ERK or JNK (Satterthwaite et al. 2000). In addition, BTK is also involved in the signaling of chemokine receptors like CXCR4 and CXCR5 (de Groter et al. 2007; Ortolano et al. 2006) (Fig. 2).

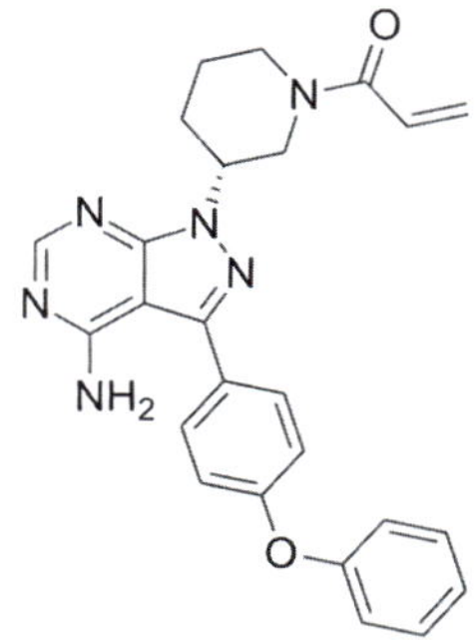

Fig. 1 Synonym, structure, chemical characteristics, and mode of action of Ibrutinib. *Synonym* PCI-32765, *molecular weight* 440.50 Da; *molecular formula* $C_{25}H_{24}N_6O_2$, *chemical name* 1-[(3R)-3-[4-amino-3-(4-phenoxyphenyl)pyrazolo[3,4-d]pyrimidin-1-yl]piperidin-1-yl]prop-2-en-1-one, *mode of action* irreversible BTK inhibitor, binds covalently to Cystein-481 in the kinase domain. Highly potent BTK inhibition at IC50 = 0.5 nM, *schedule* 420 mg p.o. once daily

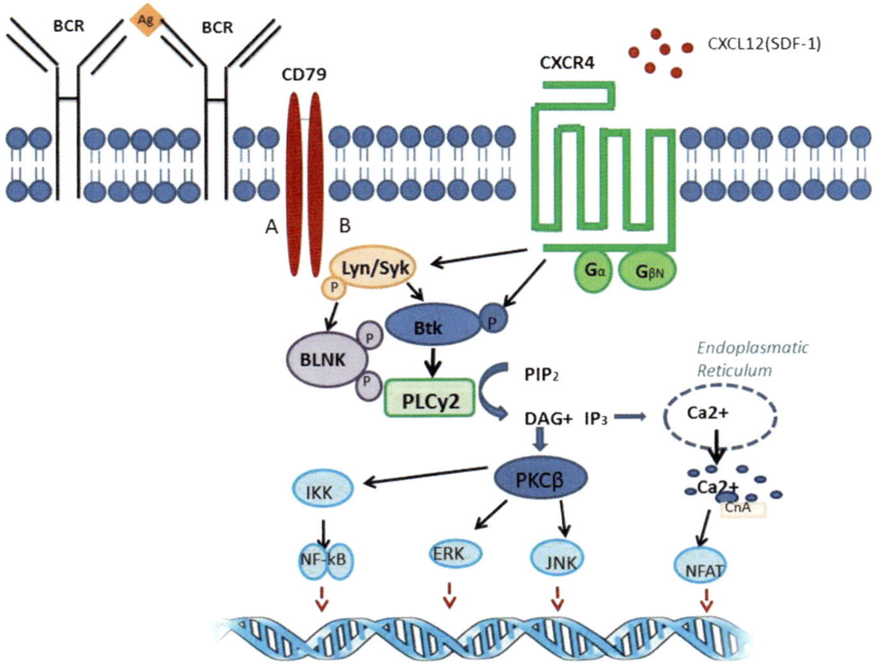

Fig. 2 BTK signaling pathways. *Abbreviations PIP2* Phosphatidylinositol 4,5-bisphosphate, *DAG* diacylglycerol, *IP3* inositol-1,4,5 trisphosphate, Ca^{2+} Calcium, *CnA* Calcineurin

BTK received its name for its role in Bruton's agammaglobulinemia, an x-linked genetic disorder which develops due to a mutation in the BTK gene. Patients suffer from an inability to generate mature B cells, which leads to severely reduced levels of Igs. They typically present with recurrent infections in early childhood. The disease was first described by Dr. Ogden Carr Bruton, a renowned pediatrician at the Walter Reed Army Hospital in Washington D.C. in 1952 (Bruton et al. 1952).

2 Preclinical Data

In 2007, a structure-based process for creating small molecules which serve as irreversible covalent inhibitors of BTK was first described by scientists at Celera Genomics (Pan et al. 2007). Of these molecules, the compound PCI-32765 was chosen for further preclinical development.

Celera Genomics was at first trying to development new compounds for treatment of rheumatoid arthritis. Therefore, the substance was initially tested in rheumatoid arthritis in vivo models. Later on, the efficacy in lymphoma models was discovered (Honigberg et al. 2010; Chang et al. 2011; di Paolo 2011). Efficacy of ibrutinib in B-cell lymphoma was first demonstrated by Honigberg et al. in spontaneous canine B-cell lymphoma. Orally administered substance induced a response in 3 out of 8 dogs treated (Honigberg et al. 2010).

Herman et al. (2011) showed that ibrutinib is able to induce apoptosis in CLL cells even in the presence of survival signals such as D40L, BAFF, TNF-α, IL-4, and IL-6. De Rooij et al. demonstrated the inhibition of CLL cell chemotaxis and integrin-mediated CLL cell adhesion by ibrutinib. These may explain the redistribution of CLL cells from the tissue to the bloodstream which can be observed after ibrutinib treatment (de Rooij et al. 2012). Ponader et al. reported the inhibition of CLL cell survival and proliferation by ibrutinib. They also showed reduced migration toward chemokines CXCL12 and CXCL13 (the ligands of CXCR 4 and 5, respectively). PCI-32765 was also shown to downregulate secretion of BCR-dependent chemokines (CCL3, CCL4) by CLL cells, both in vitro and in vivo. In an adoptive transfer TCL1 mouse model of CLL, PCI-32765 also inhibited disease progression (Ponader et al. 2012). Another study by Schwamb et al. (2012) reported ibrutinib-mediated inhibition of BCR-dependent UDP-glucose ceramide glucosyltransferase expression which in turns sensitizes CLL cells to apoptosis.

In DLCBL, Davis et al. (2010) demonstrated selective toxicity of ibrutinib in DLCBL cell lines with chronic active BCR signaling. Yang et al. (2012) reported that the substance downregulates IRF4 and syngerizes with lenalidomid in killing-activated B cell like (ABC) subtype DLBCL cells. Dasmahapatra et al. (2013) showed that coadministration of ibrutinib and bortezomib increases apoptosis in DLCBL cells and MCL cells via AKT and nuclear factor (NF)-κB (NFKB1) inactivation, downregulation of Mcl-1 (MCL1), Bcl-xL (BCL2L1), and XIAP enhanced DNA damage and endoplasmic reticulum (ER) stress, even in highly bortezomib-resistant DLBCL and MCL cells.

Tai et al. (2012) showed that PCI-32765 inhibits RANKL/M-GCSG induced phosphorylation of BTK and downstream PLC-gamma signaling in osteoclasts. Moreover, the substance also decreased chemokine and cytokine secretion by osteoclasts and bone marrow stromal cells, CLC12-induced migration of MM cells, IL6-induced growth of MM cells and in vivo MM cell growth as well as MM cell-induced osteolysis of implanted human bone chips in SCID mice (Tai et al. 2012). Rushworth et al. showed cytotoxic of ibrutinib to MM cells and synergy with bortezomib and lenalidomide chemotherapies. This is mediated via inhibitory effects on the nuclear factor-κB (NF-κB) pathway resulting in downregulation of anti-apoptotic proteins Bcl-xL, FLIP(L), and survivin leading to apoptosis (Rushworth et al. 2013).

3 Clinical Data

Still little fully published clinical data on ibrutinib exists. A phase I trial published by Advani et al. tested ibrutinib in 56 patients with relapsed or refractory B-cell malignancies of various types. Most of the observed adverse events were grade 1 or 2 with no dose-limiting toxicities. Full BTK occupancy was observed at a dose of 2.5 mg/kg and was maintained for at least 24 h. The effective half-life was only 2–3 h. An OR rate of 60 % and a CR rate of n 16 % was described (Advani et al. 2013).

In CLL patients, PCI-32765 induces lymphocytosis in the first weeks of treatment. This phenomenon is directly related to the presence of the drug, asymptomatic and temporary. It is believed that this is due to redistribution of CLL cells from solid lymphoma manifestations into the blood stream. It should not be confused with lymphocytosis due to disease progression—most experts in the field, therefore, believe that new response guidelines need to be developed in the advent of ibrutinib and similar tyrosine kinase inhibitors (Advani et al. 2013; Burger et al. 2013; Cheson et al. 2012)

In preliminary data from the PCYC 1102 trial, a phase Ib/II trial for ibrutinib in CLL/SLL patients presented at ASH 2012, Byrd et al. reported an OR rate of 68 % (10 % CR, 58 % PR) in treatment-naïve CLL patients 65 years and older ($n = 31$) and an OR rate of 71 % (2 % CR, 68 % PR) in previously treated patients ($n = 85$). A median time on treatment of 20.3 and 20.89 months, respectively, and a PFS at 26 months of 96 and 75 % were achieved (Byrd et al. 2012). Promising interim data from another phase Ib/II trial, PCYC 1108 was presented by O' Brien and colleagues on the ASCO meeting 2012. They evaluated efficacy and tolerability of the combination of ibrutinib and rituximab/bendamustin in CLL patients. The interim analysis showed an OR rate of 93 % (PR 80 %, CR 13 %, $n = 30$) with a very low rate of disease progression (O'Brien et al. 2012). Finally, Jaglowski et al. presented data from the PCYC 1109 trial evaluating the combination of ibrutinib and Ofatumomab. The OR rate was 100 % (PR 96 %, CR 4 %) in patients with CLL/SLL/PLL ($n = 24$) and 67 % in patients with Richter's transformation (all PR, $n = 3$)

(Jaglowski et al. 2012). An early evaluation of a trial by Burger et al. of rituximab in combination with ibrutinib showed an OR rate of 85 % ($n = 20$, all PR, 3 patients either persistent lymphocytosis Burger et al. 2012).

Wang and colleagues presented their first results from the PCYC 1104 trial which evaluates ibrutinib in MCL. This group observed an OR rate of 65 % in bortezomib-naïve MCL patients (CR 21 %, PR 44 %, $n = 63$) and OR rate of 72 % in those patients previously treated with bortezomib (PCR 23 %, PR 49 %, $n = 47$). The median follow-up was 9.2 months, and a median PFS of 13.9 months was reached (Wang et al. 2012).

Wilson et al. demonstrated interim results from the PCYC 1106 trial, a phase II study which evaluates ibrutinib in DLBCL. They observed preferential activity in the ABC subtype of DLBCL with an OR rate of 41 % (17 % CR, 24 % PR, $n = 29$) as opposed to the GCB subtype with an OR rate of only 5 % (PR only, $n = 20$). They also showed that the CARD11 mutation and MYD88 mutation of ABC do not respond to ibrutinib (Wilson et al. 2012).

Preliminary data from the PCYC 4753 trial by Fowler and colleagues are suggestive of activity of ibrutinib in FL. They reported an OR rate of 44 % (CR 19 %, PR 25 %, $n = 16$) and a median PFS of 13.4 months (Fowler 2012).

Vij et al. reported their first findings from the PCYC 1111 trial of ibrutinib MM. The median time on study treatment of the 13 patients enrolled so far was 3.7 months. A total of 38 % of patients had a reduction of their paraprotein. Two of the patients met criterion for MR, and one for PR during monotherapy with ibrutinib. One patient had a confirmed PR to ibrutinib dexamethasone combination treatment. Two patients completed at least 4 cycles on ibrutinib monotherapy with SD or better. Eight patients had elective addition of dexamethasone to ibrutinib for disease progression. Four of these were continuing on the combination with stable disease status (Vij et al. 2012).

4 Toxicity

The data from early stage CLL and MCL trials suggest that ibrutinib is very well tolerated. Adverse effects were typically grade 1, self-limiting, and not requiring therapy. Common side effects include but are not limited to diarrhea, nausea, fatigue, upper respiratory tract infections, rash, and edema. Treatment delays or discontinuation of therapy due to adverse effects are very rare as well as grade 3 or 4 adverse effects. Those reported are mainly infectious in nature and likely not treatment related (Byrd et al. 2012; Wang et al. 2012; Advani et al. 2013). Most notably, as opposed to conventional cytostatics, ibrutinib does not cause myelosuppression. Most patients treated even experience a marked improvement of their hematopoiesis (Byrd et al. 2012; Farooqui et al. 2012; Burger et al. 2013).

Some preclinical data prompt the assumption that ibrutinib may have a negative effect on platelet function by interfering with signaling from GPIb and the collagen receptor GPVI (Quek et al. 1998; Liu et al. 2006). However, patients suffering from Bruton's agammaglobulinemia do not have an increased risk of bleeding and the clinical data available so far does not indicated such an adverse effect. These in vitro findings should, therefore, be seen very critically in an in vivo setting.

Cases of primary resistance to ibrutinib have not been reported so far. This may, however, become a problem once ibrutinib is introduced in wider clinical practice as seen with other tyrosine kinase inhibitors.

5 Drug Interactions

Ibrutinib should be taken approximately 30 min before or 2 h after meals. The drug is a CYP 3A4/5 inhibitor. Therefore, concurrent treatment with strong CYP 3A4/5 inducers, inhibitors or substrates should be avoided. Also star fruit, grape fruit, and Seville oranges should not be eaten. For an extensive list, please refer to http://medicine.iupui.edu/clinpharm/ddis/ .

6 Summary and Perspectives

Ibrutinib is a novel covalent inhibitor of BTK. It is characterized by high selectivity for BTK and high potency. The substance has been shown to induce apoptosis of malignant B cells from various diseases. Preliminary data from ongoing phase II trials for ibrutinib in various B-cell malignancies have proven very promising so far. The substance is very well tolerable with little and mostly low-grade adverse effects and no dose-limiting toxicity. It has shown high efficacy in B-cell malignancies such as CLL, DLBCL, MCL, FL, and MM. Most notably, ibrutinib is characterized by an absence of myelosuppressive properties as opposed to conventional cytostatics. In CLL, ibrutinib causes rapid redistribution of tissue-resident CLL cells into the blood stream leading to resolution of lymphadenopathy and a temporary increase in lymphocytosis which, however, must not be confused with disease progression. This will likely prompt a revision of current response guidelines.

The definite role of ibrutinib in clinical practice will need to be determined in phase III trials, a number of which are currently in planning or have been initiated (please refer to www.clinicaltrials.gov for details). Based on the interim results from current phase II trials, the drug promises to be a powerful new weapon in the battle against B-cell malignancies both as a monotherapy and in combination with other agents.

References

Advani RH et al (2013) Bruton tyrosine kinase inhibitor ibrutinib (PCI-32765) has significant activity in patients with relapsed/refractory B-cell malignancies. J Clin Oncol 31(1):88–94

Bruton OC et al (1952) Absence of serum gamma globulins. AMA Am J Dis Child. 84(5):632–636

Burger JA et al (2012) The BTK inhibitor ibrutinib (PCI-32765) in combination with Rituximab is well tolerated and displays profound activity in high-risk chronic lymphocytic leukemia. In: Blood 120:Abstract 187

Burger JA (2013) Coming full circle: 70 years of chronic lymphocytic leukemia cell redistribution, from glucocorticoids to inhibitors of B-cell receptor signaling. Blood 121(9):1501–1509

Byrd JC et al (2012) The Bruton's tyrosine kinase (BTK) inhibitor ibrutinib (PCI-32765) promotes high response rate, durable remissions, and is tolerable in treatment naïve (TN) and relapsed or refractory (RR) chronic lymphocytic leukemia (CLL) or small lymphocytic lymphoma (SLL) patients including patients with high-risk (HR) disease: new and updated results of 116 patients in a phase Ib/II Study. Blood 120:Abstract 189

Chang BY et al (2011) The Bruton tyrosine kinase inhibitor PCI-32765 ameliorates autoimmune arthritis by inhibition of multiple effector cells. Arthritis Res Ther 13(4):R115

Cheson BD et al (2012) Novel targeted agents and the need to refine clinical end points in chronic lymphocytic leukemia. J Clin Oncol 30(23):2820–2822

Chiorazzi N et al (2005) Chronic lymphocytic leukemia. N Engl J Med 352(8):804–815

Dasmahapatra G et al (2013) The Bruton tyrosine kinase (BTK) inhibitor PCI-32765 synergistically increases proteasome inhibitor activity in diffuse large-B cell lymphoma (DLBCL) and mantle cell lymphoma (MCL) cells sensitive or resistant to bortezomib. Br J Haematol 161(1):43–56

Davis RE et al (2010) Chronic active B-cell-receptor signalling in diffuse large B-cell lymphoma. Nature 463(7277):88–92

de Gorter DJ et al (2007) Bruton's tyrosine kinase and phospholipase Cgamma2 mediate chemokine-controlled B cell migration and homing. Immunity 26(1):93–104

de Rooij MF et al (2012) The clinically active BTK inhibitor PCI-32765 targets B-cell receptor- and chemokine-controlled adhesion and migration in chronic lymphocytic leukemia. Blood 119(11):2590–2594

Di Paolo JA et al (2011) Specific BTK inhibition suppresses B cell- and myeloid cell-mediated arthritis. Nat Chem Biol 7(1):41–50

Dühren-von Minden M et al (2012) Chronic lymphocytic leukaemia is driven by antigen-independent cell-autonomous signalling. Nature 489(7415):309–312

Farooqui M et al (2012) 1789 ibrutinib (PCI 32765) rapidly improves platelet counts in chronic lymphocytic leukemia/small lymphocytic lymphoma (CLL/SLL) patients and has minimal effects on platelet aggregation. Blood 120:Abstract 1789

Fowler NH (2012) The Bruton's tyrosine kinase inhibitor ibrutinib (PCI-32765) is active and tolerated in relapsed follicular lymphoma. Blood 120:Abstract 156

Herman SE et al (2011) Bruton tyrosine kinase represents a promising therapeutic target for treatment of chronic lymphocytic leukemia and is effectively targeted by PCI-32765. Blood 117(23):6287–6296

Honigberg LA et al (2010) The Bruton tyrosine kinase inhibitor PCI-32765 blocks B-cell activation and is efficacious in models of autoimmune disease and B-cell malignancy. Proc Natl Acad Sci USA 107(29):13075–13080

Jaglowski SM, Jones JA, Flynn JM et al (2012) A phase Ib/II study evaluating activity and tolerability of BTK inhibitor PCI-32765 and ofatumumab in patients with chronic lymphocytic leukemia/small lymphocytic lymphoma (CLL/SLL) and related diseases. J Clin Oncol 30:(suppl: Abstr 6508)

Janeway et al (2005) Immunobiology, 6th edn. Garland science Publishing, New York

Liu J et al (2006) Bruton tyrosine kinase is essential for botrocetin/VWF-induced signaling and GPIb-dependent thrombus formation in vivo. Blood 108(8):2596–2603

O'Brien SM et al (2012) Combination of the Bruton's tyrosine kinase (BTK) inhibitor PCI-32765 with bendamustine (B)/rituximab (R) (BR) in patients (pts) with relapsed/refractory (R/R) chronic lymphocytic leukemia (CLL): interim results of a phase Ib/II study. J Clin Oncol 30:(suppl: Abstr 6515)

Ortolano S et al (2006) Roles for phosphoinositide 3-kinases, Bruton's tyrosine kinase, and Jun kinases in B lymphocyte chemotaxis and homing. Eur J Immunol 36(5):1285–1295

Pan Z et al (2007) Discovery of selective irreversible inhibitors for Bruton's tyrosine kinase. ChemMedChem 2(1):58–61

Ponader S et al (2012) The Bruton tyrosine kinase inhibitor PCI-32765 thwarts chronic lymphocytic leukemia cell survival and tissue homing in vitro and in vivo. Blood 119(5):1182–1189

Quek LS et al (1998) A role for Bruton's tyrosine kinase (Btk) in platelet activation by collagen. Curr Biol 8(20):1137–1140

Rushworth SA et al (2013) BTK inhibitor ibrutinib is cytotoxic to myeloma and potently enhances bortezomib and lenalidomide activities through NF-κB. Cell Signal 25(1):106–112

Satterthwaite AB et al (2000) The role of Bruton's tyrosine kinase in B-cell development and function: a genetic perspective. Immunol Rev 175:120–127

Schwamb J et al (2012) B-cell receptor triggers drug sensitivity of primary CLL cells by controlling glucosylation of ceramides. Blood 120(19):3978–3985

Stevenson FK et al (2011) B-cell receptor signaling in chronic lymphocytic leukemia. Blood 118(16):4313–4320

Tai YT et al (2012) Bruton tyrosine kinase inhibition is a novel therapeutic strategy targeting tumor in the bone marrow microenvironment in multiple myeloma. Blood 120(9):1877–1887

Vij R et al (2012) Early changes in cytokines, chemokines and indices of bone metabolism in a phase 2 study of the Bruton tyrosine kinase (Btk) inhibitor, ibrutinib (PCI-32765) in patients with relapsed or relapsed/refractory multiple myeloma (MM). Blood 120:Abstract 4039

Wang M et al (2012) Interim results of an international, multicenter, phase 2 study of Bruton's tyrosine kinase (BTK) inhibitor, ibrutinib (PCI-32765), in relapsed or refractory mantle cell lymphoma (MCL): durable efficacy and tolerability with longer follow-up. Blood 120:(Abstract 904)

Wilson WH (2012) The Bruton's tyrosine kinase (BTK) inhibitor, ibrutinib (PCI-32765), has preferential activity in the ABC subtype of relapsed/refractory de novo diffuse large B-cell lymphoma (DLBCL): interim results of a multicenter, open-label, phase 2 study. Blood 120:(Abstract 686)

Woyach JA et al (2012) The B-cell receptor signaling pathway as a therapeutic target in CLL. Blood 120(6):1175–1184

Yang Y et al (2012) Exploiting synthetic lethality for the therapy of ABC diffuse large B cell lymphoma. Cancer Cell 21(6, 19):723–737

Decitabine

Björn Hackanson and Michael Daskalakis

Abstract

Besides 5-azacytidine (azacitidine, Vidaza®), 5-aza-2′-deoxycytidine (decitabine, Dacogen®) is the most widely used inhibitor of DNA methylation, which triggers demethylation leading to consecutive reactivation of epigenetically silenced tumor suppressor genes in vitro and in vivo. Although antileukemic activity of decitabine is known for almost 40 years, its therapeutic potential in hematologic malignancies has only recently led to its approval in higher-risk MDS patients and as first-line treatment in AML patients >65 years who are not candidates for intensive chemotherapy. Several clinical trials showed promising activity of low-dose decitabine also in CML and hemoglobinopathies, whereas its efficacy in solid tumors is very limited. Clinical responses appear to be exerted both by epigenetic alterations and by induction of cell-cycle arrest and/or apoptosis. Recent and ongoing clinical trials investigate new dosing schedules, routes of administration, and combination of decitabine with other agents, including histone deacetylase inhibitors.

Contents

B. Hackanson (✉)
Freiburg, Germany
e-mail: bjoern.hackanson@uniklinik-freiburg.de

M. Daskalakis
Bern, Switzerland

U. M. Martens (ed.), *Small Molecules in Oncology*, Recent Results in Cancer Research 201, DOI: 10.1007/978-3-642-54490-3_18,

1 Introduction

Epigenetic changes play a crucial role in the development and progression of malignant diseases (Baylin et al. 1998; Baylin 2002; Hackanson et al. 2005). Epigenetic deregulation is defined as changes in gene expression mediated through mechanisms other than alterations in the DNA sequence itself. This includes DNA methylation changes, modifications of histone tails, and RNA interference (Bhalla 2005).

DNA methylation refers to the addition of a methyl group to a CpG site (Jones and Baylin 2007). These sites cluster together in areas known as CpG islands and are frequently localized in the gene promoter regions. Physiologic and aberrant DNA methylation of gene promoter regions can result in gene silencing. Hypermethylation-induced gene silencing of tumor suppressor and other cancer-related genes is one of the essential mechanisms in tumorigenesis (Esteller 2008). The rationale for the application of DNA methyltransferase inhibitors is their ability to revert hypermethylation-induced gene silencing and to restore proliferation control and apoptosis sensitivity in the malignant clone (Mund et al. 2006).

In vitro studies using cell lines have shown a time- and dose-dependent inhibition of proliferation by decitabine. At high concentrations, there is a cytotoxic effect, which may be related in part to the synthesis of alkali-labile DNA strands (D'Incalci et al. 1985). At lower concentrations, decitabine acts as a weak inducer of differentiation in myeloid leukemic cell lines (Creusot et al. 1982; Momparler et al. 1985a). Primary leukemic myeloid cells were shown by Pinto et al. (1984) to have a propensity for in vitro granulocytic or monocytic differentiation induced by decitabine. One of the early studies focused on the p15 tumor suppressor gene, which is often hypermethylated in MDS and AML patients and can be demethylated and reactivated in patients undergoing decitabine therapy (Daskalakis et al. 2002).

Several clinical trials investigating different drug-dosing schedules of decitabine have shown significant clinical benefit in the treatment of patients with MDS and AML (Yang et al. 2006; Cashen et al. 2010; Lübbert et al. 2012). In 2006, the drug has received FDA approval for the treatment of patients with MDS, and in 2012, the EMEA (European Medicines Agency) approved decitabine as first-line treatment for AML patients >65 years. Promising studies are ongoing to identify and develop new generations of DNA methyltransferase inhibitors (Yoo and Jones 2006; Kantarjian et al. 2012a, b).

2 Structure and Mechanism of Action

Decitabine was synthesized in 1964 by Sorm and coworkers (Pliml and Sorm 1964) as a classical cytostatic agent. It is a ring analog of the pyrimidine nucleoside 2′-deoxycytidine (Fig. 1). The drug is widely considered to be unstable and has therefore been handled with care. Due to deamination, the plasma half-life of decitabine is approximately 35 min (Rivard et al. 1981). Recently, the in vitro stability of decitabine in a neutral aqueous solution has been determined at different temperatures. The results indicated a considerable chemical stability (half-life time of 7 days at 4 °C, of 96 h at 20 °C and of 21 h at 37 °C), and even storing the solution at room temperature showed an effective inhibition in cytosine methylation (Stresemann and Lyko 2008).

After cellular uptake by a nucleoside-specific transport mechanism (Hubeek et al. 2005), decitabine is phosphorylated by the deoxycytidine kinase and metabolically converted into the active nucleotide for DNA methylation inhibition, 5-aza-2′-deoxycytidine-5′-triphosphate (Momparler and Derse 1979). Following incorporation of decitabine into DNA, newly hypomethylated DNA strands are synthesized (Wilson et al. 1983). Upon incorporation into DNA, decitabine forms a covalent complex with the DNA methyltransferase Dnmt 1, thereby depleting the cells of its enzymatic activity (Santi et al. 1983). Inactivation of the drug occurs through deamination by cytidine deaminase in the human liver and spleen, but also in granulocytes, intestinal epithelium, and plasma (Momparler et al. 1997). At equimolar concentrations, decitabine is at least twice as potent as azacitidine in inhibiting methylation (Creusot et al. 1982).

In a recent study, the pharmacokinetics of low-dose decitabine was evaluated in sixteen patients with MDS or AML (Cashen et al. 2008). It was concluded that the pharmacokinetics of low-dose decitabine remained unchanged from cycle to cycle. Despite repeated dosing, no systemic accumulation of the drug was observed, and the toxicity profile (transient myelosuppression) was predictable and manageable.

Regarding alternative routes of administration, Lavelle et al. (2007) investigated an oral decitabine formular recently and Kantarjian et al. (2012a, b) just recently showed clinical activity of SGI-110, a dinucleotide of decitabine which is given subcutaneously. Figure 2 summarizes schematically the regulation of gene expression by promoter methylation and the reversibility of this epigenetic mechanism by the demethylating agent decitabine.

2.1 Single-Agent Decitabine in MDS and AML

Decitabine was first used as a single agent in a phase I study in children with relapsed or refractory acute leukemia. The dose schedule of decitabine was 0.75–80 mg/kg (Rivard et al. 1981) and resulted in significant reduction in circulating blasts. In a continuation of this study, Momparler et al. (1985b) treated 27 children with acute leukemia (21 ALL, 6 AML) with a continuous infusion of

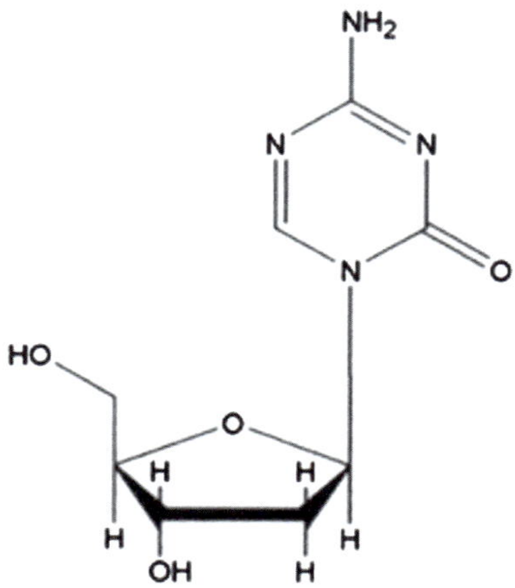

Fig. 1 Chemical structure of 5-aza-2′-deoxycytidin (decitabine, Dacogen™)

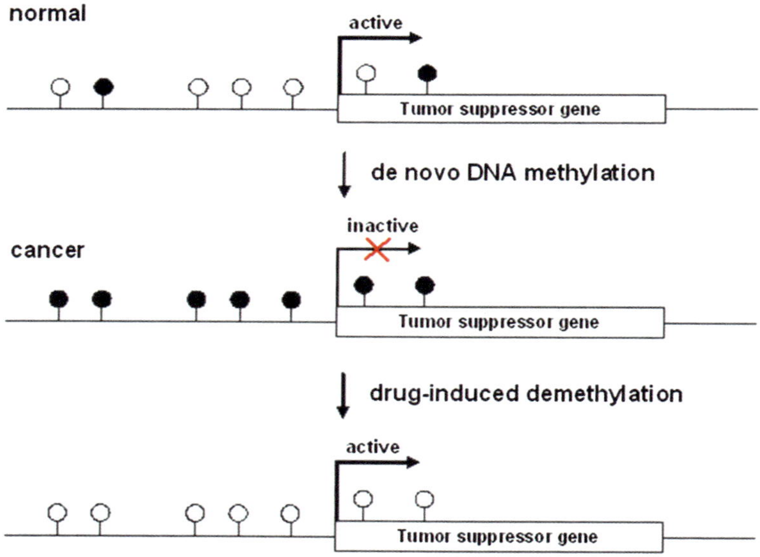

Fig. 2 Promoter methylation and gene expression

decitabine at doses ranging from 37 to 80 mg/kg over 36–60 h. In six patients (22 %), a CR was induced, and in four patients (15 %), a PR was noted. The overall objective response rate was 37 % (33 % in ALL patients, 50 % in AML patients). However, the development of the drug at these high doses was soon discontinued due to the high degree of hematologic (delayed and prolonged myelosuppression) and non-hematologic toxicities (Lübbert 2000).

Pinto et al. (1989) published results of a phase I/II trial with low doses of decitabine in elderly AML/MDS patients (median age, 74 years). This group as well as others had shown that in vitro, low-dose decitabine induced moderate differentiation in AML cell lines and primary blasts. Twenty-seven patients were treated with decitabine at 15–30 mg/m^2 for MDS and 30–90 mg/m^2 for AML, and the drug was given as a 4-h intravenous infusion 3 times daily for 3 days. After a median of two courses, three (15 %) of 20 evaluable patients had a CR, and 6 patients (30 %) achieved a PR, resulting in an overall response rate of 45 %. The median response duration was 12 weeks (range: 2–58 weeks). The median survival time of the responding patients was 19 weeks (range: 7–64 weeks). Both a reduction in peripheral blasts ("antileukemic effect") and a gradual increase in the absolute numbers of mature cells in the peripheral blood and the bone marrow, compatible with differentiation, were seen.

Since the early 1990s, Wijermans et al. (1997) conducted several large low-dose decitabine studies in elderly high-risk MDS patients. In a phase II study, a schedule of continuous infusion (72 h) with total doses of 125–225 mg/m^2 was used in 29 patients. An overall response rate of 54 % with 28 % CRs and 25 % PRs and a median response duration of 7.3 months were reported. This was followed by a multicenter phase II trial ($n = 66$) also using a three-day intravenous administration, however, over 4 h three times a day and a total dose of 135 mg/m^2 with comparable results (Wijermans et al. 2000). According to the International Prognostic Scoring System (IPSS), 3 of 5 patients (60 %) with low-risk MDS, 6 of 30 patients (20 %) with intermediate, and 10 of 26 patients (38 %) with high-risk MDS showed cytogenetic responses; cytogenetic response was associated with longer survival. Complete remissions were associated with cytogenetic remissions (Lübbert et al. 2001). Already after 2 cycles of decitabine treatment, an improvement in thrombocytopenia was noted in 63 % of the MDS patients (van den Bosch et al. 2004).

In a North American phase III trial of low-dose decitabine, 170 patients were randomized with 89 patients receiving decitabine (DAC) in a schedule of 15 mg/m^2 for a total of 9 doses over 72 h, repeated every 6 weeks, and 81 patients receiving best supportive care (BSC) (Kantarjian et al. 2006). The overall response rate in the study group was 30 % (9 % CR, 8 % PR, 13 % HI), with a median response duration of 10.3 months compared to 7 % HI in the BSC group. Notably, DAC-treated patients had a prolonged median time to progression to AML or death compared to patients receiving BSC, but this was statistically significant only for IPSS high-risk patients (all patients: 12.1 months overall survival vs. 7.8 months [$p = 0.16$]; patients with IPSS int-2/high-risk disease: 12.0 months vs. 6.8 months [$p = 0.03$]). Decitabine-treated patients (IPSS "high-risk" subgroup) had a median time to AML or death of 9.3 months compared to 2.8 months when only receiving BSC, which is a more than threefold difference ($p = 0.01$). Quality of life measures were performed and demonstrated a statistically superior quality of life during decitabine treatment regarding global health status, fatigue, and dyspnea. Severe adverse events were noted in 69 % of decitabine patients compared to 56 % of patients receiving supportive care. Specifically, 87 and 85 % of decitabine-treated patients had grade 3/4 neutropenia or thrombocytopenia, respectively, compared to 50 and 43 % on the supportive care arm. Cytopenias appeared to diminish in incidence over the first 4 courses of decitabine, but remained still frequent. This study led to the FDA approval of decitabine for the treatment of higher-risk MDS.

A European phase III trial (EORTC Leukemia and German MDS Study Groups) randomizing patients (decitabine treatment vs. best supportive care (BSC)) with almost exclusively int-2 or high-risk MDS according to IPSS included 233 patients (Lübbert et al. 2011). The median age was 70 years (range: 60–90 years). Decitabine was given as a dose of 15 mg/m^2 intravenously over 4 h three times daily for 3 days with courses repeated every 6 weeks. The median number of cycles was 4, and the overall response rate was 34 %. The median time to response (CR/PR/HI) was 0.32 years, and the response duration was 0.72 years. Decitabine lead to a significant PFS improvement (6.6 months) as compared to the BSC arm (3 months). However, the median overall survival was not significantly different between both arms [10.1 months (decitabine) vs. 8.5 months (BSC)]. It is of note that decitabine treatment was associated with improvements in patient-reported quality-of-life parameters also in this study.

In MDS patients, even after failure of previous azacitidine treatment, decitabine can still induce responses. Borthakur and colleagues treated fourteen patients with low-dose decitabine (20 mg/m^2 intravenously per day over 5 days) after failure of prior azacitidine therapy. The overall response rate was 28 % (4 patients), including a CR in 3 patients (21 %) and a HI in 1 patient (7 %) (according to the IWG criteria). The median duration of remission was 5.3 months, and the median survival time was 6 months (Borthakur et al. 2008).

For AML, two phase II studies were conducted in North America and Germany. The American study treated 55 patients with decitabine using a dosage of 20 mg/m^2/day for 5 days every 4 weeks. The complete remission rate was 24 % and another 29 % of patients showed a significant blast reduction in the bone marrow (Cashen et al. 2010). The median overall survival in this study was 7.7 months.

In the European study, 227 AML patients were treated with 15 mg/m^2/t.i.d for 3 days every 6 weeks (Lübbert et al. 2012). Thirteen percentage of patients achieved a complete remission, 13 % a partial remission, and 26 % an antileukemic effect with a significant blast reduction in the bone marrow. The median overall survival was 5.5 months and lower than in the North American study, possibly because also AML patients with leukocyte counts above 50,000/μl and a higher comorbidity index were included.

In a recent phase III trial, 485 AML patient were randomized to decitabine (20 mg/m^2/day for 5 days every 4 weeks) or treatment choice (TC) (supportive care or cytarabine 20 mg/m^2 per day as a subcutaneous injection for 10 consecutive days every 4 weeks) (Kantarjian et al. 2012a, b). The complete remission rates were 18 and 8 % for decitabine and TC, respectively, and the median overall survival showed an increase from 5 months (TC) to 7.7 months (decitabine). Interestingly, while the FDA did not approve decitabine for the treatment of AML because of the not statistically significant difference in overall survival, the EMEA

Table 1 Phase II and phase III trials of decitabine in patients with MDS

Reference	Phase	n	Age (range) years	Schedule	% responses (% CR/PR/HI)	RD (mo)	OS (mo)
Zagonel et al. (1993)	II	10	68	DAC 45 mg/m^2/day × 3 (i.v.) (= 15 mg/m^2/4 h t.i.d.); DAC 50 mg/m^2/Day × 3 (c.i.v.)	50 (40/10/0)	11	NA
Wijermans et al. (1997)	II	29	72 (58–82)	DAC 40–75 mg/m^2/day × 3 (c.i.v.)	54 (28/18/7)	7.3	10.5
Wijermans et al. (2000)	II	66	68 (38–84)	DAC 45 mg/m^2/day × 3 (i.v.) (= 15 mg/m^2/4 h t.i.d.)	49 (20/5/24)	7	15
Wijermans et al. (2005)	II	177	70 (38–89)	45–50 mg/m^2/day × 3 (i.v.) every 6 weeks	49 (24/10/14)	8.4	15
Rüter et al. (2006)	II	22	71 (51–81)	DAC 45 mg/m^2/day × 3 (i.v.) (= 15 mg/m^2/4 h t.i.d.)	14 (4/9/32)	4	27.5[b]
Kantarjian et al. (2006)	III	89[a]	70 (65–76)	15 mg/m^2/3 h t.i.d. q 3d every 6 weeks	17 (9/8/13)	10.3	14
Lübbert et al. (2011)	III	233	70 (60–90)	DAC 45 mg/m^2/day × 3 (i.v.) (= 15 mg/m^2/4 h t.i.d.)	34 (13/6/15)	8.6	10

N number of patients, *CR* complete response, *PR* partial response, *HI* hematologic improvement, *RD* median response duration, *OS* overall survival, *mo* months, *DAC* decitabine, *i.v.* intravenous infusion, *c.i.v.* continuous intravenous infusion, *q* for, *t.i.d.* three times daily, *NA* not available, [a]patients randomized to receive decitabine, [b]OS calculated from start of initial decitabine treatment

approved decitabine in the 5-day schedule (20 mg/m^2/day) for the treatment of elderly AML patients in 2012.

Table 1 depicts clinical phase II and III trials of decitabine in patients with MDS, and Table 2 summarizes clinical trials of decitabine in acute leukemia and chronic myelogenous leukemia (CML).

2.2 Combination Treatment with Decitabine in MDS and AML

The two epigenetic mechanisms DNA methylation and histone deacetylation are dynamically linked together in gene silencing (Cameron et al. 1999). Early pre-clinical studies support the view that pharmacologic targeting of both, DNA methyltransferases (DNMT) and histone deacetylases (HDAC), may result in synergistic anticancer activity (Cameron et al. 1999; Boivin et al. 2002; Garcia-Manero and Issa 2005).

Several phase I/II studies using decitabine or 5-azacytidine in combination with HDAC inhibitors have reported encouraging results (Garcia-Manero et al. 2006; Gore et al. 2006; Maslak et al. 2006; Soriano et al. 2007; Blum et al. 2007).

Table 2 Phase I, phase II, and phase III trials of decitabine in acute leukemia and chronic myelogenous leukemia

Patients	n	Age (range) years	Drug schedule	% ORR (% CR)	Reference
AML, ALL (relapsed/refractory)	22 (7, 15)	9 (2–15)	DAC 0.75–80 mg/kg (12–44 h c.i.v.)	14 (9)	Rivard et al. (1981)
AML, ALL (relapsed/refractory)	27 (6, 21)	NA (1–20)	DAC 37–80 mg/kg (36–60 h c.i.v.)	37 (22)	Momparler et al. (1985b)
AML, ALL (relapsed/refractory), CML (myeloid blast crisis)	26 (21, 2, 3)	55 (24–74)	DAC 300–500 mg/m^2 (24–120 h c.i.v.)	26 (4)	Debusscher et al. (1990)
De novo AML, AML from MDS, CML (not previously treated)	22 (12, 8, 2)	74 (62–83)	DAC 45–180 mg/m^2/d × 3 i.v. (= 15–60 mg/m^2/4 h t.i.d.)	68 (11)	Zagonel et al. (1990)
AML (not previously treated)	12	64 (47–77)	DAC 270–360 mg/m^2/d × 3 i.v. (= 90–120 mg/m^2/4 h t.i.d.)	40 (30)	Petti et al. (1993)
AML (relapsed/refractory)	5	26 (22–48)	DAC 250–500 mg/m^2 b.i.d. × 6–12	20 (0)	Richel et al. (1991)
AML (relapsed/refractory)	11	51(20–63)	DAC 125–250 mg/m^2 b.i.d. × 12, amsacrine 120 mg/m^2/d × 2	82 (73)	Richel et al. (1991)
AML (relapsed/refractory)	49	52 (18–65)	DAC 125–250 mg/m^2 b.i.d. × 12, amsacrine 120 mg/m^2/d × 2	41 (41)	Willemze et al. (1993, 1997)
AML (relapsed/refractory)	36	57 (NA)	DAC 125–250 mg/m^2 b.i.d. × 12, idarubicin 12 mg/m^2/d × 3	44(44)	Willemze et al. (1993, 1997)
AML (de novo)	8	44 (30–59)	DAC 90 mg/m^2/d × 5, daunorubicin 50 mg/m^2/d × 3	100 (100)	Schwartsmann et al. (1997)
AML (de novo and secondary)	55	74 (61–87)	DAC 20 mg/m^2 d × 5 i.v.	25 (24)	Cashen et al. (2010)
AML (de novo and secondary)	227	72 (56–86)	DAC 45 mg/m^2/day × 3 (i.v.) (=15 mg/m^2/4 h t.i.d.)	26 (13)	Lübbert et al. (2012)
AML (de novo and secondary)	242	73 (64–89)	DAC 20 mg/m^2 d × 5 i.v.	30 (16)	Kantarjian et al. (2012a, b)
CML (accelerated phase)	17	NA	DAC 50–100 mg/m^2 b.i.d. × 10	53 (0)	Kantarjian et al. (1997a, b)

(continued)

Table 2 (continued)

Patients	n	Age (range) years	Drug schedule	% ORR (% CR)	Reference
CML (Ph-positive) blastic phase (BP), accelerated phase (AP), and chronic phase (CP)	123	55 (16–78)	DAC 50–100 mg/m^2 b.i.d. × 10	BP: 28 (10) AP: 55 (23) CP: 63 (13)	Kantarjian et al. (2003)

ALL acute lymphoblastic leukemia, *AML* acute myeloid leukemia, *b.i.d.* twice daily, *c.i.v.* continuous intravenous infusion, *CML* chronic myeloid leukemia, *CR* complete remission, *DAC* decitabine, *i.v.* intravenous, *MDS* myelodysplastic syndrome, *NA* not available, *t.i.d.* three times daily

Garcia-Manero et al. (2006) treated 54 patients (AML or high-risk MDS) with low-dose decitabine (15 mg/m^2, i.v., daily for 10 days) administered concomitantly with increasing doses of VPA (50 mg/kg/day, orally, 10 days). The overall response rate (CR and PR) was 22 % (12 pts). The median duration of remission was 7.2 months, and responding patients showed a median survival time of 15.3 months. Six out of 8 responding patients also showed a cytogenetic response. Notably, responses were achieved already after a median of one cycle of treatment, which is earlier than seen with decitabine treatment alone.

In a phase I study (Blum et al. 2007) of decitabine plus VPA in 25 AML patients, the beneficial effect of VPA could not be reproduced, although responses appeared to occur earlier with the combination treatment versus single-agent decitabine. In this trial, 14 patients received decitabine alone to determine the optimal biologic dose, which was 20 mg/m^2/d (d1–10). Only 11 patients received the combination with dose-increasing VPA (d5–21). Dose-limiting encephalopathy already occurred in 2 patients at 25 mg/kg/d. Responses included 2 CRs, 2 CRis, and 2 PRs (ORR 54 %), but the authors concluded that VPA might be associated with too much toxicity in this elderly patient population.

Fiskus et al. (2009) demonstrated that the combination treatment of decitabine with the pan-HDAC inhibitor panobinostat (LBH589) targeted multiple epigenetic mechanisms resulting in antileukemic activity in AML cells in vitro.

One obstacle for a greater antitumor potential of decitabine is its rapid in vivo inactivation by the enzyme cytidine deaminase, the key enzyme in catabolism of cytosine nucleoside analogs. Besides azacytidine and decitabine, the therapeutic activity of a third cytosine nucleoside analog, pyrimidin-2-one ß-ribofuranoside (zebularine, Zeb), has been investigated (Driscoll et al. 1991; Zhou et al. 2002; Marquez et al. 2005; Flotho et al. 2009). Zebularine showed antitumor (Cheng et al. 2003, 2004) and antileukemic activity (Herranz et al. 2006; Scott et al. 2007) and is also a competitive inhibitor of the enzyme cytidine deaminase (Laliberté et al. 1992). It has been shown in murine and human leukemic cell lines that the inhibition of cytidine deaminase by zebularine enhanced the antineoplastic activity of decitabine (Lemaire et al. 2005, 2009).

Further clinical studies exploring combinations of decitabine with different HDAC inhibitors or zebularine are needed to achieve higher antitumor efficacy, find optimal dose schedules, and overcome acquired drug resistance due to DNA methylation and gene silencing.

2.3 Decitabine as a Preparative Agent for Allogeneic Stem Cell Transplantation

Giralt and colleagues conducted two studies to determine the safety and efficacy of decitabine, as a single agent or as part of a combination preparative regimen, prior to allogeneic peripheral blood progenitor cell (PBPC) transplantation. The phase I/II study protocol of single-agent decitabine prior to a second transfusion of allogeneic PBPC included 14 patients with early relapse after a first allogeneic bone marrow transplantation for AML (nine patients), CML (three patients), and ALL (two patients), respectively (Giralt et al. 1997, 1998a; Ravandi et al. 2001). Median time to relapse from initial transplantation was 6 months (range: 2–31 months). Eight patients received a total dose of 1,000 mg/m^2 decitabine (administered over 5 days), three patients received 1,250 mg/m^2, and three patients received a total dose of 1,500 mg/m^2.

In the first three patients, donor cell transfusion was performed 2 days after the end of decitabine infusion. In subsequent patients, donor stem cells were given 5 days after the last decitabine infusion, and no delayed engraftment has been observed in the responding patients. Eight of 14 patients achieved either a complete remission or a remission with partial hematologic recovery. Median time to neutrophil recovery was 13 days from donor cell transfusion (range: 10–30 days). Seven of eight patients achieving a response have relapsed. Median survival of all patients was 190 days (range: 11–1,245+ days). In patients achieving a response, the median disease-free survival was 60 days (range: 29–368+ days).

Overall, five patients were alive 176+ to 1,245+ days after transplantation, two of them in remission. Thus, salvage therapy with decitabine followed by allogeneic progenitor cell support is feasible, well tolerated, and induces CRs or hematologic responses in the majority of patients.

The other phase I/II study protocol included 23 leukemia patients prior to first allogeneic transplantation (Giralt et al. 1998b; de Lima et al. 2003), 12 patients with high-risk AML, one patient with CMMoL, one with ALL, and nine patients with CML. At the time of study enrollment, 20 patients had advanced phases of their disease, only two patients with AML were in first remission, and one patient had a late chronic phase CML. The conditioning regimen contained decitabine intravenously (3 dose levels: 400 mg/m^2 (10 patients), 600 mg/m^2 (8 patients), and 800 mg/m^2 (5 patients)) in combination with cyclophosphamide (100 mg/kg (4 patients) or 120 mg/kg (19 patients)) and busulfan (12 mg/kg, orally). In four patients transplanted according to this protocol (one with AML, three with CML in accelerated phase), the median time from leukemia diagnosis to transplantation was 5 months (range: 4–25 months). The first four patients achieved decitabine on days 7 and 8, but because of delayed neutrophil recovery beyond day 21 in three of them, the drug was given on days 11 and 10 for the subsequent patients. Two of the three patients who had graft failure needed additional donor stem cell transfusions at days 28 and 21 and recovered on days 31 and 37, respectively. Twenty-one patients achieved disease remission (CR or remission with partial hematologic recovery). Six of 23 patients (26 %) were alive at a median of 3.3 years from transplantation. The median survival was 17.2 months, and the disease-free survival was 8.9 months. Treatment-related mortality rate at 3 years was 35 %, nine patients died of disease recurrence, four patients of chronic GVHD, three patients of infections, and one patient of acute GVHD. No decitabine dose-limiting toxicity was documented, and no dose–response correlation of the three decitabine dose levels was observed.

Recently, two study groups reproduced the feasibility of an allogeneic transplantation after treatment with decitabine in MDS and AML patients (De Padua Silva et al. 2009; Lübbert et al. 2009). The outcome of 17 MDS patients with a median age of 55.5 years (range: 36–66 years) and of 15 patients with MDS ($n = 10$) or AML ($n = 5$) with a median age of 69 years (range: 60–75 years) were reported, respectively. All patients received a Fludarabin-containing conditioning regimen. De Padua Silva et al. treated eight patients with a myeloablative regimen, and nine patients with a reduced-intensity conditioning regimen, whereas Lübbert et al. treated all patients with a reduced-intensity conditioning FBM regimen. After a median follow-up of 12 months (range: 3–35 months), 11 patients were alive (eight in CR and two in PD) and six patients had died (four due to disease progression, one from acute GVHD, and one from sepsis) in De Padua Silva's study.

Stable engraftment was achieved in 14/15 patients in the German study. All 14 patients achieved a CR, with a median duration of 5 months (range: 1–51+ months). Six of these 14 patients are alive, 4 patients died from relapse and four from treatment-related complications while in CR. No increased toxicity due to the decitabine treatment has been described in both groups.

These studies suggest that decitabine is a valid alternative to standard induction chemotherapy, especially in elderly MDS/AML patients, and that this drug might improve the outcome of allogeneic transplant in MDS and AML. With this concept of "InDACtion instead of induction," the role of decitabine as a palliative drug has shifted to an agent with curative potential (Lübbert et al. 2013).

2.4 Immunomodulation with Decitabine

Epigenetic silencing plays an important role in the down-regulation of specific antigens (i.e., tumor antigens, HLA class I antigens, co-stimulatory molecules), which are involved in the immunological recognition of neoplastic cells. Among the different groups of cancer-associated antigens, cancer testis antigens (CTA) are attracting growing interest as immunotherapeutic targets. CTAs represent a family of immunogenic proteins (i.e., MAGE, BAGE, GAGE, LAGE, and NY-ESO-1) expressed in various neoplastically transformed cells and are absent in normal tissues except testis and placenta. CTAs are recognized by autologous, cytotoxic CD8(+) T lymphocytes (CTL) (Knuth et al. 2000; Bodey 2002).

The critical factor in down-regulating CTA expression in cancer cells is promoter DNA methylation, suggesting epigenetic drugs as therapeutic modulators for CTA re-expression in neoplastic cells (De Smet et al. 1999; Sigalotti et al. 2002). Several studies have shown that decitabine was consistently able to induce or up-regulate CTA expression in solid tumors and hematologic malignancies including AML, resulting in regaining immunological recognition and lysis by CTA-specific CTLs (Weber et al. 1994; Coral et al. 2002; Gattei et al. 2005; Sigalotti et al. 2004, 2005; Almstedt et al. 2010).

Recently, Oi and colleagues demonstrated that the anticonvulsant valproic acid, also acting as an HDACi, enhanced the expression of NY-ESO-1 in synergy with decitabine. After treatment, they observed significant DNA demethylation, histone H3 Lys9 demethylation, and histone re-acetylation (Oi et al. 2009).

Besides regulation of CTA expression, decitabine has been shown to increase expression of HLA class I antigens and other co-stimulatory molecules and to restore antigen-specific CTL response in vitro and in vivo (Coral et al. 2006; Calabro et al. 2005; Guo et al. 2006).

Schrump et al. (2006) designed a phase I study to investigate the maximum tolerated dose (MTD) of decitabine in patients with thoracic malignancies. No objective responses were observed, but re-expression of CTAs (NY-ESO-I, MAGE-A3, p16) was seen and antibodies to NY-ESO-I were detected post treatment in 3 patients exhibiting expression of NY-ESO-I in their tumor tissues. The MTD of decitabine was 60–75 mg/m^2.

The observation that decitabine induces or up-regulates expression of CTAs and thus may generate anti-CTA-antibodies gave impact for investigations of combined chemoimmuno-therapeutic regimens. Gollob et al. (2006) conducted a phase I trial in patients with melanoma or renal cell carcinoma to investigate the efficacy of decitabine followed by a high-dose IL2 immunotherapy. Decitabine was administered subcutaneously (daily for 5 days on weeks 1 and 2 of a 12-week cycle, escalating dosage from 0.1 to 0.25 mg/kg) before high-dose intravenous bolus IL-2. Major responses were observed in 3 of 13 melanoma patients (23 %; 1 complete response and 2 partial responses). Regarding decitabine immunomodulation, up-regulation as well as down-regulation of genes which may favor the IL2 immuno-therapy was observed.

Co-treatment of decitabine with the tyrosine kinase inhibitor gefitinib in two breast cancer cell lines (CAMA 1 and MB453) resulted in reexpression of the epidermal growth factor receptor (EGFR) and showed a significant effect on the induction of apoptosis in these cell lines (Montero et al. 2006).

After HLA-matched stem cell transplantation (SCT), a graft-versus-tumor effect leads to regression of metastatic solid tumors but is often associated with graft-versus-host disease (GVHD). GVHD is directed mainly against the multiple mismatched minor histocompatibility antigens (mHags). HA-1 is currently the best characterized mHag and particulary attractive for immunotherapy due to the restricted expression on hematopoietic cells and on some solid tumors but not on cells involved during GVHD (Hambach et al. 2008). Decitabine treatment of HA-1-negative tumor cells induced HA-1 expression and sensitized them for recognition by HA-1-specific cytotoxic T lymphocytes (Hambach et al. 2009).

Thus, epigenetic drugs are gaining increasing attention due to their immunomodulatory activity. Decitabine-induced re-expression of epigenetically silenced CTAs or mHags in hematopoietic malignancies and solid tumors presents a new strategy for tumor immunochemotherapy or as an immunotherapeutic target after allogeneic SCT.

2.5 Decitabine Treatment in Other Diseases

2.5.1 Activity of Decitabine in Patients with Acute Lymphocytic Leukemia (ALL)

Hypermethylation of multiple promoter-associated CpG islands has been frequently identified in ALL patients (Garcia-Manero et al. 2003; Roman-Gomez et al. 2004; Roman-Gomez et al. 2007; Hoshino et al. 2007). Moreover, aberrant methylation is associated with poor prognosis in childhood and adult acute lymphocytic leukemia (Shen et al. 2003; Kuang et al. 2008; Garcia-Manero et al. 2009).

Treatment of ALL-derived cell lines with decitabine results in hypomethylation and re-expression of putative tumor suppressor genes (Yang et al. 2005).

Residual DNA methylation at the time of morphologic remission of ALL might predict for worse prognosis. With these hypothesis, Yang et al. (2009) analyzed the methylation status of p73, p15, and p57(KIP2) at the time of initial remission in 199 patients with ALL (Philadelphia chromosome negative and MLL negative). In 123 patients, pretreatment samples were available and compared with remission ones. The presence of residual p73 methylation was associated with a significant lower disease-free survival and overall survival.

Recently, Yanez et al. (2009) reported a successful induction therapy with decitabine in a 10-year-old girl with refractory common B-cell ALL. The ALL was classified into standard risk and treated with the Spanish protocol for ALL (SHOP-99). One year after the end of treatment, the first relapse occured and the girl was treated with the same induction and consolidation therapy followed by autologous peripheral blood stem cell transplantation (PBSCT) in second CR. The second relapse was again treated with the same drugs in low doses, followed by an allogeneic haploidentical PBSCT from her mother in third CR. The patient never developed a graft-versus-host disease (GVHD). Getting a third relapse, the decision was made to treat the girl with decitabine (15 mg/m^2, 3 h continuous infusion, three times per day for 3 days) combined with dexamethasone (20 mg/m^2 i.v. days 1–4, 10 mg/m^2 i.v. day 5, 5 mg/m^2 i.v. day 6, and 2.5 mg/m^2 i.v. day 7). Again, a

CR was achieved and the girl underwent a second allogeneic PBSCT from her mother. Cyclosporine was used for GVHD prophylaxis, and the girl developed an extensive chronic graft-versus-host disease and remained in CR 8 months after PBSCT. Results of additional phase I and II trials investigating the activity of decitabine in patients with recurrent or refractory ALL are pending.

2.5.2 Activity of Decitabine in Patients with Chronic Myeloid Leukemia

In two of the first studies of decitabine in CML, 31 patients in myeloid blast crisis and 17 patients in accelerated phase were treated with a dose of 500–1,000 mg/m^2 administered over 5 days (Kantarjian et al. 1997a, b; Sacchi et al. 1998). Objective responses were observed in 26 % of patients in blast crisis, with a median survival of 29 weeks. One of the patients with a complete response had suppression of the Philadelphia chromosome (Ph) to 25 % of metaphases. Of 17 patients with accelerated phase, nine (53 %) responded to high-dose decitabine, with six patients achieving a second chronic phase of CML, and two showing Ph suppression. Prolonged myelosuppression was the major side effect, but no severe non-hematological toxicity was observed. During these studies, the initial decitabine dose of 1,000 mg/m^2 was, therefore, subsequently lowered to 750 mg/m^2 and to 500 mg/m^2 in order to ameliorate the prolonged myelosuppression.

In a further study, a total of 162 adult patients with the diagnosis of CML in non-lymphoid blastic phase were treated either with intensive chemotherapy ($n = 90$), with other single agents ($n = 41$), or with decitabine ($n = 31$), as described above. Decitabine showed similar objective response rates compared to intensive chemotherapy (26 % vs. 28 %), whereas other single agents showed objective response rates of 7 %. The median survival times were 29 weeks with decitabine, 21 weeks with intensive chemotherapy, and 22 weeks with other agents. Decitabine treatment emerged as an independent significant prognostic factor for survival (Sacchi et al. 1999).

Another study investigated the toxicity and activity of decitabine in all phases of CML (Kantarjian et al. 2003). One hundred and twenty-three patients with Ph-positive CML (64 blastic, 51 accelerated, and 8 chronic) and seven patients with Ph-negative CML were treated. In the first 13 patients, decitabine was given at 100 mg/m^2 over 6 h every 12 h for 5 days (1,000 mg/m^2 per course). Due to severe prolonged myelosuppression, the dose of decitabine was reduced to 75 mg/m^2 in the next 33 patients and to 50 mg/m^2 in the remaining 84 patients. Objective response rates were 28 % ($n = 18$) in patients with blastic phase (6 patients achieved a complete hematologic response (CHR), 2 achieved a partial hematologic response (PHR), 7 achieved a hematologic improvement (HI), and 3 returned to a second chronic phase (second CP)), 55 % ($n = 28$) in patients with accelerated phase (12 CHR, 10 PHR, 3 HI, and 3 second CP), and 63 % ($n = 5$) in the chronic phase patients. Four of seven patients with Ph-negative CML had objective responses (57 %). The estimated 3-year survival rate was less then 5 % for patients with blastic phase and 27 % for patients in accelerated phase. The only significant toxicity was severe and prolonged myelosuppression; febrile episodes have been described in 37 % and documented infections in 34 %.

In a phase II study, thirty-five patients with imatinib-resistant CML (12 pts in chronic phase, 17 pts in accelerated phase, and 6 pts in blastic phase) received low-dose decitabine treatment (15 mg/m^2 i.v. over 1 h daily) for a total of 10 doses (Issa et al. 2005). Thirty-four percentage of the patients achieved a complete hematologic response (CHR) and 20 % of the patients a partial hematologic response (PHR), resulting in an overall response rate of 54 %. Complete cytogenetic responses were seen in 6 patients.

In another phase II trial, the combination of low-dose decitabine and imatinib was investigated (Oki et al. 2007). Low-dose decitabine (15 mg/m^2 i.v. over 1 h daily over 5 days a week for 2 weeks) and Imatinib (600 mg/d, orally) were given in combination with 28 patients with CML (25 of whom had already known imatinib resistance). Nine patients (32 %) achieved a complete hematologic remission (CHR), one patient (4 %) had a partial hematologic remission (PHR), and two patients (7 %) had a hematologic improvement (HI). Five patients (18 %) achieved major cytogenetic responses and 3 patients minor (11 %) cytogenetic responses.

Decitabine appears to have significant activity in all CML phases; additional studies should evaluate decitabine dose schedules in tyrosine kinase inhibitor (TKI)-resistant CML, as well as combinations of decitabine and TKIs in different CML phases.

2.5.3 Activity of Decitabine in Patients with Idiopathic Myelofibrosis (IMF)

Several investigators have shown that epigenetic changes are implicated in the pathogenesis of idiopathic myelofibrosis (IMF) (Wang et al. 2002; Jones et al. 2004; Bogani et al. 2008).

In a recent phase II study, Odenike et al. (2006) could demonstrate activity of decitabine given subcutaneously (0.3 mg/kg/day on days 1–5 and days 8–12; cycles were repeated every 6 weeks) in seven patients with myelofibrosis. One patient achieved a hematological CR; another patient showed a hematologic improvement in platelet counts and a decrease in peripheral blasts.

Shi et al. (2007) investigated the treatment of peripheral blood CD34+ cells from patients with IMF with a sequential therapy of decitabine followed by a histone deacetylase inhibitor trichostatin A. Exposure to this combination therapy resulted in a reduction in the number of circulating malignant hematopoietic progenitor cells (HPCs). The proportion of JAK2V617F-positive HPCs was reduced in 83 % of the IMF patients. In two JAK2V617F-negative IMF patients, the sequential treatment led to a dramatic reduction in the number of HPCs that contained chromosomal abnormalities. Treatment of CD34+ cells of IMF patients resulted in the up-regulation of CXCR4 expression restoring the migration of these CD34+ cells in response to SDF-1alpha.

Recently, Danilov et al. (2009) reported on the successful decitabine treatment in a patient with symptomatic transfusion-dependent IMF. Despite treatment with hydroxycarbamide and lenalidomide, the patient's transfusion requirement increased further. The peripheral blood smear and a repeat bone marrow biopsy showed a disease progression, whereas the cytogenetic studies showed no evidence for t(9;22) and for the JAK2V617F mutation. After 6 cycles of the well-tolerated decitabine treatment (20 mg/m^2 for 5 days every 4 weeks), the patient's splenomegaly as well as his transfusion requirement decreased markedly.

2.5.4 Clinical Effects of Decitabine in Severe ß-Thalassemia and Sickle-Cell Disease

Epigenetic mechanisms also play an essential role in regulating globin gene expression in β-thalassemia and sickle-cell disease (SCD) (Lavelle 2004; Fathallah and Atweh 2006; Saunthararajah 2007; Fathallah 2008). An increase in the γ-globin chain synthesis leads to a lower globin chain imbalance in β-thalassemia. In SCD, the reactivation of HbF expression interferes with the polymerization of the sickle hemoglobin.

In phase I/II studies in patients with hemoglobin disorders, decitabine has shown a clinically significant increase in total and fetal hemoglobin as well as reduced red cell adhesion and endothelial damage (Koshy et al. 2000; De Simone et al. 2002; Saunthararajah et al. 2003; Saunthararajah et al. 2008). The main toxicity was transient neutropenia.

Clinical studies, investigating the efficacy of hypomethylating agents in children with SCD, are still lacking (Trompeter and Roberts 2009). Therefore, larger and longer term studies in adults are needed to confirm the short-term promising results and safety aspects of decitabine as well as to investigate new drug formulations, like an oral formulation of decitabine, which has been tested in animal models recently (Lavelle et al. 2007).

Saunthararajah et al. (2008) described an additional benefit by adding erythropoietin to decitabine treatment in four adult SCD patients. Choi et al. (2007) showed in vitro (HL-60 and T24 cancer cell lines) that hydroxycarbamide inhibits the hypomethylating activity of decitabine when given in combination, suggesting that these drugs should be used sequentially rather than concurrently.

Phase III studies are awaited to further evaluate the activity of decitabine in patients with SCD and to investigate different drug combinations modifying this severe chronic anemia (Wang 2008).

2.5.5 Efficacy of Decitabine in Patients with Solid Tumors

Anticancer activity of decitabine has also been explored in multiple clinical trials of patients with previously treated and metastasized solid tumors.

Using three 1-h infusions of 75 mg/m^2 decitabine over 24 h repeated every 5 weeks, the EORTC Early Clinical Trials Cooperative Group conducted a total of seven phase II trials with 153 patients with solid tumors. Tumor types included malignant melanoma (20), head and neck cancer (29), colorectal carcinoma (43), testicular cancer (15), renal cell carcinoma (16), non-small-cell lung cancer (8), ovarian cancer (27), and cervical cancer (17). Evaluable responses were seen in 133 patients. Of these, only two patients showed a PR: one of the 17 patients with malignant melanoma and one of the five patients with non-small-cell lung cancer (Dodion et al. 1990). The same schedule was also used in a phase II study in cervical cancer by Vermorken et al. (1991).

Two studies have revised the concept of activity of DNA methylation inhibitors in solid tumors. Momparler et al. (1997) performed a phase I/II study of decitabine in patients with metastatic non-small-cell lung cancer. Fifteen patients were treated with a single 8-h i.v. infusion of 200–660 mg/m^2 of decitabine. The major side effect was hematopoietic toxicity, necessitating a 5–6-weeks recovery period before the next treatment course. The median survival of these patients was 6.7 months, and three patients survived beyond 15 months, which suggests some clinical activity of relatively high doses of decitabine with an 8-h infusion schedule against metastatic lung cancer.

The second study was performed in 14 patients with progressive metastastic prostate cancer that was refractory to standard treatment (Thibault et al. 1998). The 1-h infusion schedule of 75 mg/m^2 three times daily, which had also been used in the EORTC studies in solid tumors, was applied. Treatment courses were repeated every 5–8 weeks to allow full recovery from myelotoxicity. Stable disease, with time to progression of over 10 weeks, was noted in two of 12 patients with evaluable responses.

Regarding combination treatment of decitabine plus chemotherapy in solid tumor patients, Schwartsmann et al. (2000) conducted a phase I trial ($n = 21$) with four dose increases of decitabine (45, 67, 90–120 mg/m^2, respectively) and a fixed dose of cisplatin (33 mg/m^2). Both agents were given on days 1–3, repeated every 3 weeks. The recommended doses for phase II trials in good and poor-risk patients were 90 mg/m^2 and 67 mg/m^2, respectively. Decitabine was given as a 2-h intravenous infusion, followed immediately by intravenous cisplatin after the end of decitabine infusion. One patient with cervical cancer showed a short-lasting partial response, and two minor regressions were described in a patient with non-small-cell lung cancer (NSCLC) and cervical cancer, respectively. Based on these data, fourteen patients with inoperable NSCLC were included in a phase II trial using the decitabine dose of 67 mg/m^2 and cisplatin with 33 mg/m^2. Only three minor responses could be described, and the median survival of patients was 15 weeks (range: 4–38 weeks).

The same combination regimen was used in another phase II trial in patients with advanced squamous cell carcinoma of the cervix. Twenty-one of 25 included patients were evaluable for tumor response, and 8 patients (38.1 %) achieved a partial response, whereas stable disease was documented in 5 patients (23.8 %). In non-irradiated metastatic tumor sites, the objective response rate was more frequent. The median progression-free survival was 16 weeks, and the median overall survival was 19 weeks (Pohlmann et al. 2002).

Samlowski et al. (2005) evaluated a 7-day continuous intravenous infusion of decitabine in 10 patients with refractory solid tumors. Decitabine was administered at 2 mg/m^2 as a continuous infusion for 168 h. Transient grade III/IV neutropenia and grade II thrombocytopenia were the only toxicities that have been observed. Measuring promoter-specific and global DNA methylation in peripheral blood cells before and after treatment, they could show significant MAGE-1 promoter demethylation and significant genomic DNA demethylation by 14 days after start of treatment; however, no objective responses were seen and seven patients progressed after two cycles of decitabine treatment.

Venturelli et al. (2007) investigated monotherapy of decitabine or vorinostat (suberoylanilide hydroxamic acid, SAHA) and the combination in human hepatocellular carcinoma (HCC)-derived cell lines and in primary human hepatocytes (PHH). The combined treatment showed enhanced antiproliferative effects in HCC-derived cells, whereas in PHH, there was no impairment of cellular integrity.

In a phase I and pharmacodynamic trial, Appleton et al. (2007) demonstrated the feasibility of combining decitabine with carboplatin at a dose and at a schedule that causes epigenetic changes in peripheral blood cells, buccal cells, and tumor biopsies. They used two separate dose increases of decitabine, the first with carboplatin fixed at area under the concentration time curve (AUC) 5 and the second with carboplatin at AUC 6. One patient with melanoma showed a partial response, and three patients had stable disease. The comparison of methylation status showed significantly less demethylation in tumor tissue after decitabine treatment compared to buccal cells and peripheral blood mononuclear cells. There was a decrease of only 3 % methylation in the tumor biopsies, which was below the threshold for resensitization to chemotherapy in other preclinical studies (Plumb et al. 2000).

A recent phase I study combining low-dose decitabine (10 mg/m^2/day for 5 days every 4 weeks) and the HDACi vorinostat in 43 patients with various advanced solid tumors and non-Hodgkin-lymphomas showed disease stabilization for more than 4 months in 29 % of patients (Stathis et al. 2011).

In summary, most of the trials investigating the activity of decitabine alone or in combination with HDACi or chemotherapeutics in solid tumors have shown rather disappointing results. However, one should keep in mind that while in MDS and AML, low-dose, multi-day, and multi-cycle decitabine treatment schedules are leading to the promising response rates, in many of the solid tumor studies dose, and schedule combinations have been used that were just recently being recognized as suboptimal. Future studies in solid tumors should investigate low-dose schedules of decitabine, by keeping toxicity low and allowing a longer exposure to the drug (several days, several cycles). Beyond others, this might lead to immunomodulatory effects, making tumor cells more sensitive to regular chemotherapeutics.

3 Toxicity

As compared to conventional chemotherapies, epigenetically active low-dose decitabine is relatively well tolerated. The major toxicity of decitabine is myelosuppression as manifested by neutropenia, thrombocytopenia, anemia, and febrile neutropenia.

Other major side effects are fever and gastrointestinal symptoms including nausea, vomiting, and diarrhea.

Very common ($\geq$1/10 patients) are fever, pneumonia, urinary tract infection, neutropenia, thrombocytopenia, anemia, headache, nausea, and diarrhea.

Common ($\geq$1/100, <1/10) are sepsis, septic shock, sinusitis, and allergic reaction.

4 Drug Interactions

There are no clinical studies evaluating drug interactions with decitabine. However, there is a likelihood of interaction with drugs that are also activated via sequential phosphorylation or that are metabolized via enzymes, which inactivate decitabine such as cytidine deaminase. Metabolic interactions mediated via cytochrome P-450 are not to be expected since decitabine is metabolized via oxidative deamination. Moreover, since decitabine exerts very little plasma protein binding, it seems unlikely that it eliminates other drugs from their plasma protein binding.

5 Biomarkers

Thus far, there exist no robust biomarkers, such as gene-specific DNA methylation or gene expression data that could predict response or prognosis upon treatment with decitabine.

Gore et al. (2006) described reversed DNA methylation of the p15 promoter in responding patients, and Garcia-Manero et al. (2006) found lower pretreatment levels of p15 methylation associated with response. Blum et al. (2010) revealed that higher expression levels of a specific microRNA, miR-29b, were associated with response to decitabine treatment. However, it seems more likely that it is rather a panel of genes than an individual gene that could provide prognostic information. Shen et al. (2010) recently showed that reduced methylation over time of a set of 10 genes (including, e.g., E-cadherin, estrogen-receptor α, OLIG2) during treatment with decitabine in MDS patients could predict clinical responses. Prospective studies are now warranted to validate the identified candidate genes as reliable biomarkers.

6 Summary and Perspectives

Epigenetic drugs represent a major improvement in the treatment modalities against hematologic malignancies. As one of the most widely used demethylating agents, decitabine has shown significant activity in MDS and AML at low-dose schedules in many clinical trials and is now the approved standard treatment for elderly AML patients who have no curative option. To improve this activity in MDS and AML, further clinical studies investigating combination regimens with other agents such as HDAC inhibitors, growth factors, all-trans-retinoic acid (ATRA), and other chemotherapeutic agents are warranted.

Further clinical studies of low-dose decitabine in CML after treatment failure of tyrosine kinase inhibitors, as well as in ALL, other hematologic diseases and in solid tumors should be conducted. For all epigenetic drugs, the optimal treatment schedules still have to be determined in monotherapy and also in combination regimens.

Moreover, further molecular studies to reveal which patients, e.g., cytogenetic subgroups or methylator-phenotypes, benefit most from the different approaches are of great importance, since thus far, no robust biomarkers for demethylating therapy have been established.

Finally, the development of new compounds with more potent hypomethylating activity is of major clinical importance. And hopefully, these new compounds and drug combinations will translate into longer overall survival.

De novo methylation of the promoter region results in inactivation of the expression of a growth regulatory gene (middle). Demethylating agent 5-aza-2′-deoxycytidine (decitabine, Dacogen^{TM}) reactivates expression of the epigenetically silenced gene by blocking the DNA methyltransferase Dnmt 1, resulting in demethylation (lower). Open circles are unmethylated CpGs; closed circles are methylated CpGs.

References

Almstedt M, Blagitko-Dorfs N, Duque-Afonso J, Karbach J, Pfeifer D, Jäger E, Lübbert M (2010) The DNA demethylating agent 5-aza-2′-deoxycytidine induces expression of NY-ESO-1 and other cancer/testis antigens in myeloid leukemia cells. Leuk Res 34:899–905

Appleton K, Mackay HJ, Judson I, Plumb JA, McCormick C, Strathdee G, Lee C, Barrett S, Reade S, Jadayel D, Tang A, Bellenger K, Mackay L, Setanoians A, Schätzlein A, Twelves C, Kaye SB, Brown R (2007) Phase I and pharmacodynamic trial of the DNA methyltransferase inhibitor decitabine and carboplatin in solid tumors. J Clin Oncol 25:4603–4609

Baylin SB, Herman JG, Vertino PM, Issa JP (1998) Alterations in DNA methylation: a fundamental aspect of neoplasia. Cancer Res 72:141–196

Baylin SB (2002) Mechanisms underlying epigenetically mediated gene silencing in cancer. Semin Cancer Biol 12:331–337

Bhalla KN (2005) Epigenetic and chromatin modifiers as targeted therapy of hematologic malignancies. J Clin Oncol 23:3971–3993

Blum W, Klisovic RB, Hackanson B, Liu Z, Liu S, Devine H, Vukosavljevic T, Huynh L, Lozanski G, Kefauver C, Plass C, Devine SM, Heerema NA, Murgo A, Chan KK, Grever MR, Byrd JC, Marcucci G (2007) Phase I study of decitabine alone or in combination with valproic acid in acute myeloid leukemia. J Clin Oncol 25:3884–3891

Blum W, Garzon R, Klisovic RB, Schwind S, Walker A, Geyer S, Liu S, Havelange V, Becker H, Schaaf L, Mickle J, Devine H, Kefauver C, Devine SM, Chan KK, Heerema NA, Bloomfield CD, Grever MR, Byrd JC, Villalona-Calero M, Croce CM, Marcucci G (2010) Clinical response and miR-29b predictive significance in older AML patients treated with a 10-day schedule of decitabine. Proc Natl Acad Sci USA 107:7473–7478

Bodey B (2002) Cancer-testis antigens: promising targets for antigen directed antineoplastic immunotherapy. Expert Opin Biol Ther 2:577–584

Bogani C, Ponziani V, Guglielmelli P, Desterke C, Rosti V, Bosi A, Le Bousse-Kerdiles MC, Barosi G, Vannucchi AM (2008) Hypermethylation of CXCR4 promotor in CD34+ cells from patients with primary myelofibrosis. Stem Cells 26:1920–1930

Boivin AJ, Momparler LF, Hurtubise A, Momparler RL (2002) Antineoplastic action of 5-aza-2′-deoxycytidine and phenylbutyrate on human lung carcinoma cells. Anticancer Drugs 13:869–874

Borthakur G, Ahdab SE, Ravandi F, Faderl S, Ferrajoli A, Newman B, Issa JP, Katarjian H (2008) Activity of decitabine in patients with myelodysplastic syndrome previously treated with azacitidine. Leuk Lymphoma 49:690–695

Calabro L, Fonsatti E, Altomonte M, Pezzani L, Colizzi F, Nanni P, Gattei V, Sigalotti L, Maio M (2005) Methylation-regulated expression of cancer testis antigens in primary effusion lymphoma: immunotherapeutic implications. J Cell Physiol 202:474–477

Cameron EE, Bachman KE, Myohanen S, Herman JG, Baylin SB (1999) Synergy of demethylation and histone deacetylase inhibition in the re-expression of genes silenced in cancer. Nat Genet 21:103–107

Cashen AF, Shah AK, Todt L, Fisher N, DiPersio J (2008) Pharmacokinetics of decitabine administered as a 3-h infusion to patients with acute myeloid leukemia (AML) or myelodysplastic syndrome (MDS). Cancer Chemother Pharmacol 61:759–766

Cashen AF, Schiller GJ, O'Donnell MR, DiPersio JF (2010) Multicenter, phase II study of decitabine for the first-line treatment of older patients with acute myeloid leukemia. J Clin Oncol 28:556–561

Cheng JC, Matsen CB, Gonzales FA, Ye W, Greer S, Marquez VE, Jones PA, Selker EU (2003) Inhibition of DNA methylation and reactivation of silenced genes by zebularine. J Natl Cancer Inst 95:399–409

Cheng JC, Weisenberger DJ, Gonzales FA, Liang G, Xu GL, Hu YG, Marquez VE, Jones PA (2004) Continuous zebularine treatment effectively sustains demethylation in human bladder cancer cells. Mol Cell Biol 24:1270–1278

Choi SH, Byun HM, Kwan JM, Issa JP, Yang AS (2007) Hydroxycarbamide in combination with azacitidine or decitabine is antagonistic on DNA methylation inhibition. Br J Haematol 138:616–623

Coral S, Sigalotti L, Altomonte M, Engelsberg A, Colizzi F, Cattarossi I, Maraskovsky E, Jager E, Seliger B, Maio M (2002) 5-aza-2′-deoxycytidine-induced expression of functional cancer testis antigens in human renal cell caricoma: immunotherapeutic implications. Cancer Res 8:2690–2695

Coral S, Sigalotti L, Colizzi F, Spessotto A, Nardi G, Cortini E, Pezzani L, Fratta E, Fonsatti E, Di Giacomo AM, Nicotra MR, Natali PG, Altomonte M, Maio M (2006) Phenotypic and functional changes of human melanoma xenografts induced by DNA hypomethylation: immunotherapeutic implications. J Cell Physiol 207:58–66

Creusot F, Acs G, Christman JK (1982) Inhibition of DNA methyltransferase and induction of Friend erythroleukemia cell differentiation by 5-azacytidine and 5-aza-2′-deoxycytidine. J Biol Chem 257:2041–2048

Danilov AV, Relias V, Feeney DM, Miller KB (2009) Decitabine is an effective treatment of idiopathic meylofibrosis (Correspondence). Brit J Haematol 145:131–132

Daskalakis M, Nguyen TT, Nguyen C, Guldberg P, Kohler G, Wijermans P, Jones PA, Lübbert M (2002) Demethylation of a hypermethylated P15/INK4B gene in patients with myelodysplastic syndrome by 5-Aza-2′-deoxycytidine (decitabine) treatment. Blood 100:2957–2964

Debusscher L, Marie JP, Dodion P, Blanc GM, Arrigo C, Zittoun R, Stryckmans P (1990) Phase-I-II trial of 5-aza-2′-deoxycytidine in adult patients with acute leukemia. In: Momparler RL, de Vos D (eds) 5-Aza-2′-deoxycytidine: preclinical and clinical studies. PCH, Haarlem, The Netherlands, pp 131–142

De Lima M, Ravandi F, Shahjahan M, Andersson B, Couriel D, Donato M, Khouri I, Gajewski J, van Besien K, Champlin R, Giralt S, Kantarjian H (2003) Long-term follow up of a phase I study of high-dose Decitabine, Busulfan, and Cyclophosphamide plus allogeneic transplantation for the treatment of patients with leukemias. Cancer 97:1242–1247
De Padua Silva L, de Lima M, Kantarjian H, Faderl S, Kebriaei P, Giralt S, Davisson J, Garcia-Manero G, Champlin R, Issa J-P, Ravandi F (2009) Feasibility of allo-SCT after hypomethylating therapy with decitabine for myelodysplastic syndrome. Bone Marrow Transplant 43:839–843
DeSimone J, Koshy M, Dorn L, Lavelle D, Bressler L, Molokie R, Talischy N (2002) Maintenance of elevated fetal hemoglobin levels by decitabine during dose interval treatment of sickle cell anemia. Blood 99:3905–3908
Smet De, Lurquin C, Lethe B, Martelange V, Boon T (1999) DNA methylation is the primary silencing mechanism for a set of germ line- and tumor-specific genes with a CpG-rich promoter. Mol Cell Biol 19:7327–7335
D'Incalci M, Covey JM, Zaharko DS, Kohn KW (1985) DNA alkali-labile sites induced by incorporation of 5-aza-2′-deoxycytidine into DNA of mouse leukemia L1210 cells. Cancer Res 45:3197–3202
Dodion PF, Clavel M, ten Bokkel Huinink W, Robinson E, Renard JF (1990) Phase-II trials with 2′-deoxy-5-azacytidine conducted by the Early Clinical Trials group of the EORTC. In: Momparler RL, de Vos D (eds) 5-Aza-2′-deoxycytidine: preclinical and clinical studies. PCH, Haarlem, The Netherlands, pp 117–124
Driscoll JS, Marquez VE, Plowman J, Liu PS, Kelley JA, Barchi JJ Jr (1991) Antitumor properties of 2(1H)-pyrimidinone riboside (zebularine) and its fluorinated analogues. J Med Chem 34:3280–3284
Esteller M (2008) Epigenetics in cancer. N Engl J Med 358:1148–1159
Fathallah H, Atweh GF (2006) DNA hypomethylation therapy for hemoglobin disorders: molecular mechanisms and clinical application. Blood Rev 20:227–234
Fathallah H (2008) DNA hypomethylation therapies and hemoglobin disorders. [An interview with Hassana Fathallah by H&O]. Clin Adv Hematol Oncol 6:806–808
Fiskus W, Buckley K, Rao R, Mandawat A, Yang Y, Joshi R, Wang Y, Balusu R, Chen J, Koul S, Joshi A, Upadhyay S, Atadja P, Bhalla KN (2009) Panobinostat treatment depletes EZH2 and DNMT1 levels and enhances decitabine mediated de-repression of JunB and loss of survival of human acute leukemia cells. Cancer Biol Ther 8:939–950
Flotho C, Claus R, Batz C, Schneider M, Sandrock I, Ihde S, Plass C, Niemeyer CM, Lübbert M (2009) The DNA methyltransferase inhibitors azacitidine, decitabine and zebularine exert differential effects on cancer gene expression in acute myeloid leukemia cells. Leukemia 23:1019–1028
Garcia-Manero G, Jeha S, Daniel J, Williamson J, Albitar M, Kantarjian HM, Issa JP (2003) Aberrant DNA methylation in pediatric patients with acute lymphocytic leukemia. Cancer 3:695–702
Garcia-Manero G, Issa JP (2005) Histone deacetylase inhibitors: a review of their clinical status as antineoplastic agents. Cancer Invest 23:635–642
Garcia-Manero G, Kantarjian HM, Sanchez-Gonzalez B, Yang H, Rosner G, Verstovsek S, Rytting M, Wierda WG, Ravandi F, Koller C, Xiao L, Faderl S, Estrov Z, Cortes J, O'brien S, Estey E, Bueso-Ramos C, Fiorentino J, Jabbour E, Issa JP (2006) Phase 1/2 study of the combination of 5-aza-2′-deoxycytidine with valproic acid in patients with leukemia. Blood 108:3271–3279
Garcia-Manero G, Yang H, Kuang SQ, O'Brien S, Thomas D, Kantarjian H (2009) Epigenetics of acute lymphocytic leukemia. Semin Hematol 46:24–32
Gattei V, Fonsatti E, Sigalotti L, Degan M, Di Giacomo AM, Altomonte M, Calabro L, Maio M (2005) Epigenetic immunomodulation of hematopoietic malignancies. Semin Oncol 32:503–510

Giralt S, Davis M, O'Brien S, Van Besien K, Champlin R, De Vos D, Kantarjian H (1997) Studies of decitabine with allogeneic progenitor cell transplantation. Leukemia 11(Suppl 1):32–34
Giralt S, Cohen A, Davis M, O'Brien S, Andersson B, Gajewski J, Khouri I, Körbling M, Champlin R, De Vos D, Kantarjian H (1998a) Phase-I/II study of decitabine with allogeneic peripheral blood stem cell transplantation for treatment of relapse after allogeneic progenitor cell transplantation. In: Symposium on methyltransferase inhibitors in hematologic malignancies, Miami, FL, Dec 1998 (abstract)
Giralt S, Cohen A, Davis M, O'Brien S, Andersson B, Gajewski J, Khouri I, Körbling M, Champlin R, de Vos D, Kantarjian H (1998b) Phase-I/II trial combining decitabine with busulfan/cyclophosphamide as a conditioning regimen for allogeneic progenitor cell transplantation. In: Symposium on methyltransferase inhibitors in hematologic malignancies, Miami, Dec 1998 (abstract)
Gollob JA, Sclambi CJ, Peterson BL, Richmond T, Thoreson M, Moran K, Dressmann HK, Jelinek J, Issa JP (2006) Phase I trial of sequential low-dose 5-aza-2′-deoxycytidine plus high-dose intravenous bolus interleukin-2 in patients with melanoma or renal cell carcinoma. Clin Cancer Res 12:4619–4627
Gore SD, Baylin S, Sugar E, Carraway H, Miller CB, Carducci M, Grever M, Galm O, Dauses T, Karp JE, Rudek MA, Zhao M, Smith BD, Manning J, Jiemjit A, Dover G, Mays A, Zwiebel J, Murgo A, Weng LJ, Herman JG (2006) Combined DNA methyltransferase and histone deacetylase inhibition in the treatment of myeloid neoplasms. Cancer Res 66:6361–6369
Guo ZS, Hong JA, Irvine KR, Chen GA, Spiess PJ, Liu Y, Zeng G, Wunderlich JR, Nguyen DM, Restifo NP, Schrump DS (2006) De novo induction of a cancer/testis antigen by 5-aza-2′-deoxycytidine augments adoptive immunotherapy in a murine tumor model. Cancer Res 66:1105–1113
Hackanson B, Guo Y, Lübbert M (2005) The silence of the genes: epigenetic disturbances in haematopoietic malignancies. Expert Opin Ther Targets 9:45–61
Hambach L, Vermeij M, Buser A, Aghai Z, van der Kwast T, Goulmy E (2008) Targeting a single mismatched minor histocompatibility antigen with tumor-restricted expression eradicates human solid tumors. Blood 112:1844–1852
Hambach L, Ling KW, Pool J, Aghai Z, Blokland E, Tanke HJ, Bruijn JA, Halfwerk H, van Boven H, Wieles B, Goulmy E (2009) Hypomethylation drugs convert HA-1-negative solid tumors into targets for stem cell-based immunotherapy. Blood 113:2715–2722
Herranz M, Martin-Caballero J, Fraga MF, Ruiz-Cabello J, Flores JM, Desco M, Marquez VE, Esteller M (2006) The novel DNA methylation inhibitor zebularine is effective against the development of T-cell lymphoma. Blood 107:1174–1177
Hoshino K, Quintás-Cardama A, Yang H, Sanchez-Gonzalez B, Garcia-Manero G (2007) Aberrant DNA methylation of the Src kinase Hck, but not of Lyn, in Philadelphia chromosome negative acute lymphocytic leukemia. Leukemia 21:906–911
Hubeek I, Stam RW, Peters GJ, Broekhuizen R, Meijerink JP, van Wering ER, Gibson BE, Creutzig U, Zwaan CM, Cloos J, Kuik DJ, Pieters R, Kaspers GJ (2005) The human equilibrative nucleoside transporter 1 mediates in vitro cytarabine sensitivity in childhood acute myeloid leukaemia. Br J Cancer 93:1388–1394
Issa JP, Gharibyan V, Cortes J, Jelinek J, Morris G, Verstovsek S, Talpaz M, Garcia-Manero G, Kantarjian HM (2005) Phase II study of low dose decitabine in patients with chronic myelogenous leukemia resistant to imatinib mesylate. J Clin Oncol 23:3948–3956
Jones LC, Tefferi A, Idos GE, Kumagai T, Hofmann WK, Koeffler HP (2004) RARbeta2 is a candidate tumor suppressor gene in myelofibrosis with myeloid metaplasia. Oncogene 23:7846–7853
Jones PA, Baylin SB (2007) The epigenomics of cancer. Cell 128:683–692
Kantarjian HM, O'Brien SM, Estey E, Giralt S, Beran M, Rios MB, Keating M, De Vos D, Talpaz M (1997a) Decitabine studies in chronic and acute myelogenous leukemia. Leukemia 11(1):35–36

Kantarjian HM, O'Brien SM, Keating M, Beran M, Estey E, Giralt S, Kornblau S, Rios MB, De Vos D, Talpaz M (1997b) Results of decitabine therapy in the accelerated and blastic phases of chronic myelogenous leukemia. Leukemia 11:1617–1620

Kantarjian HM, O'Brien S, Cortes J, Giles FJ, Faderl S, Issa JP, Garcia-Manero G, Rios MB, Shan J, Andreeff M, Keating M, Talpaz M (2003) Results of decitabine (5-aza-2′-deoxycytidine) therapy in 130 patients with chronic myelogenous leukemia. Cancer 98:522–528

Kantarjian HM, Issa JP, Rosenfeld CS, Bennett JM, Albitar M, DiPersio J, Klimek V, Slack J, de Castro C, Ravandi F, Helmer R 3rd, Shen L, Nimer SD, Leavitt R, Raza A, Saba H (2006) Decitabine improves patient outcomes in myelodysplastic syndromes: results of a phase III randomized study. Cancer 106:1794–1803

Kantarjian HM, Thomas XG, Dmoszynska A, Wierzbowska A, Mazur G, Mayer J, Gau JP, Chou WC, Buckstein R, Cermak J, Kuo CY, Oriol A, Ravandi F, Faderl S, Delaunay J, Lysák D, Minden M, Arthur C (2012a) Multicenter, randomized open-label phase III trial of decitabine versus patient choice, with physician advice of either supportive care or low-dose cytarabine for the treatment of older patients with newly diagnosed acute myeloid leukemia. J Clin Oncol 30:2670–2677

Kantarjian HM, Roboz GJ, Rizzieri DA, Stock W, O'Connell CL, Griffiths EA (2012b) Results from the dose escalation phase of a randomized phase 1-2 first-in-human (FIH) study of SGI-110, a novel low volume stable subcutaneous (SQ) second generation hypomethylating agent (HMA) in patients with relapsed/refractory MDS and AML. Blood 120: ASH annual meeting abstract number 414

Knuth A, Jäger D, Jäger E (2000) Cancer immunotherapy in clinical oncology. Cancer Chemother Pharmacol 46:S46–S51

Koshy M, Dorn L, Bressler L, Molokie R, Lavelle D, Talischy N, Hoffman R, van Overveld W, DeSimone J (2000) 2-deoxy 5-azacytidine and fetal hemoglobin induction in sickle cell anemia. Blood 96:2379–2384

Kuang SQ, Tong WG, Yang H, Lin W, Lee MK, Fang ZH, Wei Y, Jelinek J, Issa JP, Garcia-Manero G (2008) Genome-wide identification of aberrantly methylated promoter associated CpG islands in acute lymphoblastic leukemia. Leukemia 8:1529–1538

Laliberté J, Marquez VE, Momparler RL (1992) Potent inhibitors for the deamination of cytosine arabinoside and 5-aza-2′-deoxycytidine by human cytidine deaminase. Cancer Chemother Pharmacol 30:7–11

Lavelle DE (2004) The molecular mechanism of fetal hemoglobin reactivation. Semin Hematol 41:3–10

Lavelle D, Chin J, Vaitkus K, Redkar S, Phiasivongsa P, Tang C, Will R, Hankewych M, Roxas B, Singh M, Saunthararajah Y, Desimone J (2007) Oral decitabine reactivates expression of the methylated gamma-globin gene in *Papio anubis*. Am J Hematol 82:981–985

Lemaire M, Momparler LF, Bernstein ML, Marquez VE, Momparler RL (2005) Enhancement of antineoplastic action of 5-aza-2′-deoxycytidine by zebularine on L1210 leukemia. Anticancer Drugs 16:301–308

Lemaire M, Momparler LF, Raynal NJM, Bernstein ML, Momparler RL (2009) Inhibition of cytidine deaminase by zebularine enhances the antineoplastic action of 5-aza-2′-deoxycytidine. Cancer Chemother Pharmacol 63:411–416

Lübbert M (2000) DNA methylation inhibitors in the treatment of leukemias, myelodysplastic syndromes and hemoglobinopathies: clinical results and possible mechanisms of action. Curr Top Microbiol Immunol 249:135–164

Lübbert M, Wijermans P, Kunzmann R, Verhoef G, Bosly A, Ravoet C, Andre M, Ferrant A (2001) Cytogenetic responses in high-risk myelodysplastic syndrome following low-dose treatment with DNA methylation inhibitor 5-aza-2′-deoxycytidine. Br J Haematol 114:349–357

Lübbert M, Bertz H, Rüter B, Marks R, Claus R, Wäsch R, Finke J (2009) Non-intensive treatment with low-dose 5-aza-2′-deoxycytidine (DAC) prior to allogeneic blood SCT of older MDS/AML-patients. Bone Marrow Transplant 44:585–588

Lübbert M, Suciu S, Baila L, Rüter BH, Platzbecker U, Giagounidis A, Selleslag D, Labar B, Germing U, Salih HR, Beeldens F, Muus P, Pflüger KH, Coens C, Hagemeijer A, Eckart Schaefer H, Ganser A, Aul C, de Witte T, Wijermans PW (2011) Low-dose decitabine versus best supportive care in elderly patients with intermediate- or high-risk myelodysplastic syndrome (MDS) ineligible for intensive chemotherapy: final results of the randomized phase III study of the European Organisation for Research and Treatment of Cancer Leukemia Group and the German MDS Study Group. J Clin Oncol 29:1987–1996

Lübbert M, Rüter BH, Claus R, Schmoor C, Schmid M, Germing U, Kuendgen A, Rethwisch V, Ganser A, Platzbecker U, Galm O, Brugger W, Heil G, Hackanson B, Deschler B, Döhner K, Hagemeijer A, Wijermans PW, Döhner H (2012) A multicenter phase II trial of decitabine as first-line treatment for older patients with acute myeloid leukemia judged unfit for induction chemotherapy. Haematologica 97:393–401

Lübbert M, Bertz H, Müller MJ, Finke J (2013) When azanucleoside treatment can be curative: nonintensive bridging strategy before allografting in older patients with myelodysplastic syndrome/acute myeloid leukemia. J Clin Oncol 31:822–823

Marquez VE, Kelley JA, Agbaria R, Ben-Kasus T, Cheng JC, Yoo CB, Jones PA (2005) Zebularine: a unique molecule for an epigenetically based strategy in cancer chemotherapy. Ann NY Acad Sci 1058:246–254

Maslak P, Chanel S, Camacho LH, Soignet S, Pandolfi PP, Guernah I, Warrell R, Nimer S (2006) Pilot study of combination transcriptional modulation therapy with sodium phenylbutyrate and 5-azacytidine in patients with acute myeloid leukemia or myelodysplastic syndrome. Leukemia 2:212–217

Momparler RL, Derse D (1979) Kinetics of phosphorylation of 5-aza-2′-deoxycytidine by deoxycytidine kinase. Biochem Pharmacol 28:1443–1444

Momparler RL, Bouchard J, Samson J (1985a) Induction of differentiation and inhibition of DNA methylation in HL-60 myeloid leukemic cells by 5-aza-2′-deoxycytidine. Leuk Res 9:1361–1366

Momparler RL, Rivard GE, Gyger M (1985b) Clinical trial on 5-aza-2′-deoxycytidine in patients with acute leukemia. Pharmacol Ther 30:277–286

Momparler RL, Bouffard DY, Momparler LF, Dionne J, Belanger K, Ayoub J (1997) Pilot phase-I-II study on 5-aza-2′-deoxycytidine (decitabine) in patients with metastatic lung cancer. Anticancer Drugs 8:358–368

Montero AJ, Diaz-Montero CM, Mao L, Youssef EM, Estecio M, Shen L, Issa JP (2006) Epigenetic inactivation of EGFR by CpG island hypermethylation in cancer. Cancer Biol Ther 5:1494–1501

Mund C, Brueckner B, Lyko F (2006) Reactivation of epigenetically silenced genes by DNA methyltransferase inhibitors: basic concepts and clinical applications. Epigenetics 1:7–13

Odenike OM, Godwin JE, van Besien K, Huo D, Stiff PJ, Sher D, Klekowski N, Green M, Larson RA, Stock W (2006) Phase II study of decitabine in myelofibrosis with myeloid metaplasia. Blood 108: 317b (abstract 4923)

Oi S, Natsume A, Ito M, Kondo Y, Shimato S, Maeda Y, Saito K, Wakabayashi T (2009) Synergistic induction of NY-ESO-1 antigen expression by a novel histone deacetylase inhibitor, valproic acid, with 5-aza-2′-deoxycytidine in glioma cells. J Neurooncol 92:15–22

Oki Y, Kantarjian H, Gharibyan V, Jones D, O'brien S, Verstovsek S, Cortes J, Morris GM, Garcia-Manero G, Issa JP (2007) Phase II study of low-dose decitabine in combination with imatinib mesylate in patients with accelerated or myeloid blastic phase of chronic myelogenous leukemia. Cancer 109:899–906

Petti MC, Mandelli F, Zagonel V, De Gregoris C, Merola MC, Latagliata R, Gattei V, Fazi P, Monfardini S, Pino A (1993) Pilot study of 5-aza-2′-deoxycytidine (decitabine) in the treatment of poor prognosis acute myelogenous leukemia patients: preliminary results. Leukemia 7:36–41

Pinto A, Attadia V, Fusco A, Ferrara F, Spada OA, Di Fiore PP (1984) 5-Aza-2′-deoxycytidine induces terminal differentiation of leukemic blasts from patients with acute myeloid leukemias. Blood 64:922–929

Pinto A, Zagonel V, Attadia V, Bullian PL, Gattei V, Carbone A, Monfardini S, Colombatti A (1989) 5-Aza-2′-deoxycytidine as a differentiation inducer in acute myeloid leukaemias and myelodysplastic syndromes of the elderly. Bone Marrow Transplant 4(Suppl 3):28–32

Pliml J, Sorm F (1964) Synthesis of 2′-deoxy-D-ribofuranosyl-5-azacytosine. Coll Czeck Chem Commun 29:2576–2577

Plumb JA, Strathdee G, Sludden J, Kaye SB, Brown R (2000) Reversal of drug resistance in human tumor xenografts by 2′deoxy-5-azacytidine-induced demethylation of the hMLH1 gene promoter. Cancer Res 60:6039–6044

Pohlmann P, DiLeone LP, Cancella AI, Caldas AP, Dal Lago L, Campos O Jr, Monega E, Rivoire W, Schwartsmann G (2002) Phase II trial of cisplatin plus decitabine, a new hypomethylating agent, in patients with advanced squamous cell carcinoma of the cervix. Am J Clin Oncol 25:496–501

Ravandi F, Kantarjian H, Cohen A, Davis M, O'Brien S, Anderlini P, Andersson B, Claxton D, Donato M, Gajewski J, Khouri I, Korbling M, Ueno N, de Vos D, Champlin R, Giralt S (2001) Decitabine with allogeneic peripheral blood stem cell transplantation in the therapy of leukemia relapse following a prior transplant: results of a phase I study. Bone Marrow Transplant 27:1221–1225

Richel DJ, Colly LP, Kluin-Nelemans JC, Willemze R (1991) The antileukemic activity of 5-aza-2′-deoxycytidine (Aza-dC) in patients with relapsed and resistant leukemia. Br J Cancer 64:144–148

Rivard GE, Momparler RL, Demers J, Benoit P, Raymond R, Lin K, Momparler LF (1981) Phase I study on 5-aza-2′-deoxycytidine in children with acute leukemia. Leuk Res 5:453–462

Roman-Gomez J, Jimenez-Velasco A, Castillejo JA, Agirre X, Barrios M, Navarro G, Molina FJ, Calasanz MJ, Prosper F, Heiniger A, Torres A (2004) Promoter hypermethylation of cancer-related genes: a strong independent prognostic factor in acute lymphoblastic leukemia. Blood 10:2492–2498

Roman-Gomez J, Cordeu L, Agirre X, Jimenez-Velasco A, San Jose-Eneriz E, Garate L, Calasanz MJ, Heiniger A, Torres A, Prosper F (2007) Epigenetic regulation of Wnt-signaling pathway in acute lymphoblastic leukemia. Blood 8:3462–3469

Rüter B, Wijermans PW, Lübbert M (2006) Superiority of prolonged low-dose azanucleoside administration? Results of 5-aza-2′-deoxycytidine retreatment in high-risk myelodysplasia patients. Cancer 106:1744–1750

Sacchi S, Talpaz M, O'Brien S, Cortes J, Kantarjian HM (1998) Decitabine, a hypomethylating agent, is active for the treatment of chronic myelogenous leukemia (CML) in non-lymphoid blastic phase (BP). Blood 92 (Suppl 1): 252a (abstract)

Sacchi S, Kantarjian HM, O'Brien S, Cortes J, Rios MB, Giles FJ, Beran M, Koller CA, Keating MJ, Talpaz M (1999) Chronic myelogenous leukemia in nonlymphoid blastic phase: analysis of the results of first salvage therapy with three different treatment approaches for 162 patients. Cancer 86:2632–2641

Samlowski WE, Leachman SA, Wade M, Cassidy P, Porter-Gill P, Busby L, Wheeler R, Boucher K, Fitzpatrick F, Jones DA, Karpf AR (2005) Evaluation of a 7-day continuous intravenous infusion of decitabine: inhibition of promoter-specific and global genomic DNA methylation. J Clin Oncol 23:3897–3905

Santi DV, Garret CD, Barr PJ (1983) On the mechanism of inhibition of DNA-cytosine methyltransferase by cytidine analogs. Cell 83:83–89

Saunthararajah Y, Hillery CA, Lavelle D, Molokie R, Dorn L, Bressler L, Gavazova S, Chen YH, Hoffman R, DeSimone J (2003) Effects of 5-aza-2′-deoxycytidine on fetal hemoglobin levels, red cell adhesion, and hematopoietic differentiation in patients with sickle cell disease. Blood 102:3865–3870

Saunthararajah Y (2007) Decitabine and sickle cell disease: molecular therapy for a molecular disease. Pediatr Hematol Oncol 24:465–468

Saunthararajah Y, Molokie R, Saraf S, Sidhwani S, Gowhari M, Vara S, Lavelle D, DeSimone J (2008) Clinical effectiveness of decitabine in severe sickle cell disease. Br J Haematol 141:126–129

Schrump DS, Fischette MR, Nguyen DM, Zhao M, Li X, Kunst TF, Hancox A, Hong JA, Chen GA, Pishchik V, Figg WD, Murgo AJ, Steinberg SM (2006) Phase I study of decitabine-mediated gene expression in patients with cancers involving the lungs, esophagus, or pleura. Clin Cancer Res 12:5777–5785

Schwartsmann G, Fernandes MS, Schaan MD, Moschen M, Gerhardt LM, DiLeone L, Loitzembauer B, Kalakun L (1997) Decitabine (5-aza-2′-deoxycytidine; decitabine) plus daunorubicin as a first line treatment in patients with acute myeloid leukemia: preliminary observations. Leukemia 11(Suppl 1):28–31

Schwartsmann G, Schunemann H, Gorini CN, Filho AF, Garbino C, Sabini G, Muse I, DiLeone L, Mans DR (2000) A phase I trial of cisplatin plus decitabine, a new DNA-hypomethylating agent, in patients with advanced solid tumors and a follow-up early phase II evaluation in patients with inoperable non-small cell lung cancer. Invest New Drugs 18:83–91

Scott SA, Lakshimikuttysamma A, Sheridan DP, Sanche SE, Geyer CR, DeCoteau JF (2007) Zebularine inhibits human acute myeloid leukemia cell growth vitro in association with p15INK4B demethylation and reexpression. Exp Hematol 35:263–273

Shen L, Toyota M, Kondo Y, Obata T, Daniel S, Pierce S, Imai K, Kantarjian HM, Issa JP, Garcia-Manero G (2003) Aberrant DNA methylation of p57KIP2 identifies a cell cycle regulatory pathway with prognostic impact in adult acute lymphocytic leukemia. Blood 101:4131–4136

Shen L, Kantarjian H, Guo Y, Lin E, Shan J, Huang X, Berry D, Ahmed S, Zhu W, Pierce S, Kondo Y, Oki Y, Jelinek J, Saba H, Estey E, Issa JP (2010) DNA methylation predicts survival and response to therapy in patients with myelodysplastic syndromes. J Clin Oncol 28:605–613

Shi J, Zhao Y, Ishii T, Hu W, Sozer S, Zhang W, Bruno E, Lindgren V, Xu M, Hoffman R (2007) Effects of chromatin-modifying agents on CD34+ cells from patients with idiopathic myelofibrosis. Cancer Res 67:6417–6424

Sigalotti L, Coral S, Nardi G, Spessotto A, Cortini E, Cattarossi I, Colizzi F, Altomonte M, Maio M (2002) Promoter methylation controls the expression fo MAGE2, 3 and 4 genes in human cutaneous melanoma. J Immunother 25:16–26

Sigalotti L, Fratta E, Coral S, Tanzarella S, Danielli R, Colizzi F, Fonsatti E, Traversari C, Altomonte M, Maio M (2004) Intratumor heterogeneity of cancer/testis antigens expression in human cutaneous melanoma is methylation-regulated and functionally reverted by 5-aza-2′-deoxycytidine. Cancer Res 64:9167–9171

Sigalotti L, Coral S, Fratta E, Lamaj E, Danielli R, Di Giacomo AM, Altomonte M, Maio M (2005) Epigenetic modulation of solid tumors as a novel approach for cancer immunotherapy. Semin Oncol 32:473–478

Soriano AO, Yang H, Faderl S, Estrov Z, Giles F, Ravandi F, Cortes J, Wierda WG, Ouzounian S, Quezada A, Pierce S, Estey EH, Issa JP, Kantarjian HM, Garcia-Manero G (2007) Safety and clinical activity of the combination of 5-azacytidine, valproic acid, and all-trans retinoic acid in acute myeloid leukemia and myelodysplastic syndrome. Blood 110:2302–2308

Stathis A, Hotte SJ, Chen EX, Hirte HW, Oza AM, Moretto P, Webster S, Laughlin A, Stayner LA, McGill S, Wang L, Zhang WJ, Espinoza-Delgado I, Holleran JL, Egorin MJ, Siu LL (2011) Phase I study of decitabine in combination with vorinostat in patients with advanced solid tumors and non-Hodgkin's lymphomas. Clin Cancer Res 17:1582–1590

Stresemann C, Lyko F (2008) Modes of action of the DNA methyltransferase inhibitors azacytidine and decitabine. Int J Cancer 123:8–13

Thibault A, Figg WD, Bergan RC, Lush RM, Myers CE, Tompkins A, Reed E, Samid D (1998) A phase-II study of 5-aza-2′-deoxycytidine (decitabine) in hormone-independent metastatic (D2) prostate cancer. Tumori 84:87–89

Trompeter S, Roberts I (2009) Haemoglobin F modulation in childhood sickle cell disease. Brit J Haematol 144:308–316

van den Bosch J, Lübbert M, Verhoef G, Wijermans PW (2004) The effects of 5-aza-2′-deoxycytidine (decitabine) on the platelet count in patients with intermediate and high-risk myelodysplastic syndrome. Leuk Res 28:785–790

Venturelli S, Armeanu S, Pathil A, Hsieh CJ, Weiss TS, Vonthein R, Wehrmann M, Gregor M, Lauer UM, Bitzer M (2007) Epigenetic combination therapy as a tumor-selective treatment approach for hepatocellular carcinoma. Cancer 109:2132–2141

Vermorken JB, Tumolo S, Roozendaal KJ, Guastalla JP, Splinter Ted AW, Renard J (1991) 5-Aza-2′-deoxycytidine in advanced or recurrent cancer of the uterine cervix. Eur J Cancer 27:216–217

Wang JC, Chen W, Nallusamy S, Chen C, Novetsky AD (2002) Hypermethylation of the P15INK4b and P16INK4a in agnogenic myeloid metaplasia (AMM) and AMM in leukaemic transformation. Brit J Haematol 116:582–586

Wang WC (2008) The pharmacotherapy of sickle cell disease. Expert Opin Pharmacother 9:3069–3082

Weber J, Salgaller M, Samid D, Johnson B, Herlyn M, Lassam N, Treisman J, Rosenberg SA (1994) Expression of the MAGE-I tumor antigen is up-regulated by the demethylating agent 5-aza-2′-deoxycytidine. Cancer Res 54:1766–1771

Wijermans PW, Krulder JW, Huijgens PC, Neve P (1997) Continuous infusion of low-dose 5-Aza-2′-deoxycytidine in elderly patients with high-risk myelodysplastic syndrome. Leukemia 11:19–23

Wijermans PW, Lübbert M, Verhoef G, Bosly A, Ravoet C, Andre M, Ferrant A (2000) Low-dose 5-aza-2′-deoxycytidine, a DNA hypomethylating agent, for the treatment of high-risk myelodysplastic syndrome: a multicenter phase II study in elderly patients. J Clin Oncol 18:956–962

Wijermans PW, Lübbert M, Verhoef G, Klimek V, Bosly A (2005) An epigenetic approach to the treatment of advanced MDS; the experience with the DNA demethylating agent 5-aza-2′-deoxycytidine (decitabine) in 177 patients. Ann Hematol 84(Suppl 1):9–17

Willemze R, Archimbaud E, Muus P (1993) Preliminary results with 5-aza-2′deoxycytidine (DAC)-containing chemotherapy in patients with relapsed or refractory acute leukemia. The EORTC Leukemia Cooperative Group. Leukemia 7(Suppl 1):49–50

Willemze R, Suciu S, Archimbaud E, Muus P, Stryckmans P, Louwagie EA, Berneman Z, Tjean M, Wijermans P, Döhner H, Jehn U, Labar B, Jaksic B, Dardenne M, Zittoun R (1997) A randomized phase-II study on the effects of 5-aza-2′-deoxycytidine combined with either amsacrine or idarubicin in patients with relapsed acute leukemia: an EORTC Leukemia Cooperative Group phase-II study. Leukemia 11(Suppl 1):24–27

Wilson VL, Jones PA, Momparler RL (1983) Inhibition of DNA methylation in L1210 leukemia cells by 5-aza-2′-deoxycytidine as a possible mechanism of chemotherapeutic action. Cancer Res 43:3493–3496

Yanez L, Bermudez A, Richard C, Bureo E, Iriondo A (2009) Letter to the editor: Successful induction therapy with decitabine in refractory childhood acute lymphoblastic leukemia. Leukemia 23:1342–1343

Yang AS, Doshi KD, Choi SW, Mason JB, Mannari RK, Gharybian V, Luna R, Rashid A, Shen L, Estecio MR, Kantarjian HM, Garcia-Manero G, Issa JP (2006) DNA methylation changes after 5-aza-2′-deoxycytidine therapy in patients with leukemia. Cancer Res 66:5495–5503

Yang H, Hoshino K, Sanchez-Gonzalez B, Kantarjian H, Garcia-Manero G (2005) Antileukemia activity of the combination of 5-aza-2′-deoxycytidine with valproic acid. Leuk Res 29:739–748

Yang H, Kadia T, Xiao L, Bueso-Ramos CE, Hoshino K, Thomas DA, O'Brien S, Jabbour E, Pierce S, Rosner GL, Kantarjian HM, Garcia-Manero G (2009) Residual DNA methylation at remission is prognostic in adult Philadelphia chromosome-negative acute lymphocytic leukemia. Blood 113:1892–1898

Yoo CB, Jones PA (2006) Epigenetic therapy of cancer: past, present and future. Nat Rev Drug Discov 5:37–50

Zagonel V, Pinto A, Bullian PL, Sorio R, Gattei V, Curri G, De Rosa L, Attadia V, Monfardini S (1990) 5-Aza-2′-deoxycytidine as a differentiation inducer in human hemopoietic malignancies: preliminary clinical report. In: Momparler RL, de Vos D (eds) PCH 5-Aza-2′-deoxycytidine: preclinical and clinical studies. Haarlem, Netherlands, pp 165–181

Zagonel V, Lo Re G, Marotta G, Barbare R, Sardeo R, Gattei V, de Angelis V, Montardinni S, Pinto A (1993) 5-Aza-2′-deoxycytidine (decitabine) induces trilineage response in unfavourable myelodysplastic syndrome. Leukemia 7(Suppl 1):30–35

Zhou L, Cheng X, Connolly BA, Dickman MJ, Hurd PJ, Hornby DP (2002) Zebularine: a novel DNA methylation inhibitor that forms a covalent complex with DNA methyltransferases. J Mol Biol 23:591–599

5-Azacytidine/5-Azacitidine

Antonia M. S. Müller and Mareike Florek

Abstract

The hypomethylating agent 5-Azacytidine epigenetically modulates various genes, including tumor suppressor genes. For many years, the "new agent", which was first discovered in the 1960s, remained fairly unobtrusive in the rank of salvage treatment options for myelodysplastic syndromes (MDS) and acute myeloid leukemia (AML). When the significance of epigenetics in tumorigenesis became clear, 5-Azacytidine attracted new attention. Finally, it was the first drug approved for the treatment of all categories of MDS, and its survival benefit over best conventional care was confirmed. Today, in many clinical situations, when aggressive therapies including allogeneic hematopoietic cell transplantation are not an option, 5-Azacytidine is the first treatment of choice. Preliminary data on combinations of the hypomethylating agent with other new drugs are promising, and innovative strategies involving immune modulation and regenerative tissue repair hold a broad potential for future developments.

Contents

A. M. S. Müller (✉)
Division of Hematology, University Hospital Zurich, Rämistrasse 100, 8091, Zurich, Switzerland
e-mail: AntoniaMaria.Mueller@usz.ch

M. Florek
Division of Blood and Marrow Transplantation, Stanford University, Stanford, USA

U. M. Martens (ed.), *Small Molecules in Oncology*, Recent Results in Cancer Research 201, DOI: 10.1007/978-3-642-54490-3_19,

1 Introduction

5-Azacytidine (Azacitidine, Vidaza®; Pharmion Corporation) is a pyrimidine nucleoside analog that was first synthesized and shown to possess a wide range of biological effects more than 40 years ago (Sorm et al. 1964; von Hoff et al. 1976). A first wave of interest arouse when 5-Azacytidine's activity against leukemic cells was established in vitro (Li et al. 1970a; Sorm and Vesely 1964) and in vivo (Presant et al. 1975), and early clinical studies performed in the 1970s demonstrated antitumor activity in patients with acute myeloid leukemia (AML) and myelodysplastic syndrome (MDS) (von Hoff et al. 1976). Although the inhibitory effects of 5-Azacytidine on DNA methyltransferase activity were discovered shortly after (Jones and Taylor 1980), it took years until the agent attracted new attention for its hypomethylating qualities. Eventually, when it was recognized that aberrant DNA methylation is critically involved in the development of many neoplasias, including MDS (Aoki et al. 2000; Herman and Baylin 2003; Jones and Baylin 2002), trials exploring the usefulness of 5-Azacytidine in MDS were initiated (Silverman 2001; Silverman et al. 1993). Clinical efficacy, safety, a reduced risk for transformation into AML, and a beneficial impact on quality of life over best supportive were confirmed (Kornblith et al. 2002; Silverman et al. 2002). Based on these studies in May 2004 5-Azacytidine was approved by the US Food and Drug Administration (FDA) as first-line therapy for MDS of all French–American–British (FAB)-defined subtypes (Kaminskas et al. 2005a, b). In December 2008, the European Medical Agency (EMA) followed and approved 5-Azacytidine for the treatment of patients not eligible for hematopoietic cell transplantation (HCT) with: Intermediate-2-or high-risk MDS; chronic myelomonocytic leukemia (CMML) with 10–29 % bone marrow blasts without myeloproliferative disease; and World Health Organization (WHO)-classified AML with 20–30 % blasts and multilineage dysplasia. 5-Azacytidine received orphan drug designation in several markets including the European Union, the US and Japan. In 2010, the National Comprehensive Cancer Network (NCCN) upgraded 5-Azacytidine's status to a Category 1—"preferred" therapy, for high-risk MDS patients, who are most likely to progress to AML.

After a slow start from the 1960s to the early 2000s, with approval of 5-Azacytidine by the US and EU authorities, the heydays of the "not-so-novel" hypomethylating agent finally began. Today, 5-Azacytidine is well established in clinical practice and has basically replaced "best supportive care" for many patients with MDS and AML that are not eligible for induction chemotherapy and/or allogeneic HCT.

2 Structure and Mechanism of Action

2.1 Structure

5-Azacytidine (4-amino-1-b-D-ribofuranosyl 1-1,3,5 triazine-2-one or 1-b-D-ribofuranosyl-5-azacytosine; C 8 H 12 N 4 O 5; molecular weight 244) is a ring analog of the naturally occurring pyrimidine nucleoside cytidine, from which it differs only by a nitrogen in place of the fifth carbon (Bergy and Herr 1966) (Fig. 1). 5-Azacytidine is a white to off-white solid that is stable at 25 °C, not light sensitive, sparingly soluble in water, and unstable when reconstituted in aqueous solution. Hydrolytic degradation results in a 21–36 % loss over 8 h at 25–30 °C and a 2–3 % loss at 5 °C (Kaminskas et al. 2005a).

2.2 Mechanism of Action

Two main mechanisms of antineoplastic action have been identified for 5-Azacytidine, namely the capacity to (a) incorporate directly into RNA with subsequent disruption of RNA metabolism and (b) inhibit DNA methylation (Fig. 2).

(a) On uptake into cells, 5-Azacytidine is phosphorylated by several kinases (uridine cytidine-, pyrimidine monophosphate-, and diphosphate kinases) to 5-aza-2′deoxycytidine di-, and subsequently triphosphate. The ribose structure needs to be metabolized by ribonucleotide reductase (RNR) first to be integrated into DNA. Incorporation of 5-Azacytidine triphosphate into RNA occurs directly and causes a disruption of nuclear and cytoplasmic RNA metabolism with subsequent inhibition of protein synthesis (Li et al. 1970b).

(b) The second mechanism of action is the inhibition of DNA methylation by trapping DNA methyltransferases. In general, DNA methylation refers to the addition of a methyl group to the cytosine residue of a CpG site. So-called CpG islands are genomic regions with a high frequency of CG dinucleotides (the "p" in CpG notation refers to the phosphodiester bond between the cytosine and the guanine) that are typically located in proximity to promoters. The degree of methylation of CpG islands plays a role in the control of gene transcription. Usually, fully methylated sites are associated with suppression of gene expression, while hypomethylated or unmethylated CpG islands are linked to active transcription. Forming a tight-binding complex 5-Azacytidine irreversibly binds to methyltransferase, which it inhibits in its progression along the DNA duplex, and results in intracellular depletion of the enzyme. Consequently, unmethylated DNA can lead to the transcription of previously

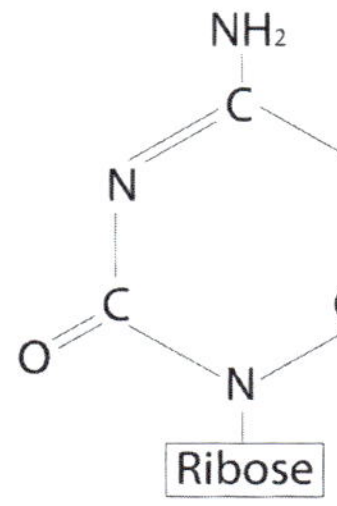

Fig. 1 Structure

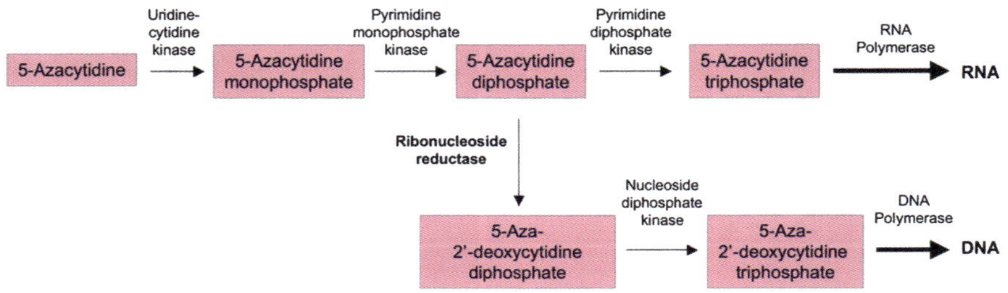

Fig. 2 Mechanism of action

quiescent genes (Jones and Taylor 1981; Taylor and Jones 1982). Already minor substitution of cytosine residues (~ 0.3 %) suffices to inactivate more than 95 % of methyltransferase activity in the cell (Creusot et al. 1982). DNA (hyper-) methylation is believed to contribute to cancer initiation and progression by silencing tumor suppressor genes and other genes critical in regulation of cell cycle, cell growth, differentiation, and apoptosis (Bird 1996). In this setting, 5-Azacytidine can restore the expression of potentially important genes by demethylating such pathologically hypermethylated regions (Silverman 2001). In addition to these modes of action, 5-Azacytidine has been reported to inhibit DNA histone acetylation, another regulatory mechanism in gene silencing (Chiurazzi et al. 1999).

2.3 Pharmacology, Bioavailability, Half-Life, Elimination, Drug–Drug Interactions

Both subcutaneous (s.c.) and intravenous (i.v.) routes are used in clinical protocols. Bioavailability of s.c. relative to i.v. 5-Azacytidine is approximately 89 %; however, there is evidence i.v. application may be associated with shorter overall survival (OS) (Martin et al. 2009). Regardless of baseline hematology laboratory values, the recommended starting dose of 5-Azacytidine is 75 mg/m^2 s.c. or i.v.

daily for 7 days, and cycles are repeated every 28 days. Alternative 5-day dosing regimens (75 mg/m^2 daily for 5 days) have been shown to achieve similar hematologic improvements in good-risk patients with MDS and possibly better tolerability (Lyons et al. 2009). Therefore, many oncologists adapted this more convenient 5-day schedule for outpatient settings, despite the lack of long-term follow-up and data on high-risk MDS patients. Because responses are often delayed, therapy should be given at least for 4–5 cycles and may be continued as long as the positive effect persists. A dose increase to 100 mg/m^2 can be considered if no beneficial effect is notable after two cycles. The maximal dose tolerated has not been formally determined; however, some early trials used daily i.v. doses of 150–200 mg/m^2 for 5 days, and even a maximum dose of 500 mg/m^2 has been given on a weekly basis to patients with solid tumors (von Hoff and Slavik 1977).

Oral formulations of 5-Azacytidine are under investigation. Their mean relative oral bioavailability (ranging from 6.3 to 20 %) and biological activity have been demonstrated in MDS and CMML patients when given at a daily dose of 480 mg for 7 days of a 28-day cycle. Kinetics of the change in DNA methylation levels after s.c. and oral 5-Azacytidine were similar, with maximum hypomethylation on day 15, and methylation levels returned to near-baseline values by the end of each cycle (Garcia-Manero et al. 2011).

5-Azacytidine is rapidly absorbed after s.c. administration with peak plasma concentrations after 30 min and a mean half-life of 41 $\pm$ 8 min. Urinary excretion is the primary route of elimination of 5-Azacitidine and its metabolites, but presumably additional extra-renal pathways for elimination exist (Chabot et al. 1983; Stresemann and Lyko 2008). Fecal excretion appears to be minimal (Marcucci et al. 2005). A formal assessment of drug—drug interactions has not been conducted as of yet, and whether the metabolism of 5-Azacytidine is affected by microsomal enzyme inducers or inhibitors remains to be clarified (Marcucci et al. 2005). Of note, RNR, which metabolizes 5-Azacytidine into the active form, is a known target of hydroxyurea. Therefore, concomitant use of both drugs can diminish efficacy of 5-Azacytidine and should be avoided, while sequential administration may be possible (Choi et al. 2007).

3 Toxicity

3.1 Safety, Side Effects, and Contraindications

Dose toxicology studies identified bone marrow, liver, kidney, and lymphoid tissues as target organs of 5-Azacytidine (Kaminskas et al. 2005a). While treatment-related mortality has been consistently low (<1 %), severe adverse side effects have been reported in ca. 60 % of 5-Azacytidine patients, consisting of thrombocytopenia, febrile neutropenia, fever, and pneumonia. Obviously, safety evaluations from the MDS trials were confounded by the pathophysiology and symptoms of the disease and their clinical resemblance to the toxicity of the drug. Other common, less serious side effects included injection site events, arthralgia, cough, dyspnea, headache, weakness, dizziness, and insomnia. Usually, adverse events occurred during the first two therapy cycles and diminished subsequently. Discontinuation of 5-Azacytidine was mostly related to myelosuppression (Silverman et al. 2002).

3.1.1 Hematologic Toxicity/Myelosuppression

Several phase I studies pointed to leukopenia (<1,500/μL) as a dose-limiting toxicity. Leukopenia was dose-related and occurred in approximately 34 % of patients, while thrombocytopenia (<100,000/μL) has been reported in 17 %. Only 4 % of patients had greater than 3 g/dL drop in hemoglobin directly attributable to the drug (von Hoff et al. 1976). In the CALG B trials, myelosuppression, either BM hypoplasia or drug-related cytopenias, required dose reduction in a third of patients (Silverman et al. 1993).

3.1.2 Gastrointestinal Toxicity

Initially, the usefulness of 5-Azacytidine was hampered by severe nausea and vomiting that accompanied rapid i.v. injection of the instable drug. Only when it became clear that the half-life of the drug at 25 °C in buffered solutions is significantly longer, infusion time could be extended and gastrointestinal toxicity could be reduced (Israili et al. 1976; Vogler et al. 1976). Split doses and s.c. administration decreased side effects slightly, and subsequent continuous infusions (150 mg/m^2/day over 120 h with fresh preparations every 4 h) were able to further improve tolerability (Lomen et al. 1975). Newer trials using the current standard dose regimen (75 mg/m^2/day over 7 days every 28 days) still revealed mild to moderate nausea and/or vomiting as the most common side effect (63 %) (Silverman et al. 1993). Diarrhea occurred in a substantial proportion of patients, but was not dose-limiting (von Hoff et al. 1976).

3.1.3 Hepatotoxicity

Liver damage appears to be unrelated to dose, schedule, or route of administration. Liver function abnormalities have been documented in 7–16 % of patients receiving 5-Azacytidine, particularly those with preexisting liver cirrhosis (Silverman et al. 2002; von Hoff et al. 1976). Hepatic comas have been reported in context with extensive liver metastasis and low baseline serum albumin levels (0.5 %) (Bellet et al. 1973). For this reason, 5-Azacytidine is contraindicated in patients with advanced hepatic malignancies.

3.1.4 Nephrotoxicity

Renal dysfunction and failure have been observed in patients receiving combination chemotherapy and/or displaying preexisting renal impairment (von Hoff et al. 1976), particularly during periods of sepsis and hypotension (Silverman et al. 2002). Since 5-Azacytidine and its metabolites are primarily excreted by the kidneys, dosage needs to be adjusted based on renal function and serum electrolytes, especially in elderly patients.

3.1.5 Other

Sporadically, in <3 % of patients, neuromuscular side effects have been documented, involving myalgia, generalized muscle tenderness, weakness, and lethargy. Other unspecific symptoms reported were fever (6 %), skin rash (2 %), stomatitis, phlebitis, and hypotension (von Hoff et al. 1976). Post-marketing interstitial lung disease, tumor lysis syndrome, injection site necrosis, and Sweet's syndrome (acute febrile neutrophilic dermatosis) have been reported, but the causal relationship to drug exposure has not been established with certainty.

3.1.6 Teratogenicity

In animal studies, 5-Azacytidine caused congenital malformations and was found to be mutagenic, clastogenic, and embryotoxic when females were dosed during gestation. The drug decreased male fertility, and preconception treatment of male rodents resulted in increased embryofetal loss in mated untreated females. Therefore, women should avoid pregnancy and men should not father a child while receiving treatment with 5-Azacytidine (Kaminskas et al. 2005b).

4 Preclinical Data

5-Azacytidine and its deoxy derivative 5-Aza-2′-Deoxycitidine were chemically synthesized and characterized in Czechoslovakia by František Šorm and his fellow investigators in the 1960s (Sorm et al. 1964). Shortly after, 5-Azacytidine was also microbiologically isolated from the fermentation beer of treptoverticillium ladakanus (Hanka et al. 1966). The new agent was shown to possess a wide range of biological effects, including antimicrobial, abortive, mutagenic, leukopenic, immunosuppressive, cytotoxic, and antineoplastic activity (von Hoff et al. 1976). Particular interest arouse when 5-Azacytidine's antitumor activity in leukemia cell lines was established (Li et al. 1970a; Sorm and Vesely 1964). In vivo studies confirmed the cytotoxicity by demonstrating a prolonged survival of mice with L1210 leukemias after administration of 5-Azacytidine (Presant et al. 1975).

Because of its capability to induce differentiation of erythroleukemic cells in vitro, and thereby alter malignant cell phenotypes (Jones and Taylor 1980), 5-Azacytidine was tested in hemoglobinopathies. Treatment attempts in patients with sickle cell anemia demonstrated an increase in fetal hemoglobin (HbF) and a decline of HbS with a slight overall increase in total hemoglobin concentration and reduced hemolysis. Similarly, patients with β-thalassemia showed increased γ-chain synthesis with significantly improved erythropoiesis, but this was not necessarily accompanied by an enhanced hemoglobin concentration (Stamatoyannopoulos 1992).

In 1980, Jones and Taylor discovered that 5-Azacytidine could inhibit DNA methyltransferase activity (Jones and Taylor 1980). Only later, when it was recognized that aberrant DNA methylation is critically involved in the development of many neoplasias, including MDS (Aoki et al. 2000; Herman and Baylin 2003;

Jones and Baylin 2002), the demethylating agents attracted new attention. Since there was no satisfactory treatment option for the majority of MDS patients, and early studies had shown responses to 5-Azacytidine, MDS offered an appropriate disease entity to study the effects of the drug on DNA methylation, gene transcription, and cell differentiation. In fact, 5-Azacytidine was the first agent that showed the potential to alter the natural course of MDS.

Next to pathological hypermethylation, there is evidence that also physiologically methylated CpG sites may be a target for methyltransferase inhibitors. Plausible data imply that a stable and permanent expression of the human transcription factor forkhead box P3 (FOXP3) in regulatory T cells might be crucial in the prevention of autoimmunity, allergy, and graft-versus-host disease after allogeneic HCT. Apparently, DNA methylation patterns in the FOXP3 locus can serve to discriminate $FOXP3^{+}$ regulatory T cells with suppressive capacity (demethylated promotor region) from activated $FOXP3^{+}$ conventional T cells that lack this protective function (methylated CpG sites) (Floess et al. 2007; Polansky et al. 2008). Experimental data support the hypothesis that inhibition of methyltransferases stabilizes transcription of FOXP3, which could result in an increase in suppressive $FOXP3^{+}$ regulatory T cells. It is conceivable that in the future hypomethylating agents might be used as a therapeutic tool for immune modulation (Nagar et al. 2008). Consistent with this idea, 5-Azacitidine has been shown to mitigate graft-versus-host disease in mice that had received a transplant of major histocompatibility complex mismatched allogeneic bone marrow and T cells. 5-Azacytidine acted by peripheral conversion of alloreactive effector T cells into $FOXP3^{+}$ regulatory T cells and epigenetic modulation of genes downstream of FOXP3 required for the suppressor function of regulatory T cells. Interestingly, graft-versus-leukemia effects appeared to be preserved under such treatment (Choi et al. 2010).

Currently, 5-Azacytidine is tested in various off-target fields. Noteworthy, findings from these preclinical studies are that the agent appears to inhibit the anti-apoptotic transcription factor NFκB, presumably via decreased phosphorylation of the upstream regulator IKKα/β, resulting in apoptosis and cell death (Fabre et al. 2008). Moreover, 5-Azacytidine has been proposed to significantly inhibit Wnt signaling, a pathway involved in oncogene expression in AML and other cancers (Chim et al. 2007; Jawad et al. 2008). Lastly, multiple studies have shown that 5-Azacytidine can induce bone marrow mesenchymal stem cells to differentiate into cardiomyogenic cells in vitro (Xing et al. 2012).

5 Clinical Use of 5-Azacytidine

5.1 Early Studies

Clinical trials using 5-Azacytidine were initiated in 1967 in Europe, and in the late 1970s in the United States. These studies investigated the application of the new agent in patients with metastatic cancer and leukemias refractory to conventional chemotherapies. In 1976, von Hoff et al. provided a comprehensive review on all preclinical and clinical data before 1975, encompassing a total of 58 protocols and reviews received at the Investigational Drug Branch of the National Institutes of Health. Eight hundred and twenty-one patients who had been treated with 5-Azacytidine, 207 of them within phase I studies, were re-evaluated. Promisingly, 5-Azacytidine revealed consistent antitumor activity in patients with AML and achieved an overall response rate of 36 % [20 % complete response (CR), 16 % partial response (PR)] in 200 patients with relapsed/refractory AML. The median duration of remission was between 15 and 19 weeks (von Hoff et al. 1976). Although these remarkable responses verified the activity of 5-Azacytidine as a single agent in AML, the drug never advanced through the US FDA review process as a leukemia therapy. In contrast to AML, both European and US experiences with 5-Azacytidine for treatment of acute lymphatic leukemia (ALL), chronic myeloid leukemia (CML), and multiple myeloma were disappointing. Likewise, clinical results of 5-Azacytidine for treatment of solid tumors failed to show any notable effects and were not encouraging at all. Few favorable responses occurred, usually of poor quality, short duration, and associated with significant toxicity (von Hoff et al. 1976).

5.2 Randomized Phase III Studies of 5-Azacytidine

MDS comprises a group of chronic BM dysfunction syndromes characterized by cytopenias of one or more blood lineages and/or an increase in bone marrow blasts. Progression of MDS is often characterized by transformation into AML. Because of their advanced age, most MDS patients are not candidates for aggressive curative therapies, such as intensive chemotherapy and allogeneic HCT, and previously had no actual treatment option superior to best supportive care (Kaminskas et al. 2005a). The discovery of the hypermethylation of the p15 INK4B gene in MDS (Christiansen et al. 2003; Uchida et al. 1997) provided the rationale for the effectiveness of 5-Azacytidine in MDS that had been observed already in the early trials of the 1970s and 1980.

When in May 2004 5-Azacytidine was the first therapeutic agent approved by the FDA for the treatment of all subtypes of MDS, this decision based on three clinical studies conducted by the Cancer and Leukemia Group B (CALG B). Two of them were single-armed (Silverman 2001; Silverman et al. 1993); the third was a controlled, randomized phase III trial (Silverman et al. 2002). 5-Azacytidine was administered at a starting dose of 75 mg/m^2/day for 7 days with 28-day cycles in all three trials. The first phase II study (protocol 8421) of the CALG B was initiated in 1984, and 49 % of 43 patients receiving 5-Azacytidine as a continuous i.v. infusion responded [12 % CR, 25 % PR, 12 % "improved" (response with less than 50 % restoration of normal blood counts and less than 50 % decreases in RBC or platelet transfusion requirements)]. The overall survival (OS) was 13.3 months, median duration of remission was 14.7 months, requirement of RBC transfusions was eliminated in 82 %, and the agent was tolerated well (Silverman et al. 1993). In the second trial (protocol 8921), 5-Azacytidine given as a s.c. bolus injection to 67 patients with high-risk MDS yielded comparable results with regard to safety and efficacy (overall response rate 53 %; CR 12 %, PR 15 %, 27 % improved) (Silverman 2001). These promising results prompted the initiation of a randomized, open-label phase III trial (protocol 9221) to compare the clinical efficacy and impact on quality of life of 5-Azacytidine with best supportive care. In 191 patients with MDS, an overall response (CR plus PR) was achieved in about 16 % (11.8–18.8 %), while there was no response in the control group. This difference between both arms was statistically highly significant. Incidence of transformation to AML decreased, and time to AML or death was considerably longer for the 5-Azacytidine group than for the supportive care group (median 21 vs. 12 months, respectively) in all age groups and all MDS subtypes (Silverman et al. 2002). The most evident benefit of a response was in transfusion-dependent patients, who lost their need for transfusion of RBC and/or platelets during CR or PR. Indicators of response, such as decrease in blast counts or increase in platelets, hemoglobin, or WBC, were observed by the fifth treatment cycle in more than 90 % of patients, and responses were long lasting (Silverman et al. 2006). In contrast to patients in the supportive care group, those receiving 5-Azacytidine experienced significant improvement in fatigue, dyspnea, physical function, positive effect, and psychological distress, which coupled with greater treatment response and delayed time to transformation to AML or death (Kornblith et al. 2002). In 2006, Silverman et al. reanalyzed the combined data from all 270 patients treated within the three CALG B trials and confirmed previous results of a CR rate of 10–17 %. The median number of cycles to first response was 3, and 90 % of responses were seen by cycle 6. The overall response rate for patients with the retrospective diagnosis of an AML, according to the new WHO classification system, was encouraging. While the CR rate of 9 % was rather moderate (vs. 0 % in the observation group), the prolongation in survival time to 19.3 months when compared with 12.9 months without specific treatment was remarkable (Silverman et al. 2006). The CALG B trials could not establish a survival benefit or delay in progression to AML as a treatment benefit for 5-Azacytidine because crossover of observation arm patients to treatment was permitted, and because the trial was insufficiently powered to detect a survival benefit.

Subsequently, the large, international, randomized, parallel group, open-label phase III 5-Azacytidine survival trial (AZA-001) demonstrated a statistically significant superior median OS of 24.5 months for 179 higher-risk MDS patients receiving 5-Azacytidine as compared to an OS of 15 months in 179 patients under conventional care [including best supportive care ($n = 105$), low-dose cytarabine ($n = 49$), or intensive chemotherapy ($n = 25$)], with a 2-year survival rate that was nearly doubled (51 vs. 26 %; $p < 0.0001$), a median time to AML transformation or death of 13 versus 7.6 months, and a CR and PR rate of 29 vs. 12 %, respectively (Fenaux et al. 2009). In all patients who responded to 5-Azacytidine (51 % CR, PR, or hematologic improvement), the median number of cycles to first response was 3 (range 1–22); 81 % and 90 % of patients achieved a first response by cycle 6 and 9, respectively (Silverman et al. 2008a). The survival benefit with 5-Azacytidine was seen across all prognostic subgroups analyzed, including those with poor, intermediate, and good-risk cytogenetics according to the international prognosis scoring system.

Several subgroup analyses of the AZA-001 trial followed the initial report:

1. 5-Azacytidine was comparably effective and significantly prolonged OS in patients who had been enrolled into the trial as FAB RAEB-T, but now meet the WHO criteria for AML (low marrow blast count of 20 to 30 %) (Fenaux et al. 2010a).
2. A particularly favorable response to 5-Azacytidine was observed in patients with alterations of chromosome 7, while those with del 5q had a poorer response rate than other high-risk MDS and AML patients (Fenaux and Ades 2009; Itzykson et al. 2008).
3. The subpopulation of elderly high-risk MDS patients ($\geq$75 years) with higher-risk MDS tolerated the agent well and experienced a significantly prolonged 2-year OS (55 % in the 5-Azacytidine group vs. 15 % in the conventional care group; $p < 0.001$) and reduced risk of death (Seymour et al. 2010).
4. 5-Azacytidine patients had significantly more and longer hematological responses, achieved more often independence of blood cell transfusions, and had prolonged OS as compared to patients given low-dose cytarabine (Fenaux et al. 2010b).
5. The difference in OS between 5-Azacytidine and intensive chemotherapy groups was not statistically significant, which the authors speculate may have been due to the small number of patients in this analysis (Fenaux et al. 2010b). Yet, a recent retrospective comparison of high-risk MDS or secondary AML patients age 60–70 receiving either an allogeneic HCT ($n = 103$) or 5-Azacytidine ($n = 75$) suggested a survival advantage for allogeneic HCT with an estimated 2-year OS of 39 % as compared to 23 % in the group given 5-Azacytidine (Platzbecker et al. 2012a).
6. Continued 5-Azacytidine therapy in responders was associated with improved responses to a higher response category in 48 % of patients (Silverman et al. 2011).
7. An analysis conducted to investigate the relationship between treatment response and OS found that achieving an overall response with 5-Azacytidine reduced risk of death by 95 % compared with achieving an overall response with the conventional care regimens ($p = 0.006$), and significantly improved OS was also observed in patients with a hematologic improvement who had never achieved CR or PR (Gore et al. 2013).

Due to the results of the AZA-001 trial, the FDA authorization was extended in August 2008, and 5-Azacytidine became the first drug approved to reflect unprecedented OS in patients with higher-risk MDS. In December 2008, 5-Azacytidine was granted marketing authorization in the EU, and the "Committee for Medicinal Products for Human Use (CHMP)" of the EMA approved the agent for treatment of adult patients who are not eligible for HCT with intermediate-2 and high-risk MDS according to IPSS; CMML with 10–29 % marrow blasts without myeloproliferative disorder; AML with 20–30 % blasts; and multilineage dysplasia (WHO classification).

5.3 Current Questions and Preliminary Results

Although 5-Azacytidine has become a commonly used drug in hematological practice, there remain critical questions to be addressed prospectively. The key points of interest involve the following distinct topics:

5.3.1 Comparison of 5-Azacytidine and Decitabine

As of today, there is no available data from randomized trials comparing the efficacy of the two hypomethylating agents. Two large meta-analyses compiled available reported outcomes of prospective studies.

Gurion et al. (2010) included 952 and analyzed 782 patients with MDS from four trials performed between 2002 and 2008 in their meta-analysis, two trials examining the effect of 5-Azacytidine and two evaluating decitabine, in comparison with conventional care (best supportive care, low-dose cytarabine or intensive chemotherapy, depending on the trial). This meta-analysis found treatment with hypomethylating agents significantly improved response rates, OS, and prolonged time to AML transformation. When subgroup analyses were performed for each type of drug, an advantage regarding OS and AML transformation was only evident for 5-Azacytidine, but no such benefit for decitabine. When Kumar et al. applied slightly different statistics on the same cohort, they observed no difference in OS in patients treated with hypomethylating agents as compared to the conventional care cohort. However, also in their subgroup analysis, 5-Azacytidine, but not decitabine, had a survival benefit over supportive care (Kumar et al. 2010).

A more recent report from the Korean AML/MDS working party retrospectively compared efficacy and safety of 5-Azacytidine and decitabine in 300 patients with MDS. While there were no significant differences between both groups regarding overall response, OS, EFS, and rate of AML transformation, in patients $\geq$65 years of age, survival was significantly better in the 5-Azacytidine group ($p = 0.017$), whereas patients given Decitabine experienced more frequent episodes of grade 3 or 4 cytopenias and infections (Lee et al. 2013).

Overall, it appears due to its better tolerability in elderly patients and those with significant comorbidities, 5-Azacytidine may have an advantage over decitabine in these patients. However, prospective randomized trials are yet to be performed to ultimately clarify which groups may benefit from one drug or the other.

5.3.2 Role of 5-Azacytidine in Patients with AML and Bone Marrow Blasts >30 %

While decitabine has been approved for treatment of AML in Europe, 5-Azacytidine is only indicated for those subsets of AML with bone marrow blasts between 20–30 % and multilineage dysplasia (formerly classified as MDS). Although 5-Azacytidine presumably is commonly used off-label to treat elderly or relapsed AML patients that cannot be offered or do not wish induction chemotherapy and/or allogeneic HCT, few prospectively acquired data are available determining the role and efficacy of the hypomethylating agent and its benefit over best supportive care in more aggressive AML with higher rate of proliferation and bone marrow infiltration.

A large retrospective analysis on the outcomes of 671 patients $\geq$65 years of age with newly diagnosed AML treated between 2000 and 2010 with intensive chemotherapy ($n = 557$) or hypomethylating agents (5-Azacytidine or decitabine; $n = 114$) revealed CR in 42 % after chemotherapy versus 28 % with epigenetic therapy ($p = 0.001$). Eight-week mortality was 18 and 11 %, respectively ($p = 0.075$). However, 2-year relapse-free survival rates (28 vs. 39 %, $p = 0.843$) and median survival (6.7 vs. 6.5 months, $p = 0.413$) were similar in both groups. Subgroup analysis within the epigenetic treatment group revealed an improved median OS for decitabine over 5-Azacytidine (8.8 vs. 5.5 months, $p = 0.03$). Multivariate analysis for the total study cohort identified older age, adverse cytogenetics, poor performance status, increased creatinine, peripheral blood blasts, bone marrow blasts, and hemoglobin, but not type of AML therapy, as independent prognostic factors for survival, leading to the overall conclusion that intensive chemotherapy and epigenetic therapy achieve similar survival rates in older patients with newly diagnosed AML (Quintás-Cardama et al. 2012).

Eighty-two AML patients (median age 72 years, 33 % secondary AML, 29 % poor risk karyotype), who were documented in a longitudinal, multicenter Italian registry and had received 5-Azacytidine as compassionate use between 06/2005 and 12/2009, were evaluated with regard to efficacy and safety of the hypomethylating agent. The overall response rate was 32 %, including 15 % CRs and 5 % CRs with incomplete blood count recovery, and responses were more frequent among previously untreated patients and those who had white blood cell counts $<10 \times 10^9$/L. For untreated patients who achieved a response, the median overall response duration was 13 months, and the 1-year and 2-years OS rates were 58 and 24 %, respectively, leading the authors to conclude that 5-Azacytidine promises to be an effective therapy for elderly patients with untreated AML and with white blood cell counts $<10 \times 10^9$/L (Maurillo et al. 2012).

A German multicenter phase I/II study demonstrated 5-Azacytidine was active and well tolerated in 40 elderly patients with newly diagnosed AML that were medically unfit for or resistant to chemotherapy. Median marrow blast infiltration was 42 %. Response (CR, PR, and hematologic improvement) was 50 % in newly diagnosed and 10 % in relapsed/refractory patients with a median time to response of 2.5 months and median duration of response of 5.9 months (Al-Ali et al. 2012).

Analyses focusing on the effect of first-line hypomethylating agents (5-Azacytidine and decitabine) in treatment for AML and high-risk MDS patients with poor prognosis due to chromosome 5 and 7 abnormalities [excluding del 5(q)] revealed 41 % of patients in the epigenetic therapy group ($n = 81$) versus 35 % in the intensive chemotherapy group ($n = 151$) achieved CRs ($p = 0.395$). The median duration of CR was 45 and 23 weeks, respectively ($p = 0.153$), and OS was superior for the hypomethylating group compared with the chemotherapy group ($p = 0.019$), suggesting that patients with chromosome 5 and 7 abnormalities benefit from epigenetic rather than aggressive therapy (Ravandi et al. 2009).

5.3.3 Role of 5-Azacytidine in Therapy-Related Myeloid Neoplasms (t-MDS and t-AML)

Therapy-related (t-) myeloid neoplasms, including t-MDS and t-AML, are associated with unfavorable clinical and biologic prognostic features, including high levels of DNA methylation. The effect of 5-Azacytidine on therapy-related MDS and AML (t-MDS/t-AML) is not well established. Recently, retrospective evaluations from the Groupe Francophone des Myelodysplasies (GFM) (Bally et al. 2013) and an Italian multicenter data collection (Fianchi et al. 2012) reported on 54 and 50 patients, respectively, with t-MDS and t-AML and their response to 5-Azacytidine. In the French data-set (42 t-MDS and 12 t-AML), most patients had a complex karyotype (71 %), as compared to 43 % in the Italian cohort. Nonetheless, both groups observed similar overall response rates for the whole cohort of 39 % and 42 %, respectively, similar to response rates observed in the French de novo MDS/AML group treated in the same program (overall response rate 45 %). However, in the French series, OS was significantly shorter in t-MDS/t-AML as compared to de novo MDS/AML (2-year OS of 14 % vs. 33.9 %, $p = 0.0005$). Multivariate analysis revealed this disadvantage was due to complex karyotype and high IPSS, and not etiology of the disease (i.e., de novo versus therapy related). Similarly, the Italian group observed significantly better OS in patients with <20 % bone marrow blasts, in normal karyotype t-AML, and when 5-Azacytidine was used as first-line treatment, and thus concluded that blasts and karyotype maintain their important prognostic role also in therapy-related myeloid neoplasias and in the era of 5-Azacytidine.

5.3.4 Role of 5-Azacytidine in Myeloproliferative Neoplasias

Few studies report on the efficacy of 5-Azacytidine in the treatment for myeloproliferative neoplasias (MPN). Since CMML was classified into the group of MDS according to the FAB (Bennett et al. 1982) and was later re-categorized into the new group of myelodysplastic/MPN according to the WHO 2008 (Orazi and Germing 2008), patients with CMML were included in the early CALGB and AZA101 trials. Yet, although 5-Azacytidine is approved by the FDA and EMA for treatment of CMML, its role remains disputed. In a compiled report on 76 CMML patients (according to WHO classification) treated with 5-Azacytidine in 3 different programs, 43 % of patients were responders (17 % CR) and had a median survival of 29 months. Increased bone marrow blast percentage and proliferative features of the disease, including splenomegaly and high WBC counts, were associated with shorter survival (Adès et al. 2013). Another retrospective analysis of 38 CMML patients treated with 5-Azacytidine revealed an overall response rate of 39 % (CR 11 %; PR 3 %; hematologic improvement of 25 %). The median OS was 12 months, and the authors concluded 5-Azacytidine was active in the treatment of CMML with acceptable toxicity (Costa et al. 2011).

In contrast, 5-Azacytidine appears to have no effects or only limited activity in primary myelofibrosis and in post-essential thrombocythemia/polycythemia vera myelofibrosis (Quintás-Cardama et al. 2008; Mesa et al. 2009).

Of note, when Philadelphia (Ph)-negative MPN transformed into MDS or AML and were treated with 5-Azacytidine, overall response rate was 52 % (24 % CR), the median response duration was 9 months, and median OS was 11 months. Prognostic factors for overall response were the underlying MPN (71 % in ET, 33 % in PV; $p = 0.016$). Interestingly, recurrence of chronic phase features of the initial MPN was observed in 39 % of the responders. Thus, 5-Azacytidine can achieve encouraging results in Ph-negative MPN after progression into AML or MDS, but response duration is usually short, and consolidation treatments have to be evaluated (Thepot et al. 2010).

5.3.5 5-Azacytidine as Maintenance Therapy

Another conceivable application for hypomethylating agents is the continuous use of low doses as a maintenance strategy in patients with remissions after more intensive types of therapy. The significance of this approach has not been fully determined as of yet, and ongoing trials seek to address this question. The first prospective phase II study assessing the feasibility and efficacy of maintenance 5-Azacytidine for older patients with high-risk MDS, CMML, or AML included patients who achieved a CR after intensive anthracycline–cytarabine-based chemotherapy and were not eligible for allogeneic HCT. Overall, 23 patients received 5-Azacytidine maintenance at a starting dose of 60 mg/m^2 s.c. for 5 days of each 28-day cycle until relapse or unacceptable toxicity. The median duration of CR was 13.5 months, with 30 % of patients maintaining a CR beyond 20 months. In addition, the group found that hypermethylation of the CDH1 promoter was associated with low CR rate, early relapse, and short OS ($p = 0.003$) (Grövdal et al. 2010).

5.3.6 5-Azacytidine for Treatment of Solid Tumors

In the 1970s, the clinical efficacy of 5-Azacytidine was tested in a wide range of solid tumors and leukemias. In contrast to leukemias, treatment results in solid tumors were generally discouraging (von Hoff et al. 1976). Nevertheless, with the late onset of success of 5-Azacytidine in MDS, groups restarted testing the efficacy of the hypomethylating agent also in solid tumors. Lin et al. reported on a phase I trial to determine the minimal effective dose and optimal dose schedule for 5-Azacytidine in combination with sodium phenylbutyrate in 27 patients with refractory, advanced solid tumors. However, the clinical response rate was disappointing and the majority of patients showed progressive disease as the best tumor response. Thus, the combination of 5-Azacytidine and phenylbutyrate was generally well tolerated and safe, yet lacked any real evidence for clinical benefit (Lin et al. 2009).

5.3.7 5-Azacytidine in Combination with Other Drug Regimens and Agents

Combinations of 5-Azacytidine for epigenetic manipulation and conventional chemotherapy regimens or other new agents are currently under investigation to improve overall response rates.

Because in vitro hypomethylation induction sensitizes cells to killing by cytarabine, and the combination is synergistic in myeloid leukemia cell lines, an adaptively randomized phase I/II study combined 5-Azacytidine and cytarabine for treatment of 34 patients with relapsed, refractory AML and previously treated high-risk MDS. While the combination administered in a concomitant fashion was safe at full doses of both drugs in this advanced AML population, it was difficult to deliver more than one cycle of therapy, and little anti-leukemic activity was seen in patients with relapsed/refractory disease. Responses seen in minimally pretreated patients were interpreted to be attributable to the fact that these patients were not exposed to prior high-dose cytarabine. Thus, the investigators concluded the combination of 5-Azacytidine and cytarabine is feasible and safe, but has limited activity in relapsed/refractory AML (Borthakur et al. 2010).

Of particular interest are combinations of the hypomethylating agent with histone deacetylase inhibitors (e.g., valproic acid and vorinostat) and lenalidomide. While no results from randomized trials testing these combinations against 5-Azacytidine alone are available, first data on dose finding, treatment schedules, and activity have been published.

Histone deacetylase inhibitors in combination with 5-Azacytidine: Since alterations in histones, specifically hypoacetylation plus subsequent chromatin remodeling, are also involved in regulating transcription and gene silencing, histone deacetylase (HDAC) inhibitors have been deemed useful combination partners for methyltransferase inhibitors (Griffiths and Gore 2008; Silverman 2001). Indeed, phase I and early phase II trials using 5-Azacytidine and HDAC inhibitors reported overall responses in the range from 20 to 50 % in patients with AML and higher-risk MDS. Time to response has been consistently one course (1–3) and appeared to be faster than the four to six courses required with single-agent 5-Azacytidine for primary response (Kuendgen et al. 2004; Soriano et al. 2007). A phase I trial testing 5-Azacytidine plus vorinostat showed that the synergistic effect is sequence-dependent, requiring exposure to the hypomethylating agent first followed by the HDAC inhibitor. The combination was well tolerated in repetitive cycles, active in both lower and higher-risk MDS/AML patients with a response superior to 5-Azacytidine alone (Silverman et al. 2008b). In a phase II multicenter study combining 5-Azacytidine and the histone deacetylase inhibitor valproic acid in 62 higher-risk MDS patients, valproic acid dosing was adjusted to reach a plasma concentration of >50 μg/mL, and then, 5-Azazytidine was added s.c. at 75 mg/m^2 for 7 days in eight monthly cycles. The median OS in the cohort was 14.4 months, and at a median follow-up of 12 months, the cumulative incidence of progression was 21 %. Of those patients who completed eight cycles, 30.7 % obtained CR or PR, and 15.4 % had a major hematologic improvement. Of note, in multivariate analyses, favorable prognostic factors for survival included valproic plasma levels $\geq$50 μ/mL, suggesting that achievement of therapeutic drug levels may indeed increase 5-Azacytidine efficacy (Voso et al. 2009). Similarly feasible was another phase II study evaluating the efficacy of combined of 5-Azacytidine, valproic acid, and all-trans retinoic acid (ATRA) in 65 patients with high-risk AML or MDS. Treatment consisted of six cycles of 5-Azacytidine and valproic acid for 7 days, followed by ATRA for 21 days ($n = 55$ AML including 13 relapsed/refractory patients, $n = 10$ MDS). CR and PR were observed in 26 % of patients, median OS was 12.4 months, and previously untreated patients had a longer OS than relapsed/refractory patients (Raffoux et al. 2010).

Lenalidomide combinations: The combination of 5-Azacytidine with thalidomide and even more so lenalidomide has attracted much attention in the past few years, as for both agents alone efficacy against myeloid neoplasias has been shown, and it was demonstrated that this combination was well tolerated without additive toxicity (phase I) (Raza et al. 2008; Sekeres et al. 2008). The scientific rationale is because both the microenvironment and cell regulatory mechanisms play a critical role in the pathophysiology and evolution of MDS; combinations of lenalidomide and 5-Azacytidine are hoped to act synergistically against the disease. Phase I studies were initiated in patients with higher-risk MDS to evaluate the possible in vivo synergism of the two agents, their maximum-tolerated dose, and to assess dose-limiting toxicity. The combination of lenalidomide and 5-Azacytidine was well tolerated and displayed encouraging clinical activity (Sekeres et al. 2010), so that phase II dosing was established as 5-Azacytidine 75 mg/m^2 daily for 5 days and lenalidomide 10 mg daily for 21 days of a 28-day cycle. Among 36 patient enrolled, the overall response rate was 72 %. CRs were obtained in 44 % of patients and lasted for a median duration of 17 months, resulting in a median OS of 37 months for complete responders and 13.6 months for the entire cohort, confirming the lenalidomide/5-Azacytidine combination is highly active in higher-risk MDS (Sekeres et al. 2012). To actually confirm the contribution of lenalidomide to response, the same study group treated 18 higher-risk MDS patients with the Lenalidomide/5-Azacytidine combination for seven cycles and then discontinued lenalidomide in eight patients who had achieved a CR, with 5-Azacytidine monotherapy continuing until disease progression. In three patients who relapsed with excess blasts on monotherapy, lenalidomide was then resumed in combination with 5-Azacytidine. All three patients recaptured a CR, which indicates that the addition of lenalidomide provides additional clinical benefit over 5-Azacytidine monotherapy (Sekeres et al. 2011).

Searching for sufficiently potent and well tolerated outpatient regimens, Pollyea et al. conducted a phase-I study to determine the maximum-tolerated dose and efficacy for sequential 5-Azacytidine and lenalidomide as remission induction and continuation therapy in elderly, previously untreated patients with AML. At the same time, they investigated the impact on global DNA methylation and bone marrow cytokines and sought biological predictors of response. Among 18 patients enrolled with a median follow-up of 8.2 months, 56 % of patients responded (CR in 44 %) with a median response duration of 6.2 months. Responders had a unique cytokine profile and a trend toward lower methylation levels in the bone marrow, confirming sequential 5-Azacytidine and lenalidomide treatment had both clinical and biological activity in previously untreated elderly AML patients. Their recommended dose and schedule were 5-Azacytidine 75 mg/m^2/day on days 1–7, lenalidomide 50 mg on days 8–28, and observation on days 29–42 (Pollyea et al. 2012).

These data were confirmed in another phase-I study using sequential or concomitant high-dose lenalidomide (50 mg daily) and 5-Azacytidine induction in patients with AML (Ramsingh et al. 2013). Phase II studies will need to clarify the best strategy for post-induction treatment with these agents, as reducing the dose of lenalidomide after the induction phase may reduce the potential for myelosuppression.

Other combinations: Before gemtuzumab ozogamicin was withdrawn from market in June 2010, the combination with the anti-CD33 immunotoxin gemtuzumab ozogamicin (Mylotarg®), which was active as a single agent in AML (Larson et al. 2002; Sievers et al. 2001), was of particular interest. Preliminary results on the combined approach of 5-Azacytidine, gemtuzumab ozogamicin, and hydroxyurea revealed a CR rate of 70 % in 20 elderly AML patients (Nand et al. 2008). In 2010, the monocloncal antibody was withdrawn from the market because a clinical trial showed the drug increased patient death and added no benefit over conventional cancer therapies.

A recent study tested the use of 5-Azacytidine in combination with sorafenib in patients with AML and mutated FMS-like tyrosine kinase-3 (FLT3)-internal tandem duplication (ITD). In 37 evaluable patients, the response rate was 46 %, including CR in 16 %, CR with incomplete count recovery in 27 %, and PR in 3 % of patients. The median time to achieve CR/CRi was 2 cycles, and the median duration of CR/CRi was 2.3 months. Sixty-four percent of patients achieved adequate (defined as >85 %) FLT3 inhibition during their first cycle of therapy, and the degree of FLT3 inhibition correlated with plasma sorafenib concentrations. The authors concluded the combination of 5-Azacytidine and sorafenib is effective for patients with relapsed AML and FLT-3-ITD (Ravandi et al. 2013).

When 5-Azacytidine was combined with etanercept in 32 patients with MDS/CMML, the overall response rate was 72 %, including 9/32 patients achieving a CR. Marrow response rates and duration were improved with 5-Azacytidine plus etanercept compared with 5-Azacytidine alone (Scott et al. 2010).

5.3.8 Azacitidine Before or After Allogeneic Hematopoietic Cell Transplantation

Allogeneic HCT is the only curative treatment option for many patients with MDS and AML, but can be offered only to selected patients with a suitable HLA-identical donor and without major comorbidities. Depending on the degree of bone marrow blast infiltration (>5 % with reduced intensity conditioning, >10 % with conventional conditioning), patients may require treatment to reduce the tumor burden prior to HCT. The role of 5-Azacytidine as an alternative treatment instead of intensive chemotherapy induction is currently studied. Moreover, 5-Azacytidine may also be effective as maintenance therapy post-HCT to reduce the risk of relapse post-HCT. Moreover, in the setting of relapsed AML and MDS post-HCT where treatment options are limited, hypomethylating agents may be effective as palliative salvage strategies.

Post-allogeneic HCT a reduced dose of 32 mg/m^2 5-Azacytidine given for 5 days every 30 days has been shown to be safe for at least 4 cycles in 45 high-risk, heavily pretreated AML/MDS patients. Two-thirds of patients were not in remission at the time of initiation of maintenance therapy, and reversible thrombocytopenia was determined to constitute the dose-limiting toxicity. Median follow-up was 20.5 months. Moreover, with a 1-year EFS and OS of 58 and 77 %, respectively, the trial also suggested this treatment may improve outcomes and that more cycles may be associated with greater benefit (De Lima et al. 2010).

The specific question of the value of 5-Azacytidine in the setting of detectable minimal residual disease following allogeneic HCT for MDS or AML was addressed in the RELAZA trial. At a median of 169 days after HCT, 20/59 prospectively screened patients were MRD-positive (as determined by decreasing CD34$^+$-donor chimerism) and therefore received four cycles of 5-Azacytidine (75 mg/m^2/day for 7 days) while still in complete hematologic remission. In total, 80 % of patients responded with increasing or stable CD34$^+$ donor chimerism in the absence of relapse. Eventually, hematologic relapse occurred in 65 % of patients with a delay of a median of 231 days after MRD detection. This small study confirmed the acceptable safety profile of preemptive 5-Azacytidine and its potential to prevent or delay hematologic relapse in patients with MDS or AML and MRD after allogeneic HSCT (Platzbecker et al. 2012b).

In the setting of overt relapse of AML or MDS after allogeneic HCT, another German single-arm multicenter phase II trial prospectively tested the combination of 5-Azacytidine and donor lymphocyte infusions (DLI) as first salvage therapy. Thirty patients received up to eight cycles 5-Azacytidine (100 mg/m^2/day, days 1–5, every 28 days) followed by DLI (from 1–5 $\times$ 10^6 to 1–5 $\times$ 10^8 CD3$^+$cells/kg) after every second 5-Azacytidine cycle. A median of three courses 5-Azacytidine were administered, 73 % of patients received DLI, achieving an overall response rate of 30 %, including CR in 23 %. The combination of 5-Azacytidine and DLI was proven to be safe and able to induce long-term remissions and thus may become an alternative treatment option for patients with AML or MDS relapsing after allogeneic HCT (Schroeder et al. 2013).

6 Conclusion and Perspective

The role of 5-Azacytidine in treatment of MDS and AML has changed dramatically over the past 5–10 years. Hypomethylating therapy has replaced best supportive care in many patients, for whom previously there was no therapy available. Moreover, there is evidence due to 5-Azacytidine's better tolerability compared with intensive chemotherapeutics, and superior response compared with low-dose chemotherapy, patients may actually benefit from this palliative treatment concept with regard to both quality of life and OS.

Despite the popularity of 5-Azacytidine as an alternative treatment option in myeloid neoplasias many questions remain to be answered, including the identification of biomarkers to predict treatment response, such as the suggested doubling of platelets after the first cycle (van der Helm et al. 2011). Particularly, because the drug is already commonly used, it is of critical importance to continue enrollment of patients into prospective, randomized trials. Currently, approximately 75 clinical studies registered under *clinicaltrials.gov* are actively recruiting and treating patients with 5-Azacytidine. The majority of these trials investigate combinations of 5-Azacytidine with lenalidomide (~20 trials), growth factors, conventional chemotherapeutics, and vorinostat; the use of 5-Azacytidine pre-, peri-, or post-allogeneic HCT; different dosing schedules; and its role for treatment of AML, as well as for other disease entities (multiple myeloma, lymphomas, and solid tumors). These trials will help to find optimized dosing and combination with other new drugs, and raise hope that MDS, AML in elderly patients, and maybe other diseases can ultimately be controlled more successfully.

References

Adès L, Sekeres MA, Wolfromm A, Teichman ML, Tiu RV, Itzykson R, Maciejewski JP, Dreyfus F, List AF, Fenaux P, Komrokji RS (2013) Predictive factors of response and survival among chronic myelomonocytic leukemia patients treated with azacitidine. Leuk Res 37:609–613

Al-Ali HK, Jaekel N, Junghanss C, Maschmeyer G, Krahl R, Cross M, Hoppe G, Niederwieser D (2012) Azacitidine in patients with acute myeloid leukemia medically unfit for or resistant to chemotherapy: a multicenter phase I/II study. Leuk Lymphoma 53:110–117

Aoki E, Uchida T, Ohashi H, Nagai H, Murase T, Ichikawa A, Yamao K, Hotta T, Kinoshita T, Saito H, Murate T (2000) Methylation status of the p15INK4B gene in hematopoietic progenitors and peripheral blood cells in myelodysplastic syndromes. Leukemia 14:586–593

Bally C, Thépot S, Quesnel B, Vey N, Dreyfus F, Fadlallah J, Turlure P, de Botton S, Dartigeas C, de Renzis B, Itzykson R, Fenaux P, Adès L (2013) Azacitidine in the treatment of therapy related myelodysplastic syndrome and acute myeloid leukemia (tMDS/AML): a report on 54 patients by the Groupe Francophone Des Myelodysplasies (GFM). Leuk Res 37:637–640

Bellet RE, Mastrangelo MJ, Engstrom PF, Custer RP (1973) Hepatotoxicity of 5-azacytidine (NSC-102816) (a clinical and pathologic study). Neoplasma 20:303–309

Bennett JM, Catovsky D, Daniel MT, Flandrin G, Galton DA, Gralnick HR, Sultan C (1982) Proposals for the classification of the myelodysplastic syndromes. Br J Haematol 51:189–199

Bergy ME, Herr RR (1966) Microbiological production of 5-azacytidine. II. Isolation and chemical structure. Antimicrob Agents Chemother (Bethesda) 6:625–630

Bird AP (1996) The relationship of DNA methylation to cancer. Cancer Surv 28:87–101

Borthakur G, Huang X, Kantarjian H, Faderl S, Ravandi F, Ferrajoli A, Torma R, Morris G, Berry D, Issa JP (2010) Report of a phase 1/2 study of a combination of azacitidine and cytarabine in acute myelogenous leukemia and high-risk myelodysplastic syndromes. Leuk Lymphoma 51:73–78

Chabot GG, Bouchard J, Momparler RL (1983) Kinetics of deamination of 5-aza-2′-deoxycytidine and cytosine arabinoside by human liver cytidine deaminase and its inhibition by 3-deazauridine, thymidine or uracil arabinoside. Biochem Pharmacol 32:1327–1328

Chim CS, Pang R, Fung TK, Choi CL, Liang R (2007) Epigenetic dysregulation of Wnt signaling pathway in multiple myeloma. Leukemia 21:2527–2536

Chiurazzi P, Pomponi MG, Pietrobono R, Bakker CE, Neri G, Oostra BA (1999) Synergistic effect of histone hyperacetylation and DNA demethylation in the reactivation of the FMR1 gene. Hum Mol Genet 8:2317–2323

Choi SH, Byun HM, Kwan JM, Issa JP, Yang AS (2007) Hydroxycarbamide in combination with azacitidine or decitabine is antagonistic on DNA methylation inhibition. Br J Haematol 138:616–623

Choi J, Ritchey J, Prior JL, Holt M, Shannon WD, Deych E, Piwnica-Worms DR, DiPersio JF (2010) In vivo administration of hypomethylating agents mitigate graft-versus-host disease without sacrificing graft-versus-leukemia. Blood 116:129–139

Christiansen DH, Andersen MK, Pedersen-Bjergaard J (2003) Methylation of p15INK4B is common, is associated with deletion of genes on chromosome arm 7q and predicts a poor prognosis in therapy-related myelodysplasia and acute myeloid leukemia. Leukemia 17:1813–1819

Costa R, Abdulhaq H, Haq B, Shadduck RK, Latsko J, Zenati M, Atem FD, Rossetti JM, Sahovic EA, Lister J (2011) Activity of azacitidine in chronic myelomonocytic leukemia. Cancer 117:2690–2696

Creusot F, Acs G, Christman JK (1982) Inhibition of DNA methyltransferase and induction of friend erythroleukemia cell differentiation by 5-azacytidine and 5-aza-2′-deoxycytidine. J Biol Chem 257:2041–2048

De Lima M, Giralt S, Thall PF, de Padua Silva L, Jones RB, Komanduri K, Braun TM, Nguyen HQ, Champlin R, Garcia-Manero G (2010) Maintenance therapy with low-dose azacitidine after allogeneic hematopoietic stem cell transplantation for recurrent acute myelogenous leukemia or myelodysplastic syndrome: a dose and schedule finding study. Cancer 116:5420–5431

Fabre C, Grosjean J, Tailler M, Boehrer S, Ades L, Perfettini JL, de Botton S, Fenaux P, Kroemer G (2008) A novel effect of DNA methyltransferase and histone deacetylase inhibitors: NFkappaB inhibition in malignant myeloblasts. Cell Cycle 7:2139–2145

Fenaux P, Ades L (2009) Review of azacitidine trials in intermediate-2-and high-risk myelodysplastic syndromes. Leuk Res 33(Suppl 2):S7–11

Fenaux P, Mufti GJ, Hellstrom-Lindberg E, Santini V, Finelli C, Giagounidis A, Schoch R, Gattermann N, Sanz G, List A, Gore SD, Seymour JF, Bennett JM, Byrd J, Backstrom J, Zimmerman L, McKenzie D, Beach C, Silverman LR (2009) International Vidaza High-Risk MDS Survival Study Group. Efficacy of azacitidine compared with that of conventional care regimens in the treatment of higher-risk myelodysplastic syndromes: a randomised, open-label, phase III study. Lancet Oncol 10:223–232

Fenaux P, Mufti GJ, Hellström-Lindberg E, Santini V, Gattermann N, Germing U, Sanz G, List AF, Gore S, Seymour JF, Dombret H, Backstrom J, Zimmerman L, McKenzie D, Beach CL, Silverman LR (2010a) Azacitidine prolongs overall survival compared with conventional care regimens in elderly patients with low bone marrow blast count acute myeloid leukemia. J Clin Oncol 28:562–569

Fenaux P, Gattermann N, Seymour JF, Hellström-Lindberg E, Mufti GJ, Duehrsen U, Gore SD, Ramos F, Beyne-Rauzy O, List A, McKenzie D, Backstrom J, Beach CL (2010b) Prolonged survival with improved tolerability in higher-risk myelodysplastic syndromes: azacitidine compared with low dose ara-C. Br J Haematol 149:244–249

Fianchi L, Criscuolo M, Lunghi M, Gaidano G, Breccia M, Levis A, Finelli C, Santini V, Musto P, Oliva EN, Leoni P, Aloe Spiriti A, D'Alò F, Hohaus S, Pagano L, Leone G, Voso MT (2012) Outcome of therapy-related myeloid neoplasms treated with azacitidine. J Hematol Oncol 5:44

Floess S, Freyer J, Siewert C, Baron U, Olek S, Polansky J, Schlawe K, Chang HD, Bopp T, Schmitt E, Klein-Hessling S, Serfling E, Hamann A, Huehn J (2007) Epigenetic control of the foxp3 locus in regulatory T cells. PLoS Biol 5:e38

Garcia-Manero G, Gore SD, Cogle C, Ward R, Shi T, Macbeth KJ, Laille E, Giordano H, Sakoian S, Jabbour E, Kantarjian H, Skikne B (2011) Phase I study of oral azacitidine in myelodysplastic syndromes, chronic myelomonocytic leukemia, and acute myeloid leukemia. J Clin Oncol 29:2521–2527

Gore SD, Fenaux P, Santini V, Bennett JM, Silverman LR, Seymour JF, Hellström-Lindberg E, Swern AS, Beach CL, List AF (2013) A multivariate analysis of the relationship between response and survival among patients with higher-risk myelodysplastic syndromes treated within azacitidine or conventional care regimens in the randomized AZA-001 trial. Haematologica 98:1067–1072

Griffiths EA, Gore SD (2008) DNA methyltransferase and histone deacetylase inhibitors in the treatment of myelodysplastic syndromes. Semin Hematol 45:23–30

Grövdal M, Karimi M, Khan R, Aggerholm A, Antunovic P, Astermark J, Bernell P, Engström LM, Kjeldsen L, Linder O, Nilsson L, Olsson A, Holm MS, Tangen JM, Wallvik J, Oberg G, Hokland P, Jacobsen SE, Porwit A, Hellström-Lindberg E (2010) Maintenance treatment with azacytidine for patients with high-risk myelodysplastic syndromes (MDS) or acute myeloid leukaemia following MDS in complete remission after induction chemotherapy. Br J Haematol 150:293–302

Gurion R, Vidal L, Gafter-Gvili A, Belnik Y, Yeshurun M, Raanani P, Shpilberg O (2010) 5-azacitidine prolongs overall survival in patients with myelodysplastic syndrome—a systematic review and meta-analysis. Haematologica 95:303–310

Hanka LJ, Evans JS, Mason DJ, Dietz A (1966) Microbiological production of 5-azacytidine. I. Production and biological activity. Antimicrob Agents Chemother (Bethesda) 6:619–624

Herman JG, Baylin SB (2003) Gene silencing in cancer in association with promoter hypermethylation. N Engl J Med 349:2042–2054

Israili ZH, Vogler WR, Mingioli ES, Pirkle JL, Smithwick RW, Goldstein JH (1976) The disposition and pharmacokinetics in humans of 5-azacytidine administered intravenously as a bolus or by continuous infusion. Cancer Res 36:1453–1461

Itzykson R, Thépot S, Fabre C, Dreyfus F, Quesnel B, Wattel E, de Botton S, Pilorge S, Dartigeas C, Stamatoullas A, Prebet T, Ojeda-Uribe M, Cheze S, Tournilhac O, Solary E, Damaj G, Tertian G, Himberlin C, Mbida RM, Beve B, Adès L, Gardin C, Fenaux P (2008) Response to azacytidine (AZA) in MDS or AML with Del 5q: current results of the french ATU program. Blood 112:2682 (abstract)

Jawad M, Russell NH, Pallis M (2008) Azacytidine and gemtuzumab ozogamicin co-operate to inhibit the Wnt pathway and increase cytotoxicity in AML. Blood 112:2991 (abstract)

Jones PA, Baylin SB (2002) The fundamental role of epigenetic events in cancer. Nat Rev Genet 3:415–428

Jones PA, Taylor SM (1980) Cellular differentiation, cytidine analogs and DNA methylation. Cell 20:85–93

Jones PA, Taylor SM (1981) Hemimethylated duplex DNAs prepared from 5-azacytidine-treated cells. Nucleic Acids Res 9:2933–2947

Kaminskas E, Farrell A, Abraham S, Baird A, Hsieh LS, Lee SL, Leighton JK, Patel H, Rahman A, Sridhara R, Wang YC, Pazdur R (2005a) Approval summary: azacitidine for treatment of myelodysplastic syndrome subtypes. Clin Cancer Res 11:3604–3608

Kaminskas E, Farrell AT, Wang YC, Sridhara R, Pazdur R (2005b) FDA drug approval summary: azacitidine (5-azacytidine, Vidaza) for injectable suspension. Oncologist 10:176–182

Kornblith AB, Herndon JE 2nd, Silverman LR, Demakos EP, Odchimar-Reissig R, Holland JF, Powell BL, DeCastro C, Ellerton J, Larson RA, Schiffer CA, Holland JC (2002) Impact of azacytidine on the quality of life of patients with myelodysplastic syndrome treated in a randomized phase III trial: a cancer and leukemia group B study. J Clin Oncol 20:2441–2452

Kuendgen A, Strupp C, Aivado M, Bernhardt A, Hildebrandt B, Haas R, Germing U, Gattermann N (2004) Treatment of myelodysplastic syndromes with valproic acid alone or in combination with all-trans retinoic acid. Blood 104:1266–1269

Kumar A, List AF, Hozo I, Komrokji R, Djulbegovic B (2010) Decitabine versus 5-azacitidine for the treatment of myelodysplastic syndrome: adjusted indirect meta-analysis. Haematologica 95:340–342

Larson RA, Boogaerts M, Estey E, Karanes C, Stadtmauer EA, Sievers EL, Mineur P, Bennett JM, Berger MS, Eten CB, Munteanu M, Loken MR, Van Dongen JJ, Bernstein ID, Appelbaum FR (2002) Antibody-targeted chemotherapy of older patients with acute myeloid leukemia in first relapse using Mylotarg (gemtuzumab ozogamicin). Leukemia 16:1627–1636

Lee YG, Kim I, Yoon SS, Park S, Cheong JW, Min YH, Lee JO, Bang SM, Yi HG, Kim CS, Park Y, Kim BS, Mun YC, Seong CM, Park J, Lee JH, Kim SY, Lee HG, Kim YK, Kim HJ; Korean Society of Haematology AML/MDS working party (2013) Comparative analysis between azacitidine and decitabine for the treatment of myelodysplastic syndromes. Br J Haematol 161:339-347

Li LH, Olin EJ, Buskirk HH, Reineke LM (1970a) Cytotoxicity and mode of action of 5-azacytidine on L1210 leukemia. Cancer Res 30:2760–2769

Li LH, Olin EJ, Fraser TJ, Bhuyan BK (1970b) Phase specifi city of 5-azacytidine against mammalian cells in tissue culture. Cancer Res 30:2770–2775

Lin J, Gilbert J, Rudek MA, Zwiebel JA, Gore S, Jiemjit A, Zhao M, Baker SD, Ambinder RF, Herman JG, Donehower RC, Carducci MA (2009) A phase I dose-finding study of 5-azacytidine in combination with sodium phenylbutyrate in patients with refractory solid tumors. Clin Cancer Res 15:6241–6249

Lomen PL, Baker LH, Neil GL, Samson MK (1975) Phase I study of 5-azacytidine (NSC-102816) using 24-hour continuous infusion for 5 days. Cancer Chemother Rep 59:1123–1126

Lyons RM, Cosgriff TM, Modi SS, Gersh RH, Hainsworth JD, Cohn AL, McIntyre HJ, Fernando IJ, Backstrom JT, Beach CL (2009) Hematologic response to three alternative dosing schedules of azacitidine in patients with myelodysplastic syndromes. J Clin Oncol 27:1850–1856

Marcucci G, Silverman L, Eller M, Lintz L, Beach CL (2005) Bioavailability of azacitidine subcutaneous versus intravenous in patients with the myelodysplastic syndromes. J Clin Pharmacol 45:597–602

Martin MG, Walgren RA, Procknow E, Uy GL, Stockerl-Goldstein K, Cashen AF, Westervelt P, Abboud CN, Kreisel F, Augustin K, Dipersio JF, Vij R (2009) A phase II study of 5-day intravenous azacitidine in patients with myelodysplastic syndromes. Am J Hematol 84:560–564

Maurillo L, Venditti A, Spagnoli A, Gaidano G, Ferrero D, Oliva E, Lunghi M, D'Arco AM, Levis A, Pastore D, Di Renzo N, Santagostino A, Pavone V, Buccisano F, Musto P (2012) Azacitidine for the treatment of patients with acute myeloid leukemia: report of 82 patients enrolled in an Italian Compassionate Program. Cancer 118:1014–1022

Mesa RA, Verstovsek S, Rivera C, Pardanani A, Hussein K, Lasho T, Wu W, Tefferi A (2009) 5-Azacitidine has limited therapeutic activity in myelofibrosis. Leukemia 23:180–182

Nagar M, Vernitsky H, Cohen Y, Dominissini D, Berkun Y, Rechavi G, Amariglio N, Goldstein I (2008) Epigenetic inheritance of DNA methylation limits activation-induced expression of FOXP3 in conventional human CD25-CD4+ T cells. Int Immunol 20:1041–1055

Nand S, Godwin J, Smith S, Barton K, Michaelis L, Alkan S, Veerappan R, Rychlik K, Germano E, Stiff P (2008) Hydroxyurea, azacitidine and gemtuzumab ozogamicin therapy in patients with previously untreated non-M3 acute myeloid leukemia and high-risk myelodysplastic syndromes in the elderly: results from a pilot trial. Leuk Lymphoma 49:2141–2147

Orazi A, Germing U (2008) The myelodysplastic/myeloproliferative neoplasms: myeloproliferative diseases with dysplastic features. Leukemia 22:1308–1319

Platzbecker U, Schetelig J, Finke J, Trenschel R, Scott BL, Kobbe G, Schaefer-Eckart K, Bornhäuser M, Itzykson R, Germing U, Beelen D, Ehninger G, Fenaux P, Deeg HJ, Adès L; German MDS Study; Cooperative Transplant Study Group; Fred Hutchinson Cancer Research Center; Groupe Francophone des Myelodysplasies (2012a) Allogeneic hematopoietic cell transplantation in patients age 60–70 years with de novo high-risk myelodysplastic syndrome

or secondary acute myelogenous leukemia: comparison with patients lacking donors who received azacitidine. Biol Blood Marrow Transplant 18:1415-1421
Platzbecker U, Wermke M, Radke J, Oelschlaegel U, Seltmann F, Kiani A, Klut IM, Knoth H, Röllig C, Schetelig J, Mohr B, Graehlert X, Ehninger G, Bornhäuser M, Thiede C (2012) Azacitidine for treatment of imminent relapse in MDS or AML patients after allogeneic HSCT: results of the RELAZA trial. Leukemia 26:381–389
Polansky JK, Kretschmer K, Freyer J, Floess S, Garbe A, Baron U, Olek S, Hamann A, von Boehmer H, Huehn J (2008) DNA methylation controls Foxp3 gene expression. Eur J Immunol 38:1654–1663
Pollyea DA, Kohrt HE, Gallegos L, Figueroa ME, Abdel-Wahab O, Zhang B, Bhattacharya S, Zehnder J, Liedtke M, Gotlib JR, Coutre S, Berube C, Melnick A, Levine R, Mitchell BS, Medeiros BC (2012) Safety, efficacy and biological predictors of response to sequential azacitidine and lenalidomide for elderly patients with acute myeloid leukemia. Leukemia 26:893–901
Presant CA, Vietti T, Valeriote F (1975) Kinetics of both leukemic and normal cell population reduction following 5-azacytidine. Cancer Res 35:1926–1930
Quintás-Cardama A, Tong W, Kantarjian H, Thomas D, Ravandi F, Kornblau S, Manshouri T, Cortes JE, Garcia-Manero G, Verstovsek S (2008) A phase II study of 5-azacitidine for patients with primary and post-essential thrombocythemia/polycythemia vera myelofibrosis. Leukemia 22:965–970
Quintás-Cardama A, Ravandi F, Liu-Dumlao T, Brandt M, Faderl S, Pierce S, Borthakur G, Garcia-Manero G, Cortes J, Kantarjian H (2012) Epigenetic therapy is associated with similar survival compared with intensive chemotherapy in older patients with newly diagnosed acute myeloid leukemia. Blood 120:4840–4845
Raffoux E, Cras A, Recher C, Boëlle PY, de Labarthe A, Turlure P, Marolleau JP, Reman O, Gardin C, Victor M, Maury S, Rousselot P, Malfuson JV, Maarek O, Daniel MT, Fenaux P, Degos L, Chomienne C, Chevret S, Dombret H (2010) Phase 2 clinical trial of 5-azacitidine, valproic acid, and all-trans retinoic acid in patients with high-risk acute myeloid leukemia or myelodysplastic syndrome. Oncotarget 1:34–42
Ramsingh G, Westervelt P, Cashen AF, Uy GL, Stockerl-Goldstein K, Abboud CN, Bernabe N, Monahan R, DiPersio JF, Vij R (2013) A phase 1 study of concomitant high-dose lenalidomide and 5-azacitidine induction in the treatment of AML. Leukemia 27:725–728
Ravandi F, Issa JP, Garcia-Manero G, O'Brien S, Pierce S, Shan J, Borthakur G, Verstovsek S, Faderl S, Cortes J, Kantarjian H (2009) Superior outcome with hypomethylating therapy in patients with acute myeloid leukemia and high-risk myelodysplastic syndrome and chromosome 5 and 7 abnormalities. Cancer 115:5746–5751
Ravandi F, Alattar ML, Grunwald MR, Rudek MA, Rajkhowa T, Richie MA, Pierce S, Daver N, Garcia-Manero G, Faderl S, Nazha A, Konopleva M, Borthakur G, Burger J, Kadia T, Dellasala S, Andreeff M, Cortes J, Kantarjian H, Levis M (2013) Phase 2 study of azacytidine plus sorafenib in patients with acute myeloid leukemia and FLT-3 internal tandem duplication mutation. Blood 121:4655–4662
Raza A, Reeves JA, Feldman EJ, Dewald GW, Bennett JM, Deeg HJ, Dreisbach L, Schiffer CA, Stone RM, Greenberg PL, Curtin PT, Klimek VM, Shammo JM, Thomas D, Knight RD, Schmidt M, Wride K, Zeldis JB, List AF (2008) Phase 2 study of lenalidomide in transfusion-dependent, low-risk, and intermediate-1 risk myelodysplastic syndromes with karyotypes other than deletion 5q. Blood 111:86–93
Schroeder T, Czibere A, Platzbecker U, Bug G, Uharek L, Luft T, Giagounidis A, Zohren F, Bruns I, Wolschke C, Rieger K, Fenk R, Germing U, Haas R, Kröger N, Kobbe G (2013) Azacitidine and donor lymphocyte infusions as first salvage therapy for relapse of AML or MDS after allogeneic stem cell transplantation. Leukemia 27:1229–1235
Scott BL, Ramakrishnan A, Storer B, Becker PS, Petersdorf S, Estey EH, Deeg HJ (2010) Prolonged responses in patients with MDS and CMML treated with azacitidine and etanercept. Br J Haematol 148:944–947

Sekeres MA, Maciejewski JP, Giagounidis AA, Wride K, Knight R, Raza A, List AF (2008) Relationship of treatment-related cytopenias and response to lenalidomide in patients with lower-risk myelodysplastic syndromes. J Clin Oncol 26:5943–5949

Sekeres MA, List AF, Cuthbertson D, Paquette R, Ganetzky R, Latham D, Paulic K, Afable M, Saba HI, Loughran TP Jr, Maciejewski JP (2010) Phase I combination trial of lenalidomide and azacitidine in patients with higher-risk myelodysplastic syndromes. J Clin Oncol 28:2253–2258

Sekeres MA, O'Keefe C, List AF, Paulic K, Afable M 2nd, Englehaupt R, Maciejewski JP (2011) Demonstration of additional benefit in adding lenalidomide to azacitidine in patients with higher-risk myelodysplastic syndromes. Am J Hematol 86:102–103

Sekeres MA, Tiu RV, Komrokji R, Lancet J, Advani AS, Afable M, Englehaupt R, Juersivich J, Cuthbertson D, Paleveda J, Tabarroki A, Visconte V, Makishima H, Jerez A, Paquette R, List AF, Maciejewski JP (2012) Phase 2 study of the lenalidomide and azacitidine combination in patients with higher-risk myelodysplastic syndromes. Blood 120:4945–4951

Seymour JF, Fenaux P, Silverman LR, Mufti GJ, Hellström-Lindberg E, Santini V, List AF, Gore SD, Backstrom J, McKenzie D, Beach CL (2010) Effects of azacitidine compared with conventional care regimens in elderly ($\geq$ 75 years) patients with higher-risk myelodysplastic syndromes. Crit Rev Oncol Hematol 76:218–227

Sievers EL, Larson RA, Stadtmauer EA, Estey E, Lowenberg B, Dombret H, Karanes C, Theobald M, Bennett JM, Sherman ML, Berger MS, Eten CB, Loken MR, van Dongen JJ, Bernstein ID, Appelbaum FR (2001) Efficacy and safety of gemtuzumab ozogamicin in patients with CD33-positive acute myeloid leukemia in first relapse. J Clin Oncol 19:3244–3254

Silverman LR (2001) Targeting hypomethylation of DNA to achieve cellular differentiation in myelodysplastic syndromes (MDS). Oncologist 6(Suppl 5):8–14

Silverman LR, Holland JF, Weinberg RS, Alter BP, Davis RB, Ellison RR, Demakos EP, Cornell CJ Jr, Carey RW, Schiffer C et al (1993) Effects of treatment with 5-azacytidine on the in vivo and in vitro hematopoiesis in patients with myelodysplastic syndromes. Leukemia 7(Suppl 1):21–29

Silverman LR, Demakos EP, Peterson BL, Kornblith AB, Holland JC, Odchimar-Reissig R, Stone RM, Nelson D, Powell BL, DeCastro CM, Ellerton J, Larson RA, Schiffer CA, Holland JF (2002) Randomized controlled trial of azacitidine in patients with the myelodysplastic syndrome: a study of the cancer and leukemia group B. J Clin Oncol 20:2429–2440

Silverman LR, McKenzie DR, Peterson BL, Holland JF, Backstrom JT, Beach CL, Larson RA (2006) Further analysis of trials with azacitidine in patients with myelodysplastic syndrome: studies 8421, 8921, and 9221 by the cancer and leukemia group B. J Clin Oncol 24:3895–3903

Silverman LR, Fenaux P, Mufti GJ, Santini V, Hellström-Lindberg E, Gattermann N, Sanz G, List AF, Gore SD, Seymour JF, Backstrom J, McKenzie D, Beach CL (2008a) The effects of continued azacitidine (AZA) treatment cycles on response in higher-risk patients (Pts) with myelodysplastic syndromes (MDS). Blood 112:227 (abstract)

Silverman LR, Verma A, Odchimar-Reissig R, LeBlanc A, Najfeld V, Gabrilove J, Isola L, Espinoza-Delgado I, Zwiebel J (2008b) A phase I trial of the epigenetic modulators vorinostat, in combination with azacitidine (azaC) in patients with the myelodysplastic syndrome (MDS) and acute myeloid leukemia (AML): a study of the New York cancer consortium. Blood 112:3656 (abstract)

Silverman LR, Fenaux P, Mufti GJ, Santini V, Hellström-Lindberg E, Gattermann N, Sanz G, List AF, Gore SD, Seymour JF (2011) Continued azacitidine therapy beyond time of first response improves quality of response in patients with higher-risk myelodysplastic syndromes. Cancer 117:2697–2702

Soriano AO, Yang H, Faderl S, Estrov Z, Giles F, Ravandi F, Cortes J, Wierda WG, Ouzounian S, Quezada A, Pierce S, Estey EH, Issa JP, Kantarjian HM, Garcia-Manero G (2007) Safety and

clinical activity of the combination of 5-azacytidine, valproic acid, and all-trans retinoic acid in acute myeloid leukemia and myelodysplastic syndrome. Blood 110:2302–2308
Sorm F, Vesely J (1964) The activity of a new antimetabolite, 5-azacytidine, against lymphoid leukaemia in Ak mice. Neoplasma 11:123–130
Sorm F, Piskala A, Cihak A, Vesely J (1964) 5-Azacytidine, a new, highly effective cancerostatic. Experientia 20:202–203
Stamatoyannopoulos JA (1992) Future prospects for treatment of hemoglobinopathies. West J Med 157:631–636
Stresemann C, Lyko F (2008) Modes of action of the DNA methyltransferase inhibitors azacytidine and decitabine. Int J Cancer 123:8–13
Taylor SM, Jones PA (1982) Mechanism of action of eukaryotic DNA methyltransferase. Use of 5-azacytosine-containing DNA. J Mol Biol 162:679–692
Thepot S, Itzykson R, Seegers V, Raffoux E, Quesnel B, Chait Y, Sorin L, Dreyfus F, Cluzeau T, Delaunay J, Sanhes L, Eclache V, Dartigeas C, Turlure P, Harel S, Salanoubat C, Kiladjian JJ, Fenaux P, Adès L; Groupe Francophone des Myelodysplasies (GFM) (2010) Treatment of progression of Philadelphia-negative myeloproliferative neoplasms to myelodysplastic syndrome or acute myeloid leukemia by azacitidine: a report on 54 cases on the behalf of the Groupe Francophone des Myelodysplasies (GFM). Blood 116:3735-3742
Uchida T, Kinoshita T, Nagai H, Nakahara Y, Saito H, Hotta T, Murate T (1997) Hypermethylation of the p15INK4B gene in myelodysplastic syndromes. Blood 90:1403–1409
van der Helm LH, Alhan C, Wijermans PW, van Marwijk Kooy M, Schaafsma R, Biemond BJ, Beeker A, Hoogendoorn M, van Rees BP, de Weerdt O, Wegman J, Libourel WJ, Luykx-de Bakker SA, Minnema MC, Brouwer RE, Croon-de Boer F, Eefting M, Jie KS, van de Loosdrecht AA, Koedam J, Veeger NJ, Vellenga E, Huls G (2011) Platelet doubling after the first azacitidine cycle is a promising predictor for response in myelodysplastic syndromes (MDS), chronic myelomonocytic leukaemia (CMML) and acute myeloid leukaemia (AML) patients in the Dutch azacitidine compassionate named patient programme. Br J Haematol 155:599–606
Vogler WR, Miller DS, Keller JW (1976) 5-Azacytidine (NSC 102816): a new drug for the treatment of myeloblastic leukemia. Blood 48:331–337
von Hoff DD, Slavik M (1977) 5-azacytidine—a new anticancer drug with significant activity in acute myeloblastic leukemia. Adv Pharmacol Chemother 14:285–326
von Hoff DD, Slavik M, Muggia FM (1976) 5-Azacytidine. A new anticancer drug with effectiveness in acute myelogenous leukemia. Ann Intern Med 85:237–245
Voso MT, Santini V, Finelli C, Musto P, Pogliani E, Angelucci E, Fioritoni G, Alimena G, Maurillo L, Cortelezzi A, Buccisano F, Gobbi M, Borin L, Di Tucci A, Zini G, Petti MC, Martinelli G, Fabiani E, Fazi P, Vignetti M, Piciocchi A, Liso V, Amadori S, Leone G (2009) Valproic acid at therapeutic plasma levels may increase 5-azacytidine efficacy in higher risk myelodysplastic syndromes. Clin Cancer Res 15:5002–5007
Xing Y, Lv A, Wang L, Yan X (2012) The combination of angiotensin II and 5-azacytidine promotes cardiomyocyte differentiation of rat bone marrow mesenchymal stem cells. Mol Cell Biochem 360:279–287

Bortezomib

Hermann Einsele

Abstract

The ubiquitin-mediated degradation of proteins in numerous cellular processes, such as turnover and quality control of proteins, cell cycle and apoptosis, transcription and cell signaling, immune response and antigen presentation, and inflammation and development makes the ubiquitin–proteosome systems a very interesting target for various therapeutic interventions. Proteosome inhibitors were first synthesized as tools to probe the function and specificity of this particle's proteolytic activities. Most synthetic inhibitors rely on a peptide base, which mimics a protein substrate, attached at a COOH terminal "warhead." Notable warheads include boronic acids, such as bortezomib and epoxy ketones, such as carfilzomib. A variety of natural products also inhibit the proteosome that are not peptide-based, most notably lactacystin, that is related to NPI-0052, or salinosporamide A, another inhibitor in clinical trials. The possibility that proteosome inhibitors could be drug candidates was considered after studies showed that they induced apoptosis in leukemic cell lines. The first proteasome inhibitor in clinical application, bortezomib showed activity in non-small-cell lung and androgen-independent prostate carcinoma, as well as MM and mantle cell and follicular non-Hodgkin's lymphoma. It is now licensed for the treatment of newly diagnosed as well as relapsed/progressive MM and has had a major impact on the improvement in the treatment of MM in the last few years.

H. Einsele (✉)
Department of Internal Medicine II, University Hospital Würzburg,
Josef-Schneider Straße 2, 97080, Wurzburg, Germany
e-mail: Einsele_h@klinik.uni-wuerzburg.de

U. M. Martens (ed.), *Small Molecules in Oncology*, Recent Results in Cancer Research 201, DOI: 10.1007/978-3-642-54490-3_20,

Contents

1 Mode of Action

Intracellular protein degradation occurs predominantly through the proteasome, which is the final common effector for the ubiquitin-dependent and most of the ubiquitin-independent proteolysis (Ciechanover 2005; Demartino and Gillette 2007). In eukaryotic cells, substrate proteins are subjected to polyubiquitination by the ubiquitin-conjugating system.

Thus, the ubiquitin–proteasome system is the major proteolytic system for non-lysosomal degradation of cellular proteins. In 2004, Aaron Ciechanover, Avram Hershko, and Irvine Rose were awarded the Nobel Prize in Chemistry for their original description of ubiquitin-mediated degradation of proteins. This recognition emphasizes the exceptional biological significance of ubiquitin-mediated degradation of proteins in numerous cellular processes, such as turnover and quality control of proteins (Goldberg 2003), cell cycle and apoptosis (Jesenberger and Jentsch 2002; Naujokat and Hoffmann 2002), transcription and cell signaling (Fuchs 2002; Muratani and Tansey 2003; Wang 2003; Wojcikiewicz 2004), immune response and antigen presentation (Kloetzel and Ossendorp 2004), and inflammation and development (Bowerman and Kurz 2006; Elliott et al. 2003).

There are two major steps in the ubiquitin–proteasome degradation pathway: Proteins are first covalently tagged with polyubiquitin chains and are then degraded by the 26 S proteasome.

The initial step of the degradation pathway, ubiquitination of proteins, involves covalent binding of the ubiquitin molecule to a lysine residue (Lys) of the substrate (Hershko and Ciechanover 1998). Ubiquitination proceeds along a cascade of enzymatic reactions, in which ubiquitin is first activated by the ubiquitin-activating enzyme E1. With the aid of an E2 ubiquitin-conjugating enzyme, ubiquitin is then covalently linked to the substrate by a specific ubiquitin ligase, E3. There is only one E1 enzyme known, several E2s, and multiple classes of E3s (Ciechanover et al. 2000). For polyubiquitination, activated ubiquitin moieties are processively transferred to the Lys 48 residue of the previously conjugated ubiquitin molecule. This process may be facilitated by a polyubiquitination factor, E4 (Koegl et al. 1999).

The second step in the degradation pathway involves proteolysis of ubiquitinated proteins by the 26 S proteasome. The 26 S proteasome is a multicatalytic protease that consists of a 20 S catalytic core and two 19 S regulatory complexes. The 19 S complex is composed of at least 19 different subunits that form a lid- and baselike structure. The lid component provides binding sites for polyubiquitinated substrates and also contains a deubiquitinating activity, which allows recycling of ubiquitin moieties on substrate degradation. The base component consists of six ATPases that form a ringlike structure and interact with the 20 S proteolytic core (Groll et al. 2000). These ATPases have chaperone function and are required for the ATP-dependent unfolding of substrates (Braun et al. 1999; Strickland et al. 2000) and the opening of the narrow entry pore of the 20 S proteasome (Kohler et al. 2001). The unfolded polypeptide chain is then inserted into the catalytic chamber of the 20 S core complex, where it is degraded into peptides of 3–25 amino acids length. Both 20 S proteasomes and their 19 S regulators are localized within the cytoplasm and nucleus of the cell and also have been colocalized with the membranes of the endoplasmic reticulum (ER) (Brooks et al. 2000).

In addition to the 19 S regulatory complexes, several components of the ubiquitin system, such as polyubiquitin-binding proteins, which presumably serve as substrate shuttles, several deubiquitinating enzymes, which are required for the removal and recycling of ubiquitin moieties, and also several E3 ligases, are associated with the 20 S proteasome, which suggests that the two steps, ubiquitination and degradation, are closely coupled and controlled within the cell (Schmidt et al. 2005).

Proteasome inhibitors were first synthesized as tools to probe the function and specificity of this particle's proteolytic activities (Vinitsky et al. 1992, 1994). Most synthetic inhibitors rely on a peptide base, which mimics a protein substrate, attached to a COOH terminal "warhead." Notable warheads include boronic acids (Adams et al. 1998), such as bortezomib (Adams et al. 1999), and epoxy ketones (Sin et al. 1999), such as carfilzomib (Kuhn et al. 2007; Demo et al. 2007; Stapnes et al. 2007). A variety of natural products also inhibit the proteasome that are not peptide-based, most notably lactacystin (Fenteany and Schreiber 1998), that is related to NPI-0052, or salinosporamide A, another inhibitor in clinical trials (Feling et al. 2003; Chauhan et al. 2005).

2 Antitumor Effects

The possibility that proteasome inhibitors could be drug candidates was considered after studies showed that they induced apoptosis in leukemic cell lines (Imajoh-Ohmi et al. 1995; Shinohara et al. 1996), including chemotherapy-resistant and radiation-resistant chronic lymphocytic leukemia cells (Delic et al. 1998). This was bolstered by findings that proteasome inhibitors induced apoptosis preferentially in transformed cells (Delic et al. 1998; Orlowski et al. 1998) and were active against an in vivo non-Hodgkin's lymphoma model (Orlowski et al.

1998). One of the early mechanisms of action attributed to proteasome inhibitors was that they repressed nuclear factor *k*B (NF-*k*B) signaling by stabilizing KB, which binds NF-*k*B and prevents its nuclear translocation (Orlowski and Baldwin 2002). Given the role of NF-*k*B in angiogenesis, cell invasion, oncogenesis, proliferation, and suppression of apoptosis, NF-*k*B inhibition was already an attractive approach to cancer therapy. Moreover, NF-*k*B inhibition induced chemosensitization, because many chemotherapeutics activated antiapoptotic NF-*k*B functions (Wang et al. 1996, 1999; Cusack et al. 2001). An especially strong rationale for targeting NF-*k*B had been worked out in multiple myeloma (MM). Adhesion of myeloma cells to bone marrow stroma induced NF-*k*B-dependent production of the antiapoptotic and growth factor interleukin-6 (Chauhan et al. 1996). Later studies documented the efficacy of proteasome inhibition against preclinical models as a single approach (Hideshima et al. 2001) and in chemosensitization and overcoming resistance (Hideshima et al. 2001, 2002; Ma et al. 2003; Mitsiades et al. 2002), with predominantly synergistic effects when bortezomib was combined with other agents.

Proteasome inhibitors are targeted because they are very potent and selective for the proteasome. Owing to their effect on proteolysis of a wide array of cellular proteins, however, they share characteristics with general cytotoxic agents, such as vinflunine, satraplatin, aurora kinase inhibitors, and epothilones, as discussed in the accompanying reviews and overview (Bennouna et al. 2008; Choy et al. 2008; Gautschi et al. 2008; Lee and Swain 2008; Teicher 2008). In that light, proteasome inhibitors have a number of important mechanisms of action beyond their effects on NF-*k*B that have been validated preclinically in cell line models (Voorhees et al. 2003; Rajkumar et al. 2005). By interfering with timely degradation of cyclins and other cell cycle regulatory proteins, proteasome inhibitors induce cell cycle arrest. Through their ability to stabilize proapoptotic proteins, such as p53 and Bax, while reducing levels of some antiapoptotic proteins, such as Bcl-2, they induce a proapoptotic state. Bortezomib-mediated programmed cell death is accompanied by c-Jun NH_2-terminal kinase induction, generation of reactive oxygen species, transmembrane mitochondrial potential gradient dissipation, release of proapoptotic mitochondrial proteins, such as cytochrome *c,* and activation of intrinsic, caspase-9-mediated apoptosis and extrinsic, caspase-8-mediated apoptosis. Other mechanisms include induction of aggresome formation, ER stress, and the unfolded protein response (Hideshima et al. 2005; Nawrocki et al. 2005a, b; Obeng et al. 2006), with the latter possibly having special relevance for MM cells, given their large basal load of immunoglobulin protein substrates. Readers interested in more detailed coverage of the mechanisms of action of proteasome inhibitors are referred to several excellent reviews (Richardson et al. 2006a, b, c, d, e; Nencioni et al. 2007).

Interestingly, the pleiotropic effects of proteasome inhibitors also result in activation of antiapoptotic pathways that may suppress antitumor activity and could be targets for chemosensitization to bortezomib. Heat-shock-response proteins have been some of the best characterized, including HSP-27 (Hideshima et al. 2004), HSP-70 (Robertson et al. 1999; Voorhees et al. 2007), and HSP-90 (Mitsiades et al.

2006). Other examples include stress-response proteins such as mitogen-activated protein kinase phosphatase-1 (Orlowski et al. 2002a, b; Small et al. 2004; Shi et al. 2006) and protein kinase B/Akt (Hideshima et al. 2006).

3 Clinical Application of Proteasome Inhibitors

Building on this solid preclinical rationale, a number of phase 1 studies have documented that bortezomib can be safely given on a variety of schedules (Aghajanian et al. 2002; Orlowski et al. 2002a, b; Papandreou et al. 2004; Cortes et al. 2004; Blaney et al. 2004; Dy et al. 2005). Early indications of activity were seen in non-small-cell lung (Aghajanian et al. 2002) and androgen-independent prostate carcinoma (Papandreou et al. 2004), as well as MM and mantle cell and follicular non-Hodgkin's lymphoma (Orlowski et al. 2002a, b). The most dramatic findings were in myeloma, in which among nine patients, all showed some clinical benefit, including one durable complete remission. Pharmacodynamic studies showed a dose-dependent 20 S proteasome inhibition in peripheral blood mononuclear cells and in limited studies of tumor tissue. However, a correlation between peripheral blood mononuclear cell proteasome inhibition and response could not be established in these small trials, which were not designed with the sample size necessary for such an analysis. Pharmacokinetic studies showed rapid bortezomib plasma clearance and tissue distribution, with an initial $t_{1/2}$ of 0.22–0.46 h, followed by a more gradual terminal elimination half-life, with $t_{1/2\beta}$ of >10 h and a large volume of distribution of >500 L. Activity against MM was confirmed with a phase 2 trial (Richardson et al. 2003) that showed a 27 % overall response rate (partial response + complete remission) in heavily pretreated patients, who received what has become the most common dose and schedule, 1.3 mg/m^2 as an i.v. bolus on days 1, 4, 8, and 11 of every 21-day cycle. Further follow-up (Richardson et al. 2006a, b, c, d, e) determined that the median duration of response was 12.7 months, the median time to progression (TTP) was 7 months, and the median overall survival (OS) was 17.0 months. A subsequent phase 3 randomized trial (Richardson et al. 2005a, b, 2007a, b) comparing dexamethasone with bortezomib showed that the latter induced a better overall response rate (43 % for bortezomib vs. 18 % for dexamethasone), a better response quality, as well as a longer median TTP (6.22 vs. 3.49 months, respectively) and OS (29.3 vs. 23.7 months, respectively). Together, these studies led to the approval of bortezomib for relapsed/refractory myeloma in patients who have progressed after at least one prior regimen.

In non-Hodgkin's lymphoma, several phase 2 studies (O'Connor et al. 2005; Goy et al. 2005; Belch et al. 2007) confirmed the activity in follicular, mantle cell, and marginal zone lymphoma. Most recently, a multicenter pivotal trial (Fisher et al. 2006) determined that the overall response rate in relapsed mantle cell lymphoma was 33 %, including 8 % complete remission/unconfirmed complete remission, with a median duration of response of 9.2 months and TTP of 6.2 months, leading to the approval of bortezomib for this indication. Activity has also been described in other B cell processes, including Waldenström's macroglobulinemia (Treon et al. 2007; Chen et al. 2007; Strauss et al. 2006; Dimopoulos et al. 2005) and amyloidosis (Wechalekar et al. 2006).

When bortezomib was being developed as a drug candidate, there was great concern that it could not be inhibited without direct consequences, because of the proteasome's vital role in cellular homeostasis. Fortunately, an acceptable therapeutic index has been documented, but patients do face the risk of some toxicities. During phase 1 studies, dose-limiting toxicities included diarrhea, fatigue, fluid retention, hypokalemia, hyponatremia, hypotension, malaise, nausea, orthostasis, sensory neuropathy, and thrombocytopenia. In the phase 2 trial of MM patients, adverse events were reported in at least 10 % included anemia, anorexia, constipation, dehydration, diarrhea, dizziness, fatigue, headache, limb pain, nausea, neutropenia, peripheral neuropathy, pyrexia, rash, thrombocytopenia, vomiting, and weakness. Subsequent studies have better characterized thrombocytopenia (Lonial et al. 2005) and neuropathy (Richardson et al. 2006a, b, c, d, e), which probably must limit dosing in the clinic. These have elucidated some of the risk factors involved in these transient, reversible effects, but a better understanding of the underlying mechanisms would be of benefit, as would the identification of biomarkers to predict efficacy or toxicity.

4 Bortezomib

Proteasome inhibition is a rational therapeutic approach both by itself and as a means to induce chemosensitization and overcome chemoresistance. As noted earlier, many cytotoxic agents activate the antiapoptotic NF-κB pathway, and blockade of this induction by proteasome inhibition enhanced their antitumor efficacy (Ma et al. 2003; Mitsiades et al. 2003). In addition, several strategies by which tumor cells survive the effects of chemotherapy can be similarly abrogated. Overexpression of Bcl-2 is one such mechanism, but proteasome inhibitors induce Bcl-2 phosphorylation and cleavage into proapoptotic fragments (Ling et al. 2002). Selection of cells overexpressing P-glycoprotein is another mechanism, but because proteasome function is needed for P-glycoprotein maturation when the proteasome is inhibited, inactive P-glycoprotein isoforms accumulate and cannot remove chemotherapeutic agents from cancer cells (Loo and Clarke 1998, 1999).

Using these rationales, bortezomib has been combined with a variety of chemotherapeutics, including carboplatin (Aghajanian et al. 2005), docetaxel (Messersmith et al. 2006), irinotecan (Ryan et al. 2006), melphalan (Berenson et al. 2006), pegylated liposomal doxorubicin (Orlowski et al. 2005a, b), and thalidomide (Barlogie et al. 2004), among others. Bortezomib has also been incorporated into more complex regimens, such as paclitaxel and carboplatin (Ma et al. 2007) and gemcitabine and cisplatin (Voortman et al. 2007). From these studies, it seems possible to conclude that bortezomib has generally been successfully combined with other agents without significantly increased toxicity and without the need for large dose adjustments.

Bortezomib (Velcade®; Millennium Pharmaceuticals Inc., Cambridge, MA, and Johnson and Johnson Pharmaceuticals, Research and Development, L.L.C., Raritan, NJ), a first-in-class proteasome inhibitor, is approved in the US and European Union for the treatment of MM patients who have received at least one prior therapy. Bortezomib was approved based on the results of the randomized, phase 3 assessment of proteasome inhibition for extending remissions (APEX) trial (Richardson et al. 2005a, b). Compared with high-dose dexamethasone, single-agent bortezomib showed superiority in terms of response rates (including CR rates), median TTP and survival and better quality of life (Richardson et al. 2005a, b; Lee et al. 2005). This study also showed that a high quality of response (100 % M-protein reduction) to bortezomib was associated with a longer duration of response (Richardson et al. 2005a, b). In addition, bortezomib was well tolerated and retained its superiority over high-dose dexamethasone in elderly patients and patients with high-risk factors such as advanced disease, more prior lines of therapy, and refractoriness to prior therapy (Richardson et al. 2007a, b). A subgroup analysis suggests that bortezomib may be more beneficial when used earlier in the course of treatment; in the APEX trial, patients with one prior line of therapy appeared to have a higher response rate, longer TTP, and longer survival following bortezomib treatment compared with patients with more than one prior line (Richardson et al. 2005a, b; Sonneveld et al. 2005). In other studies in the relapsed setting, bortezomib has been shown to be active with a similar toxicity profile in patients with chromosome 13 deletion (Sagaster et al. 2007; Jagannath et al. 2007) and in patients with renal dysfunction or renal failure requiring dialysis (Jagannath et al. 2005; Mohrbacher and Levine 2005; Chanan-Khan et al. 2007).

In addition to single-agent studies in the relapsed setting (Richardson et al. 2003, 2005a, b; Jagannath et al. 2004), bortezomib is also being investigated in a range of combination regimens with other antimyeloma agents (Richardson et al. 2006a, b, c, d, e), including steroids, melphalan, and immunomodulatory drugs (IMiDs) (Palumbo et al. 2007; Kropff et al. 2005a, b; Orlowski et al. 2005a, b, 2006; Berenson et al. 2006; Suvannasankha et al. 2006; Zangari et al. 2005; Friedman et al. 2006; Leoni et al. 2006; Hollmig et al. 2004; Biehn et al. 2007; Reece et al. 2006; Richardson et al. 2006a, b, c, d, e; Davies et al. 2006; Terpos et al. 2006; Chanan-Khan et al. 2006; Popat et al. 2006; Teoh et al. 2006). Encouragingly, despite patients having relapsed/refractory disease, high ORRs (up to 93 %) (Teoh et al. 2006) and complete response (CR)/near-complete response (nCR) rates (up to 64 %) (Teoh et al. 2006) have been reported. Bortezomib is an established component of induction therapy for patients eligible or ineligible for autologous stem cell transplantation. Bortezomib has also been incorporated into conditioning regimens before autologous stem cell transplantation, as well as into post-ASCT consolidation therapy, and in the maintenance setting. In addition, a new route of bortezomib administration, subcutaneous infusion, has recently been approved. Recently, several new agents have been introduced into the clinic, including carfilzomib, marizomib, and MLN9708, and trials investigating these "second-generation" PIs in patients with relapsed/refractory MMs have demonstrated positive results (Moreau et al. 2012).

5 Bortezomib-Based Combination Therapy for Multiple Myeloma

Owing to age or concomitant comorbidities at the time of diagnosis, more than half of the patients with MM may not be eligible for transplant; in these patients, melphalan–prednisone (MP) has remained a global standard of care for 40 years (Myeloma Trialists' Collaborative Group 1998; Cavo et al. 2002; Facon et al. 2006). MP typically results in response rates of up to 55 %; however, the CR rate is low, typically $\leq$5 % (Cavo et al. 2002; Hernandez et al. 2004; Facon et al. 2006; Palumbo et al. 2006; San Miguel et al. 2008), and the median OS is only 2–3 years (Myeloma Trialists' Collaborative Group 1998; Bladé et al. 2001; Facon et al. 2006). A large body of evidence has shown that the introduction of novel agents into frontline combination therapies improves clinical outcomes for non-transplant-eligible patients. Long-term follow-up of several of these studies is needed to fully assess the duration of response and survival benefit in this patient population.

A multicenter phase 1/2 study of 60 elderly patients (aged ^{3}65 years) ineligible for HDTSCT evaluated the addition of bortezomib to the MP regimen (VMP) (Mateos et al. 2006). Among 53 evaluable patients, VMP produced an ORR of 89 %, including a 32 % CR rate and an 11 % nCR rate. Among patients achieving CR, half of those assessed had no malignant plasma cells detectable by multiparametric flow cytometry (sensitivity level of 10^{-4}–10^{-5}), representing immunophenotypic minimal residual disease status. These response rates, among the highest reported with conventional therapy, compare very favorably with those for MP—35–53 % ORR, including a 1–9 % CR rate (Palumbo et al. 2006; Facon et al. 2006; Hernandez et al. 2004; Cavo et al. 2002). Response to VMP was rapid, with 70 % of patients responding by completion of the first cycle. VMP also compares very favorably with MP historical control data in the context of the progression-free survival (PFS) rate (91 vs. 66 %), event-free survival (EFS) rate (83 vs. 51 %), and OS rate (90 vs. 62 %) at 16 months (Mateos et al. 2006). Notably, in 33 patients for whom cytogenetic data were available, the response rates appeared comparable among patients with and without retinoblastoma gene deletion or immunoglobulin heavy-chain translocations, suggesting that the mechanism of action of bortezomib may overcome the adverse impact of these factors (Mateos et al. 2006). A median of seven cycles of therapy was administered monthly (>9 months), indicating good tolerability of the VMP regimen in this elderly population (Mateos et al. 2006). Toxicities were comparable with those seen in other major bortezomib trials.

In the large phase 3 VISTA (Velcade® as Initial Standard Therapy in MM) trial, bortezomib–MP (VMP) demonstrated superiority versus MP across all efficacy end points, including ORR by EBMT criteria (71 vs. 35 %, $p < 0.001$) and IFx-neg CR rate (30 vs. 4 %, $p < 0.001$) (San Miguel et al. 2008). Responses were more rapid and durable when compared with MP (Palumbo et al. 2008). VMP therapy significantly prolonged TTP (HR 0 48, $p < 0.001$) by approximately 50 %, when compared with MP, an improvement similar to that achieved with

HDT–SCT versus conventional chemotherapy (Attal et al. 1996). After a median follow-up of 26 months, VMP offered a substantial survival benefit when compared with MP (HR 0–644, $p > 0.0032$) (San Miguel et al. 2008). Importantly, VMP was well tolerated, with patients remaining on therapy for a median of 46 weeks (vs. 39 weeks with MP), even though patients in the bortezomib-containing arm were reported to have a higher rate of adverse events (San Miguel et al. 2008). Based on VISTA data, bortezomib has recently been approved for the treatment of all patients with MM, thus expanding the indication to include newly diagnosed (ND) patients.

The final analysis of the phase 3 VISTA trial (Velcade As Initial Standard Therapy in MM: Assessment With Melphalan and Prednisone) was conducted to determine whether the OS benefit with bortezomib–melphalan–prednisone (VMP) versus MP in patients with myeloma who were ineligible for transplantation was maintained after 5 years of follow-up and to explore the risk of second primary malignancies. A total of 682 patients received up to nine 6-week cycles of VMP or MP and were then observed every 12 weeks or less. After median follow-up of 60.1 months, there was a 31 % reduced risk of death with VMP versus MP. Sixty-three percent of VMP patients and 73 % of MP patients had received subsequent therapy. Time to next therapy was longer with VMP than with MP. Among patients who received subsequent therapies, survival from start of subsequent therapy was similar following VMP or MP. Following VMP/MP, incidence proportions of hematologic malignancies and solid tumors and exposure-adjusted incidence rates were similar and were consistent with background rates. VMP resulted in a significant reduction in risk of death versus MP that was maintained after 5 years of follow-up and despite substantial use of novel-agent-based salvage therapies. There is no emerging safety signal for second primary malignancies following VMP (San Miguel et al. 2013).

6 Treatment Options for Patients Eligible for Transplant

HDT–SCT is a standard of care in patients aged up to approximately 75 years (Kyle and Rajkumar 2004; Gertz et al. 2006). Standard induction therapies prior to HDT–SCT have included VAD (vincristine, doxorubicin, dexamethasone), DVd (VAD but with liposomal doxorubicin), and high-dose dexamethasone. Response rates are typically 40–61 % (Alexanian et al. 1990, 1992; Dimopoulos et al. 2003; Rifkin et al. 2006), and as with MP, CR rates are generally low, ranging from 3 to 13 %. A number of combinations are under investigation, utilizing conventional agents such as cyclophosphamide, doxorubicin/liposomal doxorubicin, and steroids in combination with bortezomib and an IMiD, or other novel agents. Emerging data show substantial improvements in response when compared with current standard induction regimens. However, long-term follow-up is required to fully assess the duration of response and survival benefit for these novel-agent-based regimens.

Phase 2 studies with bortezomib–dexamethasone led to the design of the IFM 2005-01 phase 3 trial, where a significantly higher post-induction ORR was achieved with bortezomib–dexamethasone versus VAD ($p < 0.0001$), which translated into a significantly higher ≥VGPR rate post-transplant (57 vs. 38 %, $p > 0\ 0003$), with fewer patients requiring a second transplant as a result. CR/nCR rates were (15 %) post-induction and (37 %) post-first-transplant in the bortezomib-containing arm (Harousseau et al. 2007, 2008). Bortezomib–dexamethasone and VAD toxicity profiles were comparable. After a median follow-up of 2 years, no OS advantage was noted; however, 2-year PFS was 69 versus 60 % in the VAD arm ($p > 0.0115$) (Harousseau et al. 2008); hence, longer follow-up is needed. A combination with cyclophosphamide (VCD) showed a very good tolerability and high efficacy as an induction regimen prior to ASCT (Knop et al. 2008).

Eligible patients with ND symptomatic MM were randomly assigned to receive induction therapy with vincristine, doxorubicin, and dexamethasone (VAD) or bortezomib, doxorubicin, and dexamethasone (PAD), followed by high-dose melphalan and autologous stem cell transplantation. Maintenance consisted of thalidomide 50 mg (VAD) once per day or bortezomib 1.3 mg/m^2 (PAD) once every 2 weeks for 2 years. The primary analysis was PFS adjusted for International Staging System (ISS) stage. CR, including near CR, was superior after PAD induction and bortezomib maintenance. After a median follow-up of 41 months, PFS was superior in the PAD arm. In multivariate analysis, OS was better in the PAD arm. Bortezomib during induction and maintenance improves CR and achieves superior PFS and OS (Sonneveld et al. 2012).

The phase 1 of pomalidomide MTD, safety, and efficacy in patients with refractory MM who have received lenalidomide and bortezomib. The study determined the maximum tolerated dose (MTD) of oral pomalidomide (4 dose levels) administered on days 1 to 21 of each 28-day cycle in patients with relapsed and refractory multiple myeloma (RRMM). After four cycles, patients who progressed or had not achieved minimal response (serum and urine M-protein reduction of ≥25 % and ≥50 %) could receive dexamethasone 40 mg per week. Safety and efficacy were evaluated. Thirty-eight patients who had received both bortezomib and lenalidomide (median 6 prior therapies) were enrolled; 63 % patients were refractory to both lenalidomide and bortezomib. There were four dose-limiting toxicities (grade 4 neutropenia) at 5 mg per day, and so the MTD was 4 mg per day. Rates of peripheral neuropathy and venous thromboembolism were low (≤5 %). Among the 38 patients enrolled (including 22 with added dexamethasone), 42 % achieved minimal response or better, 21 % achieved partial response or better, and 3 % achieved complete response. Median duration of response, PFS, and OS were 4.6, 4.6, and 18.3 months, respectively. Pomalidomide 4 mg per day on days 1 to 21 of each 28-day cycle, with or without dexamethasone (40 mg/week), has encouraging activity with manageable toxicity in RRMM, including those refractory to both lenalidomide and bortezomib (Richardson et al. 2013).

7 Next-Generation Proteasome Inhibitors

With the validation of the proteasome as a target for cancer therapy, interest has focused on the possibility that other inhibitors could offer some advantages. Two second-generation agents have entered phase 1 trials: NPI-0052 (salinosporamide A) and carfilzomib (formerly PR-171). Unlike bortezomib, which binds the proteasome in a slowly reversible manner, NPI-0052 and carfilzomib bind irreversibly, abrogating one mechanism of recovery from proteasome inhibition, namely release of the target by the drug. They both induce depolarization of the transmitochondrial membrane potential and activate caspase-8-mediated apoptosis, whereas carfilzomib also activates caspase-9. Preclinical studies have shown that both (Kuhn et al. 2007; Chauhan et al. 2005) at least partially overcome bortezomib resistance in vitro. Moreover, in a number of models, including MM (Kuhn et al. 2007; Chauhan et al. 2005) and chronic lymphocytic leukemia (Ruiz et al. 2006), these inhibitors have shown enhanced potency when compared with bortezomib, suggesting that they may have a broader spectrum of activity. Early results from phase 1 studies of carfilzomib indicate that it is well tolerated, even on a dose-intense schedule, and may have less neurotoxicity than bortezomib (Orlowski et al. 2007; Alsina et al. 2007). Evidence of antitumor activity is being seen in MM and Waldenström's macroglobulinemia, including in myeloma patients with previously bortezomib-refractory disease, and phase 2 studies are being planned.

The development of novel agents, such as immunomodulatory drugs and proteasome inhibitors, has led to a considerable increment in the response rate (RR) and outcomes for MM patients. Unfortunately, MM patients will inevitably relapse and become resistant to new drugs. This led to the continuous development of novel agents. Carfilzomib is a second-generation proteasome inhibitor, demonstrating promising results in relapsed/refractory (RR) and ND MM patients. Clinical trials (phases 1 and 2) with carfilzomib, used both as single agent or in combination with other therapies, established the MTD and recommended schedule of administration. Preliminary data showed that it had a high efficacy and a good safety profile both in RRMM and in NDMM patients. Carfilzomib seems to be effective in patients previously treated with bortezomib. Future phase 2 and 3 studies will better define the role of carfilzomib in the treatment of MM as well as its optimum dose (Pautasso et al. 2013).

The past decade has been a time of rapid progress in MM, but the future therapeutic landscape may be even more promising, as new agents are better tolerated and novel pathways are exploited. The NCCN Clinical Practice Guidelines in Oncology (NCCN guidelines) now include the proteasome inhibitor carfilzomib and immunomodulatory drug pomalidomide, which are more potent than previous generations of these drugs have been. These agents are extending progression-free and OS of patients with relapsed/refractory myeloma, as is maintenance therapy with lenalidomide after initial therapy of patients with ND disease. At the NCCN 18th Annual Conference, Dr. Kenneth C. Anderson from Dana-Farber Cancer Institute reviewed the data leading to the approval of these exciting agents, discussed the efficacy of current regimens, and described the future landscape and the exciting potential of new agents to further improve and extend the lives of patients with myeloma (Anderson 2013).

The introduction of autologous stem cell transplantation as well as novel agents such as proteasome inhibitors (bortezomib) and immunomodulatory drugs (IMiDs; thalidomide and lenalidomide) has significantly improved long-term outcome of MM patients. However, patients with high-risk disease at diagnosis had less benefit from these new strategies. In addition, myeloma patients with lenalidomide and bortezomib double-refractory disease have a very poor survival. Areas covered: Several next-generation novel agents are active in patients with double-refractory disease including carfilzomib and pomalidomide. Various monoclonal antibodies are also promising in the setting of relapsed/refractory disease, including daratumumab, elotuzumab and lorvotuzumab mertansine. This editorial will focus on the most promising next-generation novel agents for the treatment of MM. Expert opinion: Incorporation of these new novel agents in frontline therapies will lead to more effective and less toxic combination therapies. Furthermore, new diagnostic techniques such as gene-expression profiling and next-generation sequencing will hopefully result in more personalized treatments for molecularly defined subgroups (van de Donk and Lokhorst 2013).

One other study focuses on the second-generation proteasome inhibitor carfilzomib, which was recently approved by the US Food and Drug Administration for the treatment of relapsed and refractory MM patients who have received at least two prior therapies, including bortezomib and an immunomodulatory agent, and have demonstrated disease progression on or within 60 days of the completion of the last therapy. The clinical trial data lead to drug approval and provide advice for treating physicians who are now accessing this drug for patients. Carfilzomib is a potent proteasome inhibitor and effective therapy in MM with an advantageous side effect profile characterized by low rates of peripheral neuropathy and potential use in other diseases as Waldenström macroglobulinemia, lymphoma, amyloidosis, and autoimmune diseases. In MM, carfilzomib is a welcome addition to bortezomib, alkylators, corticosteroids, and the immunomodulatory drugs thalidomide and lenalidomide in the therapeutic arsenal. The results of ongoing phase 2 and multiple phase 3 trials will help to further define the role of carfilzomib in MM therapy and will help to establish the best dosing, schedule, and supportive care management that benefit these patients (Kortuem and Stewart 2013).

Another interesting target may be the immunoproteasome (Rivett and Hearn 2004), whose expression may be more tissue-restricted than the constitutive proteasome. All of the currently available inhibitors target both the constitutive and immunoproteasome isoforms, but the identification of specific immunoproteasome inhibitors (Orlowski et al. 2005a, b; Ho et al. 2007) may allow for further improvements in the therapeutic index of these drugs. As the immunoproteasome is expressed predominantly in hematopoietic tissues, it is possible that such agents could act without incurring neurotoxicity or gastrointestinal effects, among others, because those tissues express much lower levels of immunoproteasome subunits.

References

Adams J, Behnke M, Chen S et al (1998) Potent and selective inhibitors of the proteasome: dipeptidyl boronic acids. Bioorg Med Chem Lett 8:333–338
Adams J, Palombella VJ, Sausville EA et al (1999) Proteasome inhibitors: a novel class of potent and effective antitumor agents. Cancer Res 59:2615–2622
Aghajanian C, Soignet S, Dizon DS et al (2002) A phase I trial of the novel proteasome inhibitor PS341 in advanced solid tumor malignancies. Clin Cancer Res 8:2505–2511
Aghajanian C, Dizon DS, Sabbatini P et al (2005) Phase I trial of bortezomib and carboplatin in recurrent ovarian or primary peritoneal cancer. J Clin Oncol 23:5943–5949
Alexanian R, Barlogie B, Tucker S (1990) VAD-based regimens as primary treatment for multiple myeloma. Am J Hematol 33:86–89
Alexanian R, Dimopoulos MA, Delasalle K et al (1992) Primary dexamethasone treatment of multiple myeloma. Blood 80(4):887–890
Alsina M, Trudel S, Vallone M et al (2007) Phase I single agent antitumor activity of twice weekly-consecutive day dosing of the proteasome inhibitor carfilzomib (PR-171) in hematologic malignancies. Blood 110:128a (abstract 411)
Anderson KC (2013) Therapeutic advances in relapsed or refractory multiple myeloma. J Natl Compr Canc Netw 11(5 Suppl):676–679
Attal M, Harousseau JL, Stoppa AM et al (1996) A prospective, randomized trial of autologous bone marrow transplantation and chemotherapy in multiple myeloma. Intergroupe francais du myelome. New Engl J Med 335:91–97
Barlogie B, Shaughnessy JD, Tricot G et al (2004) Treatment of multiple myeloma. Blood 103:20–32
Belch A, Kouroukis CT, Crump M et al (2007) A phase II study of bortezomib in mantle cell lymphoma: the National Cancer Institute of Canada Clinical Trials Group trial IND.150. Ann Oncol 18:116–121
Bennouna J, Delord JP, Campone M, Pinel M-C (2008) Vinflunine: a new microtubule inhibitor agent. Clin Cancer Res 14:1610–1617
Berenson JR, Yang HH, Sadler K et al (2006) Phase I/II trial assessing bortezomib and melphalan combination therapy for the treatment of patients with relapsed or refractory multiple myeloma. J Clin Oncol 24:937–944
Biehn SE, Moore DT, Voorhees PM et al (2007) Extended follow-up of outcome measures in multiple myeloma patients treated on a phase I study with bortezomib and pegylated liposomal doxorubicin. Ann Hematol 86:211–216
Bladé J, San Miguel JF, Fontanillas M et al (2001) Increased conventional chemotherapy does not improve survival in multiple myeloma: longterm results of two PETHEMA trials including 914 patients. Hematol J 2:272–278
Blaney SM, Bernstein M, Neville K et al (2004) Phase I study of the proteasome inhibitor bortezomib in pediatric patients with refractory solid tumors: a Children's Oncology Group study (ADVL0015). J Clin Oncol 22:4804–4809
Bowerman B, Kurz T (2006) Degrade to create: developmental requirements for ubiquitin-mediated proteolysis during early *C. elegans* embryogenesis. Development 133:773–784
Braun BC, Glickman M, Kraft R, Dahlmann B, Kloetzel PM, Finley D, Schmidt M (1999) The base of the proteasome regulatory particle exhibits chaperone-like activity. Nat Cell Biol 1:221–226
Brooks P, Fuertes G, Murray RZ, Bose S, Knecht E, Rechsteiner MC, Hendil KB, Tanaka K, Dyson J, Rivett J (2000) Subcellular localization of proteasomes and their regulatory complexes in mammalian cells. Biochem J 346(Pt 1):155–161
Cavo M, Benni M, Ronconi S et al (2002) Melphalan-prednisone versus alternating combination VAD/MP or VND/MP as primary therapy for multiple myeloma: final analysis of a randomized clinical study. Haematologica 87:934–942

Chanan-Khan AA, Padmanabhan S, Miller KC et al (2006) Final results of a phase II study of bortezomib (Velcade) in combination with liposomal doxorubicin (Doxil) and thalidomide (VDT) demonstrate a sustained high response rate in patients (pts) with relapsed (rel) or refractory (ref) multiple myeloma. In: Updated data presented at the 2006 annual meeting of the American Society of Hematology. Blood vol 108, p 1010a

Chanan-Khan AA, Kaufman JL, Mehta J et al (2007) Activity and safety of bortezomib in multiple myeloma patients with advanced renal failure: a multicenter retrospective study. Blood 109:2604–2606

Chauhan D, Uchiyama H, Akbarali Y et al (1996) Multiple myeloma cell adhesion-induced interleukin-6 expression in bone marrow stromal cells involves activation of NF-*k*B. Blood 87:1104–1112

Chauhan D, Catley L, Li G et al (2005) A novel orally active proteasome inhibitor induces apoptosis in multiple myeloma cells with mechanisms distinct from bortezomib. Cancer Cell 8:407–419

Chen CI, Kouroukis CT, White D et al (2007) Bortezomib is active in patients with untreated or relapsed Waldenstrom's macroglobulinemia: a phase II study of the National Cancer Institute of Canada Clinical Trials Group. J Clin Oncol 25:1570–1575

Choy H, Park C, Yao M (2008) Current status and future prospect for satraplatin: an oral platinum analogue. Clin Cancer Res 14:1618–1623

Ciechanover A (2005) Intracellular protein degradation: from a vague idea thru the lysosome and the ubiquitin-proteasome system and onto human diseases and drug targeting. Cell Death Differ 12:1178–1190

Ciechanover A, Orian A, Schwartz AL (2000) Ubiquitin-mediated proteolysis: biological regulation via destruction. BioEssays 22:442–451

Cortes J, Thomas D, Koller C et al (2004) Phase I study of bortezomib in refractory or relapsed acute leukemias. Clin Cancer Res 10:3371–3376

Cusack JC Jr, Liu R, Houston M et al (2001) Enhanced chemosensitivity to CPT-11 with proteasome inhibitor PS-341: implications for systemic nuclear factor-*k*B inhibition. Cancer Res 61:3535–3540

Davies FE, Wu P, Srikanth M et al (2006) The combination of cyclophosphamide, velcade and dexamethasone (CVD) induces high response rates with minimal toxicity compared to velcade alone (V) and velcade plus dexamethasone (VD). In: Updated data presented at the 2006 annual meeting of the American Society of Hematology. Blood vol 108, p 1009a

Delic J, Masdehors P, Omura S et al (1998) The proteasome inhibitor lactacystin induces apoptosis and sensitizes chemo- and radioresistant human chronic lymphocytic leukaemia lymphocytes to TNF-α-initiated apoptosis. Br J Cancer 77:1103–1107

Demartino GN, Gillette TG (2007) Proteasomes: machines for all reasons. Cell 129:659–662

Demo SD, Kirk CJ, Aujay MA et al (2007) Antitumor activity of PR-171, a novel irreversible inhibitor of the proteasome. Cancer Res 67:6383–6391

Dimopoulos MA, Pouli A, Zervas K et al (2003) Prospective randomized comparison of vincristine, doxorubicin and dexamethasone (VAD) administered as intravenous bolus injection and VAD with liposomal doxorubicin as first-line treatment in multiple myeloma. Ann Oncol 14:1039–1044

Dimopoulos MA, Anagnostopoulos A, Kyrtsonis MC et al (2005) Treatment of relapsed or refractory Waldenstrom's macroglobulinemia with bortezomib. Haematologica 90:1655–1658

Dy GK, Thomas JP, Wilding G et al (2005) A phase and pharmacologic trial of two schedules of the proteasome inhibitor, PS-341 (bortezomib, velcade), in patients with advanced cancer. Clin Cancer Res 11:3410–3416

Elliott PJ, Zollner TM, Boehncke WH (2003) Proteasome inhibition: a new anti-inflammatory strategy. J Mol Med 81:235–245

Facon T, Mary JY, Pegourie B et al (2006) Dexamethasone-based regimens versus melphalan-prednisone for elderly multiple myeloma patients ineligible for high-dose therapy. Blood 107:1292–1298
Feling RH, Buchanan GO, Mincer TJ et al (2003) Salinosporamide A: a highly cytotoxic proteasome inhibitor from a novel microbial source, a marine bacterium of the new genus salinospora. Angew Chem Int Ed Engl 42:355–357
Fenteany G, Schreiber SL (1998) Lactacystin, proteasome function, and cell fate. J Biol Chem 273:8545–8548
Fisher RI, Bernstein SH, Kahl BS et al (2006) Multicenter phase II study of bortezomib in patients with relapsed or refractory mantle cell lymphoma. J Clin Oncol 24:4867–4874
Friedman J, Al-Zoubi A, Kaminski M et al (2006) A new model predicting at least a very good partial response in patients with multiple myeloma after cycles of velcade-based therapy. In: Updated data presented at the 2006 annual meeting of the European Hematology Association. Haematologica, vol 91, p 273
Fuchs SY (2002) The role of ubiquitin-proteasome pathway in oncogenic signaling. Cancer Biol Ther 1:337–341
Gautschi O, Heighway J, Mack PC et al (2008) Aurora kinases as anticancer drug targets. Clin Cancer Res 14:1624–1633
Gertz MA, Lacy MQ, Dispenzieri A et al (2006) High-dose chemotherapy with autologous hematopoietic stem cell transplantation in patients with multiple myeloma. Expet Rev Anticancer Ther 6:343–360
Goldberg AL (2003) Protein degradation and protection against misfolded or damaged proteins. Nature 426:895–899
Goy A, Younes A, McLaughlin P et al (2005) Phase II study of proteasome inhibitor bortezomib in relapsed or refractory B-cell non-Hodgkin's lymphoma. J Clin Oncol 23:667–675
Groll M, Bajorek M, Kohler A, Moroder L, Rubin DM, Huber R, Glickman MH, Finley D (2000) A gated channel into the proteasome core particle. Nat Struct Biol 7:1062–1067
Harousseau JL, Mathiot C, Attal M et al (2007) VELCADE/dexamethasone (Vel/D) versus VAD as induction treatment prior to autologous stem cell transplantation (ASCT) in newly diagnosed multiple myeloma (MM): updated results of the IFM 2005/01 trial. Blood 110:139a
Harousseau JL, Mathiot C, Attal M et al (2008) Bortezomib/dexamethasone versus VAD as induction prior to autologous stem cell transplantation (ASCT) in previously untreated multiple myeloma (MM): updated data from IFM 2005/01 trial. J Clin Oncol 26:455s
Hernandez JM, Garcia-Sanz R, Golvano E et al (2004) Randomized comparison of dexamethasone combined with melphalan versus melphalan with prednisone in the treatment of elderly patients with multiple myeloma. Br J Haematol 127:159–164
Hershko A, Ciechanover A (1998) The ubiquitin system. Annu Rev Biochem 67:425–479
Hideshima T, Chauhan D, Podar K et al (2001) Novel therapies targeting the myeloma cell and its bone marrow micro environment. Semin Oncol (6):607–612 (Review)
Hideshima T, Chauhan D, Richardson P et al (2002) NF-κB as a therapeutic target in multiple myeloma. J Biol Chem 277:16639–16647
Hideshima T, Podar K, Chauhan D et al (2004) p38 MAPK inhibition enhances PS-341 (bortezomib)-induced cytotoxicity against multiple myeloma cells. Oncogene 23:8766–8776
Hideshima T, Bradner JE, Wong J et al (2005) Small-molecule inhibition of proteasome and aggresome function induces synergistic antitumor activity in multiple myeloma. Proc Natl Acad Sci USA 102:8567–8572
Hideshima T, Catley L, Yasui H et al (2006) Perifosine, an oral bioactive novel alkylphospholipid, inhibits Akt and induces in vitro and in vivo cytotoxicity in human multiple myeloma cells. Blood 107:4053–4062
Ho YK, Bargagna-Mohan P, Wehenkel M, Mohan R, Kim KB (2007) LMP2-specific inhibitors: chemical genetic tools for proteasome biology. Chem Biol 14:419–430
Hollmig K, Stover J, Talamo G et al (2004) Bortezomib (Velcade™) + Adriamycin™ + thalidomide + dexamethasone (VATD) as an effective regimen in patients with refractory or

relapsed multiple myeloma (MM). In: Updated data presented at the 2004 annual meeting of the American Society of Hematology. Blood, vol 104, p 659a
Imajoh-Ohmi KT, Sugiyama S, Tanaka K, Omura S, Kikuchi H (1995) Lactacystin, a specific inhibitor of the proteasome, induces apoptosis in human monoblast U937 cells. Biochem Biophys Res Commun 217:1070–1077
Jagannath S, Barlogie B, Berenson J et al (2004) A phase 2 study of two doses of bortezomib in relapsed or refractory myeloma. Br J Haematol 127:165–172
Jagannath S, Barlogie B, Berenson JR et al (2005) Bortezomib in recurrent and/or refractory multiple myeloma. Initial clinical experience in patients with impaired renal function. Cancer 103:1195–1200
Jagannath S, Richardson PG, Sonneveld P et al (2007) Bortezomib appears to overcome the poor prognosis conferred by chromosome 13 deletion in phase 2 and 3 trials. Leukemia 21:151–157
Jesenberger V, Jentsch S (2002) Deadly encounter: ubiquitin meets apoptosis. Nat Rev Mol Cell Biol 3:112–1121
Kloetzel PM, Ossendorp F (2004) Proteasome and peptidase function in MHC-class-I-mediated antigen presentation. Curr Opin Immunol 16:76–81
Knop S, Einsele H, Bargou R et al (2008) Adjusted dose lenalidomide is safe and effective in patients with deletion (5q) myelodysplastic syndrome and severe renal impairment. Leuk Lymphoma 49(2):346–349
Koegl M, Hoppe T, Schlenker S, Ulrich HD, Mayer TU, Jentsch S (1999) A novel ubiquitination factor, E4, is involved in multiubiquitin chain assembly. Cell 96:635–644
Kohler A, Cascio P, Leggett DS, Woo KM, Goldberg AL, Finley D (2001) The axial channel of the proteasome core particle is gated by the Rpt2 ATPase and controls both substrate entry and product release. Mol Cell 7:1143–1152
Kortuem KM, Stewart AK (2013) Carfilzomib. Blood 121(6):893–897
Kropff MH, Bisping G, Wenning D et al (2005a) Bortezomib in combination with dexamethasone for relapsed multiple myeloma. Leuk Res 29:587–590
Kropff M, Bisping G, Liebisch P et al (2005b) Bortezomib in combination with high-dose dexamethasone and continuous low-dose oral cyclophosphamide for relapsed multiple myeloma. In: Updated data presented at the 2005 annual meeting of the American Society of Hematology. Blood, vol 106, p 716a
Kuhn DJ, Chen Q, Voorhees PM et al (2007) Potent activity of carfilzomib, a novel, irreversible inhibitor of the ubiquitin-proteasome pathway, against pre-clinical models of multiple myeloma. Blood 110:3281–3290
Kyle RA, Rajkumar SV (2004) Multiple myeloma. New Eng J Med 351:1860–1873
Lee JL, Swain SM (2008) The epothilones: translating from the laboratory to the clinic. Clin Cancer Res 14:1643–1649
Lee SJ, Richardson PG, Sonneveld P et al (2005) Health-related quality of life (HRQL) associated with bortezomib compared with high-dose dexamethasone in relapsed multiple myeloma (MM): results from APEX study. J Clin Oncol 23:568s
Leoni F, Casini C, Breschi C et al (2006) Low dose bortezomib, dexamethasone, thalidomide plus liposomal doxorubicin in relapsed and refractory myeloma. In: Updated data presented at the 2006 annual meeting of the European Hematology Association. Haematologica, vol 91, p 281
Ling YH, Liebes L, Ng B et al (2002) PS-341, a novel proteasome inhibitor, induces Bcl-2 phosphorylation and cleavage in association with G2-M phase arrest and apoptosis. Mol Cancer Ther 1:841–849
Lonial S, Waller EK, Richardson PG et al (2005) Risk factors and kinetics of thrombocytopenia associated with bortezomib for relapsed, refractory multiple myeloma. Blood 106:3777–3784
Loo TW, Clarke DM (1998) Superfolding of the partially unfolded core-glycosylated intermediate of human P-glycoprotein into the mature enzyme is promoted by substrate-induced transmembrane domain interactions. J Biol Chem 273:14671–14674
Loo TW, Clarke DM (1999) The human multidrug resistance P-glycoprotein is inactive when its maturation is inhibited: potential for a role in cancer chemotherapy. FASEB J 7:1724–1732

Ma MH, Yang HH, Parker K et al (2003) The proteasome inhibitor PS-341 markedly enhances sensitivity of multiple myeloma tumor cells to chemotherapeutic agents. Clin Cancer Res 3:1136–1144

Ma C, Mandrekar SJ, Alberts SR et al (2007) A phase I and pharmacologic study of sequences of the proteasome inhibitor, bortezomib (PS-341, velcade), in combination with paclitaxel and carboplatin in patients with advanced malignancies. Cancer Chemother Pharmacol 59:207–215

Mateos MV, Hernandez JM, Hernandez MT et al (2006) Bortezomib plus melphalan and prednisone in elderly untreated patients with multiple myeloma: results of a multicenter phase 1/2 study. Blood 108:2165–2172

Mateos MV, Hernandez JM, Hernandez MT et al (2007) Frontline VMP in elderly MM patients: extended follow-up. Haematologica 92:180

Messersmith WA, Baker SD, Lassiter L et al (2006) Phase I trial of bortezomib in combination with docetaxel in patients with advanced solid tumors. Clin Cancer Res 12:1270–1275

Mitsiades N, Mitsiades CS, Poulaki V et al (2002) Biologic sequelae of nuclear factor-κB blockade in multiple myeloma: therapeutic applications. Blood 99:4079–4086

Mitsiades N, Mitsiades CS, Richardson PG et al (2003) The proteasome inhibitor PS-341 potentiates sensitivity of multiple myeloma cells to conventional chemotherapeutic agents: therapeutic applications. Blood 101:2377–2380

Mitsiades CS, Mitsiades NS, McMullan CJ et al (2006) Antimyeloma activity of heat shock protein-90 inhibition. Blood 107:1092–1100

Mohrbacher A, Levine AM (2005) Reversal of advanced renal dysfunction on bortezomib treatment in multiple myeloma patients. J Clin Oncol 23:612s

Moreau P, Karamanesht II, Domnikova N, Kyselyova MY, Vilchevska KV, Doronin VA, Schmidt A, Hulin C, Leleu X, Esseltine DL, Venkatakrishnan K, Skee D, Feng H, Girgis S, Cakana A, van de Velde H, Deraedt W, Facon T (2012) Pharmacokinetic, pharmacodynamic and covariate analysis of subcutaneous versus intravenous administration of bortezomib in patients with relapsed multiple myeloma. Clin Pharmacokinet 51(12):823–829

Muratani M, Tansey WP (2003) How the ubiquitin-proteasome system controls transcription. Nat Rev Mol Cell Biol 4:192–201

Myeloma Trialists' Collaborative Group (1998) Combination chemotherapy versus melphalan plus prednisone as treatment for multiple myeloma: an overview of 6, 633 patients from 27 randomized trials. J Clin Oncol 16:3832–3842

Naujokat C, Hoffmann S (2002) Role and function of the 26 S proteasome in proliferation and apoptosis. Lab Invest 82:965–980

Nawrocki ST, Carew JS, Dunner K Jr et al (2005a) Bortezomib inhibits PKR-like endoplasmic reticulum (ER) kinase and induces apoptosis via ER stress in human pancreatic cancer cells. Cancer Res 65:11510–11519

Nawrocki ST, Carew JS, Pino MS et al (2005b) Bortezomib sensitizes pancreatic cancer cells to endoplasmic reticulum stress-mediated apoptosis. Cancer Res 65:11658–11666

Nencioni A, Grunebach F, Patrone F, Ballestrero A, Brossart P (2007) Proteasome inhibitors: antitumor effects and beyond. Leukemia 21:30–36

O'Connor OA, Wright J, Moskowitz C et al (2005) Phase II clinical experience with the novel proteasome inhibitor bortezomib in patients with indolent non–Hodgkin's lymphoma and mantle cell lymphoma. J Clin Oncol 23:676–684

Obeng EA, Carlson LM, Gutman DM et al (2006) Proteasome inhibitors induce a terminal unfolded protein response in multiple myeloma cells. Blood 107:4907–4916

Orlowski RZ, Baldwin AS (2002) NF-κB as a therapeutic target in cancer. Trends Mol Med 8:385–389

Orlowski RZ, Eswara JR, Lafond-Walker A et al (1998) Tumor growth inhibition induced in a murine model of human Burkitt's lymphoma by a proteasome inhibitor. Cancer Res 58:4342–4348

Orlowski RZ, Small GW, Shi YY (2002a) Evidence that inhibition of p44/42 mitogen-activated protein kinase signaling is a factor in proteasome inhibitor-mediated apoptosis. J Biol Chem 277:27864–27871
Orlowski RZ, Stinchcombe TE, Mitchell BS et al (2002b) Phase I trial of the proteasome inhibitor PS-341 in patients with refractory hematologic malignancies. J Clin Oncol 20:4420–4427
Orlowski RZ, Kuhn DJ, Small GW, Michaud C, Orlowski M (2005a) Identification of novel inhibitors that specifically target the immunoproteasome, and selectively induce apoptosis in multiple myeloma and other immunoproteasome-expressing model systems. Blood 106:76a (abstract 248)
Orlowski RZ, Voorhees PM, Garcia RA et al (2005b) Phase 1 trial of the proteasome inhibitor bortezomib and pegylated liposomal doxorubicin in patients with advanced hematologic malignancies. Blood 105:3058–3065
Orlowski RZ, Zhuang SH, Parekh T et al (2006) DOXIL-MMY-3001 Study Investigators. The combination of pegylated liposomal doxorubicin and bortezomib significantly improves time to progression of patients with relapsed/refractory multiple myeloma compared with bortezomib alone: results from a planned interim analysis of a randomized phase III study. In: Updated data presented at the 2006 annual meeting of the American Society of Hematology. Blood, vol 108, p 124a
Orlowski RZ, Stewart K, Vallone M et al (2007) Safety and antitumor efficacy of the proteasome inhibitor carfilzomib (PR-171) dosed for five consecutive days in hematologic malignancies: phase I results. Blood 110:127a (abstract 409)
Palumbo A, Bringhen S, Caravita T et al (2006) Oral melphalan and prednisone chemotherapy plus thalidomide compared with melphalan and prednisone alone in elderly patients with multiple myeloma: randomised controlled trial. Lancet 367:825–831
Palumbo A, Ambrosini MT, Benevolo G et al (2007) Bortezomib, melphalan, prednisone, and thalidomide for relapsed multiple myeloma. Blood 109:2767–2772
Palumbo A, Schlag R, Khuageva N et al (2008) Prolonged therapy with bortezomib plus melphalan–prednisone (VMP) results in improved quality and duration of response in the phase III VISTA study in previously untreated multiple myeloma (MM). Haematologica 93:83
Papandreou CN, Daliani DD, Nix D et al (2004) Phase I trial of the proteasome inhibitor bortezomib in patients with advanced solid tumors with observations in androgen-independent prostate cancer. J Clin Oncol 22:2108–2121
Pautasso C, Bringhen S, Cerrato C, Magarotto V, Palumbo A (2013) The mechanism of action, pharmacokinetics, and clinical efficacy of carfilzomib for the treatment of multiple myeloma. Expert Opin Drug Metab Toxicol, 9 Jul 2013 (Epub ahead of print)
Popat R, Goff L, Oakervee HE et al (2005) Changes in Mcl-1 and Bim expression with bortezomib and melphalan therapy for multiple myeloma. Blood 106:697a
Popat R, Williams C, Cook M et al (2006) A phase I/ II trial of bortezomib, low dose intravenous melphalan and dexamethasone for patients with relapsed multiple myeloma. In: Updated data presented at the 2006 annual meeting of the American Society of Hematology. Blood, vol 108, p 1011a
Rajkumar SV, Richardson PG, Hideshima T, Anderson KC (2005) Proteasome inhibition as a novel therapeutic target in human cancer. J Clin Oncol 23:630–639
Reece DE, Piza G, Trudel S et al (2006) A phase I-II trial of bortezomib plus oral cyclophosphamide and prednisone for relapsed/refractory multiple myeloma. In: Updated data presented at the 2006 annual meeting of the American Society of Hematology. Blood, vol 108, p 1009a
Richardson PG, Barlogie B, Berenson J et al (2003) A phase 2 study of bortezomib in relapsed, refractory myeloma. New Engl J Med 348:2609–2617
Richardson P, Sonneveld P, Schuster M et al (2005a) Bortezomib continues to demonstrate superior efficacy compared with high-dose dexamethasone in relapsed multiple myeloma:

updated results of the APEX trial. In: Updated data presented at the 2005 annual meeting of the American Society of Hematology. Blood, vol 106, p 715a

Richardson PG, Sonneveld P, Schuster MW et al (2005b) Bortezomib or high-dose dexamethasone for relapsed multiple myeloma. New Engl J Med 352:2487–2498

Richardson PG, Barlogie B, Berenson J et al (2006a) Extended follow-up of a phase II trial in relapsed, refractory multiple myeloma: final time-to-event results from the SUMMIT trial. Cancer 106:1316–1319

Richardson PG, Briemberg H, Jagannath S et al (2006b) Frequency, characteristics, and reversibility of peripheral neuropathy during treatment of advanced multiple myeloma with bortezomib. J Clin Oncol 24:3113–3120

Richardson PG, Jagannath S, Avigan DE et al (2006c) Lenalidomide plus bortezomib (Rev-Vel) in relapsed and/or refractory multiple myeloma (MM): final results of a multicenter phase 1 trial. In: Updated data presented at the 2006 annual meeting of the American Society of Hematology. Blood, vol 108, p 124a

Richardson PG, Mitsiades C, Ghobrial I et al (2006d) Beyond single-agent bortezomib: combination regimens in relapsed multiple myeloma. Curr Opin Oncol 18:598–608

Richardson PG, Mitsiades C, Hideshima T, Anderson KC (2006e) Bortezomib: proteasome inhibition as an effective anticancer therapy. Annu Rev Med 57:33–47

Richardson PG, Sonneveld P, Schuster M et al (2007a) Extended follow-up of a phase 3 trial in relapsed multiple myeloma: final time-to-event results of the APEX trial. Blood 110:3557–3560

Richardson PG, Sonneveld P, Schuster MW et al (2007b) Safety and efficacy of bortezomib in high-risk and elderly patients with relapsed multiple myeloma. Br J Haematol 137:429–435

Richardson PG, Siegel D, Baz R, Kelley SL, Munshi NC, Laubach J, Sullivan D, Alsina M, Schlossman R, Ghobrial IM, Doss D, Loughney N, McBride L, Bilotti E, Anand P, Nardelli L, Wear S, Larkins G, Chen M, Zaki MH, Jacques C, Anderson KC (2013) Phase 1 study of pomalidomide MTD, safety, and efficacy in patients with refractory multiple myeloma who have received lenalidomide and bortezomib. Blood 121(11):1961–1967

Rifkin RM, Gregory SA, Mohrbacher A et al (2006) Pegylated liposomal doxorubicin, vincristine, and dexamethasone provide significant reduction in toxicity compared with doxorubicin, vincristine, and dexamethasone in patients with newly diagnosed multiple myeloma: a phase III multicenter randomized trial. Cancer 106:848–858

Rivett AJ, Hearn AR (2004) Proteasome function in antigen presentation: immunoproteasome complexes, peptide production, and interactions with viral proteins. Curr Protein Pept Sci 5:153–161

Robertson JD, Datta K, Biswal SS, Kehrer JP (1999) Heat-shock protein 70 antisense oligomers enhance proteasome inhibitor-induced apoptosis. Biochem J 344:477–485

Ruiz S, Krupnik Y, Keating M et al (2006) The proteasome inhibitor NPI-0052 is a more effective inducer of apoptosis than bortezomib in lymphocytes from patients with chronic lymphocytic leukemia. Mol Cancer Ther 5:1836–1843

Ryan DP, O'Neil BH, Supko JG et al (2006) A phase I study of bortezomib plus irinotecan in patients with advanced solid tumors. Cancer 107:2688–2697

Sagaster V, Ludwig H, Kaufmann H et al (2007) Bortezomib in relapsed multiple myeloma: response rates and duration of response are independent of a chromosome 13q-deletion. Leukemia 21:164–168

San Miguel JF, Schlag R, Khuageva NK et al (2008) Bortezomib plus melphalan and prednisone for initial treatment of multiple myeloma. New Eng J Med 359:906–917

San Miguel JF, Schlag R, Khuageva NK, Dimopoulos MA, Shpilberg O, Kropff M, Spicka I, Petrucci MT, Palumbo A, Samoilova OS, Dmoszynska A, Abdulkadyrov KM, Delforge M, Jiang B, Mateos MV, Anderson KC, Esseltine DL, Liu K, Deraedt W, Cakana A, van de Velde H, Richardson PG (2013) Persistent overall survival benefit and no increased risk of second malignancies with bortezomib-melphalan-prednisone versus melphalan-prednisone in patients with previously untreated multiple myeloma. J Clin Oncol 31(4):448–455

Schmidt M, Hanna J, Elsasser S, Finley D (2005) Proteasome-associated proteins: regulation of a proteolytic machine. Biol Chem 386:725–737

Shi YY, Small GW, Orlowski RZ (2006) Proteasome inhibitors induce a p38 mitogen-activated protein kinase (MAPK)-dependent anti-apoptotic program involving MAPK phosphatase-1 and Akt in models of breast cancer. Breast Cancer Res Treat 100:33–47

Shinohara K, Tomioka M, Nakano H et al (1996) Apoptosis induction resulting from proteasome inhibition. Biochem J 317:385–388

Sin N, Kim KB, Elofsson M et al (1999) Total synthesis of the potent proteasome inhibitor epoxomicin: a useful tool for understanding proteasome biology. Bioorg Med Chem Lett 9:2283–2288

Small GW, Shi YY, Edmund NA et al (2004) Evidence that mitogen-activated protein kinase phosphatase-1 induction by proteasome inhibitors plays an antiapoptotic role. Mol Pharmacol 66:1478–1490

Sonneveld P, Richardson PG, Schuster MW et al (2005) Bortezomib at first relapse is superior to high-dose dexamethasone and more effective than when given later in relapsed multiple myeloma. Haematologica 90:146–147

Sonneveld P, Schmidt-Wolf IG, van der Holt B, El Jarari L, Bertsch U, Salwender H, Zweegman S, Vellenga E, Broyl A, Blau IW, Weisel KC, Wittebol S, Bos GM, Stevens-Kroef M, Scheid C, Pfreundschuh M, Hose D, Jauch A, van der Velde H, Raymakers R, Schaafsma MR, Kersten MJ, van Marwijk-Kooy M, Duehrsen U, Lindemann W, Wijermans PW, Lokhorst HM, Goldschmidt HM (2012) Bortezomib induction and maintenance treatment in patients with newly diagnosed multiple myeloma: results of the randomized phase III HOVON-65/ GMMG-HD4 trial. J Clin Oncol 30(24):2946–2955

Stapnes C, Doskeland AP, Hatfield K et al (2007) The proteasome inhibitors bortezomib and PR-171 have antiproliferative and proapoptotic effects on primary human acute myeloid leukaemia cells. Br J Haematol 136:814–828

Strauss SJ, Maharaj L, Hoare S et al (2006) Bortezomib therapy in patients with relapsed or refractory lymphoma: potential correlation of in vitro sensitivity and tumor necrosis factor a response with clinical activity. J Clin Oncol 24:2105–2212

Strickland E, Hakala K, Thomas PJ, DeMartino GN (2000) Recognition of misfolding proteins by PA700, the regulatory subcomplex of the 26 S proteasome. J Biol Chem 275:5565–5572

Suvannasankha A, Smith GG, Juliar BE et al (2006) Weekly bortezomib/methylprednisolone is effective and well tolerated in relapsed multiple myeloma. Clin Lymphoma Myeloma 7:131–134

Teicher BA (2008) Newer cytotoxic agents: attacking cancer broadly. Clin Cancer Res 14:1650–1657

Teoh G, Tan D, Hwang W et al (2006) Addition of bortezomib to thalidomide, dexamethasone and zoledronic acid (VTD-Z regimen) significantly improves complete remission rates in patients with relapsed/refractory multiple myeloma. In: Updated data presented at the 2006 annual meeting of the American Society of Clinical Oncology. J Clin Oncol, vol 24, p 683s

Terpos E, Anagnostopoulos A, Heath D et al (2006) The combination of bortezomib, melphalan, dexamethasone and intermittent thalidomide (VMDT) is an effective regimen for relapsed/ refractory myeloma and reduces serum levels of Dickkopf-1, RANKL, MIP-1-alpha and angiogenic cytokines. In: Updated data presented at the 2006 annual meeting of the American Society of Hematology. Blood, vol 108, pp 1010a–1011a

Treon SP, Hunter ZR, Matous J et al (2007) Multicenter clinical trial of bortezomib in relapsed/ refractory Waldenstrom's macroglobulinemia: results of WMCTG Trial 03–248. Clin Cancer Res 13:3320–3325

van de Donk NW, Lokhorst HM (2013) New developments in the management and treatment of newly diagnosed and relapsed/refractory multiple myeloma patients. Expert Opin Pharmacother 14(12):1569–1573

Vinitsky A, Michaud C, Powers JC, Orlowski M (1992) Inhibition of the chymotrypsin-like activity of the pituitary multicatalytic proteinase complex. Biochemistry 31:9421–9428

Vinitsky A, Cardozo C, Sepp-Lorenzino L, Michaud C, Orlowski M (1994) Inhibition of the proteolytic activity of the multicatalytic proteinase complex (proteasome) by substrate-related peptidyl aldehydes. J Biol Chem 269:29860–29866

Voorhees PM, Dees EC, O'Neil B, Orlowski RZ (2003) The proteasome as a target for cancer therapy. Clin Cancer Res 9:6316–6325

Voorhees PM, Chen Q, Kuhn DJ et al (2007) Inhibition of interleukin-6 signaling with CNTO 328 enhances the activity of bortezomib in preclinical models of multiple myeloma. Clin Cancer Res 13:6469–6478

Voortman J, Smit EF, Honeywell R et al (2007) A parallel dose-escalation study of weekly and twice-weekly bortezomib in combination with gemcitabine and cisplatin in the first-line treatment of patients with advanced solid tumors. Clin Cancer Res 13:3642–3651

Wang T (2003) The 26S proteasome system in the signaling pathways of TGF-beta superfamily. Front Biosci 8:d1109–d1127

Wang CY, Mayo MW, Baldwin AS Jr (1996) TNF-and cancer therapy-induced apoptosis: potentiation by inhibition of NF-*k*B. Science 274:784–787

Wang CY, Cusack JC Jr, Liu R, Baldwin AS Jr (1999) Control of inducible chemoresistance: enhanced anti-tumor therapy through increased apoptosis by inhibition of NF-kB. Nat Med 5:412–417

Wechalekar A, Gillmore J, Lachmann H, Offer M, Hawkins P (2006) Efficacy and safety of bortezomib in systemic AL amyloidosis-a preliminary report. Blood 108:42a (abstract 129)

Wojcikiewicz RJ (2004) Regulated ubiquitination of proteins in GPCR-initiated signaling pathways. Trends Pharmacol Sci 25:35–41

Zangari M, Barlogie B, Burns MJ et al (2005) Velcade (V)-thalidomide (T)-dexamethasone (D) for advanced and refractory multiple myeloma (MM): long-term follow-up of phase I-II trial UARK 2001–37: superior outcome in patients with normal cytogenetics and no prior T. In: Updated data presented at the 2005 Annual Meeting of the American Society of Hematology. Blood, vol 106, p 717a

Lenalidomide

Katja Weisel and Lothar Kanz

Abstract

Lenalidomide is an immunomodulatory drug (IMiD), which is well established and approved in the treatment of multiple myeloma (MM) and 5q-myelodysplastic syndrome (MDS). The mode of action includes immune modulation, anti-angiogenetic, anti-inflammatory, and anti-proliferative effects. Development of lenalidomide initiated a profound shift in therapeutic approaches especially toward MM. This chapter will discuss the mode of action of lenalidomide as well as its clinical applications. Important clinical phase II and III data of lenalidomide are presented. Currently, lenalidomide is not only investigated in MM and MDS, but also in malignant lymphomas and other entities.

Contents

K. Weisel (✉) · L. Kanz
Department of Oncology, Hematology and Immunology, University Hospital of Tuebingen, Otfried-Mueller-Strasse 10, 72076 Tuebingen, Germany
e-mail: katja.weisel@med.uni-tuebingen.de

U. M. Martens (ed.), *Small Molecules in Oncology*, Recent Results in Cancer Research 201, DOI: 10.1007/978-3-642-54490-3_21,

1 Introduction

Lenalidomide (Revlimid®) is an immunomodulatory drug (IMiD) which was developed as a structural analog of thalidomide, from which it differs by the addition of an amino group and the removal of one of the carbonyl groups from the phthaloyl ring system. Due to these changes, it was possible that lenalidomide minimizes the toxicity known for thalidomide, while optimizing therapeutic efficacy (Cives et al. 2012). Lenalidomide was primarily evaluated in the late 1990s. This was followed by intensive preclinical investigations. So far, lenalidomide has demonstrated substantial clinical activity in several disease states associated with significant unmet medical need (Zeldis et al. 2011). The pleiotropic biological effects of lenalidomide are the reason that this drug is in general effective as monotherapy in the treatment of MM. Proliferating malignant plasma cells is targeted by the tumoricidal effect, cell cycle arrest, disruption of tumor-microenvironment interactions, and down regulation of cytokines (Gupta et al. 2001; Mitsiades et al. 2002; Gandhi et al. 2010; Quach et al. 2012). While the relative contribution of lenalidomide-induced immune stimulation toward observed treatment responses is unclear, it is clear that lenalidomide possesses T-cell costimulatory and NK-cell activation potential (Hsu et al. 2011). This aspect of lenalidomide's function is yet to be fully explored therapeutically in MM, but seems to be particularly relevant in the setting of maintenance therapy and in the presence of minimal residual disease (MRD). Currently, synergistic tumoricidal effects are also evaluated with combination treatment of lenalidomide not only as approved with corticosteroids but also with chemotherapy or other novel therapeutic agents (Richardson et al. 2010; Larocca et al. 2012; Wang et al. 2013a, b). Currently, lenalidomide is approved by the EMA for treatment of relapsed MM and 5q-MDS. However, the drug is widely evaluated in other hematological and non-hematologic diseases such as chronic lymphatic leukemia (CLL), Hodgkin's, and non-Hodgkin's lymphoma as well as solid tumors.

2 Structure and Mechanism of Action

Lenalidomide ($C_{13}H_{13}N_3O_3$) is a synthetic compound derived by modification of the chemical structure of thalidomide ($C_{13}H_{10}N_2O_4$) (Fig. 1). Lenalidomide is rapidly absorbed following oral administration; it reaches its maximal concentration at 0.5–4 h in patients with MM and has an elimination half-life of 3 h. Approximately 30 % of plasma lenalidomide is bound to proteins and almost 70 % is excreted in the urine within 24 h, thus requiring adjustment of dosing in patients

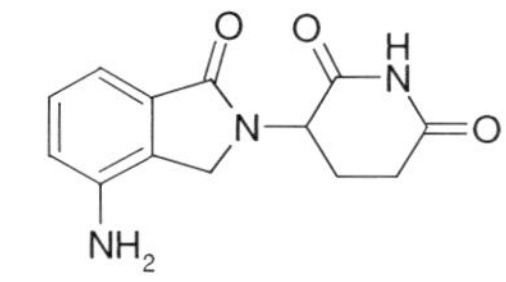

Fig. 1 Structure of lenalidomide

with renal impairment. Lenalidomide is not metabolized extensively by the P450 liver enzymes and thus does not interfere with the metabolism of other drugs (Mitsiades and Mitsiades 2004; Saloura and Grivas 2010).

Lenalidomide has a unique mechanism of action, including direct tumoricidal and immunomodulatory effects on the host microenvironment (Kotla et al. 2009). Direct tumor cytotoxicity is a result of actin polymerization and the relocalization of membrane proteins leading to cytoskeletal reorganization. Furthermore, cell cycle arrest, inhibition of autocrine cytokines, inhibition of tumor oncogenes such as *IRF4* and *C-MYC*, as well as concomitant induction of tumor suppressor genes were described (Corral et al. 1999; Xu et al. 2009; Gandhi et al. 2010; Heise et al. 2010). Myeloma cell apoptosis is induced by activation of caspases resulting in direct tumor cytotoxicity (Mitsiades et al. 2002; Gandhi et al. 2010). Multiple effects are demonstrated on the host microenvironment including the restoration of immune synapse formation, augmentation of natural-killer cell cytotoxicity, and inhibition of regulatory T cells. (Davies et al. 2001; Chang et al. 2006; Ramsay et al. 2008; Wu et al. 2008; Galustian et al. 2009). The predominant mode of action of thalidomide, tumor angiogenesis, is also seen with lenalidomide. In addition, a decrease in paracrine secretion was shown (Gupta et al. 2001; Dredge et al. 2005). During treatment with lenalidomide, the direct cytotoxic effect might lead to the rapid myeloma control, whereas the immunomodulatory effect leads to sustained and durable responses.

3 Clinical Data

Lenalidomide has shown clinical efficacy in a variety of hematological disorders, including MDS, MM, CLL, NHL, Waldenstrom's macroglobulinemia, myelofibrosis with myeloid metaplasia and primary systemic amyloidosis. In this review, single entities are selected for discussion. For solid tumors, lenalidomide has been evaluated in the management of prostate cancer, renal cell carcinoma, primary CNS tumors, and ovarian cancer.

4 Lenalidomide in Multiple Myeloma

Based on two phase I trials of lenalidomide in advanced MM, the maximum tolerated dose of lenalidomide was established as 25 mg/day (Richardson et al. 2002). Shortly after, it was shown that the in vitro synergistic tumoricidal effect with dexamethasone can be translated into the clinical setting, with additional

29 % of patients responded to the addition of dexamethasone to lenalidomide. This provided the basis for the use of the lenalidomide and dexamethasone combination in nearly all subsequent clinical trials. The role of lenalidomide in MM treatment will be elucidated for relapsed MM, as approved, and newly diagnosed MM. The emerging role of lenalidomide maintenance treatment will be discussed.

5 Lenalidomide in Relapsed Multiple Myeloma

In relapsed MM, combination treatment of lenalidomide and dexamethasone was shown to be efficacious in two large parallel phase III trials, MM-009 and MM-010, which were conducted in United States/Canada, and Europe/Australia/Israel, respectively (Dimopoulos et al. 2007; Weber et al. 2007). A recent pooled analysis of both trials after a follow-up of 48 months confirmed ongoing superiority of lenalidomide and dexamethasone compared with single-agent dexamethasone, which had served as the control arm with respect to overall response rate (ORR) and rate of complete remissions (CR) (61/15 % vs. 22/2 %, respectively; $P < 0.001$), as well as median time to progression (TTP) (13.4 months vs. 4.6 months; $P < 0.001$), and overall survival (OS) (38 months vs. 31.6 months; $P < 0.045$) (Dimopoulos et al. 2009). The most common grade 3/4 adverse events in the lenalidomide and dexamethasone arm were neutropenia (35 %) and thrombocytopenia (13 %). Interestingly, the rate of these adverse events decreased over time in patients who stayed on lenalidomide and dexamethasone therapy. At that time, as prophylactic anti-coagulation was not mandated, the rate of thromboembolic complication in the patient population on lenalidomide and dexamethasone was 16 %. Establishing obligate thromboembolic prophylaxis with the use of either aspirin or low molecular weight heparin, however, the rate of thromboembolic complication under lenalidomide and dexamethasone treatment is in the order of 2–5 %, comparable to the background incidence in patients with MM (Palumbo et al. 2008). Furthermore, the thromboembolic and infectious complications (9 %) were at least partially accounted by the use of high-dose dexamethasone in the MM-009 and MM-010 trial. When it was later found that low-dose dexamethasone given in a once-weekly schedule showed a markedly reduced rate of complications and improved tolerance, the use of reduced dexamethasone (40 mg/week) is nowadays preferred in combination with lenalidomide (Rajkumar et al. 2010).

6 Lenalidomide in Newly Diagnosed Multiple Myeloma

In newly diagnosed MM, two lenalidomide-based regimen have been evaluated in randomized phase III trials: Lenalidomide and dexamethasone as well as melphalan–prednisolone–lenalidomide (MPR). The former was evaluated in the Eastern Cooperative Oncology Group (ECOG) E4A03 study. Here, the efficacy and safety of lenalidomide (25 mg po daily, days 1–21) in combination with either conventional high-dose dexamethasone (RD; dex 40 mg po daily, days 1–4, 9–12, 17–20 every 28 days) or lower-dose dexamethasone (Rd; dex 40 mg po weekly) were evaluated. After four induction cycles, combination of lenalidomide with high-dose dexamethasone resulted in a higher overall response rate (ORR) of 79 % as compared to 68 % with the low-dose dexamethasone combination. However, the lower toxicity associated with lower-dose dexamethasone, particularly venous thromboembolisms and infections, resulted in a superior 1-year OS in the Rd arm [96 % (Rd) vs. 87 % (RD), $P < 0.0002$]. Moreover, a potentially improved immunomodulatory effect resulting to superior OS with the low-dose dexamethasone strategy arm is discussed (Gandhi et al. 2010). Patients in this study had the option of either continuing on lenalidomide and dexamethasone until disease progression or proceeding to consolidation with high-dose therapy (HDT) and autologous stem cell transplantation (ASCT). In patients not receiving HDT and ASCT, Rd given until disease progression, resulted in a 91 % ORR (57 % PR/VGPR; 22 % CR), with a 3-year PFS and OS of 50 and 79 %, respectively (Rajkumar et al. 2010).

The second lenalidomide containing regimen evaluated in newly diagnosed MM patients was following the MP Plus strategy, adding novel agents to the melphalan prednisone treatment established for more than 40 years. In the recent phase III MM015 study, patients were randomized either to nine induction cycles of MPR [melphalan 0.18 mg/kg days (D)1–4, prednisone 2 mg/kg D1–4, lenalidomide 10 mg D 1–21 for nine 28 D cycles], to MPR followed by lenalidomide (10 mg D 1–21 every 28 D) maintenance (MPR-R), or to MP. The trial was conducted in elderly MM patients not eligible for stem cell transplantation. Data analyses revealed that the addition of lenalidomide to MP during the induction phase only resulted in an unimpressive PFS benefit compared with MP (15 m vs. 12 m, respectively, $P < 0.009$). However, the MM015 trial focussed on introduction of maintenance treatment, when lenalidomide was added post-MPR induction in a 10 mg dose until disease progression or unacceptable toxicity. Here, a dramatic improvement in PFS was observed [PFS 31 m (MPR-R) vs. 13 m (MP), $P < 0.001$] (Palumbo et al. 2012). During maintenance, the sustained immunostimulatory effect of lower-dose lenalidomide monotherapy may have accounted for the improved PFS, when anti-tumor immune response becomes relevant in the presence of only minimal disease burden (Quach et al. 2012).

7 Maintenance Treatment with Lenalidomide in Multiple Myeloma After ASCT

A still open question in the management of MM is the efficacy of lenalidomide in the maintenance therapy after achieving remission following ASCT. The first fully published trial addressing this question was again by Palumbo et al. In this phase II trial, 102 previously untreated elderly MM patients received lenalidomide as a maintenance treatment after ASCT (Palumbo et al. 2010). Consolidation included four 28-day cycles of lenalidomide in combination with prednisone, followed by maintenance with lenalidomide alone until relapse. Notably, the immunofixation-negative CR improved from 38 to 66 % in patients undergoing ASCT followed by lenalidomide consolidation/maintenance therapy, as compared to bare ASCT. Furthermore, after a median follow-up of 21 months, 2-year PFS and OS rates were 69 and 86 % in lenalidomide-treated patients suggesting that lenalidomide is a feasible option in the maintenance setting for patients undergoing ASCT. Two further large phase III trials addressed the lenalidomide maintenance treatment after ASCT. A study conducted by the Cancer and Leukemia Group B compared lenalidomide with placebo as maintenance therapy after ASCT in 568 patients with newly diagnosed MM. After a median follow-up of 28 months, TTP was 48 months in the lenalidomide arm and 30.9 months in the placebo arm ($P < 0.0001$), with hazard ratio of 0.38 (95 % CI = 0.27–0.55). Although follow-up was short, a significant OS improvement was observed in the lenalidomide maintenance group, as the survival rates were 90 and 83 % for patients randomized in the lenalidomide and placebo groups, respectively. As expected, lenalidomide-receiving patients experienced mainly hematological toxicity; however, discontinuation rate due to adverse events was below 10 %. In this trial, 18 secondary malignancies were documented in the lenalidomide arm versus four in the placebo group (McCarthy et al. 2012). Similar results were obtained in the IFM 2005-02 study, which investigated lenalidomide as consolidation and maintenance treatment in young patients with non-progressive MM after a first-line ASCT. Maintenance therapy with lenalidomide improved PFS in a comparable manner as seen in the above mentioned trial. However, in contrast to the ECOG trial, in both groups, 5-year OS was not different. Again, lenalidomide was well tolerated, but an increase in the appearance of new cancers was detected, with 20 secondary malignancies in lenalidomide-receiving patients versus three in the placebo group. 5 neoplasms observed in the lenalidomide arm were not associated with MM so far (three Hodgkin's lymphomas and two acute lymphocytic leukemias) (Attal et al. 2012). The increased incidence of secondary primary malignancies (SPM) in MM patients under treatment with lenalidomide is under discussion. However, recently published pooled data demonstrated that there is no increase for solid tumors in myeloma patients on lenalidomide and a slight increase for hematological malignancies when lenalidomide is used in combination with conventional dose melphalan (Palumbo et al. 2013, abstract). So far, the benefits due to lenalidomide maintenance treatment outweigh the potential risks.

8 Lenalidomide in MDS

Initial evidence for the efficacy of lenalidomide in MDS was demonstrated in a trial of 43 patients with IPSS-classified low-risk MDS who had no response to recombinant erythropoietin or who were unlikely to benefit from conventional therapy (List et al. 2005). Overall, 20 patients had sustained red blood cell (RBC) transfusion independence, one patient had an increase in hemoglobin level of >2 g/dL, and three patients had >50 % reduction in the need for transfusions. Of particular interest was the response rate of 83 % among patients with a chromosome 5q31 deletion, a cytogenetic abnormality present in up to 30 % of MDS patients with clonal cytogenetic abnormalities (Ferrajoli et al. 2008). Durable erythroid responses were observed in a long-term analysis of six patients from this study, including four patients with a chromosome 5q31 deletion. All six patients maintained long-term transfusion independence (>4.5 years) with lenalidomide and five patients remained on therapy. The efficacy of lenalidomide was further evaluated in a large phase II study (MDS-003) of patients with IPSS-classified low- or intermediate-1-risk MDS with transfusion-dependent anemia and a chromosome 5q31 deletion (Ferrajoli et al. 2008). Among 148 patients who received lenalidomide, 67 % (95 % CI 59–74 %) no longer required transfusions, and 9 % (95 % CI 5–15 %) had at least a 50 % reduction in the number of transfusions. The response to lenalidomide was rapid and sustained, as median duration of transfusion independence had not been reached after 104-week follow-up. This study also demonstrated that lenalidomide suppressed the 5q-deletion clone. After 24 weeks of therapy, 73 % of patients had a cytogenetic response and 45 % had complete cytogenetic remission in association with sustained transfusion independence and improvement in bone marrow morphological features. These findings led to the approval of lenalidomide by the FDA for the treatment of transfusion-dependent anemia due to low- or intermediate-1-risk MDS associated with an 5q deletion with or without additional cytogenetic abnormalities (Zeldis et al. 2011). However, approval was restricted to the United States as the European Medical Agency (EMA) had concerns regarding potentially higher rates for secondary acute leukemia under lenalidomide treatment. A recent phase II study (MDS-002) investigated lenalidomide in 214 transfusion-dependent patients with low- or intermediate-1-risk MDS without a 5q deletion (Raza et al. 2008). Approximately a quarter (26 %) of patients achieved transfusion independence after a median of 4.8 weeks of treatment; median duration of transfusion independence was 41.0 weeks. At least a 50 % reduction in transfusion requirement was observed in 17 % of patients. In 2013, the EMA also has approved the use of lenalidomide for treatment of MDS with 5q deletion without additional genetic abnormalities.

9 Lenalidomide in Other Hematological Malignancies

Several clinical studies have suggested that lenalidomide has activity in chronic lymphatic leukemia (CLL) (Chanan-Khan et al. 2006; Ferrajoli et al. 2008; Badoux et al. 2011). In the first phase II study of 45 patients with relapsed/refractory CLL treated with lenalidomide, the overall response rate was 47 %, with 9 % of patients attaining a complete response (CR) (Chanan-Khan et al. 2006). In a subanalysis of patients with high-risk cytogenetics (deletions in 11q or 17p), the overall response rate was 38 %, with 19 % of patients achieving a CR (Sher et al. 2010). Median progression-free survival was 12.1 months, and the estimated 2-year survival probability was 58 %. A more recent phase II study investigated lenalidomide as frontline monotherapy in 60 elderly patients with CLL (Badoux et al. 2011). The overall response rate was 60 %, with 8 % of patients achieving a CR. In line with findings in CLL, lenalidomide has shown activity in a range of B-cell non-Hodgkin's lymphoma (NHL). In a phase II study of lenalidomide monotherapy in 49 patients with aggressive relapsed or refractory NHL, the objective response rate was 35 %, including a 12 % CR/unconfirmed-CR rate (Wiernik et al. 2008). Responses were observed in each aggressive histological subtype tested (diffuse large B cell, follicular center cell grade 3, mantle cell, and transformed lymphomas). Indeed, in a subanalysis of 15 patients with mantle cell lymphoma, the objective response rate was 53 %, with a CR rate of 20 % and median duration of response of 13.7 months (Habermann et al. 2009). In combination with rituximab, a recent phase II study in 44 patients with relapsed or refractory mantle cell lymphoma showed an ORR of 57 %. 16 (36 %) had a complete response, and nine (20 %) had a partial response. The median response duration was 18·9 months [95 % CI 17·0 months to not reached (NR)]. The median progression-free survival was 11·1 months (95 % CI 8·3–24·9 months), and the median overall survival was 24·3 months (19·8 months to NR). Main toxicity was hematological (Wang et al. 2012). The same combination of lenalidomide and rituximab was evaluated in a phase II trial, where 45 patients with relapsed or refractory diffuse large-cell B-NHL ($n = 32$), transformed lymphoma ($n = 9$) or follicular lymphoma grade 3 ($n = 4$) who had received 1–4 prior lines of treatment were evaluated. Patients received 20 mg oral lenalidomide on days 1–21 of each 28-day cycle, and intravenous rituximab (375 mg/m^2) weekly during cycle 1. Main toxicity was hematological with grade 3/4 neutropenia of 53 %, lymphopenia of 40 %, thrombocytopenia of 33 %, leukopenia of 27 %, and anemia of 18 %. With a median follow-up time of 29.1 months (range 14.7–52.0 months), ORR was 33 % and median response duration was 10.2 months. Median PFS and OS were 3.7 and 10.7 months, respectively (Wang et al. 2013).

10 Lenalidomide in Solid Tumors

Several early-stage studies have been performed to investigate the efficacy of lenalidomide in advanced solid tumors. Lenalidomide in combination with docetaxel was evaluated in a phase I study of 33 patients with advanced solid tumors (Sanborn et al. 2009). In patients evaluable for response, 69 % had stable disease and 3 % had a partial response. In a phase I study of 45 patients with eight different types of advanced refractory metastatic tumors who received lenalidomide monotherapy, stable disease was documented in 12 patients, of whom 9 had prostate cancer (Dahut et al. 2009). In a recent in vitro study, lenalidomide alone inhibited the invasion of prostate cancer cells and also enhanced the antiproliferative, proapoptotic effects of docetaxel. Among several trials of lenalidomide in prostate cancer, a phase III trial of combination lenalidomide, docetaxel, and prednisone is ongoing in castrate-resistant prostate cancer (Zeldis et al. 2011).

11 Conclusions and Future Perspectives

Development and use of lenalidomide as a novel treatment strategy in MM but also in several other, predominantly hematological malignancies opened a new understanding for pathophysiological and immunological aspects of these diseases. Clinical trials with lenalidomide established long-term treatment strategies with the goal of chronification of malignant diseases and showed enhanced therapeutic effects with other novel drugs such as monoclonal antibodies. Several interesting trials are on the way and their results are highly expected which will give us further insights into this topic and will help us to further optimize treatment strategies in the future.

References

Attal M et al (2012) Lenalidomide maintenance after stem-cell transplantation for multiple myeloma. N Engl J Med 366(19):1782–1791

Badoux XC et al (2011) Lenalidomide as initial therapy of elderly patients with chronic lymphocytic leukemia. Blood 118(13):3489–3498

Chanan-Khan A et al (2006) Clinical efficacy of lenalidomide in patients with relapsed or refractory chronic lymphocytic leukemia: results of a phase II study. J Clin Oncol 24(34):5343–5349

Chang DH et al (2006) Enhancement of ligand-dependent activation of human natural killer T cells by lenalidomide: therapeutic implications. Blood 108(2):618–621

Cives M et al (2012) Lenalidomide in multiple myeloma: current experimental and clinical data. Eur J Haematol 88(4):279–291

Corral LG et al (1999) Differential cytokine modulation and T cell activation by two distinct classes of thalidomide analogues that are potent inhibitors of TNF-alpha. J Immunol 163(1):380–386

Dahut WL et al (2009) Phase I study of oral lenalidomide in patients with refractory metastatic cancer. J Clin Pharmacol 49(6):650–660

Davies FE et al (2001) Thalidomide and immunomodulatory derivatives augment natural killer cell cytotoxicity in multiple myeloma. Blood 98(1):210–216

Dimopoulos M et al (2007) Lenalidomide plus dexamethasone for relapsed or refractory multiple myeloma. N Engl J Med 357(21):2123–2132

Dimopoulos MA et al (2009) Long-term follow-up on overall survival from the MM-009 and MM-010 phase III trials of lenalidomide plus dexamethasone in patients with relapsed or refractory multiple myeloma. Leukemia 23(11):2147–2152

Dredge K et al (2005) Orally administered lenalidomide (CC-5013) is anti-angiogenic in vivo and inhibits endothelial cell migration and Akt phosphorylation in vitro. Microvasc Res 69(1–2):56–63

Ferrajoli A et al (2008) Lenalidomide induces complete and partial remissions in patients with relapsed and refractory chronic lymphocytic leukemia. Blood 111(11):5291–5297

Galustian C et al (2009) The anti-cancer agents lenalidomide and pomalidomide inhibit the proliferation and function of T regulatory cells. Cancer Immunol Immunother 58(7): 1033–1045

Gandhi AK et al (2010) Dexamethasone synergizes with lenalidomide to inhibit multiple myeloma tumor growth, but reduces lenalidomide-induced immunomodulation of T and NK cell function. Curr Cancer Drug Targets 10(2):155–167

Gupta D et al (2001) Adherence of multiple myeloma cells to bone marrow stromal cells upregulates vascular endothelial growth factor secretion: therapeutic applications. Leukemia 15(12):1950–1961

Habermann TM et al (2009) Lenalidomide oral monotherapy produces a high response rate in patients with relapsed or refractory mantle cell lymphoma. Br J Haematol 145(3):344–349

Heise C et al (2010) Pleiotropic mechanisms of action of lenalidomide efficacy in del(5q) myelodysplastic syndromes. Expert Rev Anticancer Ther 10(10):1663–1672

Hsu AK et al (2011) The immunostimulatory effect of lenalidomide on NK-cell function is profoundly inhibited by concurrent dexamethasone therapy. Blood 117(5):1605–1613

Kotla V et al (2009) Mechanism of action of lenalidomide in hematological malignancies. J Hematol Oncol 2:36

Larocca A et al (2012) Current treatment strategies with lenalidomide in multiple myeloma and future perspectives. Future Oncol 8(10):1223–1238

List A et al (2005) Efficacy of lenalidomide in myelodysplastic syndromes. N Engl J Med 352(6):549–557

McCarthy PL et al (2012) Lenalidomide after stem-cell transplantation for multiple myeloma. N Engl J Med 366(19):1770–1781

Mitsiades CS, Mitsiades N (2004) CC-5013 (Celgene). Curr Opin Investig Drugs 5(6):635–647

Mitsiades N et al (2002) Apoptotic signaling induced by immunomodulatory thalidomide analogs in human multiple myeloma cells: therapeutic implications. Blood 99(12):4525–4530

Palumbo A et al (2010) Bortezomib as induction before autologous transplantation, followed by lenalidomide as consolidation-maintenance in untreated multiple myeloma patients. J Clin Oncol 28(5):800–807

Palumbo A et al (2012) Continuous lenalidomide treatment for newly diagnosed multiple myeloma. N Engl J Med 366(19):1759–1769

Palumbo A et al (2008) Prevention of thalidomide- and lenalidomide-associated thrombosis in myeloma. Leukemia 22(2):414–423

Palumbo A, Bringhen S, Rajkumar V, Lupparelli G, Usmani SZ, Waage A et al (2013) Second primary malignancies (SPM) in newly diagnosed myeloma (MM) patients treated with lenalidomide (Len): meta-analysis of 6,383 individual patient data (IPD). J Clin Oncol 31(suppl; abstr 8517)

Quach H et al (2012) Lenalidomide in multiple myeloma: current status and future potential. Am J Hematol 87(12):1089–1095

Rajkumar SV et al (2010) Lenalidomide plus high-dose dexamethasone versus lenalidomide plus low-dose dexamethasone as initial therapy for newly diagnosed multiple myeloma: an open-label randomised controlled trial. Lancet Oncol 11(1):29–37

Ramsay AG et al (2008) Chronic lymphocytic leukemia T cells show impaired immunological synapse formation that can be reversed with an immunomodulating drug. J Clin Invest 118(7):2427–2437

Raza A et al (2008) Phase 2 study of lenalidomide in transfusion-dependent, low-risk, and intermediate-1 risk myelodysplastic syndromes with karyotypes other than deletion 5q. Blood 111(1):86–93

Richardson PG et al (2002) Immunomodulatory drug CC-5013 overcomes drug resistance and is well tolerated in patients with relapsed multiple myeloma. Blood 100(9):3063–3067

Richardson PG et al (2010) Lenalidomide, bortezomib, and dexamethasone combination therapy in patients with newly diagnosed multiple myeloma. Blood 116(5):679–686

Saloura V, Grivas PD (2010) Lenalidomide: a synthetic compound with an evolving role in cancer management. Hematology 15(5):318–331

Sanborn SL et al (2009) Phase I trial of docetaxel given every 3 weeks and daily lenalidomide in patients with advanced solid tumors. Invest New Drugs 27(5):453–460

Sher T et al (2010) Efficacy of lenalidomide in patients with chronic lymphocytic leukemia with high-risk cytogenetics. Leuk Lymphoma 51(1):85–88

Wang L et al (2013) Bortezomib in combination with thalidomide or lenalidomide or doxorubicin regimens for the treatment of multiple myeloma: a meta-analysis of 14 randomized controlled trials. Leuk Lymphoma

Wang M et al (2012) Lenalidomide in combination with rituximab for patients with relapsed or refractory mantle-cell lymphoma: a phase 1/2 clinical trial. Lancet Oncol 13(7):716–723

Wang M et al (2013a) Oral lenalidomide with rituximab in relapsed or refractory diffuse large cell, follicular and transformed lymphoma: a phase II clinical trial. Leukemia 27(9): 1902–1909

Wang M et al (2013b) Phase 2 dose-expansion study (PX-171-006) of carfilzomib, lenalidomide and low-dose dexamethasone in relapsed or progressive multiple myeloma. Blood

Weber DM et al (2007) Lenalidomide plus dexamethasone for relapsed multiple myeloma in North America. N Engl J Med 357(21):2133–2142

Wiernik PH et al (2008) Lenalidomide monotherapy in relapsed or refractory aggressive non-Hodgkin's lymphoma. J Clin Oncol 26(30):4952–4957

Wu L et al (2008) Lenalidomide enhances natural killer cell and monocyte-mediated antibody-dependent cellular cytotoxicity of rituximab-treated CD20+ tumor cells. Clin Cancer Res 14(14):4650–4657

Xu Y et al (2009) Immunomodulatory drugs reorganize cytoskeleton by modulating Rho GTPases. Blood 114(2):338–345

Zeldis JB et al (2011) A review of the history, properties, and use of the immunomodulatory compound lenalidomide. Ann NY Acad Sci 1222:76–82

Pomalidomide

Monika Engelhardt, Ralph Wäsch, Heike Reinhardt
and Martina Kleber

Abstract

Pomalidomide (originally CC-4047 or 3-amino-thalidomide) is a derivative of thalidomide that is antiangiogenic and also acts as an immunomodulator. Pomalidomide, as the newest immunomodulatory agent (IMiD), has shown substantial in vitro antiproliferative and proapoptotic effects. In vivo studies have suggested limited cross-resistance between lenalidomide and pomalidomide, and the response of pomalidomide in relapsed and refractory (RR) multiple myeloma (MM) patients, including those who are refractory to both lenalidomide and bortezomib, has induced notable enthusiasm. Several studies have evaluated continuous (2 mg/day) or alternate (5 mg/2 day) dose schedules of pomalidomide, as well as 2 versus 4 mg schedules, and pomalidomide alone versus in combination with dexamethasone or other antimyeloma agents. Since pomalidomide plus low-dose dexamethasone has shown better responses, progression-free and overall survival than high-dose dexamethasone or pomalidomide alone, subsequent trials investigating pomalidomide combination therapy have been initiated. Among these trials combinations with alkylating agents (cyclophosphamide, bendamustin), anthracyclins (pegylated liposomal doxorubicin), proteasome inhibitors (bortezomib, carfilzomib), and various others can be found. Pomalidomide has also been assessed in AL amyloidosis, MPNs (myelofibrosis [MF]), Waldenstrom's macroglobulinemia, solid tumors (sarcoma, lung cancer), or HIV and—for AL amyloidosis and

M. Engelhardt (✉) · R. Wäsch · H. Reinhardt · M. Kleber
Hematology and Oncology, University of Freiburg, Hugstetterstr. 55,
79106 Freiburg, Germany
e-mail: monika.engelhardt@uniklinik-freiburg.de

U. M. Martens (ed.), *Small Molecules in Oncology*, Recent Results
in Cancer Research 201, DOI: 10.1007/978-3-642-54490-3_22,

MF—has already proven remarkable activity. Due to its potency, pomalidomide was approved by the US Food and Drug Administration (FDA) for RRMM in 2/2013 and has also been approved by the European Medicines Agency (EMA).

Contents

1 Structure and Mechanism of Action

The structurally related parent compound of pomalidomide, thalidomide, was originally discovered to inhibit angiogenesis in 1994 (Fig. 1). Further structure activity studies led to the first report in 2001 (D'Amato et al. 2001) that pomalidomide was able to directly inhibit both the tumor cell and vascular compartments of multiple myeloma (MM). This dual activity of pomalidomide suggested it to be more potent than thalidomide in vitro and in vivo. In subsequent studies, pomalidomide was shown to directly inhibit angiogenesis and myeloma cell growth. This dual effect is central to its activity in myeloma, whereas other pathways, such as tumor necrosis factor (TNF)-α inhibition, are of less relevance (Fig. 2): it has been shown that potent TNF-α inhibitors, including rolipram and pentoxifylline, do not inhibit myeloma cell growth nor angiogenesis (D'Amato et al. 2001). Up-regulation of IFN-γ, IL-2, and IL-10 and down-regulation of IL-6 have been reported for pomalidomide. These changes may contribute to pomalidomide's antiangiogenic and antimyeloma activities (Corral et al. 1999; Hideshima et al. 2000; Escoubet-Lozach et al. 2009; Verhelle et al. 2007) (Fig. 1). Albeit the precise molecular mechanism of action and targets through which immunomodulatory agents (IMiDs) exert their antitumor effects remains to be fully elucidated, threshold levels of cereblon (CRBN) expression are presumably important for therapy responses. Current data suggest that CRBN, a primary teratogenic target of thalidomide, is an essential requirement for IMiD activity and a possible biomarker for the clinical assessment of antimyeloma activity (Zhu et al. 2011).

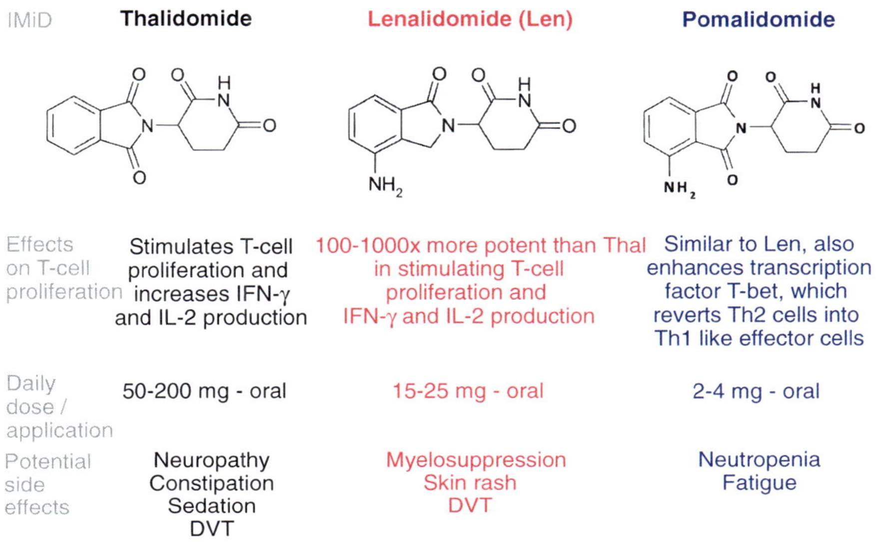

Fig. 1 Thalidomide, lenalidomide, and pomalidomide structure, immune effects, daily recommended doses, and common side effects. Albeit these 3 IMiDs are structurally similar, they are functionally different, both qualitatively and quantitatively

2 Preclinical Data

IMiDs may have antineoplastic effects by blocking signaling through nuclear factor-κB and may induce apoptosis via caspase-8/death receptor pathway. IMiDs have potent immunomodulatory properties including down-regulation of TNF, interleukin-1ß, augmentation of antimyeloma natural killer (NK) cell activity, and stimulation of cytotoxic T cells (Corral et al. 1999; D'Amato et al. 2001; Escoubet-Lozach et al. 2009; Hideshima et al. 2000; Verhelle et al. 2007; Udi et al. 2013; Waldschmidt et al. 2012) (Fig. 2). In vitro, IMiDs antagonize angiogenesis and expression of TNF-α and IL-6, while they facilitate production of IL-2 and IFN-γ and enhance T-cell and NK-cell proliferation and activity. Nevertheless, the precise mechanism of their action is not entirely revealed, but seems to include down-regulation of cytokine signaling (Görgün et al. 2010). Moreover, Görkün et al. demonstrated that the tumor suppressor molecule SOCS1 plays an important role in the tumor cell-immune cell-bone marrow (BM) microenvironment interaction in MM. Importantly, lenalidomide and pomalidomide induced epigenetic modifications of SOCS1 gene in MM cells, as well as modulated cytokine signaling via SOCS1-mediated cytokine signaling in effector cells. Therefore, characterization of the molecular mechanisms of IMiDs on immune cells in the BM environment needs to be further defined and suggest that novel immune-based targeted therapies, such as the combination of IMiDs with epigenetic modulating drugs (such as histone

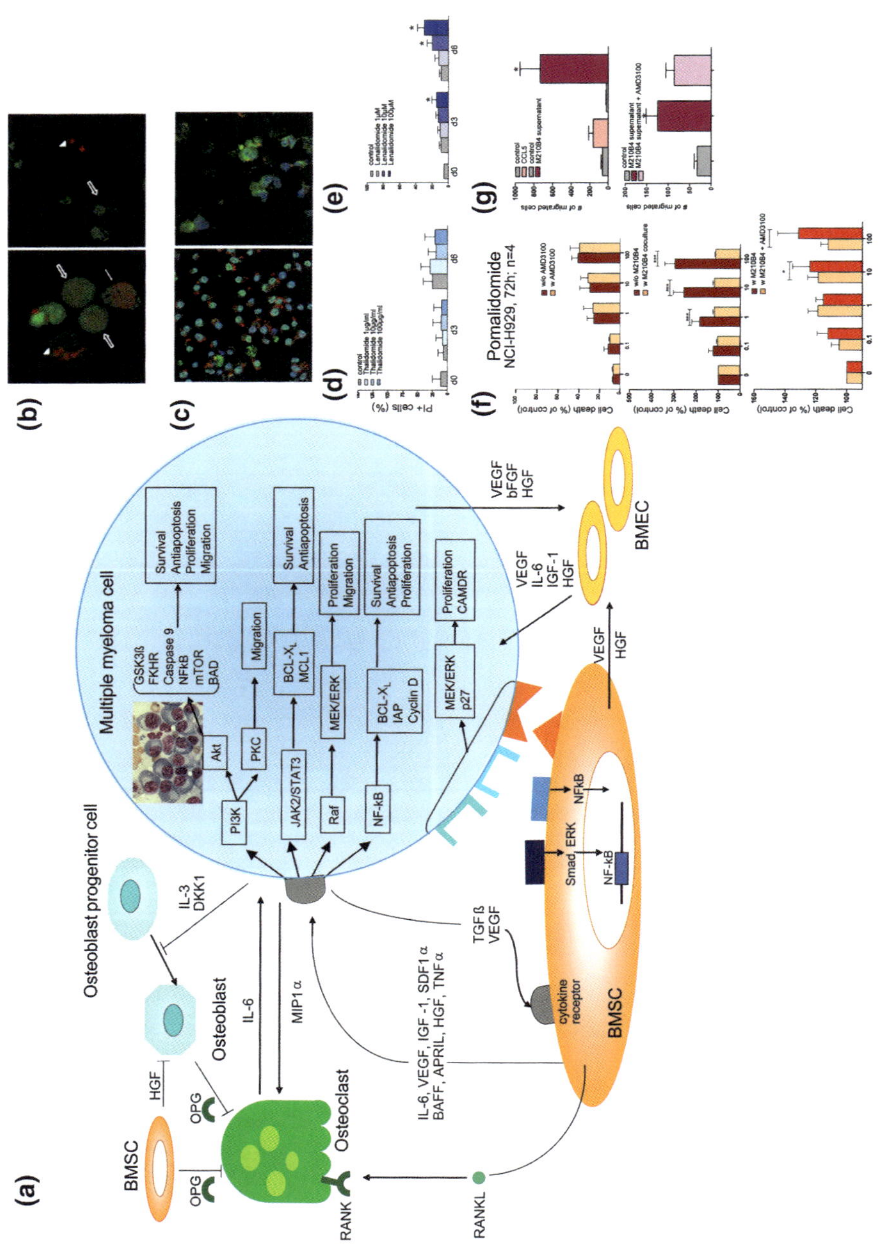
(a)
Osteoblast progenitor cell
IL-3
DKK1
Osteoblast
BMSC
HGF
OPG
OPG
RANK
Osteoclast
RANKL
IL-6
MIP1 α
IL-6, VEGF, IGF -1, SDF1 α
BAFF, APRIL, HGF, TNF α
TGF ß
VEGF
cytokine receptor
BMSC
Smad
ERK
NF-kB
NFkB
Multiple myeloma cell
PI3K
Akt
PKC
GSK3ß
FKHR
Caspase 9
NFkB
mTOR
BAD
Survival
Antiapoptosis
Proliferation
Migration
Migration
JAK2/STAT3
BCL-XL
MCL1
Survival
Antiapoptosis
Raf
MEK/ERK
Proliferation
Migration
NF-kB
BCL-XL
IAP
Cyclin D
Survival
Antiapoptosis
Proliferation
MEK/ERK
p27
Proliferation
CAMDR
VEGF
HGF
VEGF
IL-6
IGF-1
HGF
VEGF
bFGF
HGF
BMEC
(b)
(c)
(d)
PI+ cells (%)
control
Thalidomide 1µg/ml
Thalidomide 10µg/ml
Thalidomide 100µg/ml
d0
d3
d6
(e)
control
Lenalidomide 1µM
Lenalidomide 10µM
Lenalidomide 100µM
d0
d3
d6
(f)
Pomalidomide
NCI-H929, 72h; n=4
Cell death (% of control)
w/o AMD3100
w AMD3100
w/o M210B4
w M210B4 coculture
w M210B4
w M210B4 + AMD3100
(g)
# of migrated cells
control
CCL5
control
M210B4 supernatant
control
M210B4 supernatant
M210B4 supernatant + AMD3100

Fig. 2 **a** Myeloma growth within the bone marrow (BM) microenvironment is affected by osteoclasts, osteoblasts, BM stroma cells (BMSC), and endothelial cells (BMEC), which secrete cytokines and chemokines as depicted and are multiple targets of IMiDs. **b** Apoptotic changes induced by exposure of MM cells to antimyeloma agents can be visualized via confocal images, these cells coexpressing fluorescently labeled cytochrome c-GFP (*green*) and histone 2B-mCherry (*red*) and showing early and late apoptosis after antimyeloma agent treatment such as IMiDs. The release of cytochrome c is evident, as the freckled pattern (*filled white arrow*) of cytochrome c-GFP becomes diffuse (*framed white arrows*). Chromatin condensation and fragmentation (*white arrow heads*), as a typical marker for late apoptosis, are also observed. **c** Antimyeloma agents, such as IMiDs, may down-regulate CD138-expression and induce actin depolymerization and cell shape changes in vitro. Confocal images after immunocytochemistry staining with CD138-FITC, Phalloidin-594-Alexa (actin filaments), and Dapi (DNA) show CD138-down-regulation, changes in cell size, and reduction in F-actin in MM cells. **d** In vitro effect of thalidomide on cell death is less substantial after 3 and 6 days of culture despite logarithmic increases of thalidomide concentrations, whereas the effect of lenalidomide shows significant cytotoxicity. **e** Significantly increased PI-positive cells are observed on d3 with 100 μM lenalidomide and on d6 with 10 and 100 μM, as compared to the control; $*p < 0.05$. **f** Pomalidomide also induces concentration-dependent cell death increases. This is not increased with additional treatment of the CXCR4 inhibitor AMD3100, in the absence of stroma cells. With coculture of BMSCs (M210B4), MM cells' sensitivity to antimyeloma agents, such as pomalidomide, is significantly reduced; however, with addition of AMD3100 to stroma-cultured MM cells, this increases pomalidomide's toxicity and thus can restore the sensitivity to antimyeloma agent treatment. **g** Chemotaxis of MM cells can be significantly increased with M210B4 supernatant as compared to control media or CCL5 ($*p < 0.05$). In the presence of the CXCR4 inhibitor AMD3100, chemotaxis to M210B4 supernatant does decrease, however insignificantly, supporting the involvement of chemokines other than CXCL12 and chemotaxis of M210B4 not entirely being blocked by the CXCR4 inhibitor

deacetylase inhibitors and/or demethylating agents) may provide potent immunomodulatory therapies in MM. Given the new promising clinical activity of pomalidomide even in lenalidomide-refractory MM, current efforts therefore attempt to delineate direct and epigenetic mechanisms to account for important differences (Görgün et al. 2010). Several preclinical and clinical studies have also demonstrated that threshold levels of CRBN expression are important to induce response to IMiDs (Zhu et al. 2011; Schuster et al. 2012): Zhu et al. demonstrated that CRBN depletion is initially cytotoxic to human myeloma cells, but that surviving cells with stable CRBN depletion become highly resistant to both lenalidomide and pomalidomide, but not to the unrelated drugs bortezomib, dexamethasone, and melphalan. Acquired depletion of CRBN was described to be the primary genetic event of myeloma cell lines cultured to be sensitive or resistant to lenalidomide or pomalidomide. Gene expression changes induced by lenalidomide were substantially suppressed in the presence of CRBN depletion, demonstrating that CRBN is required for lenalidomide activity. Downstream targets of CRBN-included interferon regulatory factor 4 (IRF4) previously reported to be a target of lenalidomide. Patients exposed and resistant to lenalidomide had lower CRBN levels in paired samples before and after therapy, suggesting that CRBN is an essential requirement for IMiD activity and a useful biomarker for the clinical assessment of IMiDs' antimyeloma efficacy. Other recent studies have confirmed that threshold levels of CRBN expression are required for response to IMiD therapy (Schuster et al. 2012).

3 Clinical Data

The introduction of novel agents and their combination has generated major advances in MM. Nevertheless, their immediate use in first-line and subsequent therapies makes the treatment of subsequent relapses a challenge, since MM remains incurable, and patients will ultimately acquire resistance to prior agents. Once patients are no longer responsive to IMiDs and bortezomib, the prognosis is grave and new agents are needed. This outcome of relapsed disease in the current era of novel drugs has recently been described by Kumar et al.: 286 patients with relapsed MM were studied, who were refractory to bortezomib. The date, patients satisfied the entry criteria, was defined as time zero ($T(0)$). The median age at diagnosis was 58 years, and time from diagnosis to $T(0)$ was 3.3 years. Following $T(0)$, 74 % of patients ($n = 213$; Table 1) had a treatment recorded with one or more regimens (median = 1; range 0–8). The first regimen contained bortezomib in 26 % and an IMiD in 33 % of patients. A minor response or better was seen to at least one therapy after $T(0)$ in 44 %, including $\geq$ partial response in 32 %. The median OS and event-free survival from $T(0)$ were 9 and 5 months, respectively. This study impressively confirmed the poor outcome, once patients become treatment refractory and currently provides the context for interpreting trials of newer agents, such as pomalidomide combined with antimyeloma agents (Kumar et al. 2012) (Table 1).

Pomalidomide as the newest IMiD suggests at least incomplete cross-resistance among thalidomide or lenalidomide and albeit all 3 IMiDs have similar structures, they differ markedly in their potency and side effects (Fig. 1). Phase I pomalidomide results have shown tolerable side effects (Streetly et al. 2008) and phase II clinical trials for MM and MF reported promising results (Richardson et al. 2013; Leleu et al. 2013; Lacy et al. 2012; Tefferi 2011).

4 MM

In February 2013, the Food and Drug Administration (FDA) granted accelerated approval to pomalidomide for the treatment of patients with MM, who have received at least two prior therapies, including lenalidomide and bortezomib, and have demonstrated disease progression on or within 60 days of completion of the last therapy. The approval was based on the results of the CC-4047-MM-002 trial; a multicenter, randomized, open-label study in 221 patients with RRMM, who had previously received lenalidomide and bortezomib and were refractory to the last myeloma therapy (Richardson et al. 2009). The treatment arms were pomalidomide alone or pomalidomide plus low-dose dexamethasone. The efficacy results demonstrated an overall response rate of 7 % in patients treated with pomalidomide alone, and 29 % in those treated with pomalidomide plus low-dose dexamethasone. The median response duration was not evaluable in the pomalidomide monotherapy arm and was 7.4 months in the pomalidomide plus low-dose dexamethasone arm.

Table 1 Outcome after IMiDs and bortezomib (Bz; Kumar SK; Leukemia) versus pomalidomide, cyclophosphamide, and prednisone (PCP) in relapsed/refractory MM (RRMM)

	Best response				
	≥VGPR (%)	≥PR (%)	≥MR (%)	1-y PFS (%)	1-y OS (%)
Outcome after IMiDs and Bz (n = 213) Kumar et al. Leukemia 2012;26:149–157	7	24	34	25	50
All PCP patients (n = 52)	19	54	75	52	78
Relapsed after Len (n = 18)	28	67	78	63	89
Refractory to Len (n = 23)	15	47	73	48	72
Refractory to Bz (n = 15)	33	67	80	62	78
Double refractory to both Len+Bz (n = 11)	18	63	81	64	69

Abbreviations
IMiDs Immunomodulatory agents, *Len* Lenalidomide, *Bz* Bortezomib

A phase 1 dose-escalation study recently determined the maximum tolerated dose (MTD) of pomalidomide on days 1–21 of a 28-day cycle in 38 patients with RRMM (Richardson et al. 2013). Pretreatment had been substantial with a median of 6 prior therapies; including 63 % who were refractory to both lenalidomide and bortezomib. There were 4 dose-limiting toxicities (grade 4 neutropenia) at 5 mg/d, so that the MTD was specified with 4 mg/d. Among the 38 patients enrolled (including 22 with added dexamethasone), 42 % achieved minimal response or better, 21 % PR or better, and 3 % CR. Median duration of response, PFS, and OS were 4.6, 4.6, and 18.3 months, respectively.

The subsequent multicenter, phase 2 randomized study assessed 2 different pomalidomide dose schedules [4 mg for 21 vs. 28 days (21/28 vs. 28/28 cycles)] combined with dexamethasone in 84 advanced MM patients. The median number of prior therapy lines was again substantial with 5 and the overall response rate was 35 % (arm 21/28) and 34 % (arm 28/28), irrespective of the number of prior lines and level of refractoriness. Median duration of response, time to disease progression and PFS was 7.3, 5.4, and 4.6 months, respectively. At 23 months of follow-up, median OS was 14.9 months (Leleu et al. 2013). This phase 2 trial suggested that 4 mg pomalidomide—given on days 1–21 of a 28-day cycle and combined with dexamethasone—should be investigated further.

Recent results of the phase III trial, that randomized pomalidomide and low-dose dexamethasone to high-dose dexamethasone alone, have shown significant extension of PFS (median 3.6 months vs. 1.8 months; $p < 0.001$), and OS in patients taking pomalidomide and dexamethasone (Dimopoulos et al. 2012).

Moreover, the large comparative analysis of 6 sequential phase 2 trials at Mayo in 345 patients receiving pomalidomide at doses of 2 or 4 mg/d demonstrated excellent activity in relapsed MM patients (Table 2). The six cohorts consisted of: cohort 1 (n = 60): relapsed MM with 1–3 prior regimens, 2 mg dose; cohort 2 (n = 34): lenalidomide (Len)-refractory, 2 mg dose; cohort 3 (n = 35):

Table 2 Pomalidomide and low-dose dexamethasone (Pom/Dex) in relapsed MM: long-term follow-up and factors predicting outcome in 345 patients

	Pomalidomide schedule					
	2 mg relapse <3reg	2 mg Len ref	2 mg Bz/ Len ref	4 mg relapse <3 reg	4 mg relapse Bz/Len ref	4 mg relapse d1–21
	$n = 60$	$n = 34$	$n = 35$	$n = 60$	$n = 35$	$n = 120$
Confirmed response (≥PR) (%)	63	32	26	38	29	21
# of responders	39	11	9	23	10	25
Median time to response (ms)	1.7	2.0	1	1.1	1.4	1.1
Duration of response (ms)	21.3	8.2	15.6	NR	3.1	8.3
PFS (ms)	13	5	6.4	7.7	3.3	4.3
6-ms PFS (%)	73	44	54	63	37	34
OS (ms)	NR	33	16	NR	9.2	NR
6-ms OS (%)	95	85	74	92	67	74

Abbreviations
NR not reached, *ref* refractory, *reg* regimens, *d* day, *ms* months

bortezomib (Bz)/Len-refractory, 2 mg dose; cohort 4 ($n = 35$): Bz/Len-refractory, 4 mg dose; cohort 5 ($n = 60$) Len-refractory, 1–3 prior regimens, 4 mg dose; and cohort 6 ($n = 120$) Len-refractory, 4 mg dose. Pomalidomide was given orally 2 mg daily or 4 mg daily on days 1–28 (cohorts 1–5) or 1–21 (cohort 6) of a 28-day cycle with oral dexamethasone given 40 mg daily on days 1, 8, 15, and 22. 1/345 patient was ineligible and excluded from the analysis. The median age was 64 years (32–88). The median time since diagnosis was 53 months. The median number of prior therapies was 3 (1–14) and 44 % had high-risk molecular markers by mSMART criteria. Prior therapies consisted of thalidomide (52 %), lenalidomide (87 %), bortezomib (75 %), autologous stem cell transplant (70 %), and allogeneic transplant (3 %). The median follow-up was 10.4 months (5.4–34 months), with 67 % being alive and 32 % remaining progression free. The authors concluded that response rates and toxicity were similar between the 2 mg and 4 mg pomalidomide doses (Lacy et al. 2012) (Table 2).

The combination of pomalidomide and dexamethasone with cyclophosphamide in RRMM was also reported at ASH (Palumbo et al. 2012): 52 patients had received 1–3 prior lines, their median time from diagnosis was 55 months (range 15–203) and pomalidomide was administered at doses ranging from 1 to 2.5 mg/day on days 1–28, cyclophosphamide with 50 mg on alternate days and prednisone at 50 mg also every other day for 6 cycles, followed by maintenance therapy with pomalidomide/prednisone. The MTD of pomalidomide was defined as 2.5 mg/day, with impressive responses as depicted in Table 1. Other combination schedules with oral cyclophosphamide at doses of 300 or 400 mg on days 1, 8, and 15 applied with pomalidomide/dexamethasone (Baz et al. 2012), pegylated liposomal doxorubicin (Berenson et al. 2012), or carfilzomib (Shah et al. 2012) further enlarge the options to treated RRMM patients. At least one study also suggested that the addition of clarithromycin may enhance antimyeloma activity of pomalidomide plus dexamethasone: Mark et al. reported a phase 2 study that used clarithromycin 500 mg twice daily, pomalidomide 4 mg for day 1–21 of a 28-day cycle, and dexamethasone 40 mg weekly in 97 relapsed MM patients, many of whom were refractory to lenalidomide or both lenalidomide and bortezomib. They reported responses of PR or better in 53 % (Mark et al. 2012).

Albeit the dose of pomalidomide, that should be used, is a recurring question, current data suggest that either 2 mg/d continuously or 4 mg for 21 of 28 days is effective and well tolerable (Lacy 2013).

5 AL Amyloidosis

Pomalidomide/dexamethasone has shown activity in patients with immunoglobulin light-chain AL amyloidosis where patients were eligible for the prospective phase 2 trial if they had at least 1 prior regimen and reasonably preserved organ function (Dispenzieri et al. 2012): 33 patients were enrolled, with a median age of 66 years and median time from diagnosis to on study of 37 months. 82 % had cardiac involvement. The confirmed hematological response rate was 48 %, with a median time to response of 1.9 months. Organ improvement was observed in 5 patients. The median PFS and OS were 14 and 28 months, respectively. The results demonstrated the activity of pomalidomide/dexamethasone even among lenalidomide and bortezomib failures and that pomalidomide may be a beneficial treatment option in patients with previously treated AL amyloidosis.

6 Myelofibrosis

In Myelofibrosis (MF), thalidomide and lenalidomide, with or without prednisone, have shown comparable activity in alleviating anemia, splenomegaly and thrombocytopenia, with responses being induced in ~20 % each (Tefferi 2011). Treatment may be complicated by peripheral neuropathy (PNP) or severe myelosuppression in patients receiving thalidomide or lenalidomide, respectively. Therefore, another IMiD, pomalidomide, was assessed in a phase 2 trial, where ~25 % of patients with anemia responded to pomalidomide alone (2 mg/d) or pomalidomide (0.5 or 2 mg/d) combined with prednisone (Tefferi et al. 2009). In a subsequent phase 2 study of pomalidomide monotherapy (0.5 mg/d; Begna et al. 2011), anemia response was observed only in the presence of JAK2V617F (24 vs. 0 %) and was predicted by the presence of pomalidomide-induced basophilia (38 vs. 6 %) or the absence of marked splenomegaly (28 vs. 11 %). Platelet response was seen in 58 %, but the drug had limited activity on spleen size reduction. Unlike thalidomide and lenalidomide, drug-induced PNP and myelosuppression were infrequent. However, higher doses (>2 mg/d) were myelosuppressive and not necessarily better in terms of efficacy. Therefore, for MF in choosing between the 3 IMiDs, lenalidomide seems preferable in the presence of del(5q) because of the possibility of obtaining hematological and cytogenetic remission (Tefferi et al. 2007). In the absence of del(5q), pomalidomide represents an option in patients with JAK2V617F positivity without marked splenomegaly; otherwise, thalidomide plus prednisone is a reasonable alternative; albeit, of note, all 3 IMiDs should not be used in the absence of symptomatic anemia.

7 Toxicity

The most common side effects of pomalidomide reported in clinical trials have been fatigue and asthenia, neutropenia, anemia, constipation, nausea, diarrhea, dyspnea, upper respiratory tract infections, back pain, and pyrexia. In the comparative analysis of 6 sequential phase 2 trials at Mayo in 345 patients receiving pomalidomide at doses of 2 or 4 mg/d, most common toxicities (grade $\geq$3) were neutropenia (31 %), anemia (16 %), thrombocytopenia (12 %), pneumonia (8 %), and fatigue (8 %; Fig. 1). VTE was seen in 10 patients (3 %; Lacy et al. 2012). Moreover, a brief review on 2 patients who developed pulmonary toxicity related to pomalidomide was consistent with previously published reports on pulmonary toxicity related to thalidomide and lenalidomide. It was suggested that this very rare toxicity should readily be recognized by clinicians in patients with pulmonary complaints and no identifiable infectious source and that timely withdrawal of the medication leads to rapid resolution of symptoms without long-term sequelae (Geyer et al. 2011). In general, pomalidomide induces less aesthesia and neuropathy than thalidomide and is more likely to induce neutropenia than thalidomide, but this side effect is usually well manageable with a dose reduction. Subsets of MM patients, who are sensitive to the myelosuppressive effect of lenalidomide and have trouble tolerating even low doses, may do well with pomalidomide, suggesting that its myelosuppressive effect is less pronounced. Skin rash which might be observed with lenalidomide (Wäsch et al. 2012) is rarely seen with pomalidomide (Lacy 2013) (Fig. 1).

Pomalidomide is approved by the FDA and EMA with a Boxed Warning alerting patients and healthcare professionals that the drug can cause embryo-fetal toxicity and venous thromboembolism. Because of this embryo-fetal risk, pomalidomide is available only through a restricted distribution program called the POMALYST Risk Evaluation and Mitigation Strategy (REMS) Program. Prescribers must be certified with the POMALYSTREMS Program by enrolling and complying with the REMS requirements. Patients must sign a patient–physician agreement form and comply with the REMS requirements. Female patients of reproductive potential who are not pregnant must comply with the pregnancy testing and contraception requirements. Males must comply with contraception requirements. Pharmacies must be certified with the POMALYSTREMS program, must only dispense to patients who are authorized to receive pomalidomide, and comply with REMS requirements http://www.fda.gov/Drugs/InformationOnDrugs/ApprovedDrugs/ucm339286.htm.

8 Drug Interactions

Pomalidomide is metabolized by CYP1A2 and CYP3A and is a substrate for p-glycoprotein. CYP1A2 and CYP3A4 inhibitors may increase the serum concentrations of pomalidomide, whereas inducers of these enzymes may decrease pomalidomide concentrations. Current data have shown that CYP1A2 and CYP3A4 are the primary isozymes responsible for the CYP450-mediated metabolism (Hoffmann et al. 2013). Coadministration of pomalidomide with strong inhibitors of CYP1A2 (e.g., ciprofloxacin, enoxacin, and fluvoxamine), CYP3A (e.g., clarithromycin, ketoconazol, and grapefruit juice), or p-glycoprotein (e.g., azithromycin, amiodarone, and itraconazol) may increase pomalidomide exposure and should be avoided. Strong inducers of CYP1A2 (e.g., broccoli, modafinil, and nafcillin), CYP3A (carbamazepine, phenytoin, and rifampicin), or p-glycoprotein (avasimibe, rifampicin, and St.John's wort) may decrease pomalidomide plasma levels and should likewise be avoided. Cigarette smoking may reduce pomalidomide exposure via CYP1A2 induction; therefore, patients should be advised that smoking may reduce the efficacy of pomalidomide.

9 Biomarkers

Acquired depletion of CRBN has been demonstrated to be the primary genetic event of myeloma cell lines cultured to be sensitive or resistant to IMiDs. Gene expression changes induced by lenalidomide were substantially suppressed in the presence of CRBN depletion, demonstrating that CRBN is required for IMiD activity. Zhu et al. also showed that patients exposed and resistant to lenalidomide had lower CRBN levels in paired samples before and after therapy, suggesting that CRBN is an essential requirement for IMiD activity and a useful biomarker for the clinical assessment of IMiDs' antimyeloma efficacy (Zhu et al. 2011). Other recent studies have confirmed that threshold levels of CRBN expression are required for response to IMiD therapy (Schuster et al. 2012).

Across the 6 cohorts—of the sequential phase 2 trials at Mayo in 345 patients receiving pomalidomide at doses of 2 or 4 mg/d—confirmed responses of PR or better in 34 % of patients. Responses and duration of response (DOR) in those with high-risk molecular markers included the following: 17p-: 19 of 56 (34 %): DOR 8.2 months; *t*(4;14): 6 of 24 (25 %): DOR 4.8 months; *t*(14;16): 7 of 11 (64 %): DOR 9.5 months; deletion 13 by cytogenetics: 13 of 37 (35 %): DOR

8.2 months. In a multivariate analysis, LDH >ULN, number of prior regimens, and prior bortezomib therapy were predictive of a shorter time to progression and factors associated with a poor OS following initiation of pomalidomide therapy included ß2-micoglobuline levels >5.5 mg/l, LDH >ULN, number of prior regimens and prior bortezomib therapy. In general and as true for almost all anti-myeloma agents, number and types of prior regimens are the strongest predictors of pomalidomide response and survival, with best responses in patients who are the least heavily pretreated (Lacy 2013).

10 Summary and Perspectives

Although new agents have significantly improved the prognosis in MM, novel therapies are constantly needed. Pomalidomide is effective and well tolerated in patients with advanced, refractory myeloma and potentially provides an unmet clinical need in patients with previously treated MM. The use of pomalidomide and low-dose dexamethasone, and their combination with other active agents, warrants further clinical testing. Moreover, response in cytogenetically high-risk patients (Richardson et al. 2012) and those with organ impairment, such as renal insufficiency (Siegel et al. 2012), are currently confounded by low patient numbers and need to be further investigated.

References

Baz R, Shain KH, Alsina M, Nardelli LA, Nishihori T, Ochoa L, Martin T, Jagannath S, Dalton W, Sullivan DM (2012) Oral weekly cyclophosphamide in combination with pomalidomide and dexamethasone for relapsed and refractory myeloma: report of the dose escalation cohort. Blood 120:4062

Begna KH, Mesa RA, Pardanani A, Hogan WJ, Litzow MR, McClure RF, Tefferi A (2011) A phase-2 trial of low-dose pomalidomide in myelofibrosis. Leukemia 25:301–304

Berenson JR, Hilger JD, Klein LM, Eshaghian S, Nassir Y, Swift RA, Vescio R (2012) A phase 1/2 study of pomalidomide, dexamethasone and pegylated liposomal doxorubicin for patients with relapsed/refractory multiple myeloma. Blood 120:2979

Corral LG, Haslett PA, Muller GW, Chen R, Wong LM, Ocampo CJ, Patterson RT, Stirling DI, Kaplan G (1999) Differential cytokine modulation and T cell activation by two distinct classes of thalidomide analogues that are potent inhibitors of TNF-alpha. J Immunol 163:380–386

D'Amato R, Lentzsch S, Anderson KC, Rogers MS (2001) Mechanism of action of thalidomide and 3-aminothalidomide in multiple myeloma. Semin Oncol 28:597–601

Dimopoulos MA, Lacy MQ, Moreau P, Weisel KC, Song KW, Delforge M, Karlin L, Goldschmidt H, Banos A, Oriol A, Yu X, Sternas L, Jacques CJ, Zaki M, San Miguel JF (2012) Pomalidomide in combination with low-dose dexamethasone: demonstrates a significant progression free survival and overall survival advantage, in relapsed/refractory MM: a phase 3, multicenter, randomized, open-label study. Blood 120:LBA-6

Dispenzieri A, Buadi F, Laumann K, LaPlant B, Hayman SR, Kumar SK, Dingli D, Zeldenrust SR, Mikhael JR, Hall R, Rajkumar SV, Reeder C, Fonseca R, Bergsagel PL, Stewart AK, Roy V, Witzig TE, Lust JA, Russell SJ, Gertz MA, Lacy MQ (2012) Activity of pomalidomide in patients with immunoglobulin light-chain amyloidosis. Blood 119:5397–5404

Escoubet-Lozach L, Lin IL, Jensen-Pergakes K, Brady HA, Gandhi AK, Schafer PH, Muller GW, Worland PJ, Chan KW, Verhelle D (2009) Pomalidomide and lenalidomide induce p21 WAF-1 expression in both lymphoma and multiple myeloma through a LSD1-mediated epigenetic mechanism. Cancer Res 69:7347–7356

Geyer HL, Viggiano RW, Lacy MQ, Witzig TE, Leslie KO, Mikhael JR, Stewart K (2011) Acute lung toxicity related to pomalidomide. Chest 140:529–533

Görgün G, Calabrese E, Soydan E, Hideshima T, Perrone G, Bandi M, Cirstea D, Santo L, Hu Y, Tai YT, Nahar S, Mimura N, Fabre C, Raje N, Munshi N, Richardson P, Anderson KC (2010) Immunomodulatory effects of lenalidomide and pomalidomide on interaction of tumor and bone marrow accessory cells in multiple myeloma. Blood 116:3227–3237

Hideshima T, Chauhan D, Shima Y, Raje N, Davies FE, Tai YT, Treon SP, Lin B, Schlossman RL, Richardson P, Muller G, Stirling DI, Anderson KC (2000) Thalidomide and its analogs overcome drug resistance of human multiple myeloma cells to conventional therapy. Blood 96:2943–2950

Hoffmann M, Kasserra C, Reyes J, Schafer P, Kosek J, Capone L, Parton A, Kim-Kang H, Surapaneni S, Kumar G (2013) Absorption, metabolism and excretion of [14C]pomalidomide in humans following oral administration. Cancer Chemother Pharmacol 71:489–501

Kumar SK, Lee JH, Lahuerta JJ, Morgan G, Richardson PG, Crowley J, Haessler J, Feather J, Hoering A, Moreau P, LeLeu X, Hulin C, Klein SK, Sonneveld P, Siegel D, Bladé J, Goldschmidt H, Jagannath S, Miguel JS, Orlowski R, Palumbo A, Sezer O, Rajkumar SV, Durie BG (2012) International Myeloma Working Group. Risk of progression and survival in multiple myeloma relapsing after therapy with IMiDs and bortezomib: a multicenter international myeloma working group study. Leukemia 26:149–157

Lacy MQ (2013) "IM iD"eally treating multiple myeloma. Blood 121:1926–1928

Lacy MQ, Kumar SK, LaPlant BR, Laumann K, Gertz MA, Hayman SR, Buadi FK, Dispenzieri A, Lust JA, Russell S, Dingli D, Zeldenrust SR, Fonseca R, Bergsagel PL, Stewart K, Roy V, Sher T, Chanan-Khan A, Reeder C, Rajkumar SV, Mikhael JR (2012) Pomalidomide plus low-dose dexamethasone (Pom/Dex) in relapsed myeloma: long term follow up and factors predicing outcome in 345 patients. Blood 120:201

Leleu X, Attal M, Arnulf B, Moreau P, Traulle C, Marit G, Mathiot C, Petillon MO, Macro M, Roussel M, Pegourie B, Kolb B, Stoppa AM, Hennache B, Bréchignac S, Meuleman N, Thielemans B, Garderet L, Royer B, Hulin C, Benboubker L, Decaux O, Escoffre-Barbe M, Michallet M, Caillot D, Fermand JP, Avet-Loiseau H, Facon T (2013) Pomalidomide plus low-dose dexamethasone is active and well tolerated in bortezomib and lenalidomide-refractory multiple myeloma: Intergroupe Francophone du Myélome 2009-02. Blood 121:1968–1975

Mark T, Boyer A, Rossi AC, Shah M, Pearse RN, Zafar F, Pekle K, Tegnestam L, Sacris EA, Greenberg J, Speaker S, Jayabalan D, Ely SA, Coleman M, Chen-Kiang S, Niesvizky R (2012) ClaPD (clarithromycin, pomalidomide, dexamethasone) therapy in relapsed or refractory multiple myeloma. Blood 120:77

Palumbo A, Larocca A, Montefusco V, Rossi D, Carella AM, Mina R, Crippa C, Sciacca M, Galli M, Rota Scalabrini D, Marcatti M, Guglielmelli T, Giuliani N, La Verde G, Baldi I, Muccio VE, Boccadoro M, Corradini P (2012) Pomalidomide cyclophosphamide and prednisone (PCP) treatment for relapsed/refractory multiple myeloma. Blood 120:446

Richardson P, Baz R et al (2009) A phase 1/2 multi-center, randomized, open label dose escalation study to determine the maximum tolerated dose, safety and efficacy of pomalidomide alone or in combination with low-dose dexamethasone in patients with relapsed and refractory multiple myeloma who have received prior treatment that includes lenalidomide and bortezomib. Blood 114:301

Richardson P, Jakubowiak A, Bahlis NJ, Siegel DS, Chen CI, Chen M, Zaki M, Larkins G, Anderson K (2012) Treatment outcomes with pomalidomide (POM) in combination with low-dose dexamethasone (LoDex) in patients with relapsed and refractory multiple myeloma (RRMM) and Del(17p13) and/or t(4;14)(p16;q32) cytogenetic abnormalities who have received prior therapy with lenalidomide (LEN) and bortezomib (BORT). Blood 120:4053

Richardson PG, Siegel D, Baz R, Kelley SL, Munshi NC, Laubach J, Sullivan D, Alsina M, Schlossman R, Ghobrial IM, Doss D, Loughney N, McBride L, Bilotti E, Anand P, Nardelli L, Wear S, Larkins G, Chen M, Zaki MH, Jacques C, Anderson KC (2013) Phase 1 study of pomalidomide MTD, safety, and efficacy in patients with refractory multiple myeloma who have received lenalidomide and bortezomib. Blood 121:1961–1967

Schuster SR, Kortuem KM, Zhu YX, Braggio E, Shi C-X, Bruins L, Schmidt J, Ahmann G, Kumar SK, Rajkumar SV, Mikhael JR, Roy V, LaPlant BR, Laumann K, Barlogie B, Shaughnessy JD Jr, Fonseca R, Bergsagel L, Lacy MQ, Stewart K (2012) Cereblon expression predicts response, progression free and overall survival after pomalidomide and dexamethasone therapy in multiple myeloma. Blood 120:194

Shah J, Stadtmauer EA, Abonour R, Cohen AD, Bensinger WI, Gasparetto C, Kaufman JL, Lentzsch S, Vogl DT, Orlowski RZ, Kim EL, McKinley MB, Durie BGM (2012) A multicenter phase I/II trial of carfilzomib and pomalidomide with dexamethasone (Car-Pom-d) in patients with relapsed/refractory multiple myeloma. Blood 120:74

Siegel DS, Richardson PG, Baz R, Chen M, Zaki M, Anderson KC (2012) Pomalidomide (POM) with low-dose dexamethasone (LoDEX) in patients with relapsed and refractory multiple myeloma (RRMM): impact of renal function on patient outcomes. Blood 120:4072

Streetly MJ, Gyertson K, Daniel Y, Zeldis JB, Kazmi M, Schey SA (2008) Alternate day pomalidomide retains anti-myeloma effect with reduced adverse events and evidence of in vivo immunomodulation. Br J Haematol 141:41–51

Tefferi A, Lasho TL, Mesa RA, Pardanani A, Ketterling RP, Hanson CA (2007) Lenalidomide therapy in del(5)(q31)-associated myelofibrosis: cytogenetic and JAK2V617F molecular remissions. Leukemia 21:1827–1828

Tefferi A, Verstovsek S, Barosi G, Passamonti F, Roboz GJ, Gisslinger H, Paquette RL, Cervantes F, Rivera CE, Deeg HJ, Thiele J, Kvasnicka HM, Vardiman JW, Zhang Y, Bekele BN, Mesa RA, Gale RP, Kantarjian HM (2009) Pomalidomide is active in the treatment of anemia associated with myelofibrosis. J Clin Oncol 27:4563–4569

Tefferi A (2011) How I treat myelofibrosis. Blood 117:3494–3504

Udi J, Schüler J, Wider D, Ihorst G, Catusse J, Waldschmidt J, Schnerch D, Follo M, Wäsch R, Engelhardt M (2013) Potent in vitro and in vivo activity of sorafenib in multiple myeloma: induction of cell death, CD138-downregulation and inhibition of migration through actin depolymerization. Br J Haematol 161:104–116

Verhelle D, Corral LG, Wong K, Mueller JH, Moutouh-de Parseval L, Jensen-Pergakes K, Schafer PH, Chen R, Glezer E, Ferguson GD, Lopez-Girona A, Muller GW, Brady HA, Chan KW (2007) Lenalidomide and CC-4047 inhibit the proliferation of malignant B cells while expanding normal CD34+ progenitor cells. Cancer Res 67:746–755

Waldschmidt J, Wider D, Follo M, Udi J, Kleber M, Lorenz J, Ihorst G, Wäsch R, Engelhardt M (2012) Bone marrow interaction in multiple myeloma pathogenesis: phenotypical analysis, kinetics and novel therapy approaches based on CXCR4 inhibition. Blood 120:2450

Wäsch R, Jakob T, Technau K, Finke J, Engelhardt M (2012) Stevens-Johnson/toxic epidermal necrolysis overlap syndrome following lenalidomide treatment for multiple myeloma relapse after allogeneic transplantation. Ann Hematol 91:287–289

Zhu YX, Braggio E, Shi CX, Bruins LA, Schmidt JE, Van Wier S, Chang XB, Bjorklund CC, Fonseca R, Bergsagel PL, Orlowski RZ, Stewart AK (2011) Cereblon expression is required for the antimyeloma activity of lenalidomide and pomalidomide. Blood 118:4771–4779

Everolimus

Jens Hasskarl

Abstract

Everolimus (RAD001, Afinitor®) is an oral protein kinase inhibitor of the mammalian target of rapamycin (mTOR) serine/threonine kinase signal transduction pathway. The mTOR pathway regulates cell growth, proliferation, and survival and is frequently deregulated in cancer. Everolimus has been approved by the FDA and the EMA for the treatment of advanced renal cell carcinoma (RCC), subependymal giant cell astrocytoma (SEGA) associated with tuberous sclerosis (TSC), pancreatic neuroendocrine tumors (PNET), in combination with exemestane in advanced hormone-receptor (HR)-positive, HER2-negative breast cancer. Everolimus shows promising clinical activity in additional indications. Multiple phase 2 and phase 3 trials of everolimus alone or in combination are ongoing and will help to further elucidate the role of mTOR in oncology. For a review on everolimus as immunosuppressant, please consult other sources.

Contents

J. Hasskarl (✉)
Department Innere Medizin, Klinik für Innere Medizin I, Schwerpunkt Hämatologie, Onkologie und Stammzelltransplantation, Hugstetter Str. 55, 79102 Freiburg, Germany
e-mail: jens.hasskarl@uniklinik-freiburg.de

U. M. Martens (ed.), *Small Molecules in Oncology*, Recent Results in Cancer Research 201, DOI: 10.1007/978-3-642-54490-3_23,

1 Introduction

Everolimus is an analog of the naturally occurring macrolide rapamycin. Rapamycin (sirolimus) was isolated from a Streptomyces species from soil of the Easter Island (Rapa Nui) (Sehgal et al. 1975). Rapamycin is a macrolide with antifungal and immunosuppressive properties (Eng et al. 1991). The identification of the mammalian target of rapamycin (mTOR) signaling pathway spurred the development of rapamycin analogs (so-called rapalogs) in the following years (Brown et al. 1994; Sabatini et al. 1994). Several rapalogs are under clinical use, and further investigations to harness their immunosuppressive and antiproliferative potential are ongoing. These are sirolimus (rapamycin) (Sehgal 1995), temsirolimus (CCI-779) (Geoerger et al. 2001), everolimus (RAD001) (Schuler et al. 1997), and deforolimus (AP23573) (Mita et al. 2008).

Rapalogs bind to the FK506-binding protein-12 (FKBP12). This complex inhibits the mTOR, a protein kinase that regulates cell growth, proliferation, and survival (Fig. 1). mTOR can form two functionally distinct complexes that differ in their sensitivity to rapamycin (Jacinto et al. 2004). mTOR complex 1 (mTORC1) regulates translation and cell growth via phosphorylation of S6 kinase (S6K) and eukaryotic initiation factor eIF4E binding protein (4E-BP) and is very sensitive to inhibition by rapamycin. The second mTOR complex (mTORC2) is resistant to rapamycin and is involved in (re)organization of the actin cytoskeleton. mTORCs integrate signals from multiple upstream pathways and relay the information through the regulation of multiple downstream pathways (Laplante and Sabatini 2012; Houghton 2010; O'Reilly and McSheehy 2010). In essence, the mTOR pathway is activated via the phosphatidylinositol 3-kinase (PI3K) pathway and the tuberous sclerosis complex (TSC1/2) (Mak and Yeung 2004; Manning and Cantley 2003; Levine et al. 2006). Mutations in these components or in the tumor suppressor protein PTEN, a negative regulator of PI3K, may result in their dysregulation. Various preclinical models have confirmed the role of this pathway in tumor development (Manning and Cantley 2003; Podsypanina et al. 2001; Chan 2004).

There is evidence that the mTOR pathway holds several feedback loops and that it is interconnected with various other signaling pathways. Inhibition of mTORC1 by everolimus releases the inhibitory action of S6K on IRS1, allowing further activation of PI3K and compensatory activation of AKT and its downstream targets (Majumder et al. 2004). Inhibition of mTORC1 by everolimus also results in a feedback activation of the mitogen-activated protein kinase (MAPK) pathway (Carracedo et al. 2008). mTORC1 is mainly regulated by TSC1 and TSC2. Loss of function mutations of the TSC1 or TSC2 genes lead to uncontrolled signaling of mTORC1 and formation of harmatomas throughout the entire body.

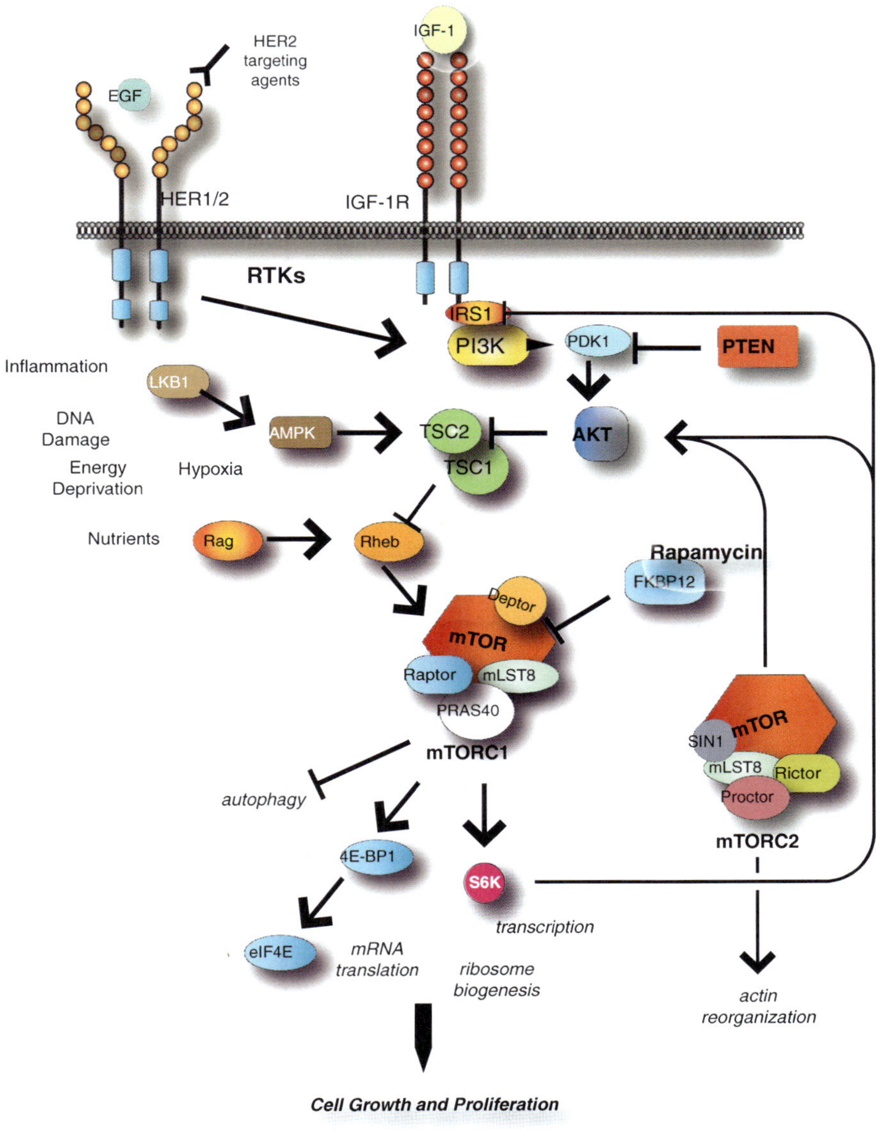

Fig. 1 The mTOR pathway [modified from Laplante and Sabatini (2012), Houghton (2010), O'Reilly and McSheehy (2010), Levine et al. (2006)]. *Deptor* DEP domain-containing mTOR-interacting protein; *EGF* epidermal growth factor; *eIF4E* Eukaryotic translation initiation factor 4E; *4E-BP* eukaryotic initiation factor 4E (eIF-4E) binding protein; *FKBP* FK506 binding protein; *HER* human epidermal growth factor receptor; *IGF(R)* insulin-like growth factor (receptor); *IRS1* insulin receptor substrate 1; *LKB1* liver kinase B1; *AMPK* adenine monophosphate-activated protein kinase, *mLST8* mammalian lethal with SEC13 protein 8; *mTOR* mammalian target of rapamycin; complex; *PDK1* 3-phosphoinositide-dependent protein kinase-1; *PI3K* Phosphatidylinositide 3-kinase; *PRAS* Proline-rich AKT1 substrate 1; *Proctor* protein observed with Rictor; *PTEN* Phosphatase and tensin homolog; *Rag & Rheb* small GTPases; *Raptor* regulatory-associated protein of mTOR; *Rictor* rapamycin-insensitive companion of mTOR; *S6K* Ribosomal protein S6 kinase; *SIN* stress-activated protein kinase interacting protein 1

From an oncologist's perspective, the PI3K/mTOR pathway is an interesting therapeutic target as it is involved in many cellular processes (Bjornsti and Houghton 2004):

- mTOR functions as a sensor of mitogens, growth factors, and energy and nutrient levels.
- mTOR facilitates G1-S cell cycle progression.
- The PI3K/mTOR/PTEN pathway is frequently dysregulated in human cancers.
- mTOR is involved in the production of pro-angiogenic factors (i.e., VEGF) and inhibition of endothelial cell growth and proliferation.
- mTOR can inactivate eukaryotic initiation factor 4E binding proteins and activate the 40S ribosomal S6 kinases, regulating protein translation, including the HIF-1 proteins.
- Oncogenic transformation may sensitize tumor cells to mTOR inhibition.

2 Structure and Mechanism of Action

Everolimus [RAD001, Afinitor® (40-O-(2-hydroxyethyl)-rapamycin)] is a derivative of rapamycin (sirolimus) (Fig. 2). It is an orally available selective inhibitor of mTOR. Like Rapamycin, it binds FKBP12 and inhibits the mTORC1 complex (Fig. 1), abrogating downstream signaling of this pathway. mTORC1 is a downstream signal transducer of the PI3K pathway, which is frequently activated in human malignancies. Everolimus, like rapamycin, does not affect the activity of mTORC2 complex. Based on its mechanism of action, everolimus is not expected induce rapid cell death but rather to slow tumor growth.

3 Preclinical Data

Everolimus and other rapalogs inhibit the proliferation of various human tumor cell lines and human umbilical vein endothelial cells in vitro. The IC_{50} (dose at which growth is inhibited by 50 %) ranges from sub-nanomolar to micromolar, depending on the cell type. In vitro everolimus reduces expression of HIF1 and VEGF, suggesting that everolimus may also act as an anti-angiogenic agent. This anti-angiogenic activity of everolimus was confirmed in vivo. Mice with primary and metastatic tumors treated with everolimus showed a significant reduction in blood vessel density when compared to controls (Lane et al. 2009). The pharmacokinetic profile of everolimus in rats and mice showed sufficient tumor penetration, above what was needed to inhibit the proliferation of endothelial cells and tumor cell lines in vitro, and below concentrations reached in humans (O'Reilly et al. 2010). Everolimus administered daily p.o. potently inhibited tumor growth in multiple different mouse and rat xenograft models.

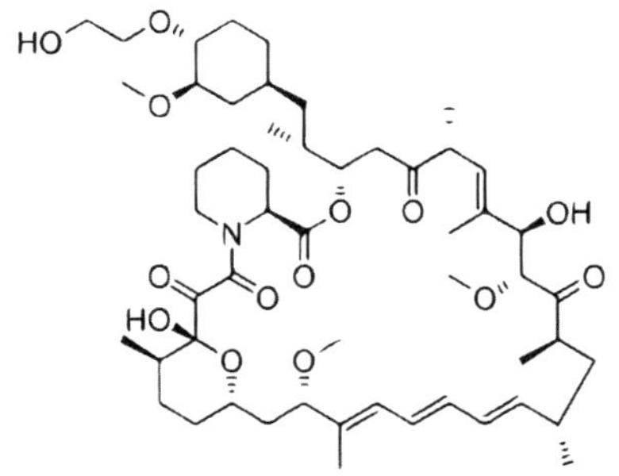

International non-proprietary name:	Everolimus
Synonyms:	RAD001
Molecular Weight:	958.2 Daltons
Molecular Formula:	$C_{53}H_{83}NO_{14}$

Chemical Name:	(1R,9S,12S,15R,16E,18R,19R,21R,23S,24E,26E,28E,30S,32S,35R)-1,18-dihydroxy-12-(1R)-2-[(1S,3R,4R)-4-(2-hydroxyethoxy)-3-methoxycyclohexyl]-1-methylethyl}-19,30-dimethoxy-15,17,21,23,29,35-hexamethyl-11,36-dioxa-4-aza-tricyclo[30.3.1.04,9] hexatriaconta-16,24,26,28-tetraene-2,3,10,14,20-pentaone
Formulations:	Four strengths of tablets (2.5 mg, 5 mg, 7.5 mg, 10 mg). Store dry at room temperature, away from heat, moisture, and light.

Source:
CSID:24747358,http://www.chemspider.com/Chemical-Structure.24747358.html (accessed 20:52, May 6, 2013)

Fig. 2 Chemical structure of everolimus

4 Clinical Data

In addition to being a potent immunosuppressive agent, everolimus is currently being investigated as an anticancer agent based on its potential to act directly on the tumor by inhibiting tumor cell growth and proliferation and indirectly by inhibiting angiogenesis (via potent inhibition of tumor cell VEGF production and VEGF-induced proliferation of endothelial cells). At time of writing 212 active interventional, investigator-initiated or industry-sponsored phase I–IV trials were registered at www.cinicaltrials.gov (Table 1). Of those, 147 trials are actively recruiting patients (35 phase I, 43 phase I/II, 50 phase II, 2 phase II/III, 9 phase III, and 8 phase IV).

4.1 Pharmacokinetics and Pharmacodynamics

In a dose-escalation study of everolimus in 92 patients with advanced cancer patients, everolimus was rapidly absorbed after oral administration, with a median time to peak blood levels (tmax) of 1–2 hours after administration. Maximum tolerated dose (MTD) was not reached. The blood concentration was dose proportional over the dose range tested while maximum blood concentration C_{max} appeared to plateau at dose levels higher than 20 mg/week (O'Donnell et al. 2008). The terminal half-life was 30 h (range, 26–38 h) similar to that in healthy volunteers. Inter-patient variability was moderate. High-fat meals alter the absorption of everolimus. Everolimus is metabolized and excreted into the feces >80 %.

Table 1 Active clinical trials with everolimus

Indication	I	I/II	II	II/III	III	IV
Advanced cancer	13	1	4			1
Brain tumors	2	5	2			
Breast cancer	1	3	15		8	2
Gastroesophageal cancer	1	3	2		2	
Hepatocellular cancer (HCC)	1	1	6		1	
GI (CRC, pancreatic cancer, BTC)		5	1			
GYN (Ovarian, endometria, cervical cancer)	2		5			
Head and neck cancer		5	2			
Acute lymphoblastic leukemia	1	1				
Acute myelogenous leukemia	1					
Lung cancer (NSCLC)	3	1				
Non-Hodgkin lymphoma (NHL)	3	10	5		1	
Hodgkin lymphoma (HL)		1	1			
Neuroendocrine tumors (NET)	4	4	7		3	2
Other (CML (uveal) melanoma, EBV-driven tumors, germ cell tumors, PKD, CUP, mesothelioma)	1	1	6	1		
Prostate cancer	2	1	5			
Kidney cancer (RCC)	1	4	19		4	3
Sarcoma		3				
Osteosarcoma		2	1			
Thyroid cancer		3	1			
Tuberous sclerosis complex (TSC)		3	1	1	3	
Urothelial cancer	1	1	2			

GI gastrointestinal cancer; *HCC* hepatocellular cancer; *CRC* colorectal cancer; *BTC* biliary tract cancer; *GYN* gynecological cancer; *NSCLC* non-small-cell lung cancer; *CML* chronic myelogenous leukemia; *EBV* Epstein–Barr virus; *PKD* polycystic kidney disease; *CUP* carcinoma of unknown primary; *RCC* renal cell carcinoma

Pharmacodynamic modeling based on S6 kinase inhibition in peripheral blood mononuclear cells suggested 5–10 mg daily to be an adequate dose to produce a high degree of sustained target inhibition (O'Donnell et al. 2008).

4.2 Clinical Development of Everolimus

Based on the mode of action, preclinical results and early clinical activity of everolimus across different tumor types, Novartis launched the WIDE (Worldwide Initiative to Develop Everolimus) program to develop everolimus in a broad range of malignancies as well as TSC. Main indications in which everolimus is developed are as follows:

- Breast cancer (BOLERO: breast cancer trials of oral everolimus).
- Gastric cancer (GRANITE: gastric antitumor trial with everolimus).
- Hepatocellular cancer (EVOLVE: everolimus for liver cancer evaluation).
- Liver cancer (EVOLVE: everolimus for liver cancer evaluation).
- Lymphoma (PILLAR: pivotal lymphoma trials of RAD001).
- Neuroendocrine tumors (RADIANT: RAD001 in advanced neuroendocrine tumors).
- Renal cell carcinoma (RECORD: renal cell cancer treatment with oral RAD001 given daily).
- TSC (EXIST: examining everolimus in a study of TSC).

The majority of these trials are in late stage, have either results or results are shortly awaited. In the following, the major indications in which everolimus has been or is being investigated, either as single agent or in combination with other agents, will be discussed.

4.2.1 Clinical Studies in Breast Cancer

Hormone-Receptor-Positive, HER2-Negative Breast Cancer

The development of everolimus in breast cancer followed a very strong lead from preclinical results, which translated nicely into early clinical activity. Proliferation of breast cancer cells is driven by the estrogen receptor (ER) and the human epidermal growth factor receptor (HER) family. The PI3K/AKT/mTOR pathway modulates these signals and can support resistance to endocrine therapy. mTORC1 activates S6K, which then can phosphorylate and activate the ER. Combination of everolimus with aromatase inhibitors inhibited proliferation and induced apoptosis in MCF7 cells (Boulay et al. 2005).

A phase I trial of everolimus in combination with letrozole reported promising clinical responses, with a manageable safety profile of the combination (Awada et al. 2008). Based on these results, a neoadjuvant, randomized phase II trial (NCT00107016) was launched. A total of 270 postmenopausal women were randomized to receive either 4 months of letrozole (2.5 mg/day) plus everolimus (10 mg/day) or letrozole plus placebo. Response rate and biomarker inhibition were higher in the everolimus arm (Baselga et al. 2009).

The BOLERO-2 trial was the logical continuation of these trials of everolimus in combination with hormonal therapy. This randomized phase III trial compared the efficacy of exemestane (25 mg/day) in combination with everolimus (10 mg/day) versus exemestane in combination with placebo. A total of 724 patients with HR-positive, advanced progressive or recurrent breast cancer who were refractory to letrozole or anastrozole were randomized 2:1 to everolimus or placebo. The primary end point was progression-free survival. Both arms were well balanced. At time of a preplanned interim analysis after 359 PFS events had been reported, median PFS was 6.9 months with exemestane plus placebo versus A total of

2.8 months with exemestane plus placebo (HR 0.43; 95 % CI 0.35–0.54; $p < 0.001$) based on local assessment, and 10.6 versus 4.1 months according to central assessment (HR 0.36; 95 % CI 0.27–0.47; $p < 0.001$) (Baselga 2012). This led to the approval of everolimus in combination with exemestane for treatment of post-menopausal women with advanced hormone-receptor (HR)-positive, HER2-negative breast cancer with recurrence or progression after treatment with letrozole or anastrozole in July 2012 by the FDA and the EMA.

Multiple other trials of everolimus in various combinations are currently active, e.g., BOLERO-4 (Open-label, Phase II, Study of Everolimus Plus Letrozole in Postmenopausal Women With ER+ Metastatic Breast Cancer), BOLERO-6 (A Phase II Study of Everolimus in Combination With Exemestane Versus Everolimus Alone Versus Capecitabine in Advance Breast Cancer), and VICTORIA (Study to Compare Vinorelbine In Combination With the mTOR Inhibitor Everolimus versus Vinorelbine monotherapy for Second-line Treatment in Advanced Breast Cancer).

HER2-Positive Breast Cancer

Preclinical studies suggested that PI3K inhibitors could overcome PTEN loss-induced resistance to trastuzumab in HER2-positive breast cancer cells in vitro and in vivo (Lu et al. 2007; Nagata et al. 2004). Clinical evidence of activity of everolimus in combination with a trastuzumab-containing regimen came from two phase I/II studies.

Study NCT00426556 was a single-arm, open-label dose-escalation trial designed to evaluate the feasibility, dose, and schedule for combining everolimus with weekly paclitaxel and trastuzumab (Andre et al. 2010). A total of 33 patients with HER2-positive advanced breast cancer previously treated with trastuzumab were treated with everolimus 5 mg/day, 10 mg/day, or 30 mg/week in combination with paclitaxel (80 mg/m^2 days 1, 8, and 15 every 4 week) and trastuzumab (2 mg/kg/week). Neutropenia (Grade 3 to 4) was the most common toxicity observed ($n = 17$ patients). On the basis of observed dose-limiting toxicities and overall safety considerations, everolimus 10 mg/day was chosen for further development. Among patients with measurable disease ($n = 27$), ORR was 44 %. Median PFS was promising (34 weeks; 95 % CI 29.1–40.7 weeks).

The second phase I/II study (NCT00426530) investigated trastuzumab and vinorelbine plus everolimus. Fifty patients with HER2-positive metastatic breast cancer pretreated with trastuzumab were enrolled in this Bayesian dose-escalation study to receive everolimus 5 mg/day, 20 mg/week, or 30 mg/week plus vinorelbine (25 mg/m^2 on day 1 and 8 every 3 week) and trastuzumab (2 mg/kg/week). Again, neutropenia (grade 3/4) was the most frequently observed toxicity (DLT), and everolimus 5 mg/day was selected for further development. Disease control was achieved in 83 % of patients; the median duration of response was 32.7 weeks for CR/PR and 38.6 weeks for SD (Jerusalem et al. 2011). Based on these results, 2 phase III trials, BOLERO-1&3 were launched.

The BOLERO-1 phase III trial (NCT00876395) is comparing the efficacy of placebo or everolimus in combination with trastuzumab and paclitaxel, as first-line therapy advanced HER2-positive breast cancer. Recruitment has been completed, and results are awaited in the near future.

The BOLERO-3 phase III trial (NCT01007942) compared the combination of trastuzumab and vinorelbine with everolimus versus trastuzumab and vinorelbine with placebo in patients with HER2-positive advanced breast cancer previously treated with a taxane and who were resistant to trastuzumab. A total of 569 patients were randomized in a 1:1 ratio and stratified by prior lapatinib use. Primary endpoint of the study was PFS. Study treatment was continued until tumor progression or intolerable toxicity. Study results were recently presented at ASCO 2013 (O'Regan R, et al. ASCO 2013, abstract #505). Arms were well balanced. The primary endpoint was PFS by local assessment. The primary efficacy analysis showed a statistically significant prolongation of median PFS from 5.8 months in the placebo arm to 7.0 months in the everolimus arm corresponding to an estimated 22 % risk reduction for PFS (HR = 0.78; 95 % CI 0.65–0.95; $p < 0.0067$). Subgroup analyses favored the everolimus arm, and no difference in global quality of life was noted. At time of the cut-off date (March 15, 2013), OS data were immature. In the light of newly available HER2-targeting treatment options like pertuzumab (Swain et al. 2013, 2012) and T-DM1 (Verma et al. 2012), the clinical implications of the BOLERO-3 results need to be carefully evaluated.

Triple Negative Breast Cancer

Data on everolimus in triple negative breast cancer might be of interest but await confirmation in larger patient cohorts (Singh et al. 2012 San Francisco Breast Cancer Symposium, abstract #108).

4.2.2 Clinical Studies in Gastric Cancer

Based on results from few smaller phase II trials, which had shown limited activity of everolimus (Doi et al. 2010; Taguchi et al. 2011; Yoon et al. 2012); GRANITE-1 (NCT00879333) was designed. Results of this phase III trial in previously treated patients with advanced gastric cancer were presented at the ASCO Gastrointestinal Cancers Symposium 2012 (J Clin Oncol 30, 2012 suppl 4; abstr LBA3). In this trial, 656 patients were randomized 2:1 to receive everolimus (10 mg/day) plus BSC or placebo plus BSC. Baseline characteristics were well balanced. The primary endpoint, prolongation of OS, was not reached. Median OS was 5.4 months with everolimus versus 4.3 months with placebo (HR 0.90; 95 % CI 0.75–1.08; $p = 0.124$). Secondary endpoints included PFS and ORR. Median PFS per local assessment was 1.7 versus 1.4 months with PBO (HR 0.66; 95 % CI 0.56–0.78; $p < 0.0001$).

4.2.3 Clinical Studies in Liver Cancer

Preclinical evidence for a possible role of mTOR in HCC came from xenograft models, in which everolimus suppressed xenograft growth, provided the rationale for investigation of everolimus in HCC (Huynh et al. 2009; Villanueva et al. 2008). One phase I/II trial in 28 patients with HCC determined 10 mg/day as recommended dose for phase II. Although possible clinical activity was noted, the trial did not reach its phase II stage (Zhu et al. 2011). One phase III study in HCC compared the efficacy of everolimus (10 mg/day) versus placebo (EVOLVE-1). In this trial, 546 patients with HCC after failure of sorafenib were randomized (2:1) to receive everolimus 7.5 mg/day or placebo. The primary endpoint of prolongation of overall survival was not met.[1]

4.2.4 Clinical Studies in Lymphoma

Preclinical results showed increased sensitivity of everolimus-treated diffuse large B-cell lymphoma (DLBCL) cells to rituximab in vitro (Wanner et al. 2006), and an increased cytotoxic effect when combined with other agents in mantle cell lymphoma (MCL) (Haritunians et al. 2007; Nishioka et al. 2008), and in other models (Crazzolara et al. 2009; Saunders et al. 2011; Xu et al. 2013).

Everolimus showed promising clinical activity as single agent in heavily pretreated Hodgkin lymphoma (HL). Of nineteen patients treated with everolimus (10 mg/day), eight patients achieved a PR and one patient achieved a CR. Median time to progression was 7.2 months (Johnston et al. 2010).

Study NCT00516412 evaluated the activity of everolimus in MCL (Renner et al. 2012). In thirty-five evaluable patients (median age 69), ORR was 20 % (95 % CI 8–37(, median PFS was 5.5 months (95 % CI 2.8–8.2). Another phase II trial investigated everolimus in 77 patients with relapsed/refractory aggressive NHL (47 DLBCL, 19 MCL, 8 FL, 3 other). Median age was 70 years, median number of prior therapies 3 (range 1–15). ORR was 30 % (95 % CI 20–41 %). ORR for patients with DLBCL was 30, 32 % for MCL and 38 % for FL. Median time to progression was 3.4 months (95 % CI 2.1–4.2), median progression-free survival was 3.0 months (95 % CI 2.1–3.9), and median overall survival was 8.1 months (95 % CI 5.3–12.5) (Witzig et al. 2011). Combination of everolimus with rituximab in 26 patients with relapsed DLBCL led to a response rate of 38 % (90 % CI 21–56). Median duration of response was 8.1 months (Barnes et al. 2013).

The PILLAR-1 trial (NCT00702052) was an open-label, single-arm, phase II study evaluating everolimus (10 mg/day) in patients with bortezomib-refractory MCL. The primary endpoint was ORR, secondary endpoints included PFS, OS, and duration of response. Preliminary results were presented at ASH 2010 (O'Connor et al. 2010) and updated at ASH 2012 (Wang et al. 2012). Full results are published in the Novartis Clinical Trial Results Database.[2] In this trial in 58 patients with heavily pretreated MCL, everolimus only showed very modest activity with an ORR of 8.6 % (90 % CI 3.5–17.3), thus failing the primary endpoint.

PILLAR-2 (NCT00790036) is an ongoing randomized, placebo-controlled phase III trial evaluating everolimus as maintenance therapy in patients with poor risk DLBCL who have achieved CR after rituximab-containing first-line therapy.

---

[1] Novartis press release http://www.novartis.com/newsroom/media-releases/en/2013/1721562.shtml.

[2] http://www.novctrd.com/ctrdWebApp/clinicaltrialrepository/displayFile.do?trialResult=8443

The primary endpoint is disease-free survival (DFS). Secondary endpoints are OS, lymphoma-specific survival, and safety.

4.2.5 Clinical Studies in Neuroendocrine tumors

Phase II Studies in NET

Two initial phase II studies were conducted in NET. The first trial conducted by J. Yao at the MD Anderson Cancer Center evaluated treatment with everolimus 5 or 10 mg/day plus depot octreotide 30 mg (LAR) every 28 days in patients with metastatic or unresectable, well-differentiated, neuroendocrine tumors (Yao et al. 2008). The overall median PFS of patients treated with octreotide LAR and everolimus was 60 weeks (95 % CI 54–66 weeks). Stratified by tumor group, median PFS of patients with carcinoid and islet cell tumors was 63 weeks (95 % CI 55–71 weeks) and 50 weeks (95 % CI 31–70 weeks), respectively (HR 1.2; 95 % CI 0.7–2.2).

An additional open-label, non-randomized phase II study in 160 patients with pancreatic neuroendocrine tumors (PNET) stratified by ongoing octreotide therapy at study entry (Yao et al. 2010). Patients who were not being treated with octreotide at study entry were assigned to Stratum 1 ($n = 115$, everolimus 10 mg/day), and patients treated with octreotide LAR for at least 3 consecutive months at study entry were assigned to Stratum 2 ($n = 45$, everolimus 10 mg/day and octreotide LAR every 28 days). Median PFS was 9.7 months (95 % CI 8.3–13.3 months) in Stratum 1, and 16.7 months (95 % CI 11.1 months-NA) in Stratum 2. Median OS in Stratum 1 was 24.9 months (95 % CI 20.2–27.1 months). Median OS had not been reached for Stratum 2 at the time of data cutoff.

Phase III Studies in NET

Two Phase III clinical trials have investigated the efficacy and safety of everolimus in NETs, the RADIANT 2&3 trials.

RADIANT-3 was an international, multicenter, double-blind, phase III study to compare the efficacy of everolimus against placebo in patents with advanced progressive PNET (Yao et al. 2011). A total of 410 patients from 18 countries were randomly assigned to receive everolimus (207 patients) or placebo (203 patients) until disease progression or intolerable toxicity. Patients assigned to placebo were allowed to crossover to everolimus upon progression. The median PFS (the primary end point) by local investigator was 11.0 months (95 % CI 8.4–13.9) in the everolimus group, as compared with 4.6 months (95 % CI 3.1–5.4) in the placebo group (HR 0.35; 95 % CI 0.27–0.45; $p < 0.001$). Median overall survival was not reached, and no significant difference between the groups was observed (HR 1.05; 95 % CI 0.71–1.55; $p = 0.59$).

Based on this trial, everolimus was approved in 2011 by the FDA for the treatment of progressive neuroendocrine tumors of pancreatic origin (PNET) in patients with unresectable, locally advanced or metastatic disease and by the EMA for the treatment of unresectable or metastatic, well- or moderately differentiated neuroendocrine tumors (NET) of pancreatic origin in adults with progressive disease.

RADIANT-2 was a prospective, randomized, double-blind, multicenter, placebo-controlled phase III study to evaluate the safety and efficacy of everolimus 10 mg/day plus octreotide LAR or matching placebo plus octreotide LAR in patients with advanced carcinoid tumor (Pavel et al. 2011). Patients enrolled had to have a progressive, advanced, well-differentiated carcinoid tumors and had to have symptoms related to carcinoid syndrome at enrollment or prior to enrollment ("functional NET"). Four hundred and twenty-nine patients with advanced functional NET were enrolled to this study worldwide, 216 were randomized to treatment with octreotide +everolimus and 213 to treatment with octreotide plus placebo. Primary endpoint was again PFS. This trial was complicated by several factors: Imbalances at baseline and opposing/conflicting results in local and central response assessment interpretations. Results as per the amended primary endpoint [PFS assessed by an independent adjudication radiology committee (IAC)] showed a 5.1-month prolongation in median PFS from 11.3 months for octreotide plus placebo to 16.4 months for octreotide plus everolimus (HR 0.77). Nevertheless, statistical significance was not reached, as the prespecified statistical boundary was missed. No statistically significant difference was evident in terms of overall survival, although numerically more deaths were reported from the everolimus treatment group (HR 1.22; 95 % CI: 0.91, 1.62; $p = 0.908$).

The RADIANT-4 trial (NCT01524783) is currently recruiting patients with advanced non-functioning NET of gastrointestinal or lung origin to compare the efficacy of everolimus + best supportive care (BSC) versus placebo + BSC. As this trial excludes patients with functional NET, somatostatin analogs are not allowed as concomitant medication. Other recruiting trials evaluating everolimus in NET are, for example, the LUNA trial (lung and thymic NET, NCT01563354) and the COOPERATE trials (gastroenteropancreatic NET, NCT01374451, NCT01263353).

4.2.6 Clinical Studies in Kidney Cancer

Based on strong preclinical rationale and early clinical results, several phase II and III trials in RCC were launched.

RECORD-1 (NCT00410124) was a randomized, double-blind, placebo-controlled phase III trial of everolimus in patients with metastatic RCC after progression on VEGF-targeted therapy. Four hundred and sixteen patients were randomized 2:1 to receive everolimus (10 mg/day) ($n = 272$) or placebo ($n = 138$). The primary endpoint was PFS, assessed by central review. Results at the second prespecified interim analysis suggested a significant difference in efficacy between arms, and the trial was stopped early after 191 PFS events had been observed. Median PFS was 4.0 months (95 % CI 3.7–5.5) versus 1.9 months (95 % CI 1.8–1.9) (Motzer et al. 2008). Final results confirmed the early results with a median PFS of 4.9 months (95 % CI 4.0–5.5) with everolimus versus 1.9 months (95 % CI 1.8–1.9) with placebo (HR 0.33; 95 % CI 0.25–0.43; $p < 0.001$). OS was similar in both arms (Median OS 14.8 vs. 14.4 months; HR 0.87; 95 % CI 0.65–1.15; $p = 0.162$) but was likely confounded by a high percentage (80 %) crossover to everolimus (Motzer et al. 2010). Based on

RECORD-1, the FDA and EMA approved everolimus for the treatment of patient with advanced RCC after failure of sunitinib or sorafenib.

The first data on combination of everolimus and bevacizumab in RCC came from trial NCT00323739 (Hainsworth et al. 2010). Eighty patients with advanced RCC (50 treatment naïve, 30 previously treated) received bevacizumab (10 mg/kg on days 1 and 15) and everolimus (10 mg/day). Median PFS in treatment naïve and previously treated patients were 9.1 and 7.1 months. Based on promising preliminary data from this trial, two larger randomized studies investigating the combination of everolimus and bevacizumab were launched.

RECORD-2 (NCT00719264) was a randomized, open-label, multicenter phase II study comparing the efficacy and safety of everolimus in combination with bevacizumab (EB) versus interferon-α in combination with bevacizumab (IB) as first-line treatment for patients with metastatic RCC. Patients were stratified according to their MSKCC risk status (favorable vs. intermediate vs. poor). Primary endpoint was PFS; secondary endpoints included OS, ORR, and duration of response, safety, and QoL. Final results for OS and safety were presented at ASCO 2013 demonstrating that EB was not superior to IB. Median OS was 27.1 months (95 % CI 19.9–35.3) in the EB arm, and 27.1 months (95 % CI 20.4–30.8) in the IB arm (HR 1.01; 95 % CI 0.75–1.34; $p = 0.96$) (Ravaud et al., ASCO 2013, abstract # 4576). Both arms showed similar PFS, response rates, and time to definitive deterioration of QoL.

The CALGB-90802 study (NCT01198158), a large randomized phase III trial, is comparing everolimus plus bevacizumab versus everolimus plus placebo after failure of ≥ 1 prior VEGFR TKI.

RECORD-3 (NCT00903175) was recently presented at ASCO 2013 (Motzer et al., ASCO 2013 abstract #4504). RECORD-3 was a randomized phase II trial comparing sequential first-line everolimus and second-line sunitinib versus first-line sunitinib and second-line everolimus in patients with metastatic RCC. Primary objective was to show PFS non-inferiority of first-line everolimus compared with first-line sunitinib. Secondary objectives included the comparison of combined PFS for the two sequences of treatment, ORR, and OS. A total of 471 treatment-naïve patients with metastatic RCC were included. The trial failed to show non-inferiority. Median PFS in first-line with everolimus was 7.85 months compared to 10.71 months with sunitinib (HR = 1.43; 95 % CI 1.15–1.77). ORR clearly favored sunitinib (26.6 %; 95 % CI 21.1–32.8) over everolimus (8 %; 95 % CI 4.9–12.2). The analysis of the combined PFS also clearly favored sunitinib as first-line. PFS in the everolimus-sunitinib arm was 21.13 months compared to 25.79 months in the sunitinib-everolimus arm (HR = 1.28; 95 % CI 0.94–1.73). Results presented clearly showed that a VEGF-TKI should be standard first-line treatment for advanced RCC, and that everolimus is a good option for second-line therapy.

The currently recruiting RECORD-4 (NCT01491672) trial will assess efficacy (PFS) of everolimus in second-line treatment of advanced RCC in three different cohorts. Patients are enrolled in one of three cohorts based upon their first-line therapy: (1) prior cytokines, (2) prior sunitinib, or (3) prior anti-VEGF therapy other than sunitinib.

4.2.7 Clinical Studies in TSC

TSC is an autosomal dominant genetic disorder that results from mutations in the TSC1 or TSC2 genes. TSC is characterized by development of benign tumors (harmatomas) throughout the body. Manifestations of TSC vary from individual to individual, ranging from mild symptoms to physical and intellectual disabilities (Orlova and Crino 2010). Approximately 1/3 of cases are inherited, whereas 2/3 are de novo mutations. TSC1 mutations appear to be more common in familial (inherited) cases of TSC, while mutations in the TSC2 gene occur more frequently in sporadic cases. Inactivating mutations in TSC1 and TSC2 release their inhibitory effect on mTORC1 and subsequent hyperproliferation. Accordingly, mTOR inhibitors were very attractive molecules to find novel treatment options for TSC. Meikle and colleagues demonstrated very good activity of rapalogs in a mouse model for TSC1 (Meikle et al. 2008), where median survival was prolonged from 33 to >100 days. Rapamycin also improved cognitive defects in a TSC2-deficient mouse model (Ehninger et al. 2008). Building on this strong preclinical rationale, an investigator-initiated phase I/II trial (NCT00411619) in children and adults with TSC suffering from subependymal giant cell astrocytomas (SEGA) was conducted. A total of 28 patients were enrolled to receive everolimus 3 mg/day. There was a clinically meaningful reduction in volume of the primary SEGA ($p < 0.001$ for baseline versus 6 months (Krueger et al. 2010). Based on these results, a full clinical development program (EXIST) was launched.

EXIST-1 was a randomized, double-blind phase III trial to assess the efficacy and safety of everolimus in patients with SEGA associated with TSC. A total of 117 patients were randomized 2:1–4.5 mg/m^2/day (titrated to achieve blood trough concentrations of 5–15 ng/ml) everolimus ($n = 78$) or placebo ($n = 39$). A total of 27 (35 %) patients in the everolimus arm had a ≥50 % reduction in SEGA volume versus none in the placebo group ($p < 0.0001$) (Franz et al. 2013).

EXIST-2 (NCT00790400) was a randomized phase III trial in adult patients with angiomyolipoma associated with TSC. A total of 118 patients were randomized 2:1 to receive everolimus 10 mg/day ($n = 79$) or matching placebo ($n = 39$). The primary endpoint was the proportion of patients with confirmed ≥50 % reduction in total volume of target angiomyolipomas relative to baseline. The angiomyolipoma response rate was 42 % (95 % CI 31–53) for everolimus versus 0 % (95 % CI 0–9) in the placebo group (Bissler et al. 2013).

Based on EXIST-1&2, everolimus was approved for treatment of adults with renal angiomyolipoma and TSC, not requiring immediate surgery, and pediatric and adult patients with TSC who have SEGA that requires therapeutic intervention but cannot be curatively resected.

There is accumulating evidence that mTOR activation might be involved not only in TSC development but also drive seizures in TSC patients (Wong 2012). EXIST-3 is a three-arm, randomized, double-blind, placebo-controlled study of the efficacy and safety of 2 trough ranges of everolimus as adjunctive therapy in patients TSC who have refractory partial-onset seizures. Patients are randomized 1:1:1 to receive either everolimus titrated to 3–7 ng/ml or to 9–15 ng/ml, or matching placebo. This multicenter study will enroll 345 patients globally, at approximately 125 sites. Participants must have a definite diagnosis of TSC based on the modified Gomez criteria and a diagnosis of partial-onset epilepsy according to the classification of the International League Against Epilepsy prior to enrollment. Primary objective is to compare the reduction in frequency of partial-onset seizures on each of 2 trough ranges of everolimus versus placebo in patients with TSC who are taking 1–3 anti-seizure drugs.

5 Toxicity

Everolimus has been investigated in over 30,000 patients in clinical studies and in post-marketing experience. In cancer patients, the main adverse events reported with everolimus were: stomatitis, non-infectious pneumonitis, infections, and renal failure. In addition, laboratory abnormalities, mainly hyperglycemia, hyperlipidemia, anemia, neutropenia, and thrombocytopenia were reported. For a recent and complete list of adverse drug reactions, please refer to your local drug label or package insert.

6 Drug Interactions

Everolimus is mainly metabolized by CYP3A4 in the liver and to some extent in the intestinal wall. Everolimus is also a substrate of P-glycoprotein (PGP). Therefore, absorption and subsequent elimination of systematically absorbed everolimus may be influenced by medications that interact with CYP3A4 and/or PGP. In vitro studies showed that everolimus is a competitive inhibitor of CYP3A4 and of CYP2D6 substrates, potentially increasing the concentrations of medicinal products eliminated by these enzymes. Strong inhibitors of CYP3A4 (azoles, antifungals, cyclosporine, erythromycin) have been shown to reduce the clearance of everolimus therapy, thereby increasing everolimus blood levels. Similarly, Rifampin, a strong inducer of CYP3A4, increases the clearance of everolimus thereby reducing everolimus blood levels. Caution should be exercised when co-administering everolimus with CYP3A4 inhibitors or inducers.

7 Biomarkers

To date, no valid predictive or prognostic biomarker for everolimus across all indications tested has been identified. S6K1 activity in peripheral blood mononuclear cells seems one of the most reliable biomarkers for target inhibition by everolimus (O'Reilly and McSheehy 2010). Hortobagyi presented a tissue-based biomarker analysis at ASCO 2013 (Abstract #505). In this retrospective exploratory analysis, 309 archival tissue samples from BOLERO-2 3230 exons of 182 oncogenes and tumor suppressor genes were analyzed using next generation sequencing. No predictive marker for response to treatment with everolimus could be identified, as treatment effect was similar in all molecular subgroups analyzed. Only a small subset of patients whose tumors showed amplification of the FGF receptors (FGFR) 1 or 2 seemed to derive smaller benefit of everolimus than patients with FGFR wild type tumors (HR 0.59, 95 % CI 0.31–1,14 vs. HR 0.36, 95 % CI 0.24–0.53, $n = 48$ vs. 114).

8 Summary and Perspectives

Everolimus is an inhibitor of the mTOR pathway, specifically mTORC1. Based on its ubiquitous expression and central role multiple cellular signaling pathways, mTOR is an interesting target for cancer therapy. So far, clinical investigations based on sound preclinical rationale have led to the approval of everolimus for the treatment of the following:

- postmenopausal women with advanced HR-positive, HER2-negative breast cancer (advanced HR+ BC) in combination with exemestane after failure of treatment with letrozole or anastrozole
- adults with progressive neuroendocrine tumors of pancreatic origin (PNET) that are unresectable, locally advanced or metastatic. The safety and effectiveness of AFINITOR in the treatment of patients with carcinoid tumors have not been established
- adults with advanced renal cell carcinoma (RCC) after failure of treatment with sunitinib or sorafenib
- adults with renal angiomyolipoma and TSC, not requiring immediate surgery
- pediatric and adult patients with TSC who have SEGA that requires therapeutic intervention but cannot be curatively resected.

Several registration trials have failed, as the data at the time of decision to move into a phase III trial were not too convincing. Nevertheless, compared to other development programs in the industry, the story if everolimus is clearly a success story. More data from phase III trials are awaited in the not too far future. Hopefully, these trials will open new treatment options for our patients.

References

Andre F et al (2010) Phase I study of everolimus plus weekly paclitaxel and trastuzumab in patients with metastatic breast cancer pretreated with trastuzumab. J Clin Oncol: Official J Am Soc Clin Oncol 28(34):5110–5115

Awada A et al (2008) The oral mTOR inhibitor RAD001 (everolimus) in combination with letrozole in patients with advanced breast cancer: results of a phase I study with pharmacokinetics. Eur J Cancer 44(1):84–91

Barnes JA et al (2013) Everolimus in combination with rituximab induces complete responses in heavily pretreated diffuse large B-cell lymphoma. Haematologica 98(4):615–619

Baselga J et al (2009) Phase II randomized study of neoadjuvant everolimus plus letrozole compared with placebo plus letrozole in patients with estrogen receptor-positive breast cancer. J Clin Oncol: Official J Am Soc Clin Oncol 27(16):2630–2637
Baselga J et al (2012a) Everolimus in postmenopausal hormone-receptor-positive advanced breast cancer. N Eng J Med 366(6):520–529
Baselga J et al (2012b) Pertuzumab plus trastuzumab plus docetaxel for metastatic breast cancer. N Eng J Med 366(2):109–119
Bissler JJ et al (2013) Everolimus for angiomyolipoma associated with tuberous sclerosis complex or sporadic lymphangioleiomyomatosis (EXIST-2): a multicentre, randomised, double-blind, placebo-controlled trial. Lancet 381(9869):817–824
Bjornsti MA, Houghton PJ (2004) The TOR pathway: a target for cancer therapy. Nat Rev Cancer 4(5):335–348
Boulay A et al (2005) Dual inhibition of mTOR and estrogen receptor signaling in vitro induces cell death in models of breast cancer. Clinical Cancer Res: Official J Am Assoc Cancer Res 11(14):5319–5328
Brown EJ et al (1994) A mammalian protein targeted by G1-arresting rapamycin-receptor complex. Nature 369(6483):756–758
Carracedo A et al (2008) Inhibition of mTORC1 leads to MAPK pathway activation through a PI3K-dependent feedback loop in human cancer. J Clin Investig 118(9):3065–3074
Chan S (2004) Targeting the mammalian target of rapamycin (mTOR): a new approach to treating cancer. Br J Cancer 91(8):1420–1424
Crazzolara R et al (2009) Potentiating effects of RAD001 (Everolimus) on vincristine therapy in childhood acute lymphoblastic leukemia. Blood 113(14):3297–3306
Doi T et al (2010) Multicenter phase II study of everolimus in patients with previously treated metastatic gastric cancer. J Clin Oncol: Official J Am Soc Clin Oncol 28(11):1904–1910
Ehninger D et al (2008) Reversal of learning deficits in a Tsc2± mouse model of tuberous sclerosis. Nat Med 14(8):843–848
Eng CP et al (1991) Inhibition of skin graft rejection in mice by rapamycin: a novel immunosuppressive macrolide. Transpl Proc 23(1 Pt 1):868–869
Franz DN et al (2013) Efficacy and safety of everolimus for subependymal giant cell astrocytomas associated with tuberous sclerosis complex (EXIST-1): a multicentre, randomised, placebo-controlled phase 3 trial. Lancet 381(9861):125–132
Geoerger B et al (2001) Antitumor activity of the rapamycin analog CCI-779 in human primitive neuroectodermal tumor/medulloblastoma models as single agent and in combination chemotherapy. Cancer Res 61(4):1527–1532
Hainsworth JD et al (2010) Phase II trial of bevacizumab and everolimus in patients with advanced renal cell carcinoma. J Clin Oncol: Official J Am Soc Clin Oncol 28(13):2131–2136
Haritunians T et al (2007) Antiproliferative activity of RAD001 (everolimus) as a single agent and combined with other agents in mantle cell lymphoma. Leukemia 21(2):333–339
Houghton PJ (2010) Everolimus. Clinical cancer research: an official journal of the American Association for Cancer Research 16(5):1368–1372
Huynh H et al (2009) RAD001 (everolimus) inhibits tumour growth in xenograft models of human hepatocellular carcinoma. J Cell Mol Med 13(7):1371–1380
Jacinto E et al (2004) Mammalian TOR complex 2 controls the actin cytoskeleton and is rapamycin insensitive. Nat Cell Biol 6(11):1122–1128
Jerusalem G et al (2011) Phase I trial of oral mTOR inhibitor everolimus in combination with trastuzumab and vinorelbine in pre-treated patients with HER2-overexpressing metastatic breast cancer. Breast Cancer Res Treat 125(2):447–455
Johnston PB et al (2010) A phase II trial of the oral mTOR inhibitor everolimus in relapsed Hodgkin lymphoma. Am J Hematol 85(5):320–324
Krueger DA et al (2010) Everolimus for subependymal giant-cell astrocytomas in tuberous sclerosis. N Eng J Med 363(19):1801–1811

Lane HA et al (2009) mTOR inhibitor RAD001 (everolimus) has antiangiogenic/vascular properties distinct from a VEGFR tyrosine kinase inhibitor. Clin Cancer Res: Official J Am Assoc Cancer Res 15(5):1612–1622

Laplante M, Sabatini DM (2012) mTOR signaling in growth control and disease. Cell 149(2):274–293

Levine AJ et al (2006) Coordination and communication between the p53 and IGF-1-AKT-TOR signal transduction pathways. Genes Dev 20(3):267–275

Lu CH et al (2007) Preclinical testing of clinically applicable strategies for overcoming trastuzumab resistance caused by PTEN deficiency. Clin Cancer Res: Official J Am Assoc Cancer Res 13(19):5883–5888

Majumder PK et al (2004) mTOR inhibition reverses Akt-dependent prostate intraepithelial neoplasia through regulation of apoptotic and HIF-1-dependent pathways. Nat Med 10(6):594–601

Mak BC, Yeung RS (2004) The tuberous sclerosis complex genes in tumor development. Cancer Invest 22(4):588–603

Manning BD, Cantley LC (2003) United at last: the tuberous sclerosis complex gene products connect the phosphoinositide 3-kinase/Akt pathway to mammalian target of rapamycin (mTOR) signalling. Biochem Soc Trans 31(Pt 3):573–578

Meikle L et al (2008) Response of a neuronal model of tuberous sclerosis to mammalian target of rapamycin (mTOR) inhibitors: effects on mTORC1 and Akt signaling lead to improved survival and function. J Neurosci: Official J Soc Neurosc 28(21):5422–5432

Mita M et al (2008) Deforolimus (AP23573) a novel mTOR inhibitor in clinical development. Expert Opin Investig Drugs 17(12):1947–1954

Motzer RJ et al (2008) Efficacy of everolimus in advanced renal cell carcinoma: a double-blind, randomised, placebo-controlled phase III trial. Lancet 372(9637):449–456

Motzer RJ et al (2010) Phase 3 trial of everolimus for metastatic renal cell carcinoma: final results and analysis of prognostic factors. Cancer 116(18):4256–4265

Motzer RJ, Barrios CH, Kim TM, Falcon S, Cosgriff T, Harker WG, Pittman KB, Sabbatini R, Rha SY, Flaig TW et al (2012) Record-3: Phase II randomized trial comparing sequential first-line everolimus (EVE) and second-line sunitinib (SUN) versus first-line SUN and second-line EVE in patients with metastatic renal cell carcinoma (mRCC). ASCO Meeting Abstracts 31(15_suppl):4504

Nagata Y et al (2004) PTEN activation contributes to tumor inhibition by trastuzumab, and loss of PTEN predicts trastuzumab resistance in patients. Cancer Cell 6(2):117–127

Nishioka C et al (2008) Blockade of mTOR signaling potentiates the ability of histone deacetylase inhibitor to induce growth arrest and differentiation of acute myelogenous leukemia cells. Leukemia 22(12):2159–2168

O'Connor OA et al (2010) PILLAR-1: preliminary results of a phase II study of mTOR inhibitor everolimus in patients with mantle cell lymphoma (MCL) who are refractory or intolerant to bortezomib. ASH Annu Meet Abstr 116(21):3963

O'Donnell A et al (2008) Phase I pharmacokinetic and pharmacodynamic study of the oral mammalian target of rapamycin inhibitor everolimus in patients with advanced solid tumors. J Clin Oncol: Official J Am Soc Clin Oncol 26(10):1588–1595

O'Reilly T, McSheehy PM (2010) Biomarker development for the clinical activity of the mTOR inhibitor everolimus (RAD001): processes, limitations, and further proposals. Transl Oncol 3(2):65–79

O'Reilly T et al (2010) Comparative pharmacokinetics of RAD001 (everolimus) in normal and tumor-bearing rodents. Cancer Chemother Pharmacol 65(4):625–639

O'Regan R, Ozguroglu M, Andre F, Toi M, Jerusalem GHM, Wilks S, Isaacs C, Xu B, Masuda N, Arena FP et al (2013) Phase III, randomized, double-blind, placebo-controlled multicenter trial of daily everolimus plus weekly trastuzumab and vinorelbine in trastuzumab-resistant, advanced breast cancer (BOLERO-3). ASCO Meeting Abstracts 31(15_suppl):505

Orlova KA, Crino PB (2010) The tuberous sclerosis complex. Ann N Y Acad Sci 1184:87–105
Pavel ME et al (2011) Everolimus plus octreotide long-acting repeatable for the treatment of advanced neuroendocrine tumours associated with carcinoid syndrome (RADIANT-2): a randomised, placebo-controlled, phase 3 study. Lancet 378(9808):2005–2012
Podsypanina K et al (2001) An inhibitor of mTOR reduces neoplasia and normalizes p70/S6 kinase activity in Pten± mice. Proc Natl Acad Sci USA 98(18):10320–10325
Renner C et al (2012) A multicenter phase II trial (SAKK 36/06) of single-agent everolimus (RAD001) in patients with relapsed or refractory mantle cell lymphoma. Haematologica 97(7):1085–1091
Sabatini DM et al (1994) RAFT1: a mammalian protein that binds to FKBP12 in a rapamycin-dependent fashion and is homologous to yeast TORs. Cell 78(1):35–43
Saunders P et al (2011) The mammalian target of rapamycin inhibitor RAD001 (everolimus) synergizes with chemotherapeutic agents, ionizing radiation and proteasome inhibitors in pre-B acute lymphocytic leukemia. Haematologica 96(1):69–77
Schuler W et al (1997) SDZ RAD, a new rapamycin derivative: pharmacological properties in vitro and in vivo. Transplantation 64(1):36–42
Sehgal SN (1995) Rapamune (Sirolimus, rapamycin): an overview and mechanism of action. Ther Drug Monit 17(6):660–665
Sehgal SN, Baker H, Vezina C (1975) Rapamycin (AY-22,989), a new antifungal antibiotic. II. Fermentation, isolation and characterization. J Antibiot 28(10):727–732
Singh JC, Stein S, Volm M, Smith JA, Novik Y, Speyer JL, Meyers M, Adams S, Omene CO, Muggia F et al (2012) Phase II trial of RAD001 plus carboplatin in patients with triple-negative metastatic breast cancer. ASCO Meeting Abstracts 30(15_suppl):e11529
Swain SM et al (2013) Pertuzumab, trastuzumab, and docetaxel for HER2-positive metastatic breast cancer (CLEOPATRA study): overall survival results from a randomised, double-blind, placebo-controlled, phase 3 study. Lancet Oncol 14(6):461–471
Taguchi F et al (2011) Efficacy of RAD001 (everolimus) against advanced gastric cancer with peritoneal dissemination. Invest New Drugs 29(6):1198–1205
Verma S et al (2012) Trastuzumab emtansine for HER2-positive advanced breast cancer. N Eng J Med 367(19):1783–1791
Villanueva A et al (2008) Pivotal role of mTOR signaling in hepatocellular carcinoma. Gastroenterology 135(6):1972–1983 (e1-11)
Wang M et al (2012) Pillar-1: multicenter phase 2 study of everolimus for patients with mantle cell lymphoma who are refractory or intolerant to bortezomib. ASH Annu Meet Abstr 120(21):2751
Wanner K et al (2006) Mammalian target of rapamycin inhibition induces cell cycle arrest in diffuse large B cell lymphoma (DLBCL) cells and sensitises DLBCL cells to rituximab. Br J Haematol 134(5):475–484
Witzig TE et al (2011) A phase II trial of the oral mTOR inhibitor everolimus in relapsed aggressive lymphoma. Leukemia 25(2):341–347
Wong M (2012) mTOR as a potential treatment target for epilepsy. Future Neurol 7(5):537–545
Xu ZZ et al (2010) Combination of rituximab and the mTOR inhibitor everolimus (RAD001) in diffuse large B cell lymphoma. Leuk Lymphoma 85(5):320–324
Yao JC et al (2008) Efficacy of RAD001 (everolimus) and octreotide LAR in advanced low- to intermediate-grade neuroendocrine tumors: results of a phase II study. J Clin Oncol: Official J Am Soc Clin Oncol 26(26):4311–4318
Yao JC et al (2010) Daily oral everolimus activity in patients with metastatic pancreatic neuroendocrine tumors after failure of cytotoxic chemotherapy: a phase II trial. J Clin Oncol: Official J Am Soc Clin Oncol 28(1):69–76
Yao JC et al (2011) Everolimus for advanced pancreatic neuroendocrine tumors. N Eng J Med 364(6):514–523

Yoon DH et al (2012) Phase II study of everolimus with biomarker exploration in patients with advanced gastric cancer refractory to chemotherapy including fluoropyrimidine and platinum. Br J Cancer 106(6):1039–1044

Zhu AX et al (2011) Phase 1/2 study of everolimus in advanced hepatocellular carcinoma. Cancer 117(22):5094–5102

Temsirolimus

Michael Schulze, Christian Stock, Massimo Zaccagnini, Dogu Teber and Jens J. Rassweiler

Abstract

Temsirolimus, an ester of sirolimus (rapamycin), selectively inhibits the kinase mammalian target of rapamycin (mTOR) and consequently blocks the translation of cell cycle regulatory proteins and prevents overexpression of angiogenic growth factors. It has been found to have antitumour activity in patients with relapsed or refractory mantle cell lymphoma (MCL). In addition, patients with advanced renal cell carcinoma (RCC) and a poor prognosis who received a once-weekly intravenous (IV) infusion of temsirolimus 25 mg experienced significant survival benefits compared with patients receiving standard interferon-α (IFN-α) therapy in a large phase III clinical study. In this study, median overall survival was 10.9 versus 7.3 months and objective response rates were 8.6 % in temsirolimus recipients versus 4.8 % IFN-α recipient group. Temsirolimus monotherapy recipients experienced significantly

M. Schulze · J. J. Rassweiler (✉)
Department of Urology SLK-Klinikum Heilbronn, Teaching Hospital
of the University of Heidelberg, Am Gesundbrunnen 20, 74074 Heidelberg, Germany
e-mail: jens.rassweiler@slk-kliniken.de

C. Stock
Department of Urology, St. Vincentius Hospital, Speyer, Germany

M. Zaccagnini
Department of Urology "U. Bracci", Policlinico Umberto I, University of Rome "La Sapienza", Rome, Italy

D. Teber
Department of Urology, University of Heidelberg, Heidelberg, Germany

U. M. Martens (ed.), *Small Molecules in Oncology*, Recent Results in Cancer Research 201, DOI: 10.1007/978-3-642-54490-3_24,

fewer grade 3 or 4 adverse events and had fewer withdrawals for adverse events than patients receiving IFN-α. The role of temsirolimus in sequential and combination therapy is yet to be found.

Contents

1 Introduction

Renal cell carcinoma (RCC) accounts for approximately 3 % of all adult malignancies and 2 % of all cancer-related deaths (Linehan et al. 2001). In US renal cell, carcinoma accounts for 2–3 % of all cancers diagnosed. Nearly 210,000 people worldwide were diagnosed with RCC in 2007, and roughly one-third of these patients presented with metastatic disease at the time of initial diagnosis (Jemal et al. 2007) with a median survival time of 10–12 months (Larkin et al. 2007).

RCC may be treated surgically for stages I–III and surgical resection (laparoscopic or open) is the mainstay for tumours that are confined to the kidney.

Most renal cell cancers (up to 85 %) are classified histologically as clear cell type. These tumours are typically (>80 %) characterized by a loss of expression of a functional von Hippel–Lindau (VHL) gene. This gene regulates protein stability of hypoxia-inducible transcription factors (HIF) (Alexandrescu and Dasanu 2006; Motzer and Bukowsky 2006). Loss of VHL function prevents the degradation of these factors and leads to their accumulation, with the subsequent increased expression of HIF-regulated proteins such as vascular endothelial growth factor (VEGF) and other angiogenic and growth-stimulating molecules.

Prior to the introduction of targeted therapies, there were limited options for systemic therapy in patients with RCC. Interleukin-2 (IL-2) and interferon-α (IFN-α) were, alone or in combination, the main treatments for metastatic renal cancer. Treatment with these agents resulted in a median survival of 12.0–17.5 months (Aass et al. 2005). Cytokine-based immunotherapy with IL-2 and IFN-α are associated with modest objective response rates of 10–15 % and substantial toxicity (Motzer and Bukowski 2006; Rosemberg et al. 1985).

A better understanding of the pathogenesis of RCC, particularly the role of tumour angiogenesis, has led to the development new therapeutic agents, with VEGF or the mammalian target of rapamycin (mTOR) being targeted (Escudier 2007).

Temsirolimus is a selective inhibitor of mTOR, a serine–threonine kinase involved in multiple tumour-promoting intracellular signalling pathways and controlling many cellular functions such as proliferation, survival, protein synthesis, and transcription of HIF-α, and it has been the first approved mTOR-targeted agent based on a phase III trial (Alexandrescu and Dasanu 2006; Hudes et al. 2007).

2 Development

Temsirolimus is a soluble ester of rapamycin, a natural product that was initially developed as an antifungal drug and then as an immunosuppressive agent, with anticancer activity noted more than 20 years ago. Rapamycin (Sirolimus, Rapamune) was isolated from the soil bacteria *Streptomyces hygroscopicus* found on Rapa Nui (commonly known as Easter Island) in the South Pacific in 1975, but its development for cancer therapeutics was not prioritized. The immunosuppressant effects of rapamycin were pursued and resulted in FDA approval in 1999 for prevention of renal allograft rejection. Laboratory studies of rapamycin starting in the early 1980s showed antitumour effects in several solid tumours.

Cell cycle inhibitor-779, now known as temsirolimus, is a derivative of rapamycin, and it was identified in the 1990s and subsequently developed as an anticancer agent (Peralba et al. 2003).

3 Structure and Mechanism of Action

Temsirolimus (Fig. 1) is a serine–threonine kinase involved in controlling many cellular functions, and it inhibits the mTOR.

The rapamycin-sensitive complex, also called mTOR complex 1 (mTORC1) (Guertin and Sabatin 2005; Martin and Hall 2005), exists in cytoplasm in a complex with three peptides: the regulatory-associated protein of mTOR (raptor), mLST8, and GhL. Regulation of mTOR pathway activation is mediated through a series of complex signalling interactions linking growth factor receptor signalling and other cell stimuli, phosphatidylinositol 3-kinase activation, and activation of the Akt/protein kinase B pathway.

mTOR phosphorylates and activates p70S6 kinase and in this way leads to enhanced translation of certain ribosomal proteins and elongation factors. This process is responsible, among other effects, for the production of hypoxia-inducible factor-1a, which regulates the transcription of genes that stimulate cell growth and angiogenesis, including VEGF (Thomas et al. 2006). When activated, mTOR is linked to increased protein synthesis by modulating elements that are important in a number of cellular processes such as stimulating and regulating the synthesis of several proteins at the translation level (phosphorylation of S6K1 and 4E-BP1); stimulating cell growth (cyclin D1) and important component of a cell cycle checkpoint for DNA replication; increasing production of the HIF-1α protein, a transcriptional regulator of angiogenic growth factors, such as VEGF and PDGF;

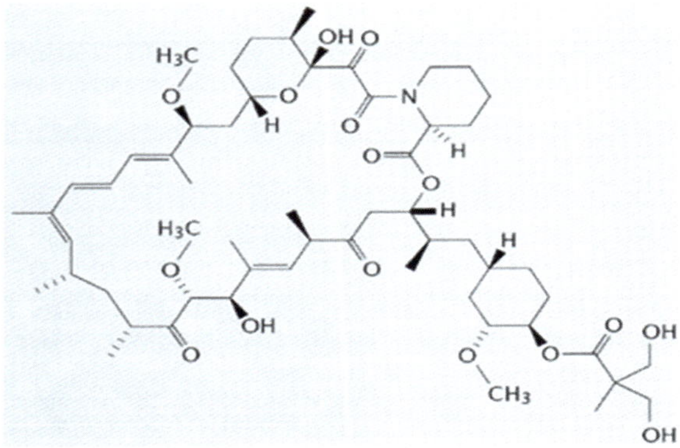

Fig. 1 Structure of temsirolimus

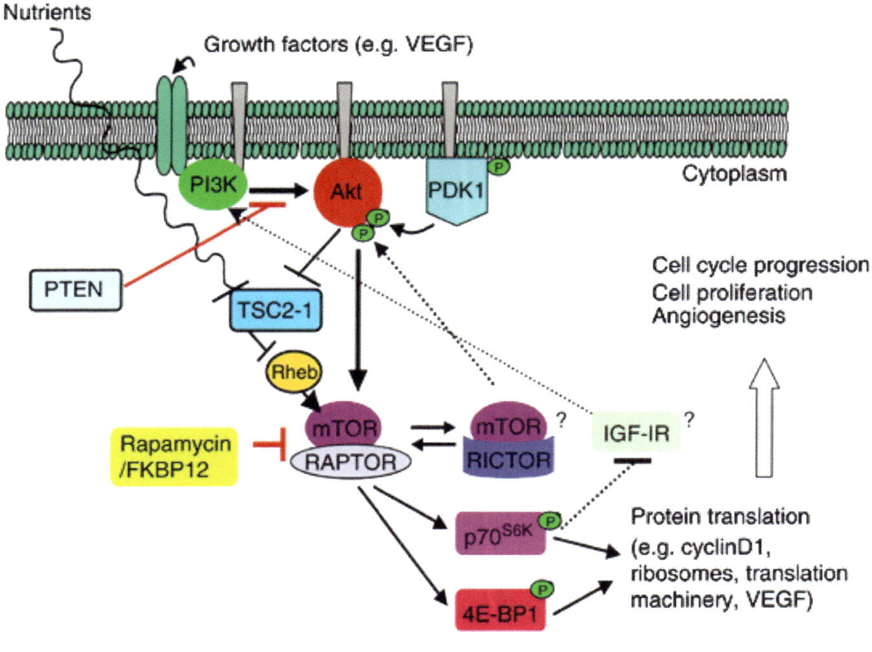

Fig. 2 PI3K/AKT/mTOR pathway showing the mTOR protein complexes, mTOR/RAPTOR and mTOR/RICTOR, and the feedback loop involving IGF-IR. *Arrows* indicate activation; *bars* indicate inhibition (Duran et al. 2006)

stimulating an increased expression of glucose and amino acid transporters, allowing the cell to take up additional metabolic fuel and extracellular nutrients. If dysregulated, the net result is uncontrolled cell growth (Fig. 2).

In cancers, signalling through mTOR is stimulated by defects in one or more of the several pathway components upstream of mTOR (growth factor receptors, PI3K, Akt, PTEN, TSC1/TSC2) or by stimulation of PI3K by mutant Ras/Raf/MAPK pathway components. In certain types of renal cell cancer and some neuroendocrine tumours, loss of function of VHL eliminates the mechanism for clearance of hypoxia-inducible factor 1α (HIF-1α), resulting in the transcription of numerous "hypoxia-associated" proteins, which drive angiogenesis and other cellular functions. HIF-1α translation is controlled by mTOR; inhibiting mTOR may be one approach to overcoming the effects of VHL loss.

Temsirolimus binds to an immuniphilin FK506-binding protein 12 KDa isoform (FKBP12) to form a complex with mTOR (Sabers et al. 1995). When mTOR is bound in this complex, it becomes unable to phosphorylate protein translation factors, as 4EBP1 and SK6 (also known as p7066 kinase), which are downstream of mTOR in the phosphatidylinositol 3-kinase (PI3K)/Akt/mTOR pathway.

The net effect of this class of compounds is inhibition of the translation of several key proteins regulating the cell cycle so that cell is blocked in the G1 phase and angiogenesis is inhibited (Hudes et al. 2007).

4 Clinical Data

Temsirolimus showed antitumour effects across a wide variety of tumour histotypes in preclinical models (Nesha et al. 2001; Podyspanina et al. 2001; Yu et al. 2001). Over the last 10 years, many series of randomized phase I–III trials have been carried out to investigate efficacy of temsirolimus in advanced RCC and in other tumours as endometrial carcinoma, breast cancer, glioblastoma multiforme, melanoma, small cell lung carcinoma, neuroendocrine carcinoma, and mantle cell lymphoma (MCL). The pivotal phase III study for temsirolimus in advanced RCC is being conducted worldwide, as well as a phase III study in MCL.

In addition, clinical studies for an oral formulation of temsirolimus in oncology (breast and prostate), multiple sclerosis, and rheumatoid arthritis indications have been conducted, but oral formulation is currently not being developed in these indications because of insufficient efficacy observed in the trials.

5 Safety and Efficacy

One phase I study evaluated toxicity, pharmacology, and preliminary activity of temsirolimus administrated daily for 5 days every 2 weeks at maximum tolerated dose of 15 mg/m^2/day in patients with advanced cancer (Hidalgo et al. 2006), demonstrating well tolerated and a preliminary evidence of antitumour activity in several advanced solid malignancies. Another phase I trial demonstrated the first evidence of antitumour activity in patients with RCC (Raymond et al. 2004).

In a randomized phase II study (Atkis et al. 2004), 111 patients with advanced refractory RCC were retrospectively classified in three groups according to Motzer's criteria (good, intermediate, and poor prognosis). They were randomly assigned to receive 25, 75, or 250 mg temsirolimus weekly to evaluate tumour response, time to tumour progression, survival and adverse events. This study brought up an objective tumour response in 7 % of patients. In addition, complete response, partial response, minor response, or stable disease $\geq$24 weeks were noted in nearly 50 % of the patients. Median time to progression was 6.0 months and median survival 15.0 months, with better survival for patients with intermediate or poor prognosis. These data seem to be encouraging comparing to 2.0 months in time to progression and median survival of 10.0 months in non-responding patients who have received IL-2- and/or IFN-α-based immunotherapy with no other treatment (Yang et al. 2003). Moreover, results from a phase II trial investigating temsirolimus in recurrent or metastatic endometrial carcinoma suggest that monotherapy with temsirolimus could be an option for the treatment of this disease for which no standard of care currently exists (Oza et al. 2005), whereas treatment with temsirolimus in patients with recurrent glioblastoma does not seem to have good activity in patients receiving 250 mg/week of temsirolimus as emerging data from two phase II trials (Galanis et al. 2005; Chang et al. 2005).

In a recent phase III, randomized, open-label, multicentre study 626 patients with metastatic RCC and three or more adverse risk features (indicators of short survival) were randomized in three arms to receive monotherapy with temsirolimus (25 mg iv q1w), monotherapy with IFN-α (18 million units three times a week) and combination therapy with temsirolimus (15 mg iv q1w) plus IFN-α (6 million units three times a week). Overall survival as primary end point was calculated. Patients treated with temsirolimus alone had a statistically longer overall survival than patients in the IFN-α monotherapy group (10.9 vs. 7.3 months, $P = 0.0069$). Secondary efficacy end points were progression-free survival, the objective response rate, and clinical benefits rate, defined as the group of patients with stable disease for at least 24 weeks or an objective response. The median progression-free survival was 3.7 months in the patients treated with temsirolimus (alone or in combination) versus 1.9 months in the arm treated with IFN-α alone and objective response rates of 4.8, 8.6, and 8.1 % in patients receiving IFN, temsirolimus, and combination therapy, respectively, did not differ significantly. By the contrast, the better rate of objective response or stable disease for at least 24 weeks was noted in temsirolimus group (32.1 %), compared with the group of combined therapy (28.1 %) and IFN alone (15.5 %) (Hudes et al. 2007).

Temsirolimus demonstrated remarkable antitumour activity in MCL a disease driven by cyclin D1 overexpression (Witzig et al. 2005a).

Patients affected by relapse of the MCL after conventional therapy or stem cell transplantation have a poor prognosis and are candidates for novel agents. A pathologic hallmark of MCL is the characteristic overexpression of cyclin D1 (CCND1). CCND1 is one of the proteins in which translation is controlled by the phosphatidylinositol 3-kinase signal transduction pathway and is downstream of the mTOR.

A phase II trial in 35 patients with MCL that had relapsed after chemotherapy and rituximab treatment indicated that temsirolimus treatment resulted in a remarkable overall response rate of 38 %, with a 3 % rate of complete remission (CR) and a 35 % rate of partial remission (PR) with a median duration of responses of 6 months (Witzig et al. 2005b).

Another phase II study with temsirolimus in MCL on 27 patients revealed an overall response rate of 41 % and a median time to progression of 6 months (Ansell et al. 2008). Results from a phase III study in 161 patients with relapsed or refractory MCL has been recently carried out and showed at the 13th Congress of the European Haematology Association (EHA) (Verhoef et al. 2008) and at the 44th Annual Meeting of the American Society of Clinical Oncology (ASCO) (Hess et al. 2008). In this randomized study, two groups of patients, receiving two different doses of temsirolimus (high-dose or low-dose temsirolimus), were compared with a third group treated with other chemo or biologic therapies (gemcitabine, fludarabine, etc.).

Objective response was 22, 6, and 2 % in the high-dose temsirolimus group, in the low-dose temsirolimus group, and in the chemo-biologic-treated group, respectively. Progression-free survival was 4.8, 3.4, and 1.9 months in the first, second, and third arms. Nevertheless, there was no significant difference in overall survival among all patients (Verhoef et al. 2008; Hess et al. 2008).

6 Side Effects

The group of Hudes et al. (2007) evaluated besides the safety and efficacy the tolerability of temsirolimus as well. More than 30 % of the patients treated by temsirolimus alone reported asthenia, rash, anaemia, nausea, and/or anorexia. The most frequently occurring grade 3 adverse events in the temsirolimus arm were asthenia (11 %), anaemia (20 %), and dyspnoea (9 %). Grade 3 or 4 asthenia were reported in 11 % of the patients in the temsirolimus group, in 26 % in the interferon group ($P < 0.001$), and in 28 % in the combination therapy group ($P < 0.001$). The proportions of patients who reported dyspnoea, diarrhoea, nausea, or vomiting were similar in all three groups. The most frequently occurring temsirolimus-related grade 3 or 4 haematological toxicities included anaemia and thrombocytopenia. Hypercholesterolaemia, hyperlipidaemia, and hyperglycaemia were also more common in the temsirolimus arm, reflecting inhibition of mTOR-mediated lipid and glucose metabolism, and generally manageable with dietary or medical management. Immunosuppression is an additional potential toxicity of temsirolimus given the known immunosuppressive effects of sirolimus, but there were not significant differences in the incidence of neutropenia, lymphopenia, or infection versus the IFN-α control arm.

Table 1 Treatment options in metastatic renal cell carcinoma (mRCC)°

RCC type	MSKCC risk group§	First-line therapy	Second-line therapy	Third-line therapy
Clear cell	Favourable or intermediate	Sunitinib [1b]	*After prior TKI*	Everolimus after prior TKI(s)
		IFN-α + Bevacizumab	• Axitinib	
			• Sorafenib	
		Pazopanib	• Everolimus	
		In selected patients: IFN-α	*After prior cytokines*	
		High-dose IL-2	• Sorafenib	
			• Axitinib	
			• Pazopanib	
	Poor	Temsirolimus		

°Guidelines on Renal Cell Carcinoma of the EAU 2012
§MSKCC risk groups
Favourable/intermediate one or two risk factors. *Poor* 3 or more risk factors determined by MSKCC
(LDH >1.5xULN) Haemoglobin below normal, corrected serum calcium >10 mg/dl, time from diagnosis to first treatment <1 year, Karnofski PS 60–70 %), number of metastatic sites

7 Conclusion and Future Perspectives

The mTOR pathway is likely critical across a broad spectrum of tumour types.

Temsirolimus has shown antitumour activity, most notably in poor-risk advanced RCC where a demonstration of overall survival benefit has been observed and promising results have been obtained in MCL and endometrial cancer.

The proof of principle that mTOR inhibitors can improve cancer patient survival has been obtained from a large randomized trial testing temsirolimus in patients with advanced poor prognostic RCC. These data led the Food and Drug Administration (FDA) to approve temsirolimus for advanced RCC in 2007. Temsirolimus is approved in the USA for the treatment of patients with advanced RCC and in Europe for first-line treatment of patients with advanced RCC and at least three of the prognostic risk factors (Table 1). The drug has shown a significant overall survival benefit and is associated with fewer withdrawals for adverse events, compared with standard IFN therapy in this patient population. Other targeted agents are now available for mRCC including combination therapy of bevacizumab with IFN-α, temsirolimus, and sorafenib (Table 2) and results are encouraging.

The lack of significant antitumour effect of temsirolimus-mediated mTOR inhibition in some tumours, especially those with predicted sensitivity based on alterations such as PTEN mutation, underline the complex interplay of multiple signalling pathways within a single tumour, and recent knowledge on the status of PTEN and PI3K/AKT/mTOR-linked pathways might help in the selection of other tumour types that will respond to mTOR inhibitors.

Table 2 Comparison of efficacy of targeted agents in the first-line treatment in patients with metastatic renal cell carcinoma

	PFS (months)	OS (months)	*p* value
Sunitinib	11.0	26.4	<0.00001
versus INF-α (Motzer et al. 2008)	5.1	21.8	
Bevacizumab + INF-α	10.2	23.3	<0.0001
versus (Escudier et al. 2007)	5.4	21.3	
Bevacizumab + INF-α	8.5	Not reached	<0.0001
versus (Rini et al. 2008)	5.2		
Temsirolimus1	5.5	10.9	<0.001
versus INF-α (Hudes et al. 2007)	3.1	7.3	
Sorafenib	5.7	Not available	Not available
versus IFN-α (part 1)	5.6		
Sorafenib (600 mg bid; part 2)	3.6		
Crossover (IFN-α—Sorafenib 400 mg bid; part 2) (Szczylik et al. 2007)	5.3		

PFS progression-free survival; *OS* overall survival

More potent or complete mTOR inhibition (e.g., through agents that inhibit both mTORC1 and mTORC2), inhibition of multiple signalling pathways simultaneously, and/or more precise molecular phenotyping of tumours to define mTOR pathway reliance are needed to build on the clinical benefits of temsirolimus observed to date.

Further studies have to prove any potential benefit of the substance in the second- or third-line treatment in poor or even favourable/intermediate risk to define the role of temsirolimus in the sequential therapy of mRCC.

On the other hand, it will be important to continue the search for predicting factors of resistance or sensitivity to mTOR inhibitors (temsirolimus and others), and it would be useful to immediately apply existing knowledge that mTOR inhibition can restore sensitivity to some existing chemotherapeutic agents in sequential therapy.

References

Aass N, De Mulder HM, Mickisch GHJ et al (2005) Randomized phase II/III trial of interferon alfa-2a with and without 13- cis –retinoic acid in patients with progressive metastatic renal cell carcinoma: the European Organization for Research and Treatment of Cancer Genito-Urinary Tract Cancer Group (EOTORC 30951). J Clin Oncol 23:4172–4178

Alexandrescu DT, Dasanu CA (2006) Kidney cancer therapy: new perspectives and avenues. Expert Opin Pharmacother 7(18):2481–2493

Ansell SM et al (2008) Low-dose, single-agent temsirolimus for relapsed mantle cell lymphoma. A phase 2 trial in the North Central Cancer Treatment Group. Cancer 113(3)

Atkins MB, Hidalgo M, Stadler WM et al (2004) Randomized phase II study of multiple dose levels of CCI-779, a novel mammalian target of rapamycin kinase inhibitor, in patients with advanced refractory renal cell carcinoma. J Clin Oncol 22:909–918

Chang SM et al (2005) Phase II study of CCI-779 in patients with recurrent glioblastoma multiforme. Invest New Drugs 23:357–361

Duran I, Kortmansky J, Singh D, Hirte H, Kocha W, Goss G, Le L, Oza A, Nicklee T, Ho J, Birle D, Pond GR, Arboine D, Dancey J, Aviel-Ronen S, Tsao MS, Hedley D, Siu LL (2006) A phase II clinical and pharmacodynamic study of temsirolimus in advanced neuroendocrine carcinomas. Br J Cancer 95(9):1148–1154

Escudier B (2007) Advanced renal cell carcinoma: current and emerging management strategies. Drugs 67(9):1257–1264

Escudier B, Pluzanska A, Koralewski P, Ravaud A, Bracarda S, Szczylik C, Chevreau C, Filipek M, Melichar B, Bajetta E, Gorbunova V, Bay JO, Bodrogi I, Jagiello-Gruszfeld A, Moore N (2007) AVOREN trial investigators. Bevacizumab plus interferon alfa-2a for treatment of metastatic renal cell carcinoma: a randomised, double-blind phase III trial. Lancet 370(9605):2103–2111

Galanis E et al (2005) Phase II trial of temsirolimus (CCI-779) in recurrent glioblastoma multiforme: a North Central Cancer Treatment Group Study. J Clin Oncol 23:5294–5304

Guertin DA, Sabatini DM (2005) An expanding role for mTOR in cancer. Trends Mol Med 11:353–361

Hess G, Verhoef G et al (2008) Phase III study of patients with relapsed, refractory mantle cell lymphoma treated with temsirolimus compared with investigator's choice therapy. In: 44th annual meeting of the American Society of Clinical Oncology (ASCO)

Hidalgo M, Buckner JC, Erlichman C et al (2006) A phase I and pharmacokinetic study of temsirolimus (CCI-779) administered intravenously daily for 5 days every 2 weeks to patients with advanced cancer. Clin Cancer Res 12:5755–5763

Hudes G, Carducci M, Tomczak P et al (2007) Temsirolimus, interferon alfa, or both for advanced renal cell carcinoma. N Engl J Med 356:2271–2281

Jemal A, Siegel R, Ward E et al (2007) Cancer statistics, 2007. CA Cancer J Clinic 57:43–66

Larkin JMG, Chowdhury S, Gore ME (2007) Drug insight: advances in renal cell carcinoma and the role of target therapies. Nat Clin Pract Oncol 4(8):470–479

Linehan WM, Zbar B, Bates SE et al (2001) Cancer of the kidney and ureter. In: DeVita VT, Hellman S, Rosenberg SA (eds) Cancer: principles and practice of oncology. Lippincott Williams & Wilkins, Philadelphia, pp 1362–1396

Martin DE, Hall MN (2005) The expanding TOR signaling network. Curr Opin Cell Biol 17:158–166

Motzer RJ, Bukowsky RM (2006) Targeted therapy for metastatic renal carcinoma. J Clin Oncol 24(35):5601–5608

Motzer RJ, Figlin RA, Hutson TE et al (2008) Overall survival with sunitinib versus interferon (IFN)-alfa as first-line treatment of metastatic renal cell carcinoma (mRCC). In: 44th annual meeting of the American Society of Clinical Oncology (ASCO)

Neshat MS, Mellinghoff IK, Tran C et al (2001) Enhanced sensitivity of PTEN-deficient tumors to inhibition of FRAP/mTOR. Proc Natl Acad Sci U S A 98:10314–10319

Oza AM et al (2005) A phase II study on temsirolimus (CCI-779) in patients with metastatic and/ or recurrent endometrial cancer. In: Proceedings of 17th symposium on molecules targets cancer therapy, Philadelphia, USA, 197 AB269, November 2005

Peralba JM, DeGraffenried L, Friedrichs W et al (2003) Pharmacodynamic evaluation of CCI-779, an inhibitor of mTOR, in cancer patients. Clin Cancer Res 9:2887–2892

Podsypanina K, Lee RT, Politis C et al (2001) An inhibitor of mTOR reduces neoplasia and normalizes p70/S6 kinase activity in Pten$\pm$ mice. Proc Natl Acad Sci US A 98:10320–10325

Raymond E, Alexandre J, Faivre S et al (2004) Safety and pharmacokinetics of escalated doses of weekly intravenous infusion of CCI-779, a novel mTOR inhibitor, in patients with cancer. J Clin Oncol 22:2336–2347

Rini BI, Halabi S, Rosenberg JE, Stadler WM, Vaena DA, Ou SS, Archer L, Atkins JN, Picus J, Czaykowski P, Dutcher J, Small EJ (2008) Bevacizumab plus interferon alfa compared with interferon alfa monotherapy in patients with metastatic renal cell carcinoma: CALGB 90206. J Clin Oncol (Epub ahead of print)

Rosemberg SA, Lotze MT, Muul ML et al (1985) Observations on the systemic administration of autologous lymphokine-activated killer cells and recombinant interleukin-2 to patients with metastatic cancer. N Engl J Med 313(23):1485–1492

Sabers CJ, Matrin MM, Brunn JJ et al (1995) Isolation of a protein target of FKBP 12-rapamycin complex in mammalian cells. J Biol Chem 270(2):815–822

Szczylik C, Demkow T, Staehler M, Rolland F, Negrier S, Hutson TE, Bukowski RM, Scheuring UJ, Burk K, Escudier B (2007) Randomized phase II trial of first-line treatment with sorafenib versus interferon in patients with advanced renal cell carcinoma: Final results. J Clin Oncol 25(suppl):Abstract 5025

Thomas GV, Tran C, Mellinghoff IK et al (2006) Hypoxia inducible factors determines sensitivity to inhibitors of mTOR in kidney cancer. Nad Med 12:122–127

Verhoef G, Hess et al (2008) Phase III study of patients with relapsed, refractory mantle cell lymphoma treated with temsirolimus compared with investigator's choice therapy. In: 13th congress of the European Hematology Association (EHA)

Witzig TE et al (2005a) Phase II trial of single-agent temsirolimus (CCI-779) for relapsed mantle cell lymphoma. J Clin Oncol 23:5347–5356

Witzig TE et al (2005b) Phase II trial of single-agent temsirolimus (CCI-779) for relapsed mantle cell lymphoma. J Clin Oncol 23:5347–5356

Yang JC, Haworth L, Sherry RM et al (2003) A randomized trial of bevacizumab, an antivascular endothelia growth factor antibody, for metastatic renal cancer. N Engl J Med 349:427–434

Yu K, Toral-Barza L, Discafani C et al (2001) mTOR, a novel target in breast cancer: the effect of CCI-779, an mTOR inhibitor, in preclinical models of breast cancer. Endocr Relat Cancer 8:249–258

Vismodegib

F. Meiss and R. Zeiser

Abstract

Vismodegib (GDC-0449, Erivedge®) is a novel small molecule antagonist of the hedgehog (Hh) pathway that binds to smoothened (SMO) and leads to inhibition of an aberrant activation of the Hh pathway. Dysregulated Hh signaling results in uncontrolled proliferation in basal cell carcinoma (BCC) and has also been found present in medulloblastoma, and many other cancers such as those of gastrointestinal tract, brain, lung, breast, and prostate. In January 2012, vismodegib became the first agent to target the Hh pathway to receive approval by the United States Food and Drug Administration (FDA) and in July 2013 approval by the European Medicines Agency (EMA) followed for the treatment of adult patients with symptomatic metastatic BCC, or locally advanced BCC inappropriate for surgery or radiotherapy. At the moment, many trials are ongoing to further investigate the role of vismodegib in other malignancies than BCC.

Contents

F. Meiss (✉)
Department of Dermatology and Venereology, Freiburg University Medical Center, Albert-Ludwigs-University, Hauptstr. 7, 79104 Freiburg, Germany
e-mail: frank.meiss@uniklinik-freiburg.de

R. Zeiser
Division of Hematology and Oncology, Department of Medicine, Freiburg University Medical Center, Albert-Ludwigs-University, Hugstetter Str. 55, 79106 Freiburg, Germany

U. M. Martens (ed.), *Small Molecules in Oncology*, Recent Results in Cancer Research 201, DOI: 10.1007/978-3-642-54490-3_25,

1 Introduction

The hedgehog (Hh) pathway is a signaling pathway involved in numerous developmental processes, including determination of cell fate, patterning, proliferation, survival, and differentiation (Varjosalo and Taipale 2008). While this pathway is inactive in most adult tissues, aberrant activation of it has been documented in a variety of malignancies (Atwood et al. 2012; McMillan and Matsui 2012). In cancers such as basal cell carcinoma (BCC), ligand-independent mechanisms lead to constitutive Hh pathway activation through mutations in components of the pathway, including patched-1 (PTCH1) or smoothened (SMO) (Rubin et al. 2005; Epstein 2008; Goppner and Leverkus 2011; Ruch and Kim 2013). Moreover, numerous other solid and hematologic tumors have been shown to harbor ligand-dependent activation of the Hh pathway by autocrine or paracrine mechanisms (Atwood et al. 2012; McMillan and Matsui 2012). Therefore, this pathway has been an attractive target for drug development and cancer therapy. While the best-characterized approach is to target the SMO receptor, other rational approaches for inhibiting the Hh pathway include inhibiting downstream components or directly binding Hh ligands. Vismodegib, a SMO antagonist, showed remarkable activity in phase I and II trials for the treatment of locally advanced and metastatic BCC (Yauch et al. 2008; Robarge et al. 2009; Von Hoff et al. 2009; LoRusso et al. 2011a, b; Sekulic et al. 2012; Tang et al. 2012; Fecher 2013; Sandhiya et al. 2013). In January 2012, vismodegib became the first agent targeting the Hh pathway to receive approval by the United States Food and Drug Administration (FDA) and in July 2013 approval by the European Medicines Agency (EMA) followed for the treatment of adult patients with symptomatic metastatic BCC, or locally advanced BCC inappropriate for surgery or radiotherapy. Despite promising preclinical data with Hh pathway inhibitors in other malignancies, the clinical benefit has been disappointing until now (LoRusso et al. 2011a, b; Atwood et al. 2012; McMillan and Matsui 2012).

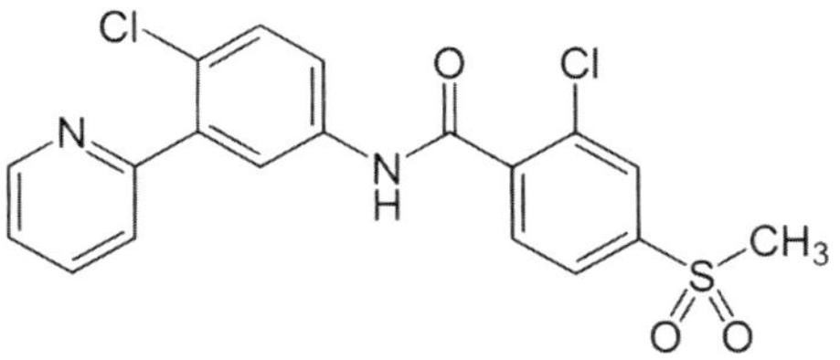

Fig. 1 Structural formula of vismodegib (GDC-0449)

2 Structure and Mechanism of Action

2.1 Structure

Structural modifications of benzimidazole led to the discovery of a functionalized 2-pyridyl amide moiety, which could inhibit the Hh pathway (Robarge et al. 2009; Wong et al. 2009). Further, optimization of pharmacokinetic and pharmacodynamic properties of this molecule finally culminated in the development of vismodegib. The chemical formula for vismodegib is $C_{19}H_{14}Cl_2N_2O_3S$ (Fig. 1). Its chemical name is 2-chloro-*N*-[4-chloro-3-(pyridin-2-yl)phenyl]-4-(methylsulfonyl)benzamide. It is a crystalline-free base with a pKa of 3.8 and a molecular weight of 421.3 g/mol. The solubility as a free base is far greater at an acidic pH (Robarge et al. 2009; Wong et al. 2009).

2.2 Mechanism of Action

Vismodegib acts by targeting the hedgehog (Hh) pathway, which is activated in most BCCs (Rubin et al. 2005; Epstein 2008; McMillan and Matsui 2012; Ruch and Kim 2013). The Hh signaling pathway is an important cascade for cellular growth and differentiation during the embryonic development (Varjosalo and Taipale 2008). The pathway was first identified in the fruit fly, Drosophila, and the name Hh was given to the pathway because of the spiky, hedgehog-like appearance of those fruit fly embryos which had mutated Hh gene (Varjosalo and Taipale 2008). Apart from the Hh ligand, the two receptor proteins involved in the cascade are patched-1 (PTCH1) and smoothened (SMO). PTCH1 is an inhibitory protein and forms an inactive complex with SMO, in the absence of Hh. When Hh binds with PTCH1 and prevents its inhibitory action, SMO becomes free to act (Fig. 2). Activated SMO is then involved in promoting the transcription of different genes, which, during the embryonic development, are responsible for cellular growth and differentiation and, in adults, are involved in tissue repair and stem cell maintenance (Rubin et al. 2005; Epstein 2008; Varjosalo and Taipale 2008; Atwood et al. 2012; McMillan and Matsui 2012; Ruch and Kim 2013).

A dysregulated Hh signaling pathway has not just been attributed to BCC, but also to medulloblastoma, and many other cancers such as those of gastrointestinal

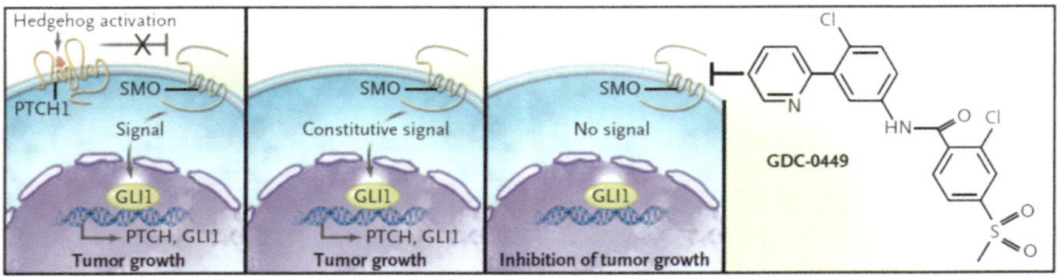

Fig. 2 Hedgehog signal transduction pathway (*left*), loss-of-PTCH1 mutations (*center*), and inhibition of smoothened homolog (SMO) signaling by GDC-0449 (*right*). Hedgehog binding to PTCH1 (*left*) relieves inhibition of SMO activation by PTCH1. In the absence of PTCH1, because of loss-of-PTCH1 mutations, SMO signaling occurs constitutively (*center*). GDC-0449 inhibits SMO signaling through direct interaction with SMO (*right*) (Von Hoff et al. 2009) (reprint with permission of Massachusetts Medical Society)

tract, brain, lung, breast, and prostate (Varjosalo and Taipale 2008; Atwood et al. 2012; McMillan and Matsui 2012). Aberrant activation of the Hh pathway has been found to cause cellular proliferation and stimulate cancer stem cells. In the stratified epithelium, this disturbs the equilibrium between cellular proliferation and cell cycle arrest, causing epidermal hyperplasia along with uncontrolled proliferation of basal cells leading to BCC (Rubin et al. 2005; Epstein 2008; Ruch and Kim 2013). Inactivation of PTCH1 or oncogenic activation of SMO is a common feature in most of the BCC. So increasing the inhibitory action of the PTCH1 or suppressing the activation of SMO can be targeted for the treatment of BCC and other tumors with hyperactivated Hh pathway. Vismodegib blocks Hh signaling by selectively inhibiting SMO and thus prevents the consequent induction of target genes and proliferation factors, leading to suppression of BCC growth (Epstein 2008; Goppner and Leverkus 2011; Fecher 2013).

3 Preclinical Data

Preclinical studies demonstrated the antitumor activity of vismodegib in mouse models of medulloblastoma and hepatocellular carcinoma and in xenograft models of colorectal and pancreatic cancer (Yauch et al. 2008; Philips et al. 2011; Atwood et al. 2012; Ferruzzi et al. 2012; McMillan and Matsui 2012).

4 Clinical Data

4.1 Vismodegib in Basal Cell Carcinoma (BCC)

Basal cell carcinoma (BCC) of the skin is the most common cancer worldwide, and its prevalence is increasing, accounting for 80 % of non-melanoma skin cancers (Rubin et al. 2005; Epstein 2008; Goppner and Leverkus 2011). Basal cell carcinoma has many clinical subtypes. In the majority of cases, BCC can be treated with surgery, cryotherapy, and laser ablation. Radiotherapy, photodynamic therapy, and topical treatment with imiquimod or 5-fluorouracil are non-surgical therapeutic options in locally circumscribed BCC (Rubin et al. 2005). But BCC can also progress to an advanced state in which surgery or radiation therapy is not considered to be helpful (locally advanced basal cell carcinoma, laBCC) (Rubin et al. 2005; Epstein 2008; Goppner and Leverkus 2011). Such lesions arise either from earlier lesions that have not been treated or from a recurrence of aggressive subtypes of BCC. Metastatic basal cell carcinoma (mBCC) is extremely rare, and the metastasis rate is believed to be less than 0.1 % (Rubin et al. 2005; Epstein 2008; Goppner and Leverkus 2011; Lo et al. 1991).

4.1.1 Phase I Trial

An open-label multicenter phase I trial was conducted in 68 patients, which included 33 patients of locally advanced (laBCC) and metastatic BCC (mBCC), to evaluate the drug's safety and tolerability (Von Hoff et al. 2009; LoRusso et al. 2011a, b). In the early stage of the trial, there were only three patients with advanced BCC (LoRusso et al. 2011a, b), but the evidence of clinical benefit in two of these, encouraged the investigators to extend the cohort, increasing the final number of BCC patients to 33 (Von Hoff et al. 2009). Patients who had metastatic disease ($n = 18$) showed an overall response rate of 50 % and those with locally advanced disease ($n = 15$) showed 60 % response rate. Safety and pharmacokinetic studies were performed for three different daily doses of 150 mg ($n = 17$), 270 mg ($n = 15$), and 540 mg ($n = 1$). The 150 mg daily dose was recommended for the phase II trials, as the higher doses did not produce higher plasma concentration of the drug and the safety profile was found to be acceptable, with no dose-limiting toxic effect (Von Hoff et al. 2009; LoRusso et al. 2011a, b).

4.1.2 Phase II Trials

A multicenter open-label phase II [Erivance BCC] study was conducted in patients with metastatic BCC (mBCC $n = 33$) and those with inoperable locally advanced BCC (laBCC $n = 63$) (Sekulic et al. 2012). A once-daily oral dose of 150 mg vismodegib was given to the patients. The objective response rate, as evaluated by independent reviewers, was 30 % in patients with mBCC and 43 % in patients with laBCC. Complete response (defined as the absence of residual basal cell carcinoma on assessment of a biopsy specimen) was seen in 13 patients (21 %) with laBCC (Sekulic et al. 2012).

Another phase II multicentric, randomized, double-blind, placebo-controlled trial ($n = 41$) tested the efficacy of vismodegib in patients with basal cell nevus syndrome (BCNS, syn: Gorlin syndrome) (Tang et al. 2012). BCNS is an autosomal dominant disorder, and the molecular basis is a mutation in the PTCH1-gene, which results clinically in numerous BCC along with other facial and skeletal abnormalities (Rubin et al. 2005; Epstein 2008; Goppner and Leverkus 2011; Tang et al. 2012). In this trial, the incidence of new BCC in the vismodegib-treated cohort was significantly lower as compared to placebo (2 vs. 29 cases per group per year). The reduction in the size of already existing BCC was also significantly greater with vismodegib than with the placebo (−65 % vs. −11 %). None of the patients on vismodegib showed progression of the BCC, and in some patients, all basal cell carcinomas showed complete clinical regression. Biopsies taken from the clinically regressed tumors could not detect any residual BCC in 83 % of the samples (Tang et al. 2012).

4.2 Vismodegib in Colorectal Cancer

Based on the observed evidence for Hh activation in human colorectal cancer (CRC) tissues (Carpenter and Lo 2012; Hong et al. 2013), preclinical Hh ligand-dependent CRC models, D5123, and 1040830 were used to test the in vivo activity of vismodegib (Wong et al. 2011). In these models, oral treatment with vismodegib at a dose of 92 mg/kg twice daily caused tumor regression (Wong et al. 2011). In these mouse xenograft models, pathway modulation was linked to efficacy of vismodegib. To test whether these preclinical findings may be translatable into the human situation, the efficacy and toxicity of vismodegib were studied in a randomized phase II trial including patients with CRC. Vismodegib was combined with FOLFOX or FOLFIRI and bevacizumab in patients with previously untreated metastatic (m)CRC (Berlin et al. 2013). In this trial, a total of 199 patients with mCRC were treated on protocol (124 FOLFOX, 75 FOLFIRI). Although Hh activity had been found in CRC, the overall response rates for placebo-treated and vismodegib-treated patients were comparable with 51 % (90 % CI 43–60) and 46 % (90 % CI 37–55), respectively. Also, the level of Hh expression in the CRC tissue did not correlate with a clinical benefit by vismodegib treatment. Overall no vismodegib-associated benefit was observed in combination with either FOLFOX or FOLFIRI. Based on the data from this clinical trial, a combination of vismodegib with FOLFOX-/FOLFIRI-based chemotherapy regimens is currently not justified in mCRC.

4.3 Vismodegib in Ovarian Cancer

In ovarian cancer (OC), aberrant activation of Hh signaling was observed to be correlated with unfavorable prognosis and the Hh pathway marker Gli1 was suggested to function as a negative prognostic marker in advanced serous OC (Ciucci et al. 2013). Consistent with the expression data, and in vitro data showing that Hh signaling pathway regulates the growth of OC spheroid forming cells (Ray et al. 2011), pharmacological inhibition of Hh signaling was shown to reduce serous OC growth in a primary xenograft model (McCann et al. 2011). Based on these preclinical data, a phase II, randomized, double-blind, placebo-controlled trial on vismodegib was performed to determine the efficacy in patients with OC in second or third complete remission as a maintenance therapy (Kaye et al. 2012).

In this clinical trial, patients with recurrent epithelial OC were treated with either vismodegib (150 mg daily) or placebo according to their randomization after completing chemotherapy (Kaye et al. 2012). The treatment was discontinued when radiographic progression or toxicity occurred (Kaye et al. 2012). One hundred and four patients were treated with vismodegib or placebo (both arms: $n = 52$), and the median PFS was 7.5 and 5.8 months, respectively. The most frequent AEs in the vismodegib arm were dysgeusia, ageusia, muscle spasms, and alopecia (Kaye et al. 2012). Grade 3/4 AEs occurred in 12 patients (23.1 %) with vismodegib and six (11.5 %) with placebo (Kaye et al. 2012). The unexpected low advantage of the vismodegib-treated group with respect to PFS could have been due to the low Hh expression, which was found only in 13.5 % of archival OC tissues.

4.4 Vismodegib in Small Lung Cell Cancer

Since therapeutic options for durable responses in patients with small cell lung cancer (SCLC) are lacking, the observation that Hh activity was present in SCLC (Watkins et al. 2003) fueled hope that a targeted disruption of this pathway could overcome therapy resistance. Using a SCLC mouse model not only an active Hh signaling pathway was described but also its pharmacological blockade inhibited the growth of mouse and human SCLC (Park et al. 2011). However, while it was shown that Hh pathway inhibition radiosensitizes non-small cell lung cancers (Zeng et al. 2013), to date no data from a large clinical trial is published for Hh inhibition in SCLC. Currently, only a phase I trial of vismodegib in patients with refractory, locally advanced solid tumors reported three patients with SCLC treated with vismodegib (LoRusso et al. 2011a, b), but a larger trial is underway.

4.5 Vismodegib in Hematologic Diseases

Inhibition of the Hh pathway was considered most promising in chronic myeloid leukemia (CML) because is was shown to be required for maintenance of myeloid cancer stem cells (Dierks et al. 2008; Zhao et al. 2009). Treatment of the BCR-ABL-positive cell line OM9;22 cells with vismodegib caused cell growth inhibition and induced apoptosis (Okabe et al. 2012). Besides these results with a cell line, vismodegib also inhibited the colony growth of Philadelphia-chromosome (Ph)-positive primary CML patient samples (Okabe et al. 2012). A combination of vismodegib and the established drug dasatinib resulted in a synergism with an increase in the cytotoxic effects of dasatinib in the presence of feeder cells in vitro (Okabe et al. 2012). A synergism was also described for the combination of ponatinib with vismodegib for therapy-resistant BCR-ABL1-positive leukemia (Katagiri et al. 2013). Also, B cell malignancies were shown to be responsive to

Hh inhibition (Dierks et al. 2007), in particular when combined with Bcl2 inhibition (Kunkalla et al. 2013). However, there is currently no clinical trial published on the efficacy of vismodegib in leukemias or lymphomas.

4.6 Vismodegib in Medulloblastoma

The ontogenesis of medulloblastoma (MB) is regulated by Sonic Hh signaling, and Gli3 as a marker of Hh pathway activity is found in MB tissues (Miyahara et al. 2013). Currently, the information on the clinical efficacy of vismodegib in MB is sparse and only a phase I trial of vismodegib in patients with different types of solid tumors reported 1 patient with MB treated with vismodegib (LoRusso et al. 2011a, b). Until more mature clinical data on vismodegib in MB are available, no statement on its potential for this tumor entity can be made.

5 Toxicity

Data of three studies (one phase I study and two phase II studies) in la/mBCC and/or BCNS patients are available, and in these studies, a total of 170 patients with la/mBCC and/or BCNS received vismodegib (Von Hoff et al. 2009; LoRusso et al. 2011a, b; Sekulic et al. 2012; Tang et al. 2012). Severe adverse effects were seen rarely, and the side effect profile of vismodegib as reported in these studies is summarized in Table 1 for 138 patients with advanced BCC (Genentech Inc. 2013). The most common side effects were muscle cramps/spasm, alopecia, dysgeusia, weight loss, and fatigue. Grade 3 or 4 fatigue was seen in 5 % of patients. Although nausea was reported in 30 % of patients, the incidence of grade 3 nausea (i.e., unable to adequately take in enough calories or fluid and potential need for parenteral nutrition, tube feedings, or hospitalization) was only 0.7 %. Only 1 patient displayed QTc interval prolongation in a phase I study, but further studies in healthy volunteers could not find an apparent relationship between the administration of vismodegib and QT prolongation (Von Hoff et al. 2009; LoRusso et al. 2011a, b; Graham et al. 2013). The phase II trial by Tang et al. was placebo-controlled (multicentric, randomized, double-blind, placebo-controlled trial tested the efficacy of vismodegib in patients with BCNS), and the adverse effects of vismodegib versus placebo could be much better outlined and illustrated under these conditions (Tang et al. 2012). In this study, patients receiving vismodegib experienced much more grade 1 and 2 dysgeusia, muscle cramps, alopecia, and weight loss compared with the placebo cohort (Tang et al. 2012). Noteworthy from this study were the patient medication discontinuation rates, after a mean of 8 months of administration, 7 of 26 (27 %) patients had discontinued therapy due to adverse effects (at the time of data cut for publication), about one year later 54 % (14 of 26) patients had discontinued the medication owing to side effects. On discontinuation, resolution of dysgeusia and muscle cramps occurred within 1 month and hair growth within 3 months (Tang et al. 2012). In the phase II study of Sekulic and coworkers, 7 fatal events were reported, including hypovolemic shock, myocardial

Table 1 Adverse reactions occurring in >10 % of advanced BCC patients (Genentech Inc. 2013)

	All aBCC[a] patients (N = 138)		
MedDRA preferred Term[b]	All grades[c] (%)	Grade 3 (%)	Grade 4 (%)
Gastrointestinal disorders			
Nausea	42 (30.4)	1 (0.7)	–
Diarrhea	40 (29.0)	1 (0.7)	–
Constipation	29 (21.0)	–	–
Vomiting	19 (13.8)	–	–
General disorders and administration site conditions			
Fatigue	55 (39.9)	7 (5.1)	1 (0.7)
Investigations			
Weight loss	62 (44.9)	10 (7.2)	–
Metabolism and nutrition disorders			
Decreased appetite	35 (25.4)	3 (2.2)	–
Musculoskeletal and connective tissue disorders			
Muscle spasms	99 (71.7)	5 (3.6)	–
Arthralgias	22 (15.9)	1 (0.7)	
Nervous system disorders			
Dysgeusia	76 (55.1)	–	–
Ageusia	15 (10.9)	–	–
Skin and subcutaneous tissue disorders			
Alopecia	88 (63.8)	–	–

[a]*aBCC* Advanced basal cell carcinoma
[b]*MedDRA* Medical Dictionary for Regulatory Activities
[c]Grading according to NCI-CTCAE v3.0

infarction, meningeal disease, and ischemic stroke (Sekulic et al. 2012). The relationship between vismodegib and these events is unknown. In this study, 57 % of the patients receiving vismodegib had at least one adverse effect and 25 % of patients with laBCC chose to discontinue therapy on their own accord, although the reason for discontinuation was not documented (Sekulic et al. 2012). The authors of this trial attributed discontinuation to either long-term, low-grade adverse effects (e.g., dysgeusia and muscle cramps) or patient perception that the maximal benefit had already been achieved by vismodegib therapy (Sekulic et al. 2012).

Besides the above-mentioned side effects and toxicities vismodegib, based on its mechanism of action is known to be teratogenic, embryotoxic, and fetotoxic (Varjosalo and Taipale 2008; Atwood et al. 2012; McMillan and Matsui 2012). In rats at maternal exposures lower than human exposures at the recommended dose of 150 mg/day, malformations included craniofacial anomalies, an open perineum, and absent or fused digits; moreover, fetal retardations and variations were also noted (Genentech Inc. 2013). Both male and female patients must be advised of this risk. In addition, before initiating treatment with vismodegib, physicians must verify a female patient's pregnancy status and must advise female patients of the need for contraception. Male patients must be informed of the potential risk of exposing their partners to vismodegib through semen (Genentech Inc. 2013).

6 Drug Interactions

The elimination of vismodegib involves several pathways. Vismodegib is predominantly excreted as an unchanged drug, but several minor metabolites are produced by cytochrome P450 isoenzymes (Genentech Inc. 2013). In parallel with safety/efficacy assessments conducted during clinical development, the drug–drug interaction (DDI) potential as well as the assessment of absorption, distribution, metabolism, and excretion has extensively been evaluated to anticipate/avoid unwanted side effects or reductions in efficacy due to concomitant drug administration (Wong et al. 2009; LoRusso et al. 2011a, b; Sharma et al. 2013). In standard in vitro assays, metabolism-based DDIs were assessed, and vismodegib had moderate potential for inhibition of cytochrome P450 (CYP) 2C8 and CYP2C9 and to a lesser extent of CYP2B6, CYP2C19, and CYP2D6. Vismodegib does not induce CYP1A2, CYP2B6, or CYP3A4/5 in cultured human hepatocytes, nor is it a strong binder of human pregnane X receptor (PXR) (Wong et al. 2009; LoRusso et al. 2011a, b; Sharma et al. 2013). Oxidative metabolites of vismodegib were primarily formed by CYP3A4/5 and CYP2C9 in vitro (Wong et al. 2009), but in vivo coadministration of CYP3A4/5 inducers and inhibitors did not alter steady-state plasma concentration (Genentech Inc. 2013; LoRusso et al. 2011a, b). In vitro studies identified vismodegib as an inhibitor/substrate (Zhang et al. 2009) of the efflux transporter P-glycoprotein, while others could not reproduce this observation (Wong et al. 2009). The clinical relevance of the effect on the P-glycoprotein therefore remains unclear, but the prescribing information indicates a potential interaction by coadministration of vismodegib and drugs inhibiting P-glycoprotein (e.g., clarithromycin, erythromycin, azithromycin) leading to an increased incidence of adverse events (Genentech Inc. 2013).

7 Summary and Perspectives

The association between PTCH1 mutations in Gorlin syndrome and aberrant pathway activity in BCC and the development of a small molecule that specifically inhibits this aberrant signaling is an exceptional example of successful translational research. Targeting the Hh pathway is a promising strategy in cancer therapy, and the efficacy of vismodegib in BCC patients has led to its approval by the FDA and the EMA for adult patients with symptomatic metastatic BCC, or locally advanced BCC inappropriate for surgery or radiotherapy. A concern in patients being treated with vismodegib is the side effect profile which, even though these side effects are mostly low grade, seems to make a long-term treatment difficult to tolerate for the patient. Side effect management should be an issue of further studies and intermittent treatment regimen could probably reduce side effects without lowering the clinical efficacy of vismodegib. An other option to lower side effects could be a "neoadjuvant" treatment regimen in which treatment duration is as short as the period until a BCC lesion can be handled by surgery again. In many other cancers, involvement of the Hh pathway has been postulated, but to date negative clinical results raise the question of the clinical significance in these tumor entities. Multiple clinical trials are ongoing at the moment addressing these questions; therefore, vismodegib and also other Hh inhibitors will be of future interest in the treatment of cancer.

References

Atwood SX, Chang AL, Oro AE (2012) Hedgehog pathway inhibition and the race against tumor evolution. J Cell Biol 199(2):193–197

Berlin J, Bendell JC, Hart LL, Firdaus I, Gore I, Hermann RC et al (2013) A randomized phase II trial of vismodegib versus placebo with FOLFOX or FOLFIRI and bevacizumab in patients with previously untreated metastatic colorectal cancer. Clin Cancer Res 19:258–267

Carpenter RL, Lo HW (2012) Hedgehog pathway and GLI1 isoforms in human cancer. Discov Med 69:105–113

Ciucci A, De Stefano I, Vellone VG, Lisi L, Bottoni C, Scambia G, Zannoni GF, Gallo D (2013) Expression of the glioma-associated oncogene homolog 1 (gli1) in advanced serous ovarian cancer is associated with unfavorable overall survival. PloS ONE 8:e60145

Dierks C, Beigi R, Guo GR, Zirlik K, Stegert MR, Manley P et al (2008) Expansion of Bcr-Abl-positive leukemic stem cells is dependent on Hedgehog pathway activation. Cancer Cell 14:238–249

Dierks C, Grbic J, Zirlik K, Beigi R, Englund NP, Guo GR, Veelken H, Engelhardt M, Mertelsmann R, Kelleher JF, Schultz P, Warmuth M (2007) Essential role of stromally induced hedgehog signaling in B-cell malignancies. Nat Med 13:944–951

Epstein EH (2008) Basal cell carcinomas: attack of the hedgehog. Nat Rev Cancer 8(10):743–754

Fecher LA (2013) Systemic therapy for inoperable and metastatic basal cell cancer. Curr Treat Options Oncol 14(2):237–248

Ferruzzi P, Mennillo F, De Rosa A, Giordano C, Rossi M, Benedetti G et al (2012) In vitro and in vivo characterization of a novel Hedgehog signaling antagonist in human glioblastoma cell lines. Int J Cancer 131(2):E33–E44

Genentech Inc, USA (2013) Erivedge® Prescribing Information. Accessed 20 Jul 2013

Goppner D, Leverkus M (2011) Basal cell carcinoma: from the molecular understanding of the pathogenesis to targeted therapy of progressive disease. J Skin Cancer 2011:650258

Graham RA, Chang I, Jin JY, Wang B, Dufek MB, Ayache JA et al (2013) Daily dosing of vismodegib to steady state does not prolong the QTc interval in healthy volunteers. J Cardiovasc Pharmacol 61(1):83–89

Hong KD, Lee Y, Kim BH, Lee SI, Moon HY (2013) Expression of GLI1 correlates with expression of lymphangiogenesis proteins, vascular endothelial growth factor C and vascular endothelial growth factor receptor 3, in colorectal cancer. Am Surg 79:198–204

Katagiri S, Tauchi T, Okabe S, Minami Y, Kimura S, Maekawa T, Naoe T, Ohyashiki K (2013) Combination of ponatinib with Hedgehog antagonist vismodegib for therapy-resistant BCR-ABL1-positive leukemia. Clin Cancer Res 19:1422–1432

Kaye SB, Fehrenbacher L, Holloway R, Amit A, Karlan B, Slomovitz B et al (2012) A phase II, randomized, placebo-controlled study of vismodegib as maintenance therapy in patients with ovarian cancer in second or third complete remission. Clin Cancer Res 18:6509–6518

Kunkalla K, Liu Y, Qu C, Leventaki V, Agarwal NK, Singh RR, Vega F (2013) Functional inhibition of BCL2 is needed to increase the susceptibility to apoptosis to SMO inhibitors in diffuse large B-cell lymphoma of germinal center subtype. Ann Hematol 92:777–787

Lo JS, Snow SN, Reizner GT, Mohs FE, Larson PO, Hruza GJ (1991) Metastatic basal cell carcinoma: report of twelve cases with a review of the literature. J Am Acad Dermatol 24(5 Pt 1):715–719

LoRusso PM, Jimeno A, Dy G, Adjei A, Berlin J, Leichman L et al (2011a) Pharmacokinetic dose-scheduling study of hedgehog pathway inhibitor vismodegib (GDC-0449) in patients with locally advanced or metastatic solid tumors. Clin Cancer Res 17(17):5774–5782

LoRusso PM, Rudin CM, Reddy JC, Tibes R, Weiss GJ, Borad MJ et al (2011b) Phase I trial of hedgehog pathway inhibitor vismodegib (GDC-0449) in patients with refractory, locally advanced or metastatic solid tumors. Clin Cancer Res 17(8):2502–2511

McCann CK, Growdon WB, Kulkarni-Datar K, Curley MD, Friel AM, Proctor JL et al (2011) Inhibition of Hedgehog signaling antagonizes serous ovarian cancer growth in a primary xenograft model. PLoS ONE 6:e28077

McMillan R, Matsui W (2012) Molecular pathways: the hedgehog signaling pathway in cancer. Clin Cancer Res 18(18):4883–4888

Miyahara H, Natsumeda M, Yoshimura J, Ogura R, Okazaki K et al (2013) Neuronal differentiation associated with Gli3 expression predicts favorable outcome for patients with medulloblastoma. Neuropathology (Epub ahead of print)

Okabe S, Tauchi T, Tanaka Y, Katagiri S, Ohyashiki K (2012) Effects of the hedgehog inhibitor GDC-0449, alone or in combination with dasatinib, on BCR-ABL-positive leukemia cells. Stem Cells Dev 21:2939–2948

Park KS, Martelotto LG, Peifer M, Sos ML, Karnezis AN, Mahjoub MR et al (2011) A crucial requirement for Hedgehog signaling in small cell lung cancer. Nat Med 17:1504–1508

Philips GM, Chan IS, Swiderska M, Schroder VT, Guy C, Karaca GF et al (2011) Hedgehog signaling antagonist promotes regression of both liver fibrosis and hepatocellular carcinoma in a murine model of primary liver cancer. PLoS ONE 6(9):e23943

Ray A, Meng E, Reed E, Shevde LA, Rocconi RP (2011) Hedgehog signaling pathway regulates the growth of ovarian cancer spheroid forming cells. Int J Oncol 39:797–804

Robarge KD, Brunton SA, Castanedo GM, Cui Y, Dina MS, Goldsmith R et al (2009) GDC-0449-a potent inhibitor of the hedgehog pathway. Bioorg Med Chem Lett 19(19):5576–5581

Rubin AI, Chen EH, Ratner D (2005) Basal-cell carcinoma. N Engl J Med 353(21):2262–2269

Ruch JM, Kim EJ (2013) Hedgehog signaling pathway and cancer therapeutics: progress to date. Drugs 73(7):613–623

Sandhiya S, Melvin G, Kumar SS, Dkhar SA (2013) The dawn of hedgehog inhibitors: vismodegib. J Pharmacol Pharmacother 4(1):4–7

Sekulic A, Migden MR, Oro AE, Dirix L, Lewis KD, Hainsworth JD et al (2012) Efficacy and safety of vismodegib in advanced basal-cell carcinoma. N Engl J Med 366(23):2171–2179

Sharma MR, Karrison TG, Kell B, Wu K, Turcich M, Geary D et al (2013) Evaluation of food effect on pharmacokinetics of vismodegib in advanced solid tumor patients. Clin Cancer Res 19(11):3059–3067

Tang JY, Mackay-Wiggan JM, Aszterbaum M, Yauch RL, Lindgren J, Chang K et al (2012) Inhibiting the hedgehog pathway in patients with the basal-cell nevus syndrome. N Engl J Med 366(23):2180–2188

Varjosalo M, Taipale J (2008) Hedgehog: functions and mechanisms. Genes Dev 22(18): 2454–2472

Von Hoff DD, LoRusso PM, Rudin CM, Reddy JC, Yauch RL, Tibes R et al (2009) Inhibition of the hedgehog pathway in advanced basal-cell carcinoma. N Engl J Med 361(12):1164–1172

Watkins DN, Berman DM, Burkholder SG, Wang B, Beachy PA, Baylin SB (2003) Hedgehog signalling within airway epithelial progenitors and in small-cell lung cancer. Nature 422 (313-7)

Wong H, Alicke B, West KA, Pacheco P, La H, Januario T, Yauch RL, de Sauvage FJ, Gould SE (2011) Pharmacokinetic-pharmacodynamic analysis of vismodegib in preclinical models of mutational and ligand-dependent Hedgehog pathway activation. Clin Cancer Res 17: 4682–4692

Wong H, Chen JZ, Chou B, Halladay JS, Kenny JR, La H et al (2009) Preclinical assessment of the absorption, distribution, metabolism and excretion of GDC-0449 (2-chloro-N-(4-chloro-3-(pyridin-2-yl)phenyl)-4-(methylsulfonyl)benzamide), an orally bioavailable systemic Hedgehog signalling pathway inhibitor. Xenobiotica 39(11):850–861

Yauch RL, Gould SE, Scales SJ, Tang T, Tian H, Ahn CP et al (2008) A paracrine requirement for hedgehog signalling in cancer. Nature 455(7211):406–410

Zeng J, Aziz K, Chettiar ST, Aftab BT, Armour M, Gajula R, Gandhi N et al (2013) Hedgehog pathway inhibition radiosensitizes non-small cell lung cancers. Int J Radiat Oncol Biol Phys 86:143–149

Zhang Y, Laterra J, Pomper MG (2009) Hedgehog pathway inhibitor HhAntag691 is a potent inhibitor of ABCG2/BCRP and ABCB1/Pgp. Neoplasia 11(1):96–101

Zhao C, Chen A, Jamieson CH, Fereshteh M, Abrahamsson A, Blum J et al (2009) Hedgehog signalling is essential for maintenance of cancer stem cells in myeloid leukaemia. Nature 458:776–779

24718745R00256

Printed in Poland
by Amazon Fulfillment
Poland Sp. z o.o., Wrocław